Penn Clinical Manual of Urology

Penn Clinical Manual of Urology

Philip M. Hanno, MD, MPH
Professor
Division of Urology
Department of Surgery
University of Pennsylvania Health System
Philadelphia, Pennsylvania

S. Bruce Malkowicz, MD
Professor of Urology
Division of Urology
Department of Surgery
University of Pennsylvania Health System
Philadelphia, Pennsylvania

Alan J. Wein, MD, PhD (hon)
Professor and Chair
Division of Urology
University of Pennsylvania School of Medicine
Chief of Urology
University of Pennsylvania Health System
Philadelphia, Pennsylvania

SAUNDERS

ELSEVIER

SAUNDERS
ELSEVIER

1600 John F. Kennedy Boulevard
Suite 1800
Philadelphia, PA 19103–2899

PENN CLINICAL MANUAL   ISBN-13: 978-1-4160-3848-1
OF UROLOGY

Library of Congress Cataloging-in-Publication Data

Penn clinical manual of urology / [edited by] Philip M. Hanno, Alan J. Wein, S. Bruce Malkowicz. – 1st ed.
    p. ; cm.
  Includes bibliographical references.
  ISBN 1-4160-3848-5
  1. Urology–Handbooks, manuals, etc.   I. Hanno, Philip M.   II. Wein, Alan J.
III. Malkowicz, S. Bruce.   IV. Campbell-Walsh urology.   V. Title: Clinical manual of urology.
  [DNLM: 1. Urogenital Diseases.   2. Urology–methods. WJ 100 P412 2007]
RC872.9.P46 2007
616.6–dc22   2006026913

Acquisitions Editor: Rebecca Schmidt Gaertner
Editorial Assistants: Suzanne Flint, Elizabeth Hart
Project Manager: Bryan Hayward
Design Direction: Gene Harris

Working together to grow
libraries in developing countries
www.elsevier.com | www.bookaid.org | www.sabre.org

ELSEVIER   BOOK AID International   Sabre Foundation

Printed in China
Last digit is the print number: 9 8 7 6 5 4 3 2 1

Dedication

To our families, who cheerfully suffer us daily, and to all our residents, past and present, who represent a never ending source of knowledge, intellectual honesty, and pride.

Table of Contents

Preface

It has been over 20 years since we first put together a basic urology text designed for the busy student and house officer studying this fascinating and evolving area of medicine and surgery. The *Penn Clinical Manual of Urology* reflects our latest effort to present a useful introductory text. Rather than provide a heavily referenced compendium, we have striven to present a framework upon which program directors can build an educational foundation that will reflect their individual practices and allows their methods to be placed in the perspective of the urologic field in general. We believe the book also will appeal to other providers who routinely see patients with urologic problems: the primary care physician, gynecologist, nurse practitioner, and urologic nurse specialist.

Each of the contributors has been carefully selected, and all are superb clinicians and educators with experience in teaching medical students and residents didactically and in the clinic and operating room. All have been affiliated with the Penn urology program currently or in the past, hence the designation of the text. Although the practices and philosophy of the University of Pennsylvania Division of Urology will no doubt be evident in the exposition, more so in some sections than others, we have tried to keep "dogma" to a minimum, and thus allow program directors to add their input without the intellectual disruption (to the reader) of major disagreements. Algorithms, suggested readings, and self assessment questions are a part of each chapter.

From the physical examination to the MR urogram, and from the identification and treatment of testicular torsion to screening for prostate cancer and robotic prostatectomy, we have tried to encapsulate this fast-moving field. Urology incorporates a blend of medicine and surgery, traditional and extremely high-tech procedures, and acute care and long-term follow-up. Our goal has been to present the material in such a way that it will be comprehended by the novice, but also comprehensive enough for the chief resident doing a quick board review. Hopefully it will find a place not only on the office desk, but also on the clinic desk and in the house staff coat pocket.

We thank our contributors and our publisher for making this volume possible. We hope the *Penn Manual* will prove to be a trusted resource and ready reference.

Philip Hanno
Bruce Malkowicz
Alan Wein

List of Contributors

Andrew C. Axilrod, MD
Clinical Assistant Professor and Director, Male Sexual Health
Department of Urology
University of Pennsylvania Health System
Philadelphia, Pennsylvania
19: Male Sexual Dysfunction

Marc P. Banner, MD
Professor Emeritus
Department of Radiology
University of Pennsylvania Health System
Philadelphia, Pennsylvania
3: Diagnostic and Interventional Uroradiology

Ashok K. Batra, MD, FACS
Director
Division of Clinical Evaluation and Pharmacology/
  Toxicolcogy
Office of Cellular, Tissue, and Gene Therapy
Center for Biologic Evaluation and Research
Rockville, Maryland
6: Specific Infections of the Genitourinary Tract

Kerem H. Bortecen, MD, PhD
Fellow in Multi-Organ Transplantation
Department of Surgery
University of Pennsylvania Health System
Philadelphia, Pennsylvania
23: Renal Transplantation

Douglas A. Canning, MD
Professor
Division of Urology
Department of Surgery
University of Pennsylvania Health System
Director, Pediatric Urology
The Children's Hospital of Philadelphia
Philadelphia, Pennsylvania
28: Congenital Anomalies

Jeffrey P. Carpenter, MD
Professor
Department of Vascular Surgery

University of Pennsylvania Health System
Philadelphia, Pennsylvania
24: Renovascular Hypertension

Michael C. Carr, MD, PhD
Assistant Professor
Department of Surgery
University of Pennsylvania Health System
Urologist
Children's Hospital of Philadelphia
Philadelphia, Pennsylvania
26: Pediatric Oncology

Pasquale Casale, MD
Assistant Professor
Division of Urology
University of Pennsylvania Health System
Department of Urology
Children's Hospital of Philadelphia
Philadelphia, Pennsylvania
28: Congenital Anomalies

Ricardo E. Dent, MD
Medical Officer
Center for Drug Evaluation and Research
Division of Anesthesia, Analgesia, and Rheumatology
Rockville, Maryland
6: Specific Infections of the Genitourinary Tract

George W. Drach, MD
Professor
Division of Urology
Department of Surgery
University of Pennsylvania Health System
Attending Urologist
Department of Surgery
VA Medical Center
Philadelphia, Pennsylvania
29: Geriatric Urology

Pinaki R. Dutta, MD, PhD
Department of Radiation Oncology
University of Pennsylvania Health System
Philadelphia, Pennsylvania
17: Radiation Therapy

Thomas J. Guzzo, MD
Instructor
Division of Urology
Department of Surgery
University of Pennsylvania Health System
Philadelphia, Pennsylvania
18: Retroperitoneal Diseases

Philip M. Hanno, MD, MPH
Professor
Division of Urology
Department of Surgery
University of Pennsylvania Health System
Philadelphia, Pennsylvania
4: Lower Urinary Tract Infections in Women and Pyelonephritis; 7: Painful Bladder Syndrome (Interstitial Cystitis)

Jagajan Karmacharya, MD
Fellow
Department of Vascular Surgery
University of Pennsylvania Health System
Philadelphia, Pennsylvania
24: Renovascular Hypertension

Ira J. Kohn, MD
Delta Medix Urology
Scranton, Pennsylvania
9: Urologic Emergencies

Thomas F. Kolon, MD
Department of Urology
Children's Hospital of Philadelphia
Philadelphia, Pennsylvania
25: Disorders of Sexual Development

Alexander Kutikov, MD
Instructor
Division of Urology
Department of Surgery
University of Pennsylvania Health System
Philadelphia, Pennsylvania
22: Disorders of the Adrenal Gland

Steve Lebovitch, MD
Resident
Department of Urology
Temple University Hospital

Philadelphia, Pennsylvania
5: Prostatitis and Lower Urinary Tract Infections in Men

David I. Lee, MD
Chief
Section of Urology
Penn Presbyterian Medical Center
Philadelphia, Pennsylvania
1: Laparoscopic Anatomy, Laparoscopy, and Robotic-Assisted Laparoscopic Surgery; 14: Benign Prostatic Hyperplasia and Related Entities

S. Bruce Malkowicz, MD
Professor of Urology
Division of Urology
Department of Surgery
University of Pennsylvania Health System
Philadelphia, Pennsylvania
15: Adult Genitourinary Cancer—Prostate and Bladder; 18: Retroperitoneal Diseases

James F. Markmann, MD, PhD
Associate Professor
Division of Transplantation Surgery
Department of Surgery
University of Pennsylvania Health System
Philadelphia, Pennsylvania
23: Renal Transplantation

Michael J. Metro, MD
Attending Physician
Director of Traumatic and Reconstructive Urology
Department of Urology
Albert Einstein Medical Center
Jefferson Health System
Assistant Clinical Professor
Department of Urology
Philadelphia College of Osteopathic Medicine
Philadelphia, Pennsylvania
11: Urethral Stricture Disease

M. Louis Moy, MD
Assistant Professor
Division of Urology
Department of Surgery
University of Pennsylvania Health System

Philadelphia, Pennsylvania
13: Voiding Function and Dysfunction; Urinary Incontinence

John J. Pahira, MD
Professor
Department of Urology
Georgetown University Hospital
Washington, District of Columbia
8: Nephrolithiasis

Shane S. Parmer, MD
Attending Physician
Department of Vascular Surgery
Camden Clark Memorial Hospital
Parkersburg, West Virginia
24: Renovascular Hypertension

Millie Pevzner, MD
Department of Urology
Georgetown University Hospital
Washington, District of Columbia
8: Nephrolithiasis

Michel A. Pontari, MD
Professor of Urology
Department of Urology
Temple University School of Medicine
Philadelphia, Pennsylvania
5: Prostatitis and Lower Urinary Tract Infections in Men

Parvati Ramchandani, MD
Associate Professor and Chief, Genitourinary Radiology
Department of Radiology
University of Pennsylvania Health System
Philadelphia, Pennsylvania
3: Diagnostic and Interventional Uroradiology

Eric S. Rovner, MD
Associate Professor
Department of Urology
Medical University of South Carolina
Charleston, South Carolina
12: Urinary Fistula

Ricardo F. Sánchez-Ortiz, MD
Assistant Professor of Urology
University of Puerto Rico School of Medicine

Adjunct Professor of Urology
The University of Texas MD Anderson Cancer Center
Guaynabo, Puerto Rico
16: Renal, Testicular, and Penile Cancer

Abraham Shaked, MD, PhD
Chief
Division of Transplantation Surgery
Penn Transplant Center
University of Pennsylvania Health System
Philadelphia, Pennsylvania
23: Renal Transplantation

Ariana L. Smith, MD
Chief Resident
Department of Urology
University of Pennsylvania Health System
Philadelphia, Pennsylvania
19: Male Sexual Dysfunction

Howard M. Snyder III, MD
Division of Pediatric Urology
Children's Hospital of Philadelphia
Philadelphia, Pennsylvania
26: Pediatric Oncology

Paul J. Turek, MD
Professor and Endowed Chair, Urologic Education
Department of Urology, Obstetrics, Gynecology &
    Reproduction Sciences
Director, Male Reproductive Laboratory
Department of Urology
University of California, San Francisco
San Francisco, California
20: Male Fertility and Sterility

Keith N. Van Arsdalen, MD
Director, Male Infertility
Professor of Urology
Division of Urology
Department of Surgery
University of Pennsylvania Health System
Philadelphia, Pennsylvania
2: Signs and Symptoms: The Initial Examination

David J. Vaughn, MD
Associate Professor of Medicine
Division of Hematology/Oncology
Department of Medicine

Abramson Family Research Cancer Center
University of Pennsylvania Health System
Philadelphia, Pennsylvania
*15: Adult Genitourinary Cancer—Prostate and Bladder;
16: Renal, Testicular, and Penile Cancer*

Alan J. Wein, MD, PhD (hon)
Professor and Chair
Division of Urology
University of Pennsylvania School of Medicine
Chief of Urology
University of Pennsylvania Health System
Philadelphia, Pennsylvania
*13: Voiding Function and Dysfunction; Urinary
Incontinence; 14: Benign Prostatic Hyperplasia and Related
Entities; 15: Adult Genitourinary Cancer—Prostate
and Bladder*

Jeffrey P. Weiss, MD, FACS
Clinical Associate Professor
James Buchanan Brady Department of Urology
Weill Medical College of Cornell University
Associate Attending Physician
Department of Urology
The New York Presbyterian Hospital
Delta Medix Urology
Scranton, Pennsylvania
9: Urologic Emergencies

Hunter Wessells, MD, FACS
Professor
Department of Urology
University of Washington
Chief
Department of Urology
Harborview Medical Center
Seattle, Washington
10: Urinary and Genital Trauma

Richard Whittington, MD
Professor
Department of Radiation Oncology
University of Pennsylvania Health System
Chief
Department of Radiation Oncology
VA Medical Center
Philadelphia, Pennsylvania
17: Radiation Therapy

Jonathan L. Wright, MD, MS
Resident
Department of Urology
University of Washington School of Medicine
Seattle, Washington
10: Urinary and Genital Trauma

Heidi Yeh, MD
Instructor
Department of Surgery
University of Pennsylvania School of Medicine
Philadelphia, Pennsylvania
23: Renal Transplantation

Stephen A. Zderic, MD
Professor of Urology
Division of Pediatric Urology
Children's Hospital of Philadelphia
Philadelphia, Pennsylvania
27: Pediatric Voiding Function and Dysfunction

Edward Zoltan, MD
Instructor
Division of Urology
Department of Surgery
University of Pennsylvania Health System
Philadelphia, Pennsylvania
21: Sexually Transmitted Disease

Laparoscopic Anatomy, Laparoscopy, and Robotic-Assisted Laparoscopic Surgery

David I. Lee, MD

INTRODUCTION

Since the advent of laparoscopy in urology with diagnostic laparoscopy for the cryptorchid testes, pelvic lymphadenectomy by Schuessler in 1991, and major organ ablative (kidney) by Clayman in 1991, the overall adoption curve was relatively slow. Recently, with increasing experience and improved technology, laparoscopic urology has become well accepted and is being increasingly utilized by urologists.

LAPAROSCOPIC ANATOMY

During the initial learning curve for urologists into laparoscopy, a significant hurdle that needs to be overcome is the adjustment from an environment that is both tactile and visual to a surgical field that is very limited in a tactile sense and a visual field that is magnified but two dimensional.

Renal Anatomy

Certainly all urologists are familiar with the anatomy of the kidney and the surrounding structures. However, the transperitoneal approach that is most commonly used for laparoscopy is a perspective that is initially foreign. The retroperitoneal approach is used by some clinicians; however, the anatomic landmarks can be even less distinct at times and the working space is more limited. As patients are typically placed in either a rolled flank or full flank position, the visual orientation must also be so adjusted. On the right side, the liver will immediately come into view and typically drapes over at least half of the kidney. The right colon should immediately be identified to establish its course in

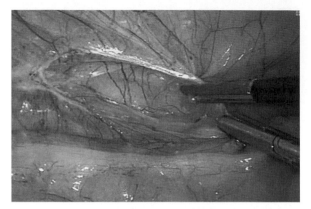

FIGURE 1-1. Dividing the white line of Toldt.

preparation of incision of the white line of Toldt (Figure 1-1). Once the colon is reflected medially, the surgeon should pay close attention to fat layers as they slide over one another during this maneuver. In most cases the mesenteric fat will be easily identified as separate from the underlying Gerota's fascia and the perinephric fat. One helpful landmark just caudal to the kidney is the psoas muscle that often comes into easy view once the colon is reflected. Overlying the psoas muscle will also be the genitofemoral nerve. Central in the psoas is also the psoas tendon. Medial to these structures will lay the gonadal vein and the ureter (Figure 1-2). If dissection around the kidney is difficult early on, the ureter can be mobilized at this point and then followed to the lower pole of the kidney.

In the region of the kidney itself, the colon must be medially rotated to expose the renal hilar region. This will in most cases require incision of the mesentery around the liver to gain sufficient room. **Once the colon is out of the way, the first significant structure that is noted on the medial surface of the kidney is the duodenum. This must be Kocherized to gain access to the hilum.** The next major structure oriented on a horizontal plane then becomes the inferior vena cava. Careful dissection along this structure then reveals the insertion of the gonadal vein, the main renal vein, and the adrenal vein from caudal to cranial. Then very commonly, the renal artery lies directly posterior to the renal vein (Figure 1-3). Often the ureter can be mobilized and used to lift the kidney upward; this can more easily expose the renal artery behind the vein. Once the main hilar

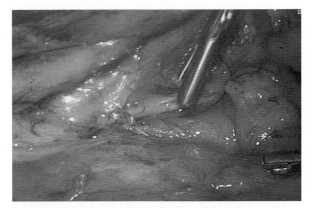

FIGURE 1-2. View of the ureter and adjacent gonadal vein during right laparoscopic nephrectomy.

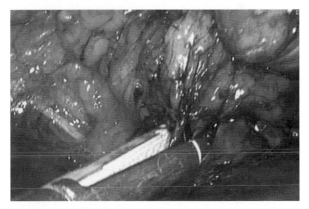

FIGURE 1-3. Stapler placed on renal artery with renal vein and vena cava anteriorly.

structures have been divided, access can then be obtained to the adrenal gland that will lie just medial to the upper pole of the kidney (Figure 1-4). **The adrenal vein drains directly into the vena cava and must be clearly identified if the adrenal gland is to be resected.**

On the left side the spleen lies anterior and superior to the kidney. There is a very consistent adhesion in the region of the left colon to the side wall just inferior to the spleen. This is usually the point at which the left colon mobilization is begun. After the colon is reflected medially in a similar

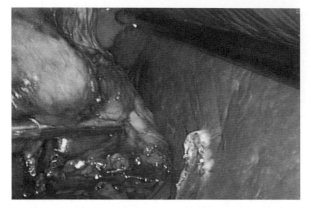

FIGURE 1-4. Adrenal vein being dissected off the upper pole of the right kidney.

fashion to the right side, the same landmarks can be found. However, the left gonadal vein can be much more useful, and dissection along this structure leads directly to the left renal vein. As dissection proceeds toward the hilum, it is often useful to obtain adequate space around the top of the kidney. **This can be accomplished by performing a very high dissection of the splenic attachments off the sidewall or by incision of the mesentery of its splenic attachments.** It is the author's preference to mobilize the spleen as much as possible to avoid inadvertent tearing of the capsule. Mobilization of the spleen will also move the tail of the pancreas out of the way as well. This structure can be very close to the upper pole of the kidney.

As a mirror image to the right side, the aorta will be the dominant structure crossing horizontally across the bottom of the dissection field. If dissection across the hilum is difficult in cases of xanthogranulomatous pyelonephritis (XGP) and the like, the dissection plane can be directed to the aorta and this can be followed over its left lateral surface to find the renal artery. **As the hilum is approached along the course of the gonadal vein it is also important to remember the venous tributaries of the left renal vein. The adrenal vein, the ascending lumbar vein, and the gonadal vein all consistently drain into the renal vein.** More often than not each one of these veins is mobilized and divided before dissection of the renal artery is approached. If an adrenalectomy alone is targeted, then the adrenal vein is ligated and the adrenal can be easily dissected off the anteromedial surface of the kidney.

Pelvic Anatomy

In approaching the pelvis for laparoscopic urology, most often the patients will be placed in a supine position and then converted to a Trendelenburg position to allow gravity to retract the bowels into the upper abdomen. This maneuver allows beautiful visualization of important pelvic structures. The usual landmarks to be initially identified for orientation are the medial umbilical ligaments and the internal inguinal rings. In a thinner patient, the Foley catheter tip will often be seen on the anterior surface of the abdomen. Most posterior the rectum can be seen diving caudally. On the anterior surface of this rectovesical pouch, there are two peritoneal arches. In males, the seminal vesicles and vasa lie deep to the inferior fold. Once identified and depending on the operation planned, incisions in the peritoneum are created. During radical prostatectomy, some clinicians prefer to incise in the anterior rectovesical pouch to commence the seminal vesicle dissection. It is my preference to use this incision only in cases of cystectomy after lymphadenectomy. Both radical prostatectomy and lymphadenectomy are commenced by incision of the peritoneum lateral to the medial umbilical ligament down to a point medial to the internal inguinal rings in the direction of the vasa. The vasa can then be divided if preferred. This incision is carried to the transversalis fascia fibers; the plane along these fibers then can be followed down to the pubis, which is a reliable landmark. If lymphadenectomy is to be performed, the iliac vein should then be skeletonized and the packet developed off the pelvic side wall. The packet can then be further mobilized to the obturator nerve, excised, and delivered. For an extended lymph node dissection for bladder cancer, the vas should be divided and the iliac artery and vein should be skeletonized (Figure 1-5). This dissection plane can then be carried proximally all the way to the bifurcation of the iliacs. The ureter will be encountered and can be mobilized and left intact until definitive dissection is performed.

For prostatectomy, the bladder can be dropped by incision across both medial umbilical ligaments. This provides access to the space of Retzius, which can be further widened by blunt dissection. Careful dissection distally uncovers fully the arch of the pubis (Figure 1-6). Superficial fat overlying the prostate and bladder can be mobilized to visualize the endopelvic fascia and puboprostatic ligaments. Further anatomic landmarks for laparoscopic radical prostatectomy are described in a later section. For cystectomy, once the

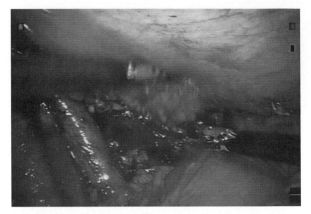

FIGURE 1-5. View of dissected iliac artery and vein during lymphadenectomy for robotic cystectomy.

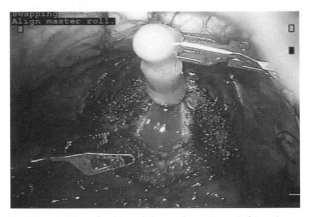

FIGURE 1-6. View of pubis and dissected prostatovesical junction.

lymphadenectomy portion is completed, the posterior bladder pedicle is then facilitated by the dissection of the branches of the internal iliac artery. Ligation of the major branches of this artery and completion of the division of the peritoneum along the inferior peritoneal fold of the rectovesical pouch allow posterior dissection of the bladder and even prostate away from the rectum. Once this plane is firmly established, a lateral plane around the more lateral aspect of the prostate will lead to visualization of the endopelvic fascia. Clear visualization of this plane affirms sufficient dissection posterior and lateral to the bladder; the space of Retzius can then be entered in the manner as described previously.

GENERAL CONSIDERATIONS

Before a laparoscopic procedure is contemplated, certain foundation steps must be taken. **One of the foremost of these is ensuring that the operating room (OR) has all the necessary equipment that may be remotely necessary for the completion of the procedure at hand.** Table 1-1 lists a set of basic equipment that is necessary for a laparoscopic procedure. All OR staff involved in the case should be well trained in the use and troubleshooting of laparoscopic equipment such as the insufflator and the suction device. The surgeon's assistant, whether this person is another urologist or some other assistant, should have an excellent understanding of the laparoscopic camera as this job can literally "make or break" the case.

Another foundation step is confirming that the anesthesiologist is well versed with the potential physiologic challenges that are unique to laparoscopy such as acid-base disturbances, pulmonary and cardiac changes, urine output (typically decreases), and gas embolism. Initial insufflation may cause a vagal response that is ameliorated by temporarily decreasing the pneumoperitoneum. As decreases in urine output are expected, fluids generally should not be aggressively given as this may cause postoperative fluid overload. However, in cases of donor nephrectomy, low-dose dopamine and/or mannitol can help maintain urine output that is crucial for optimization of the donor organ. Avoidance of nitrous oxide is helpful as it has been reported that this accumulates in the bowel causing distention and potential explosion if the bowel is violated.

Finally, the importance of patient selection cannot be overstated. As surgeon experience increases, more difficult patients and tumors can be approached successfully. **However, early on it is prudent to select average build patients without previous surgery with smaller tumors (especially in regard to nephrectomy). Despite all these preparations, conversion to an open procedure should not be considered a failure.** Conversion is to be expected at some point in the learning curve of every laparoscopic surgeon. Laparoscopy is performed to reduce patient morbidity; however, sometimes this is best achieved with conversion to a more familiar approach. Again, with increasing experience, conversion will become exceedingly rare.

Table 1-1: Basic Laparoscopic Instrument Set

Disposable Equipment

5-mm Endoshears
12-mm multifire laparoscopic stapler with reloads
10-mm clip applier
Trocars—5 mm (3) and 12 mm (4) (axially dilating clear ports)
Laparoscopic entrapment sac
Veress needles (150 mm)
CO_2 insufflation tubing
10 sponges (Raytex)
5-mm ultrasonic scalpel

Nondisposable Equipment

Endoholder
Suction irrigator, extra long, 5 mm
Laparoscope: 10-mm 0-degree and a 10-mm 30-degree lens
  and a 5-mm 0-degree lens
3, atraumatic, nonlocking 5-mm smooth tip (duckbill)
  grasping forceps
4, traumatic (toothed), locking, 5-mm grasping forceps
5-mm hook electrode
5-mm and 10-mm PEER retractors
5-mm needleholders
10-mm soft curved angled forceps (Maryland dissector)
10-mm right angle dissector
Carter Thomason needle suture grasper and closure cones
  (Inlet Medical)

Available but not Opened Equipment

Disposable Hasson trocar 12-mm blunt tip
3–0 cardiovascular silk (RB-1 needle) and 0-Vicryl sutures for
  fascial closure
Lapra-ty clips and 10 mm Laparo-Ty clip applier (Ethicon)
Gauze rolls (5) (Carefree Surgical Specialties)
10-mm Satinsky clamp with flexible port (Aesculap)

LAPAROSCOPIC ACCESS

The basis of laparoscopy begins with insufflation of the abdomen with carbon dioxide gas. Modern insufflators with high flow capabilities are excellent at maintaining and quickly refilling the belly with carbon dioxide even in the face of frequent suctioning and small gas leaks from around trocars. The establishment of pneumoperitoneum can be accomplished in several different ways. The author prefers the Veress needle. With experience this is a rapid, easily reproducible, and safe technique for insufflation. Typically, a small skin incision is made at a planned port site. The Veress needle can then be placed perpendicular to the abdominal fascia. The needle should be held along the shaft similar to a dart to maximize feel of the needle popping through the layers of the abdomen. After two distinct pops are felt, a syringe is attached to the needle and gentle aspiration is performed to rule out return of succus or blood. Then, a small amount of fluid is injected and aspiration of the fluid is attempted. If the fluid can be withdrawn, the needle is likely not in the peritoneal cavity but rather in a potential space just outside. If there is no return, the syringe is removed. If the fluid level in the needle drops, the carbon dioxide tubing can be attached to the needle and insufflation is begun. The pressure should be less than 9 mm Hg if placement is correct. Once the pressure reaches 15 mm Hg, the ports can be placed. Alternatively an open, Hasson type approach can be used. This involves a slightly more generous incision over the trocar site. The subcutaneous tissue is dissected away from the fascia. The fascia is then grasped with towel clamps and a suture is placed on either side of the planned incision. The fascial incision is created under direct vision and the peritoneum is also visualized and opened. The Hasson trocar is then placed and tied to the fascia by the preplaced sutures. These sutures can then be later used to close the fascia. Once the primary trocar is placed the remaining trocars can be placed under direct visualization of the abdominal wall with the laparoscope.

When exiting the abdomen, it is important to first decrease the pneumoperitoneum pressure in the abdomen to 5 mm Hg. This will allow any potential significant venous bleeding to become apparent. Careful visualization of the bed of the dissection should be performed with irrigation to wash out any clots. Once hemostasis is satisfactory, the trocars should also be removed under direct laparoscopic vision so that any port site bleeding is immediately recognized. If there is bleeding that is refractory to cautery, then a suture can be placed to tie off the bleeding port site. A Carter Thomason device or other suture passer can be used to correctly place this stitch (Figure 1-7). Once tied, the laparoscope is used to confirm hemostasis. Once the ports are removed, any port sites that held bladed trocars

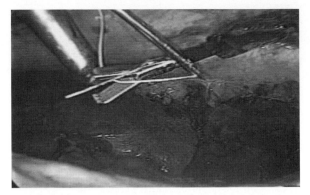

FIGURE 1-7. Laparoscopic view of suture passer placed into abdomen with suture.

larger than 10 mm should be closed at the fascial layer with suture. However, the author now uses only nonbladed dilating trocars. These are only closed if used in the midline. Even 12-mm trocars placed off the midline are not typically closed.

ROBOTICS

A significant step in the development of equipment for laparoscopic urology is the use of robotics. Robotic surgical systems, including the AESOP and DaVinci Surgical Systems (Intuitive Surgical, Sunnyvale, CA), are being employed more frequently. The AESOP robot manipulates a laparoscopic camera under voice control. Currently, the support from Intuitive Surgical for the AESOP is gradually being phased out. The DaVinci Surgical System is a more sophisticated system. The benefits that this platform provides are three-dimensional visual systems, proprietary wristed instruments, motion scaling, and improved ergonomics. The DaVinci consists of three primary components: the patient-side cart, the vision system, and the surgeon's console. The patient-side cart has three or four arms that are attached to the specialized robotic laparoscopic trocars that are positioned by the surgeon (Figure 1-8). The robotic arms then translate the movements of the console surgeon to the attached instruments. A binocular viewer enables the surgeon to see the three-dimensional video image transmitted from the double-headed camera. Foot pedals allow the surgeon to independently move the camera, activate cautery, and reset the instruments to

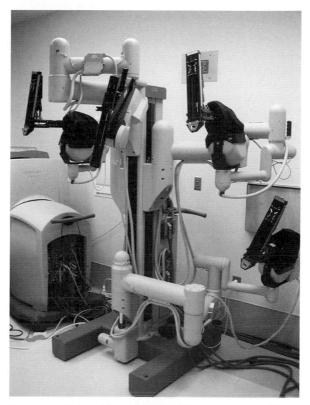

FIGURE 1-8. Patient side cart with fourth arm component of the DaVinci Surgical System (Intuitive Surgical, Sunnyvale, CA).

comfortable working positions as needed. These advantages of the robot have applied themselves seamlessly to radical prostatectomy. The robot is also applicable to pyeloplasty and radical cystectomy. A large variety of other cases have also been performed robotically.

LAPAROSCOPIC RENAL SURGERY

Since Ralph Clayman's report in 1991, laparoscopic nephrectomy has evolved and is becoming a standard of care for removal of malignant or benign kidneys in the United States. Experience from Johns Hopkins has now shown 10-year equivalence between laparoscopic and open nephrectomy in regard to cancer control.

Laparoscopic Radical Nephrectomy

Indications

Patients with evidence of renal malignancy without involvement of tumor thrombus of the inferior vena cava are candidates for laparoscopic nephrectomy. **With increasing experience, tumors upward of 15 cm in size and thrombus involvement limited to the renal vein can be managed laparoscopically.**

Preparation

Informed consent is obtained which includes the possibility of conversion to open nephrectomy. Standard lab work including liver function studies, serum calcium, and alkaline phosphatase is obtained. The computed tomography (CT) scan should be carefully examined for signs of renal vein involvement or lymphadenopathy. A chest x-ray (CXR) should also be obtained to rule out occult chest disease or metastasis. A formal bowel preparation is not performed. Perioperative antibiotics and heparin are administered. General anesthesia is administered and an orogastric tube and Foley catheter are placed. **The patient is usually placed in a 70-degree flank position with the table very slightly flexed.**

Instrumentation

Standard laparoscopic instrumentation is utilized. The author prefers certain devices to aid the expeditious performance of this case. The PEER retractor (J. Jamner Surgical, Hawthorne, NY) is an excellent atraumatic retractor that is especially useful when combined with an Endoholder (Codman, Raynham, MA), a self-retaining laparoscopic retractor (Figure 1-9). The combination of these instruments can provide excellent lateral retraction of the kidney during dissection of the renal hilum. Control of the hilum itself is usually obtained by individual firings of a laparoscopic stapler with vascular tissue load (Ethicon Endo-Surgery, Cincinnati, OH). The effectiveness of this stapler is maximized when the tissue to be stapled is compressed between the jaws for at least 10 seconds. This compression allows better staple formation and improved hemostasis.

A laparoscopic entrapment sac should be at the ready. Either the LapSac (Cook Urological, Bloomington, IN) or EndoCatch II (US Surgical Corp., Norwalk, CT) should be employed. The LapSac is impermeable and should be the only sac used when morcellation is to be performed.

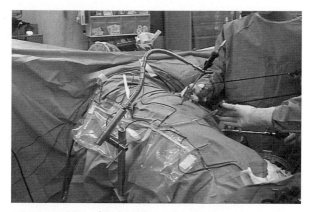

FIGURE 1-9. View of Endoholder used for laparoscopic retraction.

The EndoCatch II has an easily deployable ring that facilitates organ entrapment but is used to deliver intact specimens. If hand-assisted nephrectomy is to be performed, a hand-assist device such as the Gelport (Applied Medical, Rancho Santa Margarita, CA) should be available.

Operative Steps

Once access and pneumoperitoneum are established, the working trocar and hand-assist device should be placed. Figure 1-10 shows suggested left and right standard laparoscopic port positions; many variations in port placement exist.

For a right-sided nephrectomy, the following steps are generally followed. The colon is visualized and the white line of Toldt is incised. This incision is extended into the lower abdomen and cranially over the kidney to the triangular ligament of the liver. A counterincision is then created off this line caudal to the liver to allow the hepatic flexure of the colon to fall further medially. The ureter can then be dissected and divided; lateral upward retraction then exposes the lower pole of the kidney. En bloc dissection of the Gerota's fascia lifting the kidney off the psoas provides an easy plane to follow toward the hilum of the kidney. Once the hilum is approached, the duodenum should be Kocherized. The inferior vena cava is followed cranially until the renal vein is encountered. A right-angle instrument is usually passed behind the renal vein to ensure adequate dissection. The artery is then completely dissected to ensure adequate room for the stapler or placement of clips. **If the surgeon**

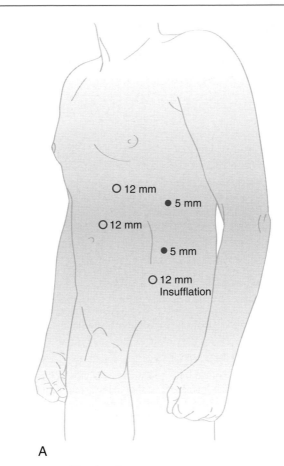

A

FIGURE 1-10. (Continued)

elects clips, at least three titanium clips should be placed on the stay side of the artery. Once the artery is divided, the vein is stapled. Following the dissection plane of the vena cava, the adrenal can be spared or excised en bloc. If it is to be removed, the adrenal vein must be carefully ligated. If it is to be spared, then the medial capsule of the kidney should be exposed and followed along its contour to the upper pole. Once the upper pole is reached, then the posterolateral attachments of the kidney are divided.

The left kidney is approached in a similar fashion. After reflection of the colon, the ureter can be divided; **however,**

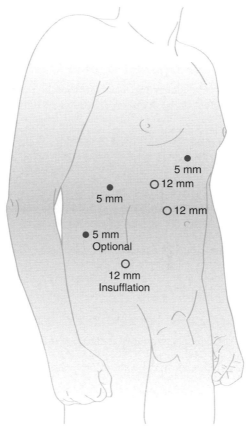

B

FIGURE 1-10. Diagram of laparoscopic port placement for left- (**A**) and right- (**B**) sided standard laparoscopic nephrectomy.

the gonadal vein is a consistent landmark that can be traced directly to the renal vein. Sufficient mobilization of the spleen is mandatory to allow easy access to the hilum and upper pole. Once the renal vein is identified, all tributaries must be identified and ligated. The artery is then dissected and divided; the vein is stapled. The upper pole and lateral and posterior attachment dissections are completed. The freed kidney is then placed in the laparoscopic entrapment sac. We prefer to make a small Gibson-type counterincision to remove the kidney whole.

Once the kidney is removed, the pneumoperitoneum of 5 mm Hg is reestablished to inspect the surgical bed for bleeding. Once hemostasis is satisfactorily established, the ports are removed under direct vision and the port sites are closed.

Retroperitoneal Approach

Alternatively, the kidney may be approached in a retroperitoneal fashion. Initial trocar placement is performed off the tip of the 12th rib. The thoracolumbar fascia is pierced and a dilating balloon is placed to develop the working space. A Hasson trocar is placed in the initial dilation port and accessory ports are placed. Proper balloon dissection allows immediate visualization of the psoas. More careful visualization often reveals the pulsations of the renal hilum or aorta/vena cava. **Gerota's fascia is then incised longitudinally 1 to 2 cm above the psoas to allow access to the hilum with the artery presenting first.** Once the hilum is controlled, the remaining renal attachments are divided. The kidney is placed in a laparoscopic entrapment sac. A Pfannenstiel incision can then be created and blunt dissection is used to connect the extraperitoneal planes to remove the kidney.

Postoperative Care

Patients are typically transferred to the floor after recovery in the postanesthesia care unit. Usual pain medication consists of ketorolac intravenous (IV) with an oral narcotic for breakthrough pain. Early ambulation is encouraged. Diet is resumed with a clear diet and advanced as tolerated. Discharge is planned for the night of postoperative day 1 or early day 2.

Results

Representative results for laparoscopic nephrectomy include mean OR times of between 2 and 4 hours. Typical reported hospital stays range from 1.6 to 3.5 days. Estimated blood loss is 100 to 300 mL. Complications rates range from 0% to 6% for major and 0% to 32% for minor. As stated earlier, cancer recurrence data reveal no differences between the open and laparoscopic approaches.

Laparoscopic Partial Nephrectomy

Indications

Tumors of less than 4 cm in a favorable location are amenable to partial nephrectomy. Long-term outcomes have demonstrated cancer control equivalence between radical and partial nephrectomy. Complex cysts of the kidney (Bosniak class 3 or higher) may also be approached in this fashion.

Preparation

The preparation for a laparoscopic partial nephrectomy is very similar to that of a radical nephrectomy. A CT scan with thin cuts through the kidney or a magnetic resonance imaging (MRI)/magnetic resonance angiography (MRA) should be performed to evaluate for depth of tumor in the kidney. If the tumor is small and very exophytic, a wedge excision may be performed. However, deeper tumors near the collecting system almost certainly mandate temporary hilar occlusion. Renal hilar anatomy can also be defined to determine vessel orientation and presence of multiple vessels. Some surgeons place a retrograde ureteral catheter to test for watertightness of collecting system repair if this is anticipated.

Instrumentation

If hilar clamping is anticipated, the laparoscopic bulldog clamps or a laparoscopic Satinsky clamp should be ready. Sutures suitable for collecting system repair should also be available. If a wedge resection is to be performed, some surgeons prefer an ultrasonic dissector. Finally, equipment to obtain hemostasis should be at the ready. Usually an argon beam coagulator (Conmed Corp, Utica, NY) or the Tissuelink (Tissuelink, Dover, NH) is used for initial hemostasis followed by a hemostatic agent such as Tisseel or Floseal (Baxter, Deerfield, IL). Laparoscopic ultrasound may be useful as well particularly for endophytic tumors that may be very difficult to find visually.

Operative Steps

Typically, anterior or lateral tumors are approached transperitoneally, whereas posteriorly placed tumors are approached retroperitoneally. The dissection steps for mobilization of the kidney are identical to that for laparoscopic radical nephrectomy. Once the region of the kidney involving the tumor is visualized, the capsule of the kidney around the tumor is exposed. This careful dissection should reveal the tumor's contour. The capsule is then scored to leave a small margin around the tumor. If hilar control is necessary, this should be prepared (Figure 1-11). Some surgeons also purposefully cool the kidney either by

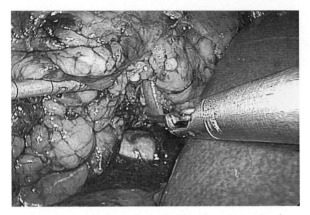

FIGURE 1-11. Laparoscopic view of bulldog clamp being placed on renal artery.

surrounding the kidney with a plastic bag with ice slush or via an intrarenal cooling technique accomplished by retrograde irrigation of the kidney with ice-cold solution. After clamping the artery and/or vein, the tumor is dissected out of the kidney using either ultrasonic shears or scissors with or without cautery. Some advocate as much as a 1-cm margin around the tumor, whereas others are more comfortable with a smaller 2- to 3-mm margin as nearly all of these tumors have a pseudocapsule. The tumor once excised is immediately placed in a laparoscopic entrapment sac and sent to pathology for a frozen section of the margin. Steps are taken to achieve hemostasis. The author prefers use of the Tissuelink with coverage of the bed with a fibrin glue/Surgicel patch. Another technique involves the placement of sutures through the parenchyma of the kidney similar to reconstruction during open partial nephrectomy. These sutures are then tied over a Surgicel patch. These steps are taken to achieve a closure similar to an open partial nephrectomy. Care must also be taken to rule out collecting system violation that would require suture repair. Once hemostasis is obtained and all suturing is completed, a drain is placed via one of the port sites.

Postoperative Care

The postoperative care is identical to that of laparoscopic radical nephrectomy. The drain is removed if no significant fluid is seen a few hours after Foley catheter removal to rule out significant urine leak.

Results

In one of the largest series (n = 223) of laparoscopic partial nephrectomy, Kavoussi reported a mean tumor size of 2.6 cm and mean operating room (OR) time of 186 minutes. Mean estimated blood loss (EBL) was 385 mL with a transfusion rate of 7%. There was no relationship between creatinine and warm ischemia time. The overall positive margin rate was 3.5% with more than 30% of the tumors being benign on final pathology.

Laparoscopic Nephroureterectomy

Indications

Transitional cell carcinoma (TCC) of the upper urinary tract is best treated by nephroureterectomy. As the recommendation for adjuvant treatment of TCC requires accurate pathologic staging, intact extraction of the surgical specimen is mandatory. Hand-assisted laparoscopy is therefore commonly used for this procedure. **The optimal method of bladder cuff removal is still debated; some advocate a standard laparoscopic approach to the kidney with the bladder cuff being done open to also allow kidney removal.**

Preparation

The preparation of the patient should be similar to that of laparoscopic radical nephrectomy.

Instrumentation

Specifically for the nephrectomy portion of the procedure, the instrumentation would be similar to that of laparoscopic radical nephrectomy. Differences in instrumentation would result from the requirements for the distal cuff portion.

Operative Steps

The operative technique for the renal dissection was outlined previously. Once the kidney is devascularized, attention is turned into the pelvis and the ureter is mobilized to the bladder. Here the techniques will depend on the individual surgeon's preference. Some prefer an open cuff removal, especially if there was no hand port incision created. The lower quadrant Gibson type incision for access to the ureter is also ideal for removal of the kidney.

Another option that has been used by Gill and colleagues is the needlescopic approach. In this method, cystoscopy is initiated to rule out bladder tumor and to fill the bladder with irrigant. Two needlescopic (2 mm) trocars are inserted into the bladder. A ureteral catheter is passed through an Endoloop into the ureter. A resectoscope with Collins' knife is use to score around the ureter. Using needlescopic retraction, the ureter is disarticulated and the Endoloop is closed tightly around the ureter as the catheter is withdrawn. Others perform a cystoscopic disarticulation prior to laparoscopic dissection followed by early clipping of the distal ureter. This allows the surgeon to "pluck" the ureter from above. Finally, Clayman and colleagues have used a technique in which the ureter is dissected laparoscopically into the bladder hiatus. Once the ureter appears to be dissected as deeply into the bladder as possible, the ureter is stapled. Once the laparoscopic portion is completed, the patient undergoes cystoscopy. If staples are clearly seen in the bladder, then the procedure is completed. If a ureteral tunnel remains, a ureteral catheter is placed up the ureter as far as possible. A Collins' knife is then used to unroof the ureteral tunnel with the catheter as a guide. Staples should be visualized and then gently coagulated on the surface to ablate any remaining malignant cells.

Postoperative Care

Patients are again treated in a similar fashion to that of laparoscopic radical nephrectomy. If a "pluck" technique or needlescopic technique is used, the bladder must be drained with a Foley catheter for at least 7 days.

Results

Representative results include OR times of 2.5 to 5.5 hours. Mean blood loss is 350 mL. Hospital stay has been around 4.5 days. Complication rates average around 10%.

Laparoscopic Pyeloplasty

Indications

Modern series of laparoscopic pyeloplasty have reported success rates equaling the open counterpart. There certainly exists a significant learning curve to this operation with the need for complex laparoscopic tying and suturing skills. However, in specialized centers, laparoscopic pyeloplasty is the preferred method of treating ureteropelvic junction obstruction. Patients with either primary or secondary ureteropelvic junction (UPJ) obstruction may be treated. Patients with anatomic abnormalities such as horseshoe kidney, duplication, and pelvic kidneys have been successfully treated.

Preparation

Many surgeons routinely screen patients with UPJ obstruction with a CT angiogram to detect crossing vessels. This may help guide treatment options, especially if a patient is willing to undergo an endopyelotomy in the absence of crossing vessels. Another method of accurately detecting crossing vessels is the endoluminal ultrasound. However, this usually needs to be performed under anesthesia and is combined with ureteroscopy. Some surgeons prefer to place a stent at the time of operation, others prefer 1 week in advance, and others not at all. Those who prefer not to stent believe that the stent causes some inflammation, which may make dissection more difficult. More times than not, however, patients do have a stent placed preoperatively for pain control reasons.

Instrumentation

For those facile at laparoscopic suturing, a pair of laparoscopic needle drivers is sufficient instrumentation. However, the Endostitch (USS, Norwalk, CT) is a 10-mm laparoscopic tool that has a needle that is passed back and forth between opposable jaws. The needles come attached to sutures in a variety of types and sizes. This can greatly facilitate the suturing process for surgeons still expanding their laparoscopic skills. The DaVinci Surgical System is an extremely useful tool for laparoscopic pyeloplasty. The author prefers to perform all pyeloplasties from beginning to end with robotic assistance.

Operative Steps

The ports are placed after the establishment of pneumoperitoneum with the patient in the 70-degree flank position. A ureteral stent can be placed preoperatively if desired. If the robot is to be used, it is docked at this point. However, there are some surgeons who prefer to perform the dissection laparoscopically and then dock the robot for the reconstructive portion of the procedure. Once the laparoscopic dissection portion is begun, careful inspection of the operative field is prudent. In patients with very large hydronephrotic systems, the pelvis may be easily visible through the mesentery. If so, a small window can be created through the mesentery to access the UPJ. However, if there is any question as to the location of the ureter, the colon should be dissected off the side wall as for laparoscopic nephrectomy. After reflection of the colon, the upper ureter should be identified. Often it can be found through an incision in the Gerota's fascia of the lower pole of the kidney. **The ureteral dissection must not compromise the blood supply as the UPJ is reached. A crossing vessel should be evident if present. Complete mobilization of the vessels from the UPJ and ureter is mandatory to allow transposition of the UPJ.** Once the dissection is completed, the orientation of the ureter should be fixed in mind as the ureter is divided. The stent if present will be identified. It is often helpful to spatulate before complete transection of the ureter. Once the ureter is divided the stent should be removed from the pelvis and transposition of the ureter and pelvis to the anterior surface of the vessels should be performed. After the pelvis is spatulated and/or tailored if necessary, the back wall of the UPJ repair is completed. The repair can be performed in either a running or interrupted fashion (Figure 1-12). After completion of the back wall, the stent is replaced into the pelvis. Alternatively, if there was no stent at the outset, it can be placed now in an antegrade fashion. A glidewire can be placed down one of the trocars and into the ureter. A stent that is slightly longer than necessary is placed over the wire until the distal curl is at the UPJ. If this method is used, it is prudent to check for the curl of the stent in the bladder cystoscopically at the end of the case. After the anterior wall repair is completed, a drain is left in place and the abdomen is exited.

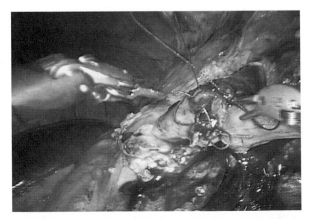

FIGURE 1-12. Laparoscopic view of front wall closure during robotic pyeloplasty.

Postoperative Care

The postoperative care is similar to that of a partial nephrectomy. The Foley catheter is usually removed early in the morning of postoperative day 1. If there is no increase in the output of the JP drain, the drain is removed in the afternoon and discharge is planned for the night or the next morning.

Results

Representative series of laparoscopic pyeloplasty demonstrate mean OR time of 2 to 4 hours. EBL is 100 to 200 mL. Hospital stay of 1 to 3 days is noted. Radiographic improvement of obstruction is seen in at least 90% of patients.

Laparoscopic Donor Nephrectomy

Indications

Patients deemed suitable candidates for kidney donation may be offered a laparoscopic donor nephrectomy. Certainly, benefits of less postoperative pain, shorter hospital stays, and quicker recovery are attractive for many potential donors. Data are accumulating that suggest that warm ischemia times and graft function are equivalent.

Preparation

Donors should be extensively screened according to institutional standards as well as those of the American Society of Transplant Physicians. Typical tests required in the workup include ABO histocompatibility and human leukocyte antigen (HLA) crossmatching. Hepatitis B and C, syphilis, human immunodeficiency virus (HIV), cytomegalovirus (CMV), and varicella must be screened for. A renal angiography plus intravenous pyelogram (IVP) or three-dimensional CT angiography are mandatory to clearly delineate the vascular anatomy of the kidney.

Instrumentation

The laparoscopic instrumentation should be identical to that of a laparoscopic radical nephrectomy. However, the transplant team will be ready for preparation of the kidney for the recipient. The anesthesiologist should also have all necessary medication for preparation of the kidney including heparin, mannitol, and furosemide. Papaverine should be available for the surgeon for application to the artery to prevent vasospasm.

Operative Steps

The operative steps are somewhat similar to a left-sided radical nephrectomy. However, mobilization of the kidney without significant dissection of the ureter is imperative to the success of the operation. Therefore, the upper pole of kidney is usually dissected first from within Gerota's fascia until the kidney can rest on the spleen. **Dissection of the ureter is accomplished by taking a wide band of tissue starting with the gonadal vein and sweeping this laterally. This gentle sweeping is continued until the psoas is clearly visualized.** The dissection plane is then carried back toward the hilum. A complete hilar dissection is performed while maintaining the lateral attachments of the kidney. Lasix and mannitol are administered. The extraction site, usually a Pfannenstiel incision or a hand-assist port, should be prepared. The transplant team is notified and the ureter and gonadal vessel are transected. The remaining kidney attachments are lysed and the renal vessels are ligated after the administration of heparin sulfate. The kidney is secured in the preplaced entrapment sac and the kidney is extracted. The patient is given protamine and the extraction site is closed. The renal bed is inspected for bleeding and, if satisfactory, the abdomen is exited.

Postoperative Care

The postoperative care is identical to that after a laparoscopic radical nephrectomy.

Results

Several comparative studies between open and laparoscopic donor nephrectomy reveal significantly shorter length of stay and shorter time to full activity and return to work. Early data regarding graft function, incidence of rejection, and ureteral complications are comparable between the open and laparoscopic groups.

Laparoscopic Cyst Decortication

Indications

The usual indication for laparoscopic cyst decortication for patients with autosomal dominant polycystic kidney disease (ADPKD) is chronic debilitating pain. Many of these patients are on chronic narcotic regimens. Other consequences of ADPKD are hypertension, renal failure, early satiety, and shortness of breath.

Preparation

The preparation of the patient is the same as that for laparoscopic nephrectomy.

Instrumentation

The use of a laparoscopic ultrasound probe is very helpful to find all cysts on the surface of the kidney. Otherwise instrumentation is that for laparoscopic nephrectomy.

Operative Steps

The approach should be to treat all "detectable" peripheral and perihilar cysts. As many cysts as possible should be decorticated and drained. Often greater than 500 cysts may be treated in a single procedure (Figure 1-13). A careful dissection of the renal hilum should also be performed. Hemostasis is obtained by electrocautery and use of the argon beam coagulator. At the end of the procedure, the kidney should be re-examined with a laparoscopic ultrasound to detect any remaining cysts within a few millimeters of the renal surface. On completion of cyst drainage, the kidney can be sutured to the retroperitoneal musculature (i.e., nephropexy) to preclude renal torsion.

Postoperative Care

The postoperative care of these patients can be quite challenging as their pain threshold has been altered by the chronic

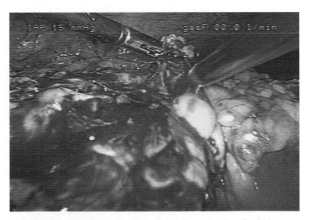

FIGURE 1-13. Laparoscopic view of cyst decortication for kidney affected by ADPKD.

pain that they have endured. Additionally, some patients after cyst decortication experience pain out of proportion to the procedure; this has been related to cyst fluid spillage. In either case, pain medication requirements will be significant in this period.

Results

In the largest series to date regarding laparoscopic cyst decortication, OR times were 5 hours. An average of 220 cysts were treated. With a follow-up of 32 months, the pain relief was durable. **Strikingly, however, hypertension improved and renal function stabilized.**

LAPAROSCOPIC PELVIC LYMPHADENECTOMY

Indications

This operation, which was once a fertile training ground for urologists familiarizing themselves with laparoscopy, has become much less frequently performed with the decreased utilization of the procedure overall. Patients who are at high risk of lymph node involvement are offered this procedure to rule out metastasis; if negative, this is usually followed by definitive local treatment.

Preparation

Informed consent is obtained, which includes the possibility of conversion to open lymph node dissection. A formal bowel preparation is not performed. Perioperative antibiotics and heparin are administered. General anesthesia is administered and a Foley catheter is placed. The patient is usually placed supine on the OR table but secured so that the bed can be placed into the Trendelenburg position and tilted from side to side.

Instrumentation

Standard laparoscopic instrumentation is all that is necessary.

Operative Steps

The important landmarks to identify are the internal inguinal rings and the medial umbilical ligaments. The initial incision in the peritoneum is created along the lateral edge of the medial umbilical ligament. The incision is carried down along the ligament toward the internal inguinal ring and the vas deferens. This opening can then be deepened until the pubis is seen. Lateral dissection along the pubis will then lead toward the lymph node packet. Careful observation will reveal the pulsations of the external iliac vein and/or artery. Dissection down onto the vein leads to a clear plane that carries the surgeon down to the bony pelvic sidewall. Care must be taken to avoid bleeding of small variable tributaries of the vein. Dissection of the packet is started distally toward the node of Cloquet and carried along the vein and pelvic sidewall. The packet is dissected off the medial aspect of the pubis; further blunt dissection reveals the obturator nerve. The remaining nodal packet is excised and sent for pathologic examination. Judicious cautery or a hemostatic agent can control any small amount of oozing.

Postoperative Care

Patients can usually be discharged the same day of the procedure with a minimum amount of pain.

Results

Comparative studies between open and laparoscopic pelvic lymph node dissection (PLND) have revealed similar numbers of lymph nodes retrieved with a slightly longer OR time (150–200 minutes vs. 100–150 minutes). Hospital stays were much shorter (1 vs. 5 days).

LAPAROSCOPIC AND ROBOTIC RADICAL PROSTATECTOMY

Indications

Although standard laparoscopic approaches to radical prostatectomy have been very successfully applied at very experienced centers, robotic-assisted radical prostatectomy is outstripping this procedure in growth and utilization. The benefits of the robotic platform have been previously discussed. Patients with preoperative evaluation suggesting organ confined disease are candidates for laparoscopic prostatectomy. There are exceptionally few patients who cannot undergo a robotic prostatectomy in regard to size of patient or prostate. The author has performed robotic prostatectomy for patients as large as 350 lb and prostate sizes as large as 250 g.

Preparation

Patients are usually prepared in a very similar fashion to laparoscopic nephrectomy. Positioning in the OR involves a Trendelenburg position, which can sometimes be rather severe. Some surgeons use shoulder bolsters to help prevent sliding toward the head of the table. If robotic prostatectomy is to be performed, the legs of the patient are usually split and lowered to allow the patient side cart to approach the patient from the feet. The author prefers the use of spreader bars as opposed to stirrups as this eases positioning of the patient and helps prevent slippage of the patient toward the head.

Instrumentation

Obviously if robotic prostatectomy is performed, then all adequate robotic support equipment should be available. It is often very helpful to employ a bariatric length suction cannula during these cases. This allows the surgeon or assistant to always have easy reach of the very deepest portions of the pelvis. We also prefer to use a laparoscopic vascular stapler for stapling the dorsal venous complex. Suture suitable for the anastomosis should be available.

Operative Steps

Port placement for robotic prostatectomy is shown in Figure 1-14. A representative figure for laparoscopic prostatectomy is seen in Figure 1-15. Once the ports are placed and the robot is docked if necessary either an anterior or posterior approach can be performed. If a posterior approach is used, the vas deferens and seminal vesicles are dissected completely first. Next, the bladder is dropped from the anterior abdominal wall by incision of the peritoneum. If the anterior approach is used, this is the first step. Some surgeons, however, prefer a retroperitoneal approach. This would involve balloon dilation of the retroperitoneal space of Retzius via the midline line port prior to secondary port placement. This step essentially drops the bladder from the anterior abdominal wall.

   Once the bladder is dropped, the anterior bladder and prostate come into view. The pubis is the first landmark that should be definitively defined. The fat from the medial edge of the pubis is bunched toward the superficial dorsal venous complex. This complex is usually divided with bipolar cautery. This whole fat packet then can be rolled cranially

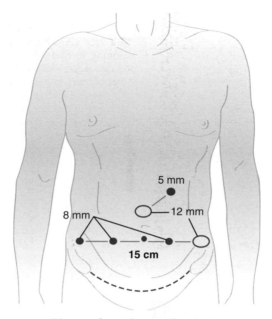

FIGURE 1-14. Diagram of port placement for robotic prostatectomy.

to the bladder neck. The author prefers to excise this whole packet of adipose tissue and deliver it from the abdomen.

The endopelvic fascia is then incised from the base of the prostate to the puboprostatic ligaments. The levator muscles are then visualized and gently dissected from the lateral surfaces of the prostate. Very fine muscle fibers can be dissected off the lateral surfaces of the apex of the prostate and lateral edges of the dorsal venous complex. The puboprostatic ligaments are then sharply divided. The dorsal venous complex and can be ligated, either using a suture ligature or the laparoscopic stapler (Figure 1-16).

The bladder neck dissection is then performed next. A number of different methods exist to perform this dissection. We prefer to begin by wiggling the Foley catheter so that the bladder neck can be identified. **If it does not move in a straight up-and-down fashion, this usually indicates the presence of a median lobe component.** Once the bladder neck area is visualized, lateral dissection is performed that drops the lateral portions of the bladder away from the prostate. As the bladder neck is approached, there are usually whitish longitudinal fibers that can be thinned

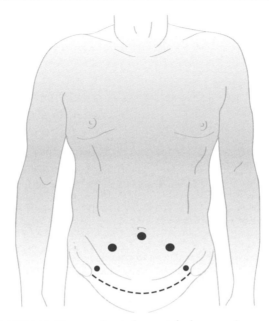

FIGURE 1-15. Diagram of port placement for laparoscopic prostatectomy.

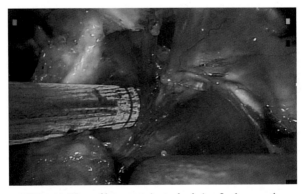

FIGURE 1-16. View of laparoscopic stapler being fired across the dorsal venous complex.

from a lateral to medial direction. Further dissection in the proper plane usually allows entry into the bladder neck very near the prostatovesical junction. The thickness of the muscle wall of bladder will help the surgeon to maintain the correct thickness posteriorly. Once the bladder is dropped away, the vas deferens and seminal vesicles are dissected if not performed earlier. If the posterior approach was utilized, these structures can simply be pulled through the newly created window. Once dissection is complete, these structures are used as retraction handles for the later dissection.

The vas deferens are then pulled anteriorly and the Denonvilliers fascia is incised. The rectum is then dropped away from the posterior side of the prostate. This dissection plane is taken as distally and laterally as possible. The use of any cautery is minimized from this point forward. Some surgeons prefer at this point to create an incision in the lateral prostatic fascia to begin to separate the neurovascular bundle (Figure 1-17). **Once accomplished, attention is then turned back to the base of the prostate and the pedicles are divided with clips, bipolar energy, or ultrasonic energy. A newer technique is to place a laparoscopic bulldog clamp on the pedicle, which is then sharply divided. Any bleeding points are then suture ligated at the completion of the prostate dissection.** Great care is taken to definitively visualize the apex during dissection especially posterior to the urethra. Preservation of urethral length is crucial for continence preservation. Once the prostate has been detached, it is immediately placed into a laparoscopic entrapment sac.

The anastomosis is then performed either with interrupted sutures or a running anastomosis. A Foley catheter

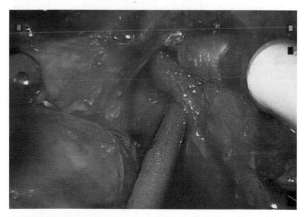

FIGURE 1-17. Laparoscopic view of right apical dissection with spared neurovascular bundle seen on the right.

is placed to irrigate the anastomosis for water tightness. A drain can be left at this point. A lymph node dissection may also be performed at the preference of the surgeon.

Postoperative Care

Patients are usually transferred to the floor or from the recovery unit. Patients are typically ambulated the night of postoperative day 1 and given a clear liquid diet. If they continue to ambulate and are taking regular food, by the next morning they are planned for discharge.

Results

Representative series of laparoscopic prostatectomy quote OR times of 200 to 280 minutes. Mean estimated blood loss is 150 to 400 mL. Complication rates have been reported between 11% and 30%. Robotic prostatectomy data demonstrate slightly shorter operative times, less blood loss, and lower complication rates than laparoscopic prostatectomy. Positive margin rates, continence data, and potency data are comparable to open radical prostatectomy.

LAPAROSCOPIC RADICAL CYSTECTOMY

Indications

Muscle invasive bladder cancer has been traditionally treated by open radical cystectomy with ileal conduit or neobladder formation. Laparoscopic approaches have been performed for both the bladder extirpative and bowel reconstructive portions. Many surgeons who performed these procedures are commonly performing the bladder portion laparoscopically, whereas the bowel reconstruction is performed through a mini-laparotomy from which the bladder specimen was retrieved.

Preparation

After a complete metastatic workup, patients are prepared for surgery with a complete mechanical bowel preparation. Preoperative and enterostomal nursing visitation is required for proper placement of the postoperative appliance.

Instrumentation

The instrumentation is similar to that of laparoscopic prostatectomy.

Operative Steps

After placement of ports and docking of the robot if applicable, the dissection is commenced by incising along the lateral aspect of the medial umbilical ligament to expose the external iliac artery and vein in a manner similar to the pelvic lymphadenectomy. The author's preference is to perform the lymphadenectomy at this point. The dissection plane is opened posteriorly toward the bifurcation of the iliac vessels. The vasa should be divided. The ureter will then be encountered and should be completely mobilized where it lies over the iliac vessels. The complete dissection of the iliac vessels then allows the lymphadenectomy to be performed. Ureteral mobilization should be carried as cranially as possible. Once the lymphadenectomy is complete, the origin of the superior vesical artery off the internal iliac should be visible; this will lead to the dissection of the bladder pedicle. The peritoneum deep in the cul-de-sac is incised and the rectum is dropped away from the posterior bladder. It is important to carry this dissection plane as distally as possible to facilitate later prostatic dissection. Dissection lateral to the bladder should be carried to the endopelvic fascia. Once this layer is well visualized, the pedicle of the bladder may be divided with a vessel sealing device or a laparoscopic stapler. Once the pedicle is dissected as distally as possible, the bladder may be dropped off the anterior abdominal wall. The endopelvic fascia is incised and the dorsal venous complex is divided. A clip or tie should be placed around the urethra before division to prevent any urine contamination. Mid to apical posterior prostate attachments may be divided sharply and visualized by side to side rotation of the specimen. The specimen is placed into a laparoscopic entrapment sac and placed out of the way in the upper abdomen. The bowel segments are then carefully examined for use of the reconstruction portion. Although there are reports of totally intracorporeal bowel reconstruction, we prefer to perform this portion through a small open incision from which the bladder is to be removed. **Before removal, the bowel segments are meticulously marked with sutures to ensure proper orientation of the bowel segment as orientation can be confused once the bowel is pulled upward through a very small incision. The ureters are also tagged with very long sutures.** The left ureter is passed behind the sigmoid colon over the sacral promontory to the right side. The open incision is made to remove the bladder. The bowel segments and ureters are pulled upward and the rest of the operation is completed in an open fashion.

Postoperative Care

Patients may be transferred to the floor unless they suffer from significant preoperative medical problems. A nasogastric tube is placed but is usually removed postoperative day 1. Patients are ambulated the first postoperative day and given sips of clears until evidence of bowel function returns.

Results

The experience with laparoscopic cystectomy is still fairly limited. Overall it seems that patients do have less pain and may have a quicker return of bowel function. Vallencien and colleagues reported on 84 cases with a mean of 18 months of follow-up. They reported a mean OR time of 280 minutes with a mean EBL of 550 mL. All surgical margins were negative and no port site recurrences have been noted. Robotically, Menon has reported on 24 patients who underwent cystectomy and diversion. The cystectomy portion and urinary diversion ranged in time from 110 to 170 minutes and 120 to 180 minutes, respectively. The blood loss ranged from 100 to 300 mL and patients were discharged from the hospital in 3 to 5 days.

CONCLUSIONS

Laparoscopic and robotic-assisted urologic surgery is now becoming routine in many centers and may become standard of care. As operative experience continues to grow so will the applications. As such, the benchmark results of open surgery are being approached and even in some cases surpassed while patient morbidity continues to improve.

SELF-ASSESSMENT QUESTIONS

1. Discuss the laparoscopic anatomy of the kidney and the pelvis.
2. Discuss the general and specialized instrumentation that is needed for laparoscopy.
3. Discuss the important aspects of establishment of pneumoperitoneum and exiting the abdomen.
4. Discuss the general procedural steps of the more commonly performed urologic laparoscopic procedures.
5. Discuss the general outcomes after commonly performed laparoscopic procedures.

SUGGESTED READINGS

1. Cathelineau X, Arroyo C, Rozet F, et al: Laparoscopic assisted radical cystectomy: the Montsouris experience after 84 cases. *Eur Urol* 47:780–784, 2005.
2. Clayman RV, Kavoussi LR, Soper NJ, et al: Laparoscopic nephrectomy. *N Engl J Med* 324:1370–1371, 1991.
3. Guillonneau B, el-Fettouh H, Baumert H, et al: Laparoscopic radical prostatectomy: oncological evaluation after 1,000 cases at Montsouris Institute. *J Urol* 169:1261–1266, 2003.
4. Hemal AK, Abol-Enein H, Tewari A, et al: Robotic radical cystectomy and urinary diversion in the management of bladder cancer. *Urol Clin North Am* 31:719–729, 2004.
5. Jarrett TW, Chan DY, Charambura TC, et al: Laparoscopic pyeloplasty: the first 100 cases. *J Urol* 167:1253–1256, 2002.
6. Lee DI, Andreoni CR, Rehman J, et al: Laparoscopic cyst decortication in autosomal dominant polycystic kidney disease: impact on pain, hypertension, and renal function. *J Endourol* 17:345–354, 2003.
7. Link RE, Bhayani SB, Allaf ME, et al: Exploring the learning curve, pathological outcomes and perioperative morbidity of laparoscopic partial nephrectomy performed for renal mass. *J Urol* 173:1690–1694, 2005.
8. Matin SF, Gill IS: Recurrence and survival following laparoscopic radical nephroureterectomy with various forms of bladder cuff control. *J Urol* 173:395–400, 2005.
9. Menon M, Tewari A, Peabody JO, et al: Vattikuti Institute prostatectomy, a technique of robotic radical prostatectomy for management of localized carcinoma of the prostate: experience of over 1100 cases. *Urol Clin North Am* 31:701–717, 2004.
10. Patel V: Robotic-assisted laparoscopic dismembered pyeloplasty. *Urology* 66:45–49, 2005.
11. Permpongkosol S, Chan DY, Link RE, et al: Long-term survival analysis after laparoscopic radical nephrectomy. *J Urol* 174:1222–1225, 2005.
12. Schuessler WW, Vancaillie TG, Reich H, et al: Transperitoneal endosurgical lymphadenectomy in patients with localized prostate cancer. *J Urol* 145:988–991, 1991.
13. Shalhav AL, Dunn MD, Portis AJ, et al: Laparoscopic nephroureterectomy for upper tract transitional cell cancer: the Washington University experience. *J Urol* 163:1100–1104, 2000.
14. Wein AJ, Kavoussi LR, Novick AC, et al: *Campbell's Urology*. 9th ed. Elsevier Science, Philadelphia, 2007.

Chapters:

C H A P T E R 2

Signs and Symptoms: The Initial Examination

Keith N. Van Arsdalen, MD

I. BACKGROUND

A. Definition

Urology is a surgical specialty devoted to the study and treatment of disorders of the genitourinary tract of the male and the urinary tract of the female. In addition to the surgical correction of acquired and congenital abnormalities, the urologist is often involved with the diagnosis and treatment of many "medical" disorders of the genitourinary tract.

B. Importance to Other Branches of Medicine

1. Approximately 15% of patients initially presenting to a physician will have a urologic complaint or abnormality.
2. There is a wide overlap with other specialties and frequent interaction with other physicians, including family practitioners, internists, pediatricians, geriatricians, endocrinologists, nephrologists, neurologists, obstetricians and gynecologists, and general, vascular, and trauma surgeons.
3. It is important that all physicians be aware of the specific diagnostic and therapeutic measures that are available within this specialty.

II. UROLOGIC MANIFESTATIONS OF DISEASE

A. Direct

The most obvious manifestations of urologic disease are those signs and symptoms that are directly related to the urinary tract of the male and female or to the genitalia of the male. Hematuria and scrotal swelling are examples in this category.

37

B. Manifestations Referred to or from Other Organ Systems

1. Symptoms from the genitourinary tract may be referred to other areas within the genitourinary tract or to contiguous organ systems.
   a) A stone in the kidney or upper ureter may produce ipsilateral testicular pain.
   b) This same stone may be associated with symptoms of nausea and vomiting.
   c) The gastrointestinal (GI) tract is probably the most common site to manifest symptoms from primary urologic problems. This is most probably due to the common innervation of these systems as well as the close direct relationship between the various component organs.
2. Primary urologic disorders may also be manifest in different organ systems and by seemingly unrelated signs and symptoms. Bone pain and pathologic fractures secondary to metastatic carcinoma arising in the genitourinary tract are examples.
3. Similarly, primary disease in other organ systems may result in secondary urologic signs and symptoms that initially lead the patient to the urologist. Diabetes may be detected by finding glucosuria in a patient presenting with frequency and nocturia. Other signs and symptoms mimicking urologic disease are related to inflammatory or neoplastic processes arising in the
   a) Lower lobes of the lungs
   b) GI tract
   c) Female internal genitalia

C. Systemic

Fever, weight loss, and malaise can be nonspecific systemic manifestations of acute and chronic inflammatory disorders, renal failure, and genitourinary carcinoma with or without metastases.

D. Asymptomatic

Finally, it should be remembered that localized or extensive disease may exist within the genitourinary tract without any signs or symptoms being manifest.

1. Renal calculi or neoplasms may be found during other examinations. Up to 60% of renal masses are detected incidentally.

2. Sixty percent of prostate cancers are currently detected secondary to prostate-specific antigen (PSA) elevations only without palpable abnormalities of the prostate.
3. Far-advanced renal deterioration may occur prior to the detection of silent reflux or obstruction.

III. HISTORY

A. Symptoms

1. A symptom is any departure from normal appearance, function, or sensation as experienced by the patient. Symptoms are reported to the physician or uncovered by careful history taking, with varying degrees of importance and/or significance attached to each symptom by both parties.
   a) The chief complaint, history of the present illness, and past medical history are delineated in a standard fashion.
   b) The character, onset, duration, and progression of the symptom are carefully defined. It is important to note what factors exacerbate or ameliorate the problem.
2. Urologic symptoms are generally related to
   a) Pain and discomfort
   b) Alterations of micturition
   c) Changes in the gross appearance of the urine
   d) Abnormal appearance and/or function of the external genitalia

B. Pain

1. Pain within the genitourinary tract generally arises from distention or inflammation of a part or parts of the genitourinary system. Pain can be experienced directly in the involved organ or referred as noted previously. Referred pain is a relatively common symptom of genitourinary disease.
2. Renal pain
   a) The kidney and its capsule are innervated by sensory fibers traveling to the T10-L1 aspect of the spinal cord.
   b) The etiology of renal pain may be due either to capsular distention or inflammation or to distention of the renal collecting system.
   c) Renal pain can be a dull, aching sensation felt primarily in the area of the costovertebral angle or pain of a sharp colicky nature felt in the area of the flank, with radiation around the abdomen into the groin and

ipsilateral testicle or labium. The latter is due to the common innervation.

d) The nature of the primary disease process within the kidney often determines the type of sensation that is experienced and depends on the degree and rapidity of capsular and/or collecting system distention.

3. Ureteral pain

a) The upper ureter is innervated in a similar fashion to that described previously for the kidney. Therefore, upper ureteral pain has a similar distribution to that of renal pain.

b) The lower ureter, however, sends sensory fibers to the cord through ganglia subserving the major pelvic organs. Therefore, pain derived from the lower ureter is generally felt in the suprapubic area, bladder, penis, or urethra.

c) The most common etiologic mechanism for ureteral pain is sudden obstruction and ureteral distention.

d) Acute renal and ureteral colic are among the most severe types of pain known to humankind.

4. Bladder pain

a) Pain within the bladder may be derived from retention of urine with overdistention or from inflammatory processes.

b) The pain of overdistention is generally felt within the suprapubic area, resulting in severe local discomfort.

c) The pain due to bladder inflammation is generally felt as a sharp, burning pain that is often referred to the tip of the penile urethra in males and the entire urethra in females.

5. Prostate pain

a) Sensory fibers from the prostate mostly enter the sacral aspect of the spinal cord.

b) Prostate pain is most commonly due to acute inflammation and is generally perceived as discomfort in the lower back, rectum, and perineum.

c) Irritative symptoms arising from the bladder may overshadow the purely prostate symptoms.

6. Penile pain

a) Penile and urethral pain are generally directly related to a site of inflammation.

7. Scrotal pain

a) Pain within the scrotum generally arises from disorders of the testis and or epididymis.

b) The most common etiologic factors include trauma, torsion of the spermatic cord, torsion of the appendix testis or appendix epididymis, and acute inflammation, particularly epididymitis. The pain in these cases is generally of rapid onset, if not sudden, and severe in nature.

c) Hydroceles, varicoceles, and testicular tumors can also be associated with scrotal discomfort but are generally of a more insidious nature and less severe in most cases.

C. Alterations of Micturition

1. Definitions and problems
   a) A variety of specific terms have been developed to describe alterations related to the act of micturition. This section defines a variety of these terms.
   b) It must be emphasized that a variety of disease processes can result in similar symptoms at the level of the lower urinary tract, and although these terms are used to describe specific symptoms in this area, they do not necessarily pertain to specific etiologies.
2. Changes in urine volume
   a) *Anuria* and *oliguria* are terms that refer to the varying degrees of decreased urinary output that may be secondary to prerenal, renal, or postrenal factors. In all cases, it is essential to rule out urethral and/or ureteral obstruction as postrenal causes for these problems.
   b) *Polyuria* refers to an increase in the volume of urine excreted on a daily basis. The etiologic mechanisms include increased fluid intake, exogenous or endogenous diuretics, and abnormal states of central or peripheral osmoregulation.
3. Irritative symptoms
   a) *Dysuria* is a term that refers simply to painful or difficult urination. The burning sensation that occurs during micturition associated with either bladder, urethral, or prostatic inflammation is generally used synonymously. This discomfort is generally felt in the entire urethra in females and in the distal urethra in males.
   b) *Strangury* is a subtype of dysuria in which intense discomfort accompanies frequent voiding of small amounts of urine.
   c) *Frequency* refers to the increased number of times one feels the need to urinate. This can be secondary to a true decrease in bladder capacity from a loss of

elasticity or edema due to inflammation or secondary to a decrease in the effective bladder capacity due to a failure of the bladder to empty completely with persistence of a large amount of residual urine.

d) *Nocturia* is essentially the nighttime equivalent of urinary frequency, that is, there is a decreased real or effective bladder capacity that forces the patient to arise at night to urinate.

e) *Nycturia* refers to the excretion of larger volumes of urine at night than during the day and is secondary to mobilization of dependent fluid that accumulated when the patient was in the upright position. Nycturia can result in nocturia even in the presence of a normal bladder capacity if large quantities of fluid are mobilized.

f) *Urgency* refers to the sudden, severe urge to void that may or may not be controllable.

g) The irritative symptoms noted previously are most commonly associated with inflammation of the lower urinary tract, that is, bladder and prostate. Acute bacterial infections probably represent the most common etiologic mechanism. It should be noted, however, that the irritative symptoms may be secondary to the presence of a foreign body, nonspecific inflammation, radiation therapy or chemotherapy, neoplasms, and neurogenic bladder dysfunction.

h) The term overactive bladder refers to the symptoms of frequency and urgency, with or without urge or reflex incontinence, in the absence of local pathologic or metabolic factors that would account for these symptoms. The urodynamic-based definition of overactive bladder requires the demonstration of involuntary bladder contractions.

4. Bladder outlet obstructive symptoms

a) *Hesitancy* refers to the prolonged interval necessary to voluntarily initiate the urinary stream.

b) *Straining* refers to the need to increase intra-abdominal pressure to initiate voiding.

c) *Decreased force* and *caliber* of the urinary stream refer to the physical changes of the urinary stream that may be noted due to increased urethral resistance.

d) *Terminal dribbling* refers to the prolonged dribbling of urine from the meatus after the completion of micturition.

e) *Sense of residual urine* is the complaint of a sensation of incomplete emptying of the bladder that the patient recognizes after micturition.

f) *Prostatism.* All of the previous symptoms may be noted with any type of bladder outlet obstruction, that is, secondary to benign prostatic hypertrophy (BPH), prostate carcinoma, or urethral stricture disease. The most common cause of these symptoms, however, is benign prostatic enlargement, and hence this complex of symptoms has often been referred to as prostatism.

g) *Urinary retention.* Acute urinary retention may be associated with severe suprapubic discomfort. Alternatively, the chronic retention of urine within the bladder may occur on a gradual basis due to progressive obstruction and bladder decompensation, and large amounts of urine may be retained with minor changes in symptomatology.

h) *Interruption* of the urinary stream. Sudden painful interruption of the urinary stream can be secondary to the presence of a bladder calculus that ball valves into the bladder neck causing abrupt blockage of the urinary flow.

i) *Bifurcation* of the urinary stream. The symptom of a double stream or spraying of the urinary stream can be secondary to urethral stricture disease or can occur intermittently without any obvious pathology.

5. Incontinence

a) *True* or *total incontinence* occurs when there is constant dribbling of urine from the bladder. It may be due to the configuration of the bladder, such as with extrophy or epispadias, to ectopia of the ureteral orifices distal to the bladder neck in females, or to a fistula, usually between the bladder and the vagina. The most common cause, however, is secondary to injury to the sphincter mechanisms of the bladder neck and urethra due to trauma, surgery, or childbirth. Neurogenic disorders affecting the bladder outlet can also have similar effects.

b) *False* or *overflow incontinence* is seen with total bladder decompensation in which the bladder acts as a fixed reservoir and the only outflow of urine is an overflow phenomenon with constant dribbling through the bladder outlet.

c) *Urgency incontinence* results when the sensation of urgency becomes so severe that involuntary bladder emptying occurs. This is commonly secondary to severe inflammation of the urinary bladder. This type of incontinence can also be due to involuntary bladder contractions without inflammation (see previous definition of overactive bladder).

d) *Stress incontinence* is secondary to distortion of the normal anatomic relationship between the bladder and the urethra such that sudden increases in intra-abdominal pressure (laughing, straining, etc.) are transmitted unequally to the bladder and the urethra, resulting in elevated bladder pressure without a concomitant rise in urethral pressure. Most commonly, this is related to laxity of the pelvic floor, particularly following childbirth, but it may also be noted in women who have not had children. It is also a frequent sequel of radical prostatectomy surgery for prostate cancer.

e) It is important to differentiate the various types of incontinence as each is treated differently. Historical factors are very important in separating these different entities.

6. *Enuresis* refers to involuntary urination and bed-wetting that occurs during sleep.

7. Quantification of voiding symptoms

a) The AUA Symptom Index (internationally known as the IPSS) is a self-administered questionnaire consisting of seven questions relating to symptoms of prostatism (Table 2-1). The IPSS includes a quality of life question to assess the degree of bother experienced by the patient.

b) Symptoms are classified as mild (0–7), moderate (8–19), or severe (20–35).

c) The symptom score is an integral part of the clinical practice guidelines for treatment planning and follow-up for BPH management.

d) The symptom score is not specific for or diagnostic of BPH. It can be used in men and women for general assessment of voiding symptoms.

D. Changes in the Gross Appearance of the Urine

1. Cloudy urine

a) Cloudy urine is most commonly due to the benign process of precipitation of phosphates in an alkaline urine (phosphaturia). This may be noted after meals or after consumption of large quantities of milk and is generally intermittent in nature. Patients are otherwise asymptomatic. Acidification of the urine with acetic acid at the time of urinalysis causes prompt clearing of the specimen.

Table 2-1: The AUA Symptom Index						
Question	Not at All	Less Than 1 Time in 5	Less Than Half the Time	About Half the Time	More Than Half the Time	Almost Always
1. During the last month or so, how often have you had a sensation of not emptying your bladder completely after you finished urinating?	0	1	2	3	4	5
2. During the last month or so, how often have you had to urinate again less than 2 hours after you finished urinating?	0	1	2	3	4	5
3. During the last month or so, how often have you found you stopped and started again several times when you urinated?	0	1	2	3	4	5
4. During the last month or so, how often have you found it difficult to postpone urination?	0	1	2	3	4	5

(Continued)

Table 2-1:—Cont'd

Question	Not at All	Less Than 1 Time in 5	Less Than Half the Time	About Half the Time	More Than Half the Time	Almost Always
5. During the last month or so, how often have you had a weak urinary stream?	0	1	2	3	4	5
6. During the last month or so, how often have you had to push or strain to begin urination?	0	1	2	3	4	5
7. During the last month, how many times did you most typically get up to urinate from the time you went to bed at night until the time you got up in the morning?	None	1 Time	2 Times	3 Times	4 Times	5 or More Times
	0	1	2	3	4	5

AUA symptoms score = sum of questions 1 to 7.

    b) *Pyuria* refers to the finding of large quantities of white blood cells that cause urine to have a cloudy appearance. Microscopic examination of the urine sample will demonstrate the inflammatory nature that is usually secondary to an infection.

    c) *Chyluria* refers to the presence of lymph fluid mixed with the urine. It is an unusual cause of cloudy urine.

2. *Pneumaturia* refers to the passage of gas along with urine while voiding. There may be associated pyuria or frank fecal contamination of the urine, as this phenomenon is almost exclusively due to the presence of a fistula between the GI and urinary tracts. On occasion, the presence of a gas-forming infection within the urinary tract can produce similar symptoms, although this is very unusual.

3. Hematuria

    a) The passage of bloody urine is always alarming, and generally the patient makes a prompt visit to the physician. Investigation is always warranted, including a properly performed urinalysis to be certain that the red discoloration of the urine is indeed secondary to the presence of blood. For a differential diagnosis of the causes of red urine, see the following section.

    b) Although hematuria is always a danger signal, a clue to its significance may lie in whether there is associated pain or whether the bleeding is essentially painless. Pain that occurs in association with cystitis or passage of a urinary tract calculus may indicate that the bleeding is in fact benign in nature. Painless hematuria, however, is always believed to be secondary to a urinary tract neoplasm until proven otherwise. This differentiation is not infallible, and therefore all urinary tract bleeding warrants investigation to be certain that there is not an associated neoplasm in addition to the more obvious cause for painful bleeding.

    c) The probable site of bleeding within the urinary tract may be ascertained by determining whether the bleeding is initial (at the beginning of the stream only), terminal (at the end of the stream only), or total (throughout the entire stream). Initial hematuria generally indicates some type of anterior urethral bleeding that is flushed out by the initial passage of the bladder urine through the urethra. Terminal hematuria is often secondary to posterior urethral, bladder neck, or trigone bleeding and is noted when the bladder finally compresses these areas at the end of micturition. Total hematuria indicates that the bleeding occurs at the level of the bladder or above, such that all of the urine is mixed with blood and is therefore bloody throughout the entire stream.

4. *Colored urine* may result from a variety of foods, medications, and medical disorders. The colors may range from almost clear to black, with all other colors of the spectrum noted in between. (See Table 2-4 for common causes of colorful urine.)

E. Abnormal Appearance and/or Function of the Male External Genitalia

1. Sexual dysfunction
2. Infertility
3. Penile problems
   a) *Cutaneous lesions.* A variety of exophytic and ulcerative lesions may be noted by the patient. The relationship of the onset of these lesions to recent sexual activity should be explored. The physical characteristics of these lesions should be noted at the time of physical examination. The combination of historical and physical factors, as well as associated physical findings such as adenopathy, will provide a working diagnosis for the treatment of these lesions.
   b) *Penile curvature.* Bending of the penis, particularly during erection, is noted in association with scarring and fibrosis of the tunica albuginea. These plaque-like structures may be noted on physical examination. The process is essentially idiopathic and has been referred to as Peyronie's disease. Congenital curvature is usually in a ventral direction and is not associated with fibrosis or formation of a plaque.
   c) *Urethral discharge.* The character of the urethral discharge should be described as well as its onset in relation to sexual activity as noted previously. The presence of the discharge should be confirmed on physical examination and a microscopic examination performed and a culture obtained.
   d) *Bloody ejaculate.* Like hematuria, this is also a frightening experience that usually causes the patient to seek prompt attention. This problem, however, is generally secondary to benign congestion and/or inflammation of the seminal vesicles. The process is usually self-limited or treatable with antibiotics and does not initially require an extensive evaluation.

4. Scrotal problems
   a) *Cutaneous lesions.* The hair-bearing skin of the scrotum is susceptible to the variety of skin diseases that can occur anywhere else on the body. Fungal infections and venereal warts may also be noted commonly.
   b) *Scrotal swelling* and *masses.* The presence of scrotal swelling and/or a scrotal mass may be noted incidentally by the patient while bathing or performing a self-examination or due to the presence of associated discomfort. A variety of lesions can produce unilateral or bilateral scrotal enlargement. These range from normal structures that are misinterpreted by the patient to testicular neoplasms. The differential diagnosis is as noted in Table 2-2. A combination of historical information, particularly with regard to onset of the mass, progression, and associated pain, and the physical examination is helpful in differentiating some of the more confusing lesions. (See section on physical examination and Table 2-3.)

Table 2-2: Causes of Scrotal Swelling	
Structure Involved	**Pathology**
Scrotal wall	Hematoma
	Urinary extravasation
	Edema from cardiac, hepatic, or renal failure
Testis	Carcinoma
	Torsion of testes or appendix testis
Epididymis	Epididymitis
	Tumor
	Torsion of appendix epididymis
Spermatic cord	Hydrocele surrounding testis of involving cord only
	Hematocele
	Hernia
	Varicocele
	Lipoma

Table 2-3: Differential Diagnosis of Scrotal Discomfort and Solid Mass Lesions

	Torsion	Epididymitis	Tumor
Age	Birth to 20 years	Puberty to old age	15 to 35 years
Pain			
Onset	Sudden	Rapid	Gradual
Degree	Severe	Increasing severity	Mild or absent
Nausea/ vomiting	Yes	No	No
Examination			
Testis	Swollen	Normal early	Mass
Epididymis	together and both tender	Swollen, tender	Normal
Spermatic cord	Shortened	Thickened, often tender as high as inguinal canal	
Urinalysis	Normal	Often infection	Normal

IV. THE PHYSICAL EXAMINATION

A. General Information

1. The problems delineated in the history will determine how extensive the physical examination should be. A complete physical examination is obviously necessary for someone who will undergo some type of urologic surgery; in most instances, however, a limited examination of the genitourinary tract is usually sufficient at the time of the initial examination.

2. The commonly taught techniques of physical examination, including inspection, palpation, percussion, and auscultation, are also used during the urologic examination. Each has varying degrees of usefulness depending on the organ being evaluated. Particular aspects of the physical examination will be noted later.

B. Kidneys and Flanks

1. *Inspection.* Inspection of the flanks is best carried out with the patient in the sitting or standing position facing straight ahead and the examiner located behind the patient facing the area in question. Scoliosis may be evident in the patient with an inflammatory process directly or indirectly involving the psoas muscle with resultant spasm. Bulging of the flank may be noted if there is an underlying mass, although this is only evident in most cases if the mass is extremely large or the patient is very thin. Edema of the flank may be noted if there is an underlying inflammatory process.

2. *Palpation* and *percussion.* A method of bimanual renal palpation has been described with the patient in the supine position (Figure 2-1). The examiner lifts the flank by placing one hand beneath this area and subsequently palpates deeply beneath the ipsilateral costal margin anteriorly. This technique is successful in children and thin adults but generally yields little information under most

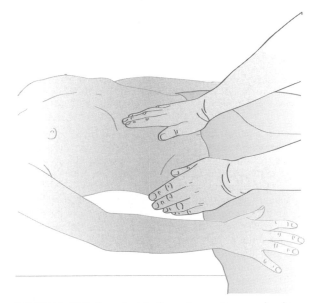

FIGURE 2-1. With the patient in the supine position, one hand is used to raise the flank while the abdominal hand palpates deeply beneath the costal margin. (From Van Arsdalen K: Signs and symptoms: the initial examination. In Hanno P, et al: *Clinical Manual of Urology.* McGraw Hill, 2001, F2-1.)

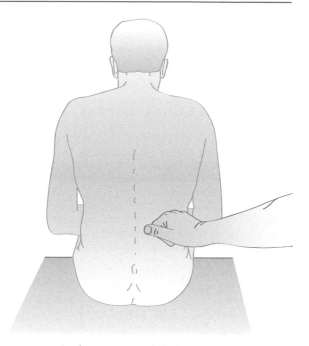

FIGURE 2-2. Gentle percussion with the heel of the hand in the angle between the lumbar vertebrae and the 12th rib is useful in eliciting underlying tenderness due to obstruction or inflammation. (From Van Arsdalen K: Signs and symptoms: the initial examination. In Hanno P, et al: *Clinical Manual of Urology.* McGraw Hill, 2001, F2-2.)

other circumstances. A large mass may be palpable. Percussion is a useful technique, particularly in the area of the costovertebral angle, to elicit tenderness due to underlying capsular inflammation or distention (Figure 2-2).

3. *Auscultation.* This technique is particularly useful in evaluating patients with possible renovascular hypertension. An underlying bruit may be noted in the area of the costovertebral angle due to renal artery stenosis, aneurysm formation, or arteriovenous malformation.

4. *Transillumination.* This technique, which may differentiate a solid from a cystic mass in neonates or infants, has largely been replaced by ultrasonography, which defines these lesions much more clearly.

C. Abdomen and Bladder

1. *Inspection.* The abdominal and bladder examinations are best carried out with the patient in the supine position.

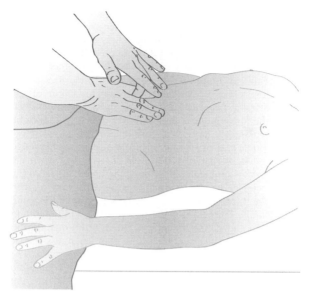

FIGURE 2-3. Percussion over the bladder may be particularly useful when palpation is difficult due either to obesity or failure of the patient to relax during the examination. The bladder may be percussed if it contains greater than 150 mL of urine in the adult. (From Van Arsdalen K: Signs and symptoms: the initial examination. In Hanno P, et al: *Clinical Manual of Urology.* McGraw Hill, 2001, F2-3.)

The full or overdistended bladder may be visible on general inspection of the abdomen with the patient in this position.

2. *Palpation* and *percussion.* It is generally possible to palpate or percuss the bladder above the level of the symphysis pubis if it contains 150 mL or more of urine (Figure 2-3). It should be remembered that in the child, the bladder *may* be percussible or palpable with much smaller volumes of urine due to the fact that it is more of an intra-abdominal organ in the child than the true pelvic organ it is in the adult.

D. Penis

1. *Inspection.* Inspection of the penis will reveal obvious lesions of the skin and will define whether the patient has been circumcised. If the patient has been circumcised, the glans penis and meatus can be inspected

directly. In the uncircumcised patient, the foreskin as well as the glans and meatus should then be inspected. The number and position of ulcerative and/or exophytic lesions should be noted if they are present. The position and size of the urinary meatus should be defined.

a) *Foreskin.* Phimosis is present when the orifice of the foreskin is constricted preventing retraction of the foreskin over the glans. Paraphimosis is present when the foreskin, once retracted over the glans, cannot be replaced to its normal position covering the glans.

b) *Penile meatus.* The normal meatus should be located at the tip of the glans. Hypospadias is present when the meatus opens anywhere along the ventral aspect of the penis or in the perineum. Epispadias is present when the meatus is located on the dorsal aspect of the penis.

2. *Palpation.* Palpation of the penile shaft is important to identify and define the limits of areas of fibrous induration that may be found in patients with Peyronie's disease who complain of penile curvature during erection. The urethra should also be palpated for areas of induration that may be associated with periurethritis and urethral stricture disease. The urethra can also be "stripped" from the penile-scrotal junction toward the meatus to look for a urethral discharge that can then be collected for microscopic examination and culture.

E. Scrotum and Scrotal Contents

1. *Inspection.* The inspection of the scrotum and the remainder of this portion of the physical examination are best carried out with the patient initially in the standing position. Lesions of the scrotal skin are readily evident in this position. The examiner also generally notes that if two testicles are present, one usually hangs lower than the other. In most cases, the left testicle is lower than the right. In cases of congenital absence or failure of descent of one or both testicles, the involved side may demonstrate hypoplastic scrotal development. It is always important to note the presence or absence of the testes. Scrotal masses and the "bag of worms" appearance of an underlying large varicocele may be identified on initial inspection.

2. *Palpation.* The contents of each hemiscrotum should be palpated in an orderly fashion. First, the testes should be examined, then the epididymides, then the cord structures, and finally, the area of the external inguinal ring to check for the presence of an inguinal hernia (Figure 2-4).

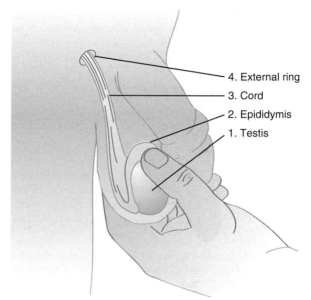

4. External ring
3. Cord
2. Epididymis
1. Testis

Palpate in sequence: 1. testis 2. epididymis - head, body, tail 3. cord 4. external ring

FIGURE 2-4. Palpation of the scrotal contents should be carried out in an orderly, routine fashion. One should begin palpating the testes, followed by the epididymides, the cord structures, and finally the external rings. Palpating each structure from side to side is useful for detecting differences in testicular size and identifying varicoceles. All of the scrotal structures may be examined between the thumb and the index and middle fingers. (From Van Arsdalen K: Signs and symptoms: the initial examination. In Hanno P, et al: *Clinical Manual of Urology.* McGraw Hill, 2001, F2-4.)

   a) Each testis should be in the dependent portion of the scrotum when the patient is relaxed and in a warm environment. The long axis of the testicle should be in a vertical direction and the size of the testis should normally be greater than or equal to 4 cm in adult males.

   b) Each epididymis is adherent to the posterolateral aspect of the testicle. The head of the epididymis is noted to be near the superior pole of the testicle, the body of the epididymis near the middle portion of the testicle, and the tail of the epididymis represents the most inferior aspect of this structure. The examiner should palpate each portion of the epididymis looking primarily for areas of tenderness or induration.

    c) The spermatic cord varies somewhat in thickness and often this depends on the presence or absence of what has been termed a "lipoma of the cord." The examiner should be particularly attentive to the presence or absence of enlarged venous structures (i.e., a varicocele). If a varicocele is detected, the patient should also be examined in the supine position to be certain that the varicocele decompresses. If it does not, one must suspect inferior vena cava or renal vein obstruction. Changes in the size of the cord between the standing and the supine positions or when using the Valsalva maneuver with the patient in the upright position indicate the presence of a small varicocele. The vas deferens should be palpated. This structure normally has the thickness of a pencil lead and has a distinct, smooth firmness.

    d) Finally, with the patient in the standing position, palpation of the inguinal canal may be carried out. Increasing intra-abdominal pressure by asking the patient to cough or by using the Valsalva maneuver will help to define the presence of an inguinal hernia.

3. Abnormal scrotal masses and transillumination (Figures 2-5 and 2-6).

    a) The presence of an abnormal mass within the scrotum is best defined by careful palpation. It should be noted whether the mass arises from the testicle, is contained within the testicle, arises from the epididymis, is located in the cord, or tends to surround most of the scrotal structures. It is important to note the character of the mass, that is, whether it is hard, firm, or cystic in nature.

    b) All scrotal masses should be transilluminated and this can be accomplished with a small penlight. Any mass that radiates a reddish glow of light through the lesion represents a cystic, fluid-filled structure. Caution is advised in defining the benignity of these lesions, however, in that benign and malignant lesions can coexist. A hydrocele surrounding a testicular tumor is a not uncommon example.

    c) See Table 2-3 for a differential diagnosis of scrotal masses.

F. The Rectum and Prostate

1. *Position.* A variety of positions have been described for performing a digital rectal examination (DRE). Having the patient lie on the examining table in the lateral

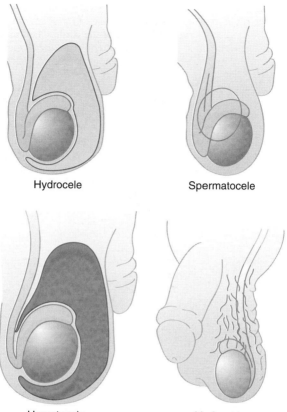

FIGURE 2-5. A variety of fluid-filled masses develop within the scrotum. Hydroceles and spermatoceles (and occasionally bowel in the hernia sac) will transilluminate. Hydrocele fluid is contained within the tunica vaginalis and essentially surrounds the testicle. A spermatocele generally occurs above or adjacent to the upper pole of the testis and represents a cyst of the rete testis or epididymis. A hematocele is a collection of blood within the tunica vaginalis due usually to trauma or surgery. Occasionally bleeding will occur spontaneously associated with bleeding disorders. A varicocele represents dilated veins of the pampiniform plexus as discussed in the text. Hematoceles and varicoceles will not transilluminate. (From Van Arsdalen K: Signs and symptoms: the initial examination. In Hanno P, et al: *Clinical Manual of Urology.* McGraw Hill, 2001, F2-5.)

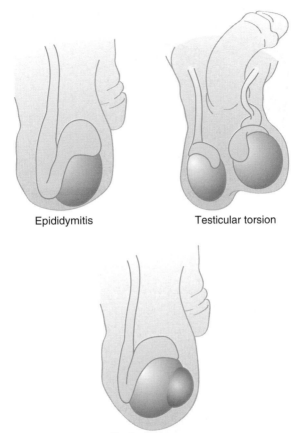

Epididymitis   Testicular torsion

Testicular tumor

FIGURE 2-6. Solid scrotal masses may be painful or painless and may involve the testis, epididymis, or both. (From Van Arsdalen K: Signs and symptoms: the initial examination. In Hanno P, et al: *Clinical Manual of Urology.* McGraw Hill, 2001, F2-6.)

decubitus position with the legs flexed at the hips and knees and the uppermost leg pulled higher toward the chest than the lowermost leg creates a comfortable position for the patient and the examiner (Figure 2-7). Alternatively, the patient can bend over the examining table while in the standing position so that the weight of his upper body rests on his elbows. The lateral decubitus position typically allows for deeper penetration of the rectum to feel the prostate in obese patients or to feel

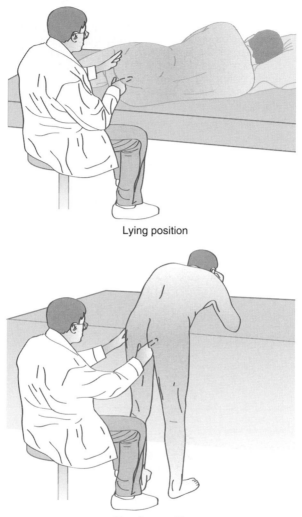

Lying position

Standing position

FIGURE 2-7. Two positions are illustrated for performing the digital rectal examination. (From Van Arsdalen K: Signs and symptoms: the initial examination. In Hanno P, et al: *Clinical Manual of Urology.* McGraw Hill, 2001, F2-7.)

the top of large glands. Probably more important than the position, however, is that the gloved examining finger be adequately lubricated and slow, gentle pressure be applied as the finger traverses the anal sphincter. A rectal examination can be an extremely painful or a painless experience depending on the skill and patience of the examiner. It is important at the time of the examination not only to palpate the prostate gland but to palpate the entire inside of the rectum in search of other abnormalities.

2. *Prostate.* During the rectal examination, the posterior aspect of the prostate is palpated (Figure 2-8). The

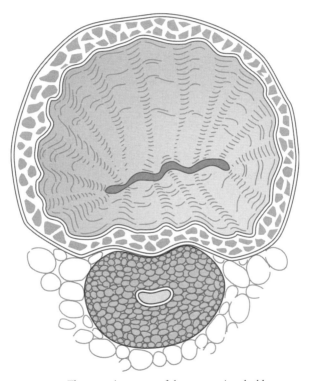

FIGURE 2-8. The posterior aspect of the prostate is palpable on rectal examination. The surface is normally smooth, rubbery, and approximately 4 × 4 cm in size. The median furrow may be lost with diffuse enlargement of the gland and the lateral sulci may be either accentuated or obscured. Deviations from normal contour, consistency, or size should be carefully described. Stating that an area is "hard" implies that one is suggesting the presence of carcinoma. The seminal vesicles are not normally palpable. *Remember:* Check the entire rectum. Do not miss an occult rectal carcinoma. (From Smith DR: *General Urology,* 11th ed. Lange, Los Altos, 1984, p. 40.)

significance of this part of the general physical examination cannot be overemphasized. Most types of prostate carcinoma begin in the posterior lobe of the prostate, which is very accessible to the examining finger.

a) The prostate gland is normally a small, walnut-sized structure with a flattened, heart-shaped configuration. There is a median furrow, which runs down the longitudinal axis of the prostate. There are two lateral sulci, where the rectal mucosa folds back on itself after reflecting off the prostate. The consistency of the normal prostate is generally described as "rubbery" in nature and has been likened to the consistency of the thenar eminence when one opposes the thumb and fifth finger.

b) Abnormal consistency of the prostate may be noted on rectal examination and includes nodular abnormalities that can be raised or within the substance of the prostate, areas of induration that can suggest malignancy, or areas of bogginess or fluctuance that can be associated with abscess formation.

c) Prostatic massage can be carried out to express prostatic secretions into the urethral lumen. These secretions may then be collected directly if they happen to drain through the penile meatus or by having the patient void a small amount of urine directly into a container immediately following the massage. Prostatic massage is generally carried out in a methodical fashion to strip the entire gland from a lateral to a medial aspect bilaterally.

3. *Seminal vesicles.* Under normal conditions, the seminal vesicles are not palpable. They can become evident on a rectal examination, however, if they are enlarged due to obstruction or inflammation.

G. The Vaginal Examination

1. *Inspection.* The vaginal examination is best performed with the patient in the relaxed lithotomy position. Inspection of the vulva may reveal a variety of venereal and nonvenereal lesions. The urinary meatus should be identified and its position and size noted. An erythematous tender lesion arising from the meatus may represent a benign urethral caruncle or possibly a urethral carcinoma. The character of the vaginal mucosa at the introitus should be noted. The examiner *may* also note the presence of a cystocele or a rectocele while examining the patient in this position. These structures may be

accentuated with increases in intra-abdominal pressure such as occur with coughing or straining. In fact, this maneuver may elicit some leakage of urine in patients with stress urinary incontinence.

2. *Palpation.* Palpation of the urethra to the level of the bladder neck and trigone may be accomplished during examination of the anterior vaginal wall. Bimanual palpation is useful to define the internal genitalia and to define further the size and consistency of the urinary bladder.

V. THE URINALYSIS AND CULTURE

A. Collection

Proper collection and prompt examination of the urine are essential to gain the most information from the routinely collected specimen.

1. Males
   a) A midstream urine collection is most commonly obtained in men for routine examination. With this technique, the male patient is instructed to retract the foreskin if he is uncircumcised and to gently cleanse the glans. He begins to urinate into the toilet, subsequently inserting a sterile glass container into the urinary stream to collect a urine sample. The container is then removed and the act of voiding is completed.
   b) A variety of other collection techniques afford more information with regard to localization of infection within the urinary tract. Four such specimens may be obtained and analyzed separately by routine microscopic evaluation as well as culture techniques. These have been designated the VB-1, VB-2, EPS, and VB-3 specimens, according to Stamey. The VB-1 is the initial 5 to 10 mL of the stream, which contains bladder urine mixed with urethral contents that are initially washed from the urethra. The VB-2 specimen is essentially the midstream portion of the collection. The EPS specimen represents the expressed prostatic secretions following prostatic massage. Finally, the VB-3 specimen represents a small voided specimen that mixes bladder urine with the contents contained in the urethra immediately following the expression of prostatic secretions. This collection is particularly useful if inadequate amounts of secretion from the prostate are actually expressed during the prostatic massage. The value of these cultures for

localization of urinary tract infection is that the VB-1 represents urethral flora, the VB-2 represents bladder flora, and the EPS and VB-3 represent prostatic flora.

2. Females

   a) The midstream urine collection in females is somewhat more difficult to accomplish and is often considered to be inadequate for even the most routine examination. With this technique, the vulva is cleansed and the stream is initiated into the toilet with subsequent insertion of a collecting container as described previously for the male. If this specimen is grossly contaminated or appears infected, then one of the collection methods noted later may be necessary to differentiate these two possibilities. However, if the collection has been done with reasonable care and the specimen is essentially negative on microscopic examination, then this technique is generally considered adequate.

   b) A more proper method of midstream urine collection has been described in which the patient is placed in the lithotomy position and then asked to void. The nurse holds the labia apart to prevent contamination and collects a midstream specimen. This is often awkward, if not difficult, for both the patient and the nurse and this method of collection is not recommended.

   c) If there is any question with regard to the problem of contamination versus infection of the midstream specimen as noted previously, then catheterization to obtain a true bladder specimen is the preferred technique. An examiner should not hesitate to use this method to properly categorize a patient's problem.

3. Children

   a) Percutaneous suprapubic aspiration of urine from neonates and infants is a particularly useful method of obtaining a truly uncontaminated specimen of urine from the bladder. With this technique, the suprapubic area is cleansed with an antiseptic solution and percutaneous aspiration is performed with a fine-gauge needle. The specimen can then be examined for urinalysis and sent for culture.

   b) A variety of sterile plastic bags with adhesive collars are available that surround the male and female infant's genitalia. They are particularly useful for routine screening urinalysis, but as with the collection of midstream specimens from women, it may be difficult at times to differentiate a truly infected urine from a contaminated specimen due to this collection technique.

c) Older boys and girls may have urine collected in a fashion similar to that described previously for their adult counterparts. One is generally quite hesitant, however, to catheterize young boys due to the possibility of urethral trauma. It is easier and safer to perform this in girls and may be used if necessary.

B. Physical Aspects of the Urine

1. *Color.* The color of the urine is generally a clear light yellow, but a wide range of colors has been described, as noted earlier. The changes in color can be secondary to foods and medications, as well as intrinsic disease processes. Table 2-4 describes the etiologic factors in relationship to abnormal urine color.
2. *pH.* The normal pH of urine ranges from 4.5 to 8.0. Urine is described as having an acid pH if it ranges between 4.5 and 5.5. It is referred to as having an alkaline pH if it ranges between 6.5 and 8.0.
3. *Specific gravity.* The specific gravity can be determined in the office by relatively simple techniques and gives some idea of the concentrating ability of the kidneys and their ability to excrete waste products. A variety of substances within the urine, such as intravenous contrast material, can detract from the value of this test. The osmolality of the urine is a better indicator of renal function but requires standard laboratory methods.

C. Dipstick Tests

1. A variety of dipsticks are available to evaluate the urine sample. These consist of short plastic strips with small pads that are impregnated with a variety of reagents that react with abnormal substances within the urine.
2. In addition to determination of urinary pH, the most sophisticated dipsticks now contain reagents for the determination of the following:
   a) Protein
   b) Glucose
   c) Ketones
   d) Urobilinogen
   e) Bilirubin
   f) Blood
   g) Hemoglobin
   h) Leukocytes
   i) Nitrites

Table 2-4:	Common Causes of Colorful Urine
Colorless	Very dilute urine
	Overhydration
Cloudy/milky	Phosphaturia
	Pyuria
	Chyluria
Red	Hematuria
	Hemaglobin/myoglobinuria
	Anthrocyanin in beets and blackberries
	Chronic lead and mercury poisoning
	Phenolphthalein (in bowel evacuants)
	Phenothiazines (Compazine, etc.)
	Rifampin
Orange	Dehydration
	Phenazopyridine (Pyridium)
	Sulfasalazine (Azulfadine)
Yellow	Normal
	Phenacetin
	Riboflavin
Green-blue	Biliverdin
	Indicanuria (tryptophan indole metabolites)
	Amitriptyline (Elavil)
	Indigo carmine
	Methylene blue
	Phenols (IV cimetidine [Tagamet] IV promethazine [Phenergan], etc.)
	Resorcinol
	Triampterene (Dyrenium)
Brown	Urobilinogen
	Porphyria
	Aloe, fava beans, and rhubarb
	Chloroquine and primaquine
	Furazolidone (Furoxone)
	Metronidazole (Flagyl)
	Nitrofurantoin (Furadantin)
Brown-black	Alcaptonuria (homogentisic acid)
	Hemorrhage
	Melanin
	Tyrosinosis (hydroxyphenylpyruvic acid)
	Cascara, senna (laxatives)
	Methocarbamol (Robaxin)
	Methyldopa (Aldomet)
	Sorbitol

D. Microscopic Examination

1. A small portion of the collected urine sample is placed in a test tube and centrifuged at approximately 5000 rpm for 5 minutes. The supernate is then poured from the tube and the remaining sediment is resuspended in the small quantity of urine that drains back down the side of the tube to the sediment. A drop of the resuspended sediment is placed on a glass slide followed by a cover slip.
2. The wet specimen described previously is then examined under low and high power for the presence and number of epithelial cells, red blood cells, white blood cells, bacteria, and casts.

E. Urine Culture

1. If a urine culture is desired, it should be promptly plated in the office or sent immediately to the laboratory to prevent overgrowth of bacteria and falsely elevated bacterial counts.
2. The value of localization cultures has been noted previously.

VI. BLOOD TESTS

A. Panel 7 (or Similar Designation)

1. Serum electrolytes (Na, K, Cl, CO_2) are useful indicators of maintenance of homeostasis for which the kidney plays a significant role.
2. Glucose levels in the serum may be variable relative to the presence of glucosuria.
   a) Diabetes is a significant risk factor for voiding and sexual dysfunction.
3. Blood urea nitrogen (BUN) and creatinine are indicators of renal function.

B. PSA Level

1. PSA is a protein kinase produced, essentially uniquely, by the prostatic epithelium.
   a) It is a normal component of the ejaculate responsible for liquification of the semen.
   b) Normally found in very low levels in serum (0–4.0 ng/mL).
2. Causes of PSA elevation
   a) Prostate cancer
   b) BPH

    c) Prostatitis (acute and chronic)

    d) Instrumentation (catheterization, cystoscopy, biopsy)

    e) Urinary retention

    f) Vigorous prostatic massage, probably little elevation for routine DRE

3. PSA as a tumor marker

    a) Limitations due to prostate organ specific but not cancer specific.

    b) Substantial overlap of values for men with prostate cancer and benign conditions (see previous).

    c) Absolute value greater than 10 ng/mL has more than 60% predictive risk of prostate cancer.

    d) Sixty percent of current prostate cancer diagnoses are made due to an elevated PSA level.

    e) Useful marker for following efficacy of treatment for prostate cancer.

4. Recommendations

    a) Yearly PSA and DRE for all men older than 50 years old

    b) Yearly PSA and DRE starting at 40 years old for blacks and all men with a positive family history of prostate cancer

VII. INSTRUMENTATION

A. General Information

The instrumentation and procedures to be described later can be commonly performed in the office setting under local anesthesia. Some of these techniques, such as cystourethroscopy, placement of retrograde catheters, and biopsy of the prostate, may also be performed with regional or general anesthesia.

B. Urethral Catheters

1. *Straight catheters.* The standard straight, red, or Robinson catheter is useful for office catheterization when an indwelling catheter is not warranted. It is useful for collecting relatively uncontaminated specimens directly from the bladder as noted previously.

2. *Standard balloon* or *Foley catheter.* This type of catheter has a double lumen that permits drainage of urine through the larger lumen and inflation of a balloon located at the tip of the catheter. This allows it to be retained within the urinary bladder. This type of catheter is useful following certain operative procedures on the urinary tract and

for establishing temporary, constant urinary drainage, to monitor urine output or for relief of bladder outlet obstruction. These catheters generally have 5- and 30-mL balloons, but the amount of water placed in these balloons is not precisely critical as each will hold significantly more than its stated volume.

3. *Coude catheters.* Red Robinson catheters or balloon retention catheters may each be specially constructed to have a "coudé-tip configuration." This is essentially a curved tip that allows passage of the catheter beyond certain urethral, prostatic, or bladder neck impediments that may preclude passage of a straight catheter due to impingement of the catheter tip on these lesions.

4. *Three-way irrigation catheters.* This type of catheter has a triple lumen that has an irrigation port, a drainage port, and a port for inflating the balloon used for retention of the catheter within the bladder. Three-way irrigation catheters are particularly useful following transurethral resection of the prostate and in cases of gross hematuria to irrigate the bladder and prevent formation and retention of clots.

5. *Technique of catheter insertion.* Insertion of a urethral catheter by the physician for either diagnostic or therapeutic reasons always involves sterile technique. Gloves should be applied and the glans and meatus of the male and the vulva and meatus of the female are then prepared with an antiseptic skin preparation solution. The catheter is then well-lubricated with sterile jelly and inserted gently into the meatus. Prior to inflation of the balloon, if a retention catheter is used, it must be certain that the tip of the catheter is within the urinary bladder and that urine is obtained. In cases in which urine does not flow freely from the end of the catheter, it is important to irrigate the catheter gently prior to inflation of the balloon to prevent inflation within the urethra. Hematuria and/or sepsis may be noted if this occurs. The catheter is then pulled gently to seat the balloon at the level of the bladder neck. It is then attached to a drainage bag with sterile technique.

C. Urethral Sounds and Filiforms and Followers

1. *General information.* These two types of instruments are often used to evaluate the urethra in cases of urethral stricture disease or for other reasons that preclude passage of a urethral catheter. They may be used in both a diagnostic and therapeutic fashion by the skilled urologist who is familiar with their use.

2. *Urethral sounds.* These metal objects come in a variety of sizes and shapes. They must be passed carefully to prevent disruption of the lower urinary tract. They are never inserted with force and must pass smoothly into the urinary bladder, where rotation of the tip of the sound is confirmed with each passage.

3. *Filiforms* and *followers.* These instruments are also useful for establishing access to the urinary bladder and dilating urethral strictures. The tiny filiform aspect of this set is used to gain access initially to the urinary bladder. These filiforms have different shapes at their tip that allow them to be manipulated through or around a variety of abnormal urethral configurations. It may be necessary to pass several filiforms simultaneously before access can be gained to the bladder. Once it is established that one of these filiforms has passed easily into the bladder, the follower can then be attached to the protruding threaded end and passed as a unit with the filiform into the bladder. Using serially larger followers, it is possible to dilate the urethra. Each follower has an eye in the end and a hollow center so that the urine can be obtained as the follower is passed. In cases of severe urethral stricture disease, it may be best to leave the follower in place prior to insertion of a Foley catheter. If the urethra dilates easily, the followers can be removed and a Foley catheter inserted immediately.

D. Cystourethroscopy and Associated Techniques

1. Equipment

   a) The standard rigid cystourethroscope consists of a sheath, bridge, and lighted telescope for visualization. An irrigation port is attached to the sheath that allows gravity-directed inflow of fluid to distend the urethra and bladder and aid in visualization. The bridge essentially attaches the telescope to the sheath and may contain a variety of working ports through which urethral catheters, biopsy forceps, and alligator forceps may be passed. The lighted telescopes generally have 30- and 70-degree viewing angles that allow complete inspection within the bladder.

   b) Flexible cystoscopes, like flexible endoscopes for GI endoscopy and bronchoscopy, consist of many tiny fiberoptic bundles organized with a deflection mechanism to allow movement of the tip. The flexible scope has an advantage for male patient comfort in that it conforms to, rather than straightens, the natural

curves of the lower urinary tract. Its limitations relate
to field of view and ease of working instrumentation.

2. Technique of insertion

   a) *Males.* Insertion of the cystourethroscope into the
   male is best performed under direct vision following
   antiseptic preparation and draping. The cystourethroscope is assembled and a flow of fluid is obtained.
   The instrument is then introduced into the meatus
   and passed under direct vision through the anterior
   urethra. Some narrowing and voluntary constriction
   of the external sphincter may be noted, but this is
   passed with slow gentle pressure. With the patient in
   the lithotomy position, it is necessary to lower the
   eyepiece of the rigid scope to redirect the tip of the
   instrument beneath the symphysis pubis, through
   the prostate, and into the bladder. The bladder can
   then be emptied and inspected with both lenses. With
   the flexible cystoscope, the patient can remain supine
   and the tip directed by manipulation of the deflecting
   mechanism. Flexible cystoscopy can be performed at
   the bedside if necessary, such as in an intensive care
   unit (ICU) setting.

   b) *Females.* The female patient is also placed in the
   lithotomy position. After proper cleansing and
   draping, the cystourethroscope can be inserted into
   the bladder either under direct vision or with the
   obturator in the cystoscope sheath taking care to
   follow the course of the urethra that may be
   deviated due to associated pathology such as a
   cystocele. Once again, the bladder is inspected with
   both lenses and the urethra is inspected with the
   30-degree lens.

3. Procedures

   a) *Inspection.* In most cases, the urethra and bladder are
   merely inspected under local anesthesia with these
   endoscopic techniques in the office setting. This
   allows the urologist to ascertain the presence or
   absence of urethral pathology, degree of anatomic
   obstruction, and state of the bladder mucosa and
   underlying musculature. It is also possible to note
   the presence or absence of efflux from the ureteral
   orifices as well as to judge their location and configuration. At the time of inspection of the bladder,
   bladder urine can be obtained for culture or cytology.
   The bladder can also be washed by barbotage techniques and the washings sent for cytology.

b) *Bladder biopsies.* These may be taken under local anesthesia using cold cup biopsy forceps. Generally, however, there is some degree of associated discomfort and if biopsies are necessary, they are usually best performed under regional or general anesthesia to ensure an adequate specimen.

c) *Retrograde ureteral catheterization.* The placement of small (sizes 4 to 7 F) ureteral catheters may be performed without difficulty under local anesthesia. These catheters can be passed just within the ureteral orifice for retrograde injection of contrast or to the level of the kidney for relief of obstruction within the ureter, to obtain renal washings, or for the injection of contrast material for radiographic studies. They can be removed immediately or left temporarily in place.

d) A variety of resectoscopes and specialized endoscopes are available to perform more sophisticated procedures on the urethra, bladder, and prostate as well as the ureter and kidney. These are therapeutic rather than diagnostic procedures and require regional or general anesthesia. Their use is not considered further herein.

E. Ultrasound Evaluation of the Urinary Tract

1. *General information.* Small, portable ultrasound machines are available from a number of manufacturers. These are increasingly being used in urologists' offices and on hospital floors, in addition to radiology departments, to evaluate the urinary tract and to guide diagnostic procedures. Probes that have different frequencies and different configurations are designed to evaluate specific areas and aspects of the urinary tract.

2. *Renal ultrasonography.* The kidney can be evaluated for mass lesions, hydronephrosis, or the presence of stones or stone fragments.

3. *Abdominal ultrasonography.* Abdominal masses and the lower urinary tract, especially the bladder, can be imaged. Built-in computer programs allow computation of ultrasound-determined residual urine volumes. This makes a determination of bladder emptying possible without catheterization.

4. *Ultrasonography of the external genitalia.* This may be used to evaluate scrotal masses to determine whether they are cystic or solid and their relationship to the testicle and epididymis. Special Doppler probes are useful in evaluating penile blood flow in cases of erectile failure and in

confirming the presence of venous reflux in suspected varicoceles.

5. *Transvaginal ultrasonography.* This may be useful in evaluating the lower urinary tract in cases of incontinence and voiding dysfunction.

6. *Transrectal ultrasonography.* This technique is most frequently used to evaluate the prostate relative to carcinoma, although it may also be used to evaluate the benign prostate with regard to size and to look for abnormalities in cases of ejaculatory dysfunction. At this time, the indications for transrectal ultrasonography of the prostate are in the assessment of prostate nodules that are palpable on the DRE, to look for abnormalities associated with elevated PSA levels, and for needle localization for biopsy of the prostate. It must be emphasized that there are no specific ultrasonographic findings that definitely differentiate carcinoma of the prostate from benign lesions.

F. Percutaneous Suprapubic Cystostomy

1. In instances of urinary retention when it is not possible to traverse the urethra into the bladder, various types of percutaneous suprapubic tubes may be placed with or without ultrasound guidance.

2. Equipment
   a) Percutaneous needle-guided catheters consist of a plastic drainage tube with a retention device (Malecot design or balloon) surrounding a sharpened metal trocar that is passed as a unit. These are typically smaller in caliber than the trocar-sheath devices described later.
   b) A peel-away sheath around a metal or plastic trocar may be passed into the bladder. After removal of the trocar, up to a 16-F catheter can be advanced into the bladder and the balloon inflated. The peel-away configuration of the sheath allows it to be removed without dislodging or damaging the catheter.

3. Technique
   a) The abdomen must be carefully examined for evidence of prior surgery or scars.
   b) The bladder must be palpable or percussible.
   c) With prior surgery or obesity, ultrasound examination of the suprapubic area should be performed.
   d) The skin is anesthetized and a small incision is made, generally in the midline, two fingerbreadths above the pubis.

e) A spinal needle may be passed in the anticipated direction of the bladder to confirm the location of the bladder and the appropriate direction of the tract.

f) The needle catheter device or the trocar sheath device is then passed with fairly swift but gentle pressure directly posteriorly into the bladder. The trocar is removed once urine is obtained leaving either the retention device in place or allowing passage of a separate catheter as noted previously.

G. Needle Biopsy of the Prostate

1. *General information.* Needle biopsy techniques are the most accurate means of determining whether a prostate nodule or other area of abnormality is benign or malignant.

2. *Techniques.* The prostate can be sampled by either a transrectal or transperineal approach. To be accurate, the tip of the needle must enter the area of concern. Localization may be by digital direction but is now done almost exclusively by ultrasound guidance. Use of ultrasonography in combination with needles placed through a port in the probe has clearly improved the accuracy of this procedure and improved patient tolerance.

   a) Spring-loaded thin-core biopsy needles are available that may be passed directly through a channel or guide in the ultrasound probe such that the tip may be seen as it enters the lesion of concern. These cores are obtained for sectioning, and despite the use of a transrectal approach in most cases, there appears to be little risk of sepsis.

   b) Vim-Silverman and Tru-Cut needles obtain thicker cores of tissue for standard pathologic sectioning and examination. These are wide bore and, even with local anesthesia, are associated with significant patient discomfort and higher rates of urosepsis. These needles are used infrequently now.

   c) Skinny-needle aspiration obtains cells for cytologic evaluation and is well tolerated but lacks preservation of architecture and precise accuracy of sampling.

VIII. SUMMARY

The surgical subspecialty of urology deals with a well-defined organ system within the body. The urologist diagnoses and treats a wide variety of medical and surgical disorders that may have local or systemic ramifications for the patient.

The history, physical examination, and urinalysis serve as the cornerstones of the initial evaluation of these patients. In addition, a variety of unique diagnostic and therapeutic instruments are available for use in the office or outpatient setting to aid in caring for those with urologic diseases. The frequency with which these problems are seen by generalists and other specialists necessitates that all practitioners have some familiarity with this field.

SELF-ASSESSMENT QUESTIONS

1. A primary irritative process in what structure may cause pain in the ipsilateral testicle?
2. What is the significance of painless versus painful hematuria?
3. Name four causes of scrotal swelling.
4. What is the difference between phimosis and paraphimosis?
5. What is the normal role of PSA in the semen?

SUGGESTED READINGS

1. Barry MJ, Fowler FJ, O'Leary MP, et al: The American Urological Association symptom index for benign prostatic hyperplasia. *J Urol* 148:1549, 1992.
2. Carter HB: Instrumentation and cystoscopy. In: Walsh PC, Retik AB, Vaughn ED Jr, Wein AJ, eds. *Campbell's Urology,* 8th ed. Saunders, Philadelphia, 2002, p. 111.
3. Gerber GS, Brendler CB: Evaluation of the urologic patient: History, physical examination, and urinalysis. In: Walsh PC, Retik AB, Vaughn ED Jr, Wein AJ, eds. *Campbell's Urology,* 8th ed. Saunders, Philadelphia, 2002, p. 83.
4. Scott W, Burns P, Brown JL, Hammer L: Ultrasound evaluation of the urinary tract. In: Pollack HM, McClennan BL, eds. *Clinical Urography.* Saunders, Philadelphia, 2000, pp. 388–472.
5. Stamey TA: *Pathogenesis and Treatment of Urinary Tract Infections.* Williams & Wilkins, Baltimore, 1980.
6. Thompson I, Carroll P, Coley C, et al: The PSA best practices policy of the American Urological Association. *AUA update series XX.* American Urological Association, Houston, 2001.

Diagnostic and Interventional Uroradiology

Parvati Ramchandani, MD and
Marc P. Banner, MD

DIAGNOSTIC URORADIOLOGY

The urinary tract can be evaluated by conventional plain film radiography, ultrasonography (US), computed tomography (CT), magnetic resonance imaging (MRI), radionuclide studies, and evolving techniques such as positron emission tomography (PET). In this chapter, the role of these different imaging modalities in the management of patients is addressed.

Intravenous Urography

The intravenous urogram (IVU), also referred to as excretory urogram (EU) or intravenous pyelogram (IVP), was the basic diagnostic radiologic study to evaluate the upper urinary tract for many decades. Its role in the assessment of many urologic conditions is now more limited due to the advantages offered by cross-sectional imaging modalities. IVU requires intravenous (IV) injection of radiographic contrast medium, followed by a sequence of films.

Indications

1. Hematuria (macroscopic and microscopic). IVU provides evaluation of both the renal parenchyma and the collecting system in patients with gross or microscopic hematuria. However, the role of IVU in these patients is increasingly being questioned. CT is indisputably more sensitive for detecting renal masses compared to an IVU; although large masses are identifiable on an IVU, it is well recognized that renal masses smaller than 2 cm are often missed on an IVU (Figure 3-1). The sensitivity of CT urography (CTU) in detecting urothelial abnormalities as compared to IVU currently remains unknown and is a subject of intensive study.

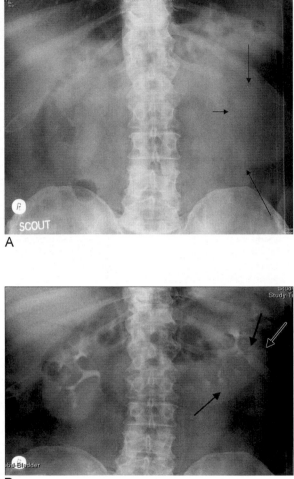

FIGURE 3-1. (Continued)

       CT is also more sensitive than IVU in detecting uro-
lithiasis—small stones and those that are faintly opaque
are often not detectable on an IVU (Figure 3-2).
2. Upper urinary tract surveillance in patients with a history
of a urothelial malignancy such as bladder cancer or positive urine cytology (Figure 3-3).

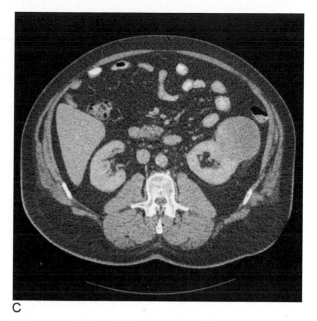

C

FIGURE 3-1. **A–C.** Renal cell carcinoma. **A** and **B** show a large mass arising from the anterior aspect of the left kidney *(arrows)* on an IVU. **C.** CT scan in same patient demonstrates the mass well.

3. Preoperative evaluation for select endourologic procedures such as endopyelotomy. However, CT is increasingly being used even for this indication as three-dimensional (3-D) reconstructions can be performed with high spatial resolution, allowing display of the vascular structures and their relationship to the collecting system. Additionally, the collecting system can also be displayed in a manner similar to that seen on an IVU.

4. Postoperative evaluation following urologic procedures (Figure 3-4).

5. Complicated or unusual urinary tract infections (including tuberculosis).

6. Stone disease. Patients who present with acute renal colic are best evaluated with noncontrast CT (no oral or IV contrast is necessary), which is acknowledged to be the most sensitive and specific study to exclude an obstructing ureteral calculus as the cause of the abdominal pain. This is addressed further in the section on CT. IVUs are no

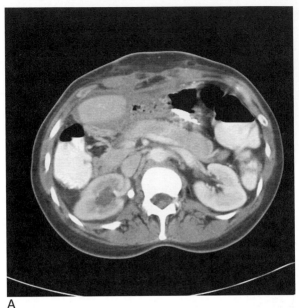

A

FIGURE 3-2. (Continued)

longer considered the study of choice in a patient with suspected renal colic, as small and faintly opaque stones may not be discernible on an IVU, making it difficult to establish a conclusive diagnosis of stone induced renal colic. Further, in patients with high grade ureteral obstruction, it can take up to 24 hours for the collecting system and ureter to opacify densely enough to determine the level of ureteral obstruction.

IVU continues to have a role in the management of patients with known stone disease, to help determine the best therapy for an individual patient and in follow-up after treatment with shockwave lithotripsy (SWL), ureteroscopy, or percutaneous methods.

Radiographic Iodinated Contrast Agents

Radiographic contrast media (CM) consist of three atoms of iodine attached to a benzene ring. In the developed world, newer nonionic agents that are either of low osmolarity (low osmolarity contrast media, LOCM) or of iso-osmolarity

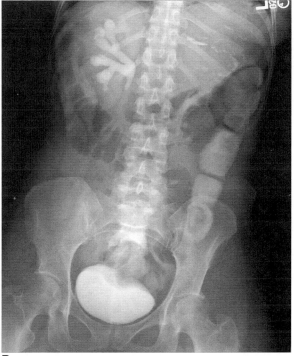

B

FIGURE 3-2. **A** and **B.** Acute renal colic due to a right proximal ureteral calculus. **A.** CT scan demonstrates a large calculus in the proximal right ureter. The right nephrogram is delayed indicating that the obstruction is urodynamically significant. **B.** Abdominal film obtained immediately after the CT scan shows impaired drainage of the dilated right collecting system due to the stone. Although well seen on CT, the stone was nonopaque on plain abdominal radiographs. It is important to keep in mind that even radio-opaque stones will not be visible in a collecting system that is filled with contrast.

are generally used for intravascular administration. Contrast agents used in the past were of high osmolarity (high osmolarity contrast media, HOCM) and are referred to as ionic contrast agents. Multiple studies have shown that the frequency of reactions is lower with the LOCM as compared to the HOCM when given intravenously, in both the general population and in patients at higher risk for contrast

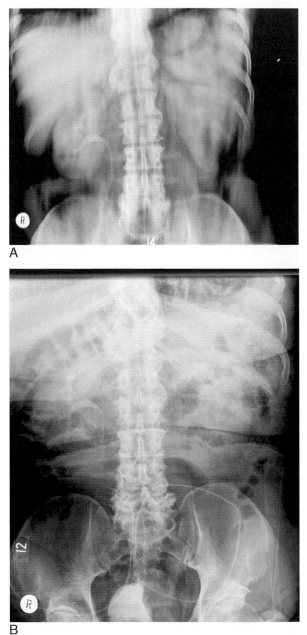

A

B

FIGURE 3-3. (Continued)

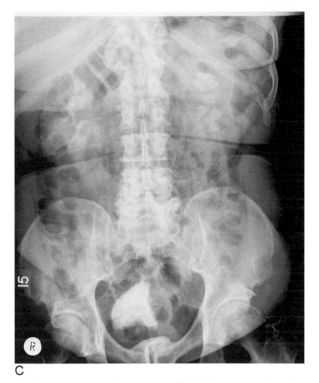

C

FIGURE 3-3. **A–C.** IVU in a patient with bladder cancer undergoing upper tract evaluation. **A.** Nephrotomogram shows delayed excretion from the left kidney due to obstructing bladder tumor. **B.** Right collecting system and ureter are normal but the left collecting sytem is not opacified yet; the delay in opacification is due to the obstruction caused by the bladder tumor, which is seen as asymmetry on the left side of the bladder. **C.** 15 minutes after contrast injection, the dilated left collecting system is just beginning to opacify. The left wall bladder tumor is clearly seen. However, it is important to note that IVU and cystography are insensitive in detection of bladder cancer.

reaction. Although the cost of nonionic contrast has decreased over the last decade, LOCM are still two to three times more expensive than HOCM.

The majority of injected contrast is excreted almost entirely by glomerular filtration. A small amount may be bound to serum albumin and is then excreted by the liver and biliary system, and referred to as vicarious excretion.

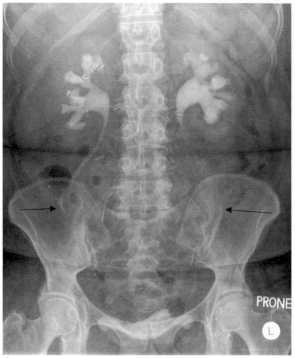

A

FIGURE 3-4. (Continued)

Patients with renal insufficiency or obstruction frequently have vicarious excretion (Figure 3-5).

Technique of IVU

1. Patient preparation. A thorough bowel preparation helps in optimal visualization of the urinary tract by eliminating obscuring fecal material in the bowel. Fluids are withheld overnight for better opacification of the collecting system and to optimize renal concentration of the contrast medium. An empty stomach is also helpful in the event of vomiting after contrast administration, which is more common with the use of HOCM.
2. A plain film of the abdomen (also known as scout film, preliminary film, "KUB"—kidney ureters, and bladder film, abdominal "flat plate") is obtained. This is an essential component of every radiographic examination of

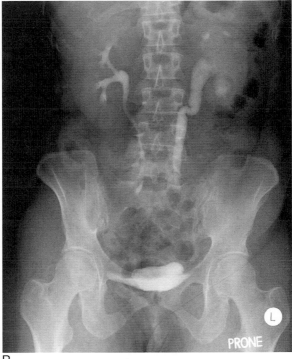

B

FIGURE 3-4. **A.** Follow-up IVU in a patient with retroperitoneal fibrosis who underwent ureterolysis and intraperitonealization. This prone film demonstrates residual fullness of the collecting systems, particularly on the left. The lateral bowing of the lumbar and sacral ureters is a characteristic finding after intraperitonealization of the ureters. **B.** Preoperative IVU demonstrates hydronephrosis, more marked on the left, with normally positioned ureters.

the genitourinary (GU) tract. Urinary tract calculi can be identified only on the KUB as most urinary calculi are obscured by excreted contrast, which has the same radiographic density as calculi. Important finding such as soft tissue masses, calcifications, and bony changes will also be disclosed on the preliminary film.

3. Contrast administration. CM can be administered intravenously as a rapid bolus injection; slow, steady injection; or drip infusion. This is more often an individual preference rather than a matter of scientific selection. At our

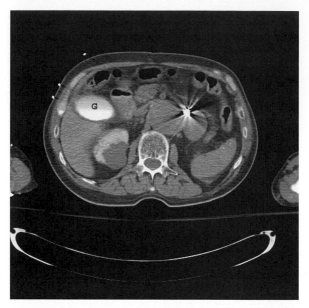

FIGURE 3-5. Contrast induced nephrotoxicity in patient with a
solitary right kidney, who received multiple contrast loads for
cardiac catheterization. The left kidney was removed for benign
disease many years ago. Noncontrast CT scan demonstrates that the
right kidney has a dense, persistent nephrogram from contrast given
48 hours previously. Note vicarious excretion of contrast into the
gallbladder (G). The abdominal aorta is aneurysmal.

institution, patients receive 1 mL contrast per pound of
body weight, to a maximum of 150 mL.
4. Filming sequence (Figure 3-6). Immediately after the
contrast has been injected, nephrotomograms are made
to visualize the renal parenchyma (nephrographic phase)
and assess for renal masses. Within 3 minutes, contrast is
usually visible in the collecting systems and several films
are taken to visualize the calyces, pelves, and ureters (pye-
lographic phase). Films of the bladder (often including a
postvoiding film) conclude the examination.

Contraindications

1. Pre-existing renal insufficiency. The administration of IV
contrast to patients with pre-existing renal insufficiency
places them at risk for worsening of their renal function
(contrast induced nephrotoxicity, CIN). Diabetic patients

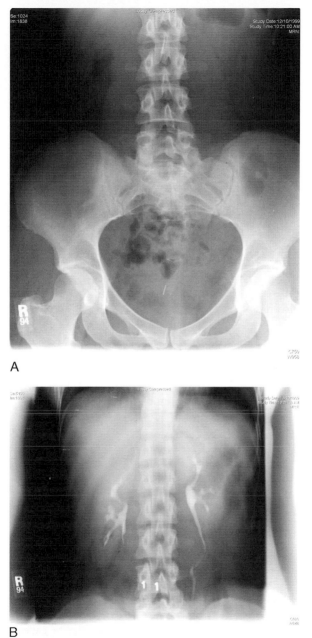

FIGURE 3-6. (Continued)

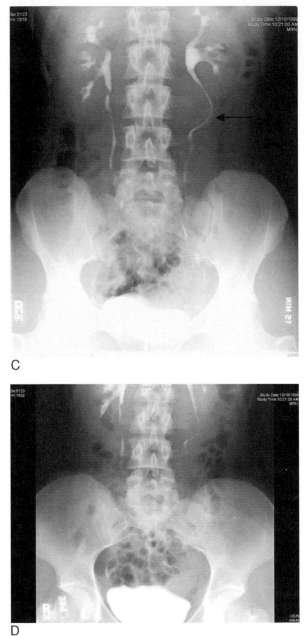

C

D

FIGURE 3-6. (Continued)

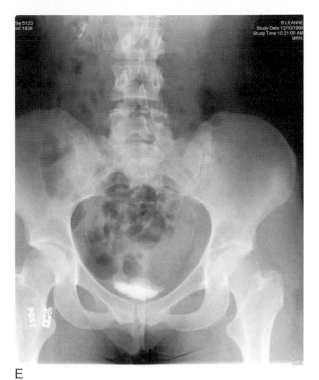

E

FIGURE 3-6. (Continued)

with renal failure due to diabetic nephropathy are more vulnerable to this complication, and if CIN occurs, it may be irreversible in these patients. Thus, in patients with pre-existing renal insufficiency, radiologic evaluation of the urinary tract should consist of renal parenchymal evaluation with US or MRI and urothelial evaluation by a combination of cystoscopy (for urinary bladder assessment) and retrograde pyelography (to evaluate the urothelium of the pyelocalyceal systems and ureters). IVU is contraindicated in patients with renal insufficiency, as are other studies requiring parenteral administration of radiographic contrast.

2. Relative contraindications

   a) Multiple consecutive contrast studies. Patients who receive closely repeated doses of IV contrast are at greater risk for CIN. This risk is greater than the

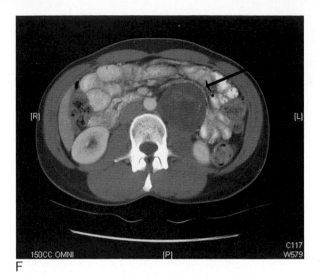

F

FIGURE 3-6. **A–F.** IVU in young woman with microhematuria.
A. Scout film demonstrates no abnormality. **B.** Selected
nephrotomogram demonstrates no renal mass. Several
nephrotomograms are required to demonstrate the kidneys in their
entirety—not all are included here. **C.** Excretory phase demonstrates
normal collecting systems but displacement of the left ureter
(arrow), suggesting the presence of a retroperitoneal mass.
D. Prevoid film of the bladder again demonstrates left ureteral
displacement but no obstruction or bladder abnormality.
E. Postvoid film demonstrates good emptying of the bladder.
F. CT scan was recommended to evaluate the ureteral displacement
and demonstrates a large retroperitoneal mass *(arrow),* which
proved to be a schwannoma.

combined risk of two random contrast examinations. It is best to separate any two studies requiring parenteral contrast administration by at least
24 hours and preferably by 48 hours, during which
time the patient should be thoroughly hydrated (see
Figure 3-5).
b) In patients with a documented allergic reaction to contrast such as urticaria (hives), cutaneous and subcutaneous edema (angioedema), upper airway (laryngeal)
edema, bronchospasm, and hypotension with tachycardia, the indications for contrast administration
should be carefully considered and other alternative
studies performed, if possible. If the decision to give

contrast to such patients is made, premedication with corticosteroids and antihistamines is essential, and such patients should be given LOCM, as discussed previously. One example of a premedication regimen in clinical use for an elective examination is prednisone 50 mg orally, given 12, 6, and 1 hour before the examination, and diphenhydramine 50 mg 1 hour before the examination, orally or by intramuscular injection. Patients have to be cautioned about the drowsiness that accompanies diphenhydramine administration and should not undertake activities such as driving or other dangerous tasks. For emergent contrast administration, 200 mg hydrocortisone is given intravenously immediately and then every 4 hours until the examination is complete.

c) Patients at increased risk for adverse reactions include those with a history of prior contrast reactions (four times increased risk) or a history of allergies or asthma (two to three times increased risk) as compared to patients who do not have such histories. Premedicating such patients prior to contrast administration is prudent. Symptoms of nausea, vomiting, or sensation of heat after contrast administration are considered to be side effects of the contrast and not allergic reactions; such symptoms are much less common with LOCM than with HOCM. Shellfish allergy has no particular significance for contrast administration and is managed the same way as other non-contrast allergies, for example, allergy to bee sting, penicillin, and peanut.

d) Multiple myeloma was long considered a risk factor for CIN with the cause believed to be precipitation of protein-contrast aggregates in the renal tubules. However, it is now thought that myeloma does not increase the risk of CIN if the patient is well hydrated.

e) In patients with cardiac disease, CM administration can cause worsening of congestive heart failure, due to the osmotic load.

f) Patients who are on metformin, an oral hypoglycemic agent (trade names Glucophage, Glucovance, Avandamet, Metaglip, etc.), should discontinue the drug when they receive contrast and not resume taking their medication until their renal function is documented to be normal 48 hours after the contrast administration. Although metformin itself does not have an adverse effect on renal function, patients who develop renal failure on the drug (possibly due

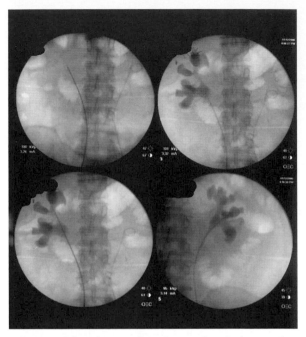

FIGURE 3-7. Bilateral retrograde pyelograms done in the operating room with portable fluoroscopy equipment, which limits image resolution. There is mild bilateral hydronephrosis due to retroperitoneal fibrosis; patient had renal insufficiency that precluded intravenous contrast administration.

> to contrast administration or other causes) can rarely develop lactic acidosis that can be fatal.
> g) Delayed reactions, defined as those occurring more than 1 hour after contrast administration, can be seen with all contrast agents, occur in 0.5–23% of patients, and tend to be skin reactions.

Retrograde Pyeloureterography (RPG)

Indications

1. To investigate lesions of the renal collecting system and ureter that cannot be adequately defined by IVU or CTU.
2. To visualize the collecting systems and ureters when IVU is contraindicated (renal insufficiency, severe prior contrast reaction) (Figure 3-7).

3. To demonstrate the collecting systems and ureters in their entirety when IVU or CTU fails to do so.
4. To visualize the ureteral stump remaining after nephrectomy in a patient with hematuria or positive urinary cytology.

Contraindications

1. Untreated urinary tract infection.
2. Patients who cannot or should not be cystoscoped (e.g., patients recovering from recent bladder or urethral surgery).

Technique

1. Preliminary cystoscopy is required.
2. A ureteral orifice is identified and catheterized with a catheter, usually 5 F. The catheter is advanced to the renal pelvis and contrast is instilled. The same contrast agents employed for IVU or CT are used for retrograde pyelography. To opacify the ureter alone, the ureteral orifice is occluded with a bulb occlusion catheter and contrast injected while a film is obtained.
3. Films—a preliminary KUB film is essential. After contrast injection, films are obtained to delineate unopacified or poorly seen portions of the collecting system or ureter in question. If obstruction is suspected, a film is also obtained several minutes after removal of the ureteral catheter to evaluate the drainage of the collecting system.
4. The use of fluoroscopy is an important adjunct to RPG. In most hospital settings, however, this requires the placement of a ureteral catheter in the cystoscopy suite and the subsequent transport of the patient to the radiology department for catheter injection.
5. RPG may be impossible in some patients, such as those with very larger prostates, in whom the gland overlies the ureteral orifices, preventing proper catheter placement. At times, even though the orifice is identifiable, it may not be possible to catheterize it, such as may occur with tortuous ureters or after ureteral reimplantation.

Complications

1. Perforation of the ureter is uncommon. When it does occur, there is usually no serious sequela. Contrast extravasation outside the collecting system does not usually result in any harm. In some cases of perforation associated with a large amount of urine leakage, diversion of urine with a ureteral stent may be required for a few weeks.

2. A too vigorous injection of contrast material in an infected urinary tract may disseminate bacteria into the bloodstream as well as into the kidney, causing bacteremia and rarely pyelonephritis. This risk increases in the presence of a urinary tract obstruction. Fortunately, the normal antegrade flow of urine is usually enough to wash out any bacteria that may have been introduced during the procedure. Patients usually receive prophylactic periprocedural antibiotics as well.

3. Absorption of contrast agent can occur if there is perforation of the collecting system or pyelosinus extravasation due to overdistention. In patients truly allergic to CM, the retrograde approach does not obviate a systemic contrast reaction, although reactions are much less common than after IV injection. Patients with a history of contrast allergy should receive premedication with corticosteroids and antihistamines.

Antegrade Pyelography

Indications

1. To visualize the urothelium of the upper urinary tract when an IVU is unsatisfactory and RPG cannot be done.

2. In patients with history of urothelial malignancy and high grade obstruction of a collecting system, an antegrade pyelogram may be the only way to evaluate the urothelium of the collecting system and ureter. Contrast excretion in an obstructed system is impaired, and thus IV contrast administration for either an IVU or CTU will not depict the collecting system well enough to exclude upper urinary tract urothelial lesions.

3. In patients with renal transplants who have azotemia in association with a dilated collecting system, antegrade pyelogram can help determine whether the transplant collecting system is obstructed or not. The ureteroneocystostomy created to drain a renal transplant is often difficult to cannulate cystoscopically.

Contraindication

1. Bleeding diathesis.

Technique

The renal pelvis is percutaneously punctured with a 20- or 21-gauge thin-walled needle from a posterior or posterolateral approach. Localization is provided by means of contrast excreted after an IV injection or with US in dilated collecting systems. Contrast is injected and films are exposed under fluoroscopic control.

Complications

These are similar to a percutaneous nephrostomy (PCN).

1. Inadvertent puncture of neighboring structures may occur. Although puncture of the renal vein, kidney, parenchyma, or liver and spleen is possible, few if any, complications result because of the small size of the needle.
2. Some extravasation usually occurs with many antegrade pyelograms. However, the puncture site is very small and rapidly seals after the needle has been removed.
3. Entry into the nondilated collecting system may be difficult and time consuming and, on rare occasions, may fail completely.

Cystography

Indications

1. Suspected bladder trauma. Bladder opacification by contrast excreted during an IV injection for an IVU or CT is unreliable in assessment for bladder ruptures. The bladder should be opacified by means of a catheter placed in the bladder until a detrusor contraction is elicited to reliably exclude a bladder rupture.
2. Evaluation of fistulas involving the urinary bladder (Figure 3-8).
3. Evaluation of healing following bladder or distal ureteral surgery.

Contraindications

There are no contraindications to cystography itself. When a patient has sustained significant pelvic trauma, the integrity of the urethra must first be established before passing a ureteral catheter. This may often require that retrograde urethrography precede cystography.

Technique

1. After a preliminary KUB, a urethral catheter is passed and CM is instilled into the bladder. Films of the filled bladder are made in multiple projections. The bladder is then allowed to empty through the catheter, after which a drainage film is obtained. The post-drainage film is extremely important, as small leaks from the posterior wall may be

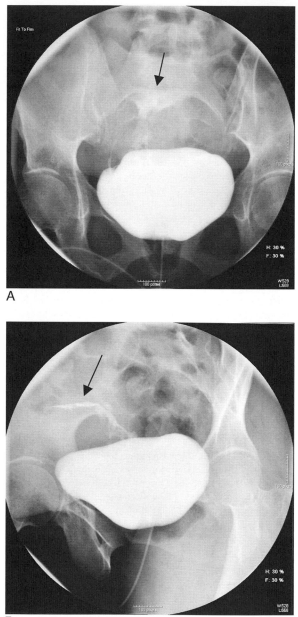

A

B

FIGURE 3-8. **A** and **B.** Frontal and oblique views of cystogram in a woman with vaginal leakage a few weeks after cesarean section delivery. There is opacification of the uterus *(arrow)* from the urinary bladder.

obscured by a contrast filled bladder and be visible only after the bladder has been drained of contrast.

2. Cystography may also be performed through an existing cystostomy tube or via suprapubic puncture.

Complications

1. Complications of cystography are rare. Excessively forceful injection may result in disruption of a fresh suture line.

Modifications of Cystography

CT Cystogram

Because most patients with significant abdominal or pelvic trauma undergo a CT scan for evaluation, the addition of a CT cystogram to assess the bladder is helpful in patients with significant pelvic injury. After the initial set of CT images have been obtained, diluted contrast is injected through an indwelling Foley catheter and scanning is repeated through the pelvis. Most published reports indicate that CT cystograms and conventional cystograms have comparable sensitivity in detecting bladder injury. An advantage of CT is that the patient does not have to be turned into different projections (an obvious advantage in patients with pelvic fractures) for optimal evaluation, and a post-drain film is unnecessary because the entire bladder is well seen on a CT.

When evaluating a patient for a suspected fistula involving the bladder, a CT cystogram helps in demonstrating the fistula well. CT is the most sensitive imaging technique in patients with suspected colovesical fistulas due to complications of diverticulitis.

Voiding Cystourethrogram (VCUG)

This study demonstrates the anatomy of the lower urinary tract during micturition and allows assessment for vesicoureteral reflux.

Indications

1. Recurrent urinary tract infections, especially in children, in whom reflux is not uncommon.
2. Evaluation of the posterior urethra in the male and the entire urethra in the female. VCUG is used to evaluate urethral stricture disease, posterior urethral valves in the infant male, and the postoperative urethra (Figure 3-9). In the female, it is a primary method of visualizing urethral diverticula.

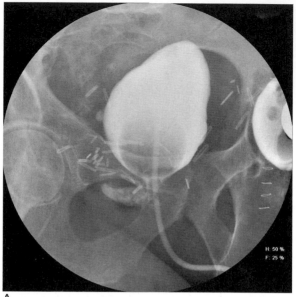

A

FIGURE 3-9. (Continued)

3. Evaluation of certain voiding dysfunctions (e.g., detrusor-external sphincter dyssynergia, neurogenic bladder). VCUG can be combined with simultaneous pressure-flow recordings for a study known as videourodynamics.
4. For the evaluation of an ectopic ureter thought to insert into the urethra. Reflux into such ectopic ureters is fairly common.

Contraindication

1. Acute urinary tract infection.

Technique

1. This procedure is best performed under fluoroscopic control.
2. The bladder is catheterized and filled with water-soluble CM. HOCM is usually used for this study as a large amount of contrast is required (300–600 mL) and adverse reactions to contrast injection into the bladder are uncommon. When the patient has a strong desire to void, the catheter is withdrawn and the patient voids. Fluoroscopic images are obtained during voiding and an estimate of the completeness of bladder

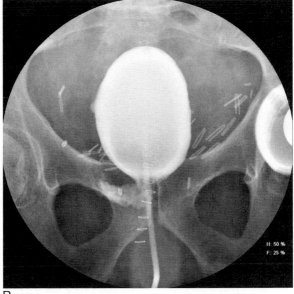

B

FIGURE 3-9. VCUG 10 days after radical retropubic prostatectomy demonstrates leak from the right posterior aspect of the anastomosis. Study done a week later showed healing of the leak. **A.** Left posterior oblique view. **B.** Frontal view.

emptying is made. In patients who have undergone recent bladder neck or urethral surgery, voiding around an indwelling urethral catheter is initially performed to look for contrast extravasation. If none is seen fluoroscopically, the urethral catheter may be removed and another void documented fluoroscopically.

3. Although the bladder is filled with the patient recumbent, voiding is usually performed with the patient standing.

Complications

These are the same as those listed under cystography.

Retrograde Urethrogram (RUG)

Purpose

To provide detailed visualization of the anterior urethra in the male. The procedure has little or no application in the female. On a RUG, the posterior urethra is incompletely visualized

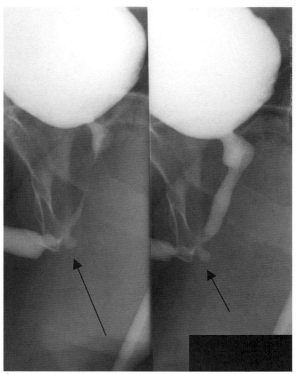

A

FIGURE 3-10. (Continued)

because the closed external urethral sphincter resists the retrograde flow of contrast into the posterior urethra. Complete
evaluation of the anterior and posterior urethra in a male
requires both a VCUG and a RUG (Figure 3-10). Although
the anterior urethra is seen on a VCUG, a diseased anterior
urethra is better demonstrated on a RUG.

Indications

1. Detailed delineation of suspected or known urethral
   stricture (most common indication).
2. Suspected urethral trauma. RUG should be routinely performed before attempting passage of a urethral catheter
   in a male patient with a pelvic fracture.
3. Demonstration of urethral diverticula, fistulas, and
   neoplasms.

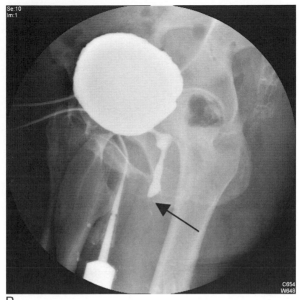

B

FIGURE 3-10. (Continued)

Contraindications

1. Acute urethritis, as discussed later.
2. Patients who are allergic to contrast should be pretreated. LOCM should be used in this situation.

Technique

1. A Foley catheter is placed with sterile technique and the Foley balloon is inflated in the fossa navicularis.
2. LOCM is then injected and radiographic images of the fully distended urethra are taken.

Complications

Reflux/intravasation of contrast from the urethra into the surrounding corpus spongiosum can occur during RUG. Such reflux is usually minimal and without clinical consequence except in the presence of urethritis when bacteria may be forced into the bloodstream. In patients with venereal warts, the procedure should not be performed until the

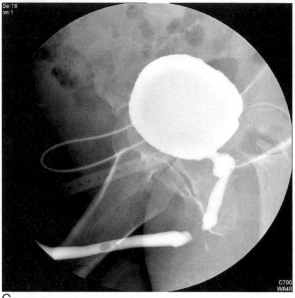

C

FIGURE 3-10. Straddle injury. **A.** VCUG through a suprapubic catheter demonstrates irregularity of the bulbar urethra at injury site *(arrow)*. **B.** VCUG demonstrates urethral occlusion at injury site *(arrow)* 5 weeks later. **C.** Combined VCUG and RUG help in assessing the length of occlusion more optimally.

active infection has been controlled, to avoid spreading the infection to the urethra. Spongiosal intravasation is more apt to occur in patients with high grade urethral strictures.

Loopogram and Pouchogram

Anastomosis of the ureters to an isolated intact segment of ileum or transverse colon (loop) or to a detubularized large or small bowel segment (pouch) is the most common method of establishing permanent urinary diversion (Figure 3-11). The isolated bowel loop serves as a conduit to propel urine outward toward the stoma in a continuous, rhythmic, isoperistaltic way. A urine collection bag is applied to the stoma. The detubularized pouch, on the other hand, lacks the contractility to propel urine to the outside, thus functioning as a continent reservoir rather than a conduit.

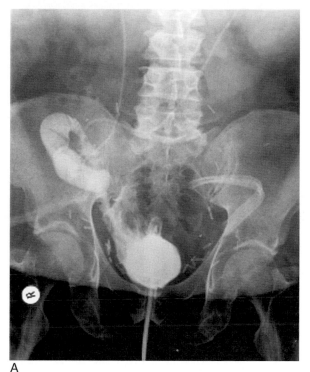

A

FIGURE 3-11. (Continued)

Pouches can be connected to a cutaneous stoma or be anastomosed to the urethra (orthotopic diversion). Cutaneous continent pouches require intermittent catheterization for emptying while patients with orthotopic pouches void by increasing abdominal pressure to empty the pouch. Radiologic examination of urinary diversions is referred to as loopography or pouchography.

Indications

1. To evaluate the bowel conduit or reservoir for suspected intrinsic disease (e.g., filling defect, anastomotic or other leaks, loop stenosis), capacity, or peristaltic activity.
2. To visualize the upper urinary tract by reflux. Reflux is normal with ileal conduits but unpredictable in continent

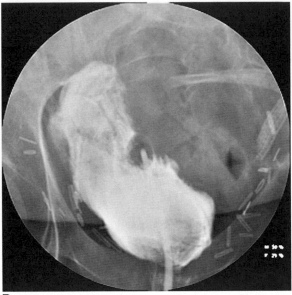

B

FIGURE 3-11. Normal examination of a Studer pouch 3 weeks after surgery. **A.** Early filling allows better visualization of the afferent limb than when the pouch is fully distended (**B**).

diversions. If a patient with a continent diversion requires urothelial evaluation beyond that provided by an IVU or CTU, antegrade pyelogram is usually the next step.
3. To evaluate patients with loop diversion whose upper urinary tracts show deterioration on serial IVUs or ultrasonogram (i.e., worsening hydronephrosis, renal calculi, renal scarring) or whose renal function is diminishing. In such patients the absence of reflux from the ileal loop into the ureters may indicate uretero-ileal obstruction.

Contraindications

1. There are no contraindications to the retrograde study of a urinary conduit or reservoir other than active urinary tract infection. Because the urinary tract of patients with urinary diversions is usually colonized with bacteria, prophylactic antibiotics are administered prior to the procedure to prevent bacteremia.

Technique

1. Following a KUB, the stoma of an ileal conduit is catheterized with a 14- or 16-F Foley catheter with aseptic technique. The balloon is inflated just below the anterior abdominal wall and the conduit is filled with LOCM until the ileum is well distended. Fluoroscopic images are obtained with particular attention given to the presence or absence of reflux. Images of the collecting systems and ureters are obtained to evaluate for urothelial abnormalities. The catheter is then removed and the conduit and upper urinary tracts evaluated for emptying.

2. A continent urinary pouch or reservoir is also evaluated fluoroscopically. The stoma (for a cutaneous diversion) or urethra (for an orthotopic diversion) is catheterized and a Foley catheter placed into the reservoir. The reservoir is opacified with CM to capacity, which varies with time. At maturity, it should accommodate several hundred milliliters of fluid. Filling defects and leaks are documented, if present. Nonopaque mucus in the reservoir is an expected finding.

Although many pouches do not normally allow for ureteral reflux, reflux may be observed with a Studer pouch, in which the ureters are anastomosed to an isoperistaltic afferent loop of ileum, which drains into a detubularized ileal pouch (see Figure 3-11). Although reflux does not occur in a normally functioning Studer pouch, the elevated intraluminal pressures generated during retrograde pouch opacification will fill the isoperistaltic afferent limb and diverted ureters.

Complications

Pyelonephritis may accompany forceful reflux of infected urine.

Angiography

Angiography refers to the radiologic study of both the arterial and venous systems. Studies pertinent to the study of the urinary tract include the following:

1. Arterial: aortography, renal arteriography, adrenal arteriography.
2. Venous: inferior venacavography, renal phlebography, adrenal phlebography, gonadal phlebography.

Indications for Renal Arteriography

1. To evaluate for suspected renal artery stenosis (RAS). RAS is a cause of potentially reversible hypertension

and renal insufficiency, particularly in elderly patients. Many screening tests have been used in an effort to non-invasively diagnose RAS, and currently, CT angiography and MR angiography are the most frequently used imaging techniques; the latter is preferred in patients with renal insufficiency to avoid the risks of CIN. Patients with significant truncal stenosis of the renal artery and fibro-muscular dysplasia are treated with angioplasty. Lesions at the renal artery ostia are resistant to angioplasty and require primary stenting. Randomized trials that compared renal artery angioplasty with best medical therapy do not indicate that angioplasty is a convincingly superior treatment. Large trials are currently under way in Europe to conclusively evaluate the value of treating RAS.

2. Neoplasms. Since the development of CT and MRI, angiography is almost never used in the diagnosis of renal masses. It is still used occasionally for the preoperative embolization of large, hypervascular renal cell carcinomas and for prophylactic embolization of angiomyolipomas that are larger than 4 cm in size, to prevent spontaneous hemorrhage.

3. Renal trauma. Most traumatic parenchymal and vascular lesions can be satisfactorily imaged by CT. Angiography is usually reserved to demonstrate an arterial bleeder or arteriovenous communication prior to embolization.

4. For the evaluation (and potential ablation) of vascular abnormalities such as aneurysms and arteriovenous malformations (AVMs) suspected on other imaging studies.

5. To provide a preoperative arterial "road map" when there is a high risk of anomalous vascular supply such as in a horseshoe kidney or an ectopic kidney. Currently, CT angiography or MR angiography is preferred to catheter angiography for this indication.

6. In the preoperative evaluation of potential renal donors. CT angiography and MR angiography have supplanted catheter angiography in most institutions for this indication as well.

Indications for Adrenal Gland Angiography

1. Ablation of adrenal function by embolization or overinjection of the adrenal veins.

2. For adrenal vein sampling to diagnose functioning adrenal tumors.

Indications for Gonadal Phlebography

1. Gonadal phlebography is valuable in evaluating varicoceles and in treating them by means of venous occlusion with balloons, coils, or sclerosing agents.

2. High-resolution CT and MRI are preferred to gonadal phlebography to search for a nonpalpable undescended testis.

Radionuclide Imaging

Radionuclide imaging is used to assess renal vascular perfusion, renal function, and obstruction. Examples of some of the radiopharmaceuticals frequently employed for GU imaging are ^{131}I-ortho-iodohippurate, ^{99m}Tc-glucoheptonate, ^{99m}Tc-DTPA, ^{99m}Tc-DMSA, ^{99m}Tc-MAG$_3$, and ^{67}Ga citrate.

Indications

1. Assessment of renal function. Following a bolus injection of radionuclide, computer analysis of radioactivity plotted against time allows analysis of blood clearance rates to determine the glomerular filtration rate and effective renal function. Ascertaining the relative function of the kidneys is especially important when decisions regarding nephrectomy versus salvage operation must be made in patients with renal malignancies. In cases of severe hydronephrosis, split renal functions before and after a period of nephrostomy drainage may show a surprising degree of renal functional improvement in the previously obstructed kidney.
2. Hypertension. Differential renal blood flow studies (performed before and after the administration of an angiotensin-converting enzyme [ACE] inhibitor such as captopril) detect approximately 85% of cases of renal vascular disease. Difficulties with isotope screening in hypertension include problems in distinguishing unilateral renovascular lesions from unilateral renal parenchymal disease and problems recognizing bilateral vascular stenoses. The accuracy of the examination is decreased in patients with renal insufficiency and with chronic use of ACE inhibitors.
3. Evaluation of renal transplant failure. Isotopic methods of imaging the kidney are very helpful in evaluating renal transplant complications including obstruction, extravasation, and stenosis of the arterial anastomosis. Differentiation between acute tubular necrosis and transplant rejection is a more difficult task.
4. Questionable or intermittent obstruction. The presence of intermittent obstruction, especially at the ureteropelvic junction (UPJ), is often difficult to evaluate and confirm. Using radionuclide methods, the rate of emptying of the collecting system after a diuretic challenge (washout or

Lasix renogram) can be evaluated and compared to standard emptying profiles. A normal kidney puts out more than 76% of the activity that enters it within 20 minutes.

5. Evaluate for urine leak. Small urinary leaks in patients who cannot receive iodinated contrast can be detected readily with radionuclide studies. Renal transplant patients with impaired renal function and suspected urinary leak are the classic cases in which radionuclide studies are very helpful in evaluating for urinary leak.

6. Evaluate for vesicoureteral reflux. VCUG is used for initial evaluation of suspected reflux in children, so that the anatomy of the lower urinary tract can also be assessed, a task not possible with radionuclide imaging. However, radionuclide cystogram is the follow-up procedure of choice for proven reflux, as it is more sensitive than VCUG and imposes less of a radiation burden on the patient. Using agents such as ^{99m}Tc-DMSA, the renal scarring, which is often the consequence of reflux, can also be demonstrated.

7. The "acute" scrotum. When testicular torsion is suspected, a radionuclide flow study of the scrotum will demonstrate the viability of the testis and compare its perfusion to the opposite side. Increased nuclide perfusion favors epididymitis over torsion.

8. Inflammatory lesions. Inflammatory lesions of any organ result in abnormal uptake of ^{67}Ga citrate. Gallium scanning is useful in uncovering occult inflammatory foci in or around the kidneys or in confirming the presence of a clinically atypical infection. Other agents such as ^{111}In, which can be fixed to leukocytes, may also be used.

9. Adrenal gland. ^{131}I-metaiodobenzylguanidine (MIBG), an adrenal medullary imaging agent, can readily and easily localize pheochromocytomas. Cholesterol analogues (^{131}I-NP-59) have also been synthesized and have proved helpful in localizing hyperfunctioning and hypofunctioning adrenal lesions.

10. PET scanning. In urogenital imaging, the most widely used tracer is ^{18}F-fluorodeoxyglucose (FDG), which is taken into cells through glucose transporters. Many tumors have increased glucose uptake and therefore concentrate FDG. FDG is normally excreted by the kidneys through urine, which limits its utility in evaluating the kidneys. Modern machines have a CT scanner incorporated into the PET machine, allowing accurate localization of sites of increased uptake.

FDG-PET scanning is used in restaging testicular cancer after chemotherapy, as it appears to be more accurate than CT for detecting recurrence. To date, FDG-PET has not shown much value in the evaluation of prostate or bladder cancer.

11. Prostascint scanning. Prostascint (capromab pendetide) is a monoclonal antibody to the prostatic surface membrane antigen that is thought to occur only at the surface of metabolically active prostate cells. Localization of the agent is slow and requires imaging at 72 or 96 hours after injection. At present, this agent is not helpful in initial staging but may be of some value in localizing recurrent disease.

Contraindications

Radionuclides should not be administered during pregnancy. There are no other contraindications to the use of radionuclide studies for diagnostic purposes.

Technique

Techniques vary depending on the information desired. In general, a tracer dose of radioactive isotope bound to a specific pharmaceutical agent is administered and the patient is placed beneath a gamma camera where images (scans, scintigrams) are generated at intervals depending on the information sought. For flow studies, images are taken as frequently as every few seconds. For anatomic information, images are obtained by accumulating counts for several minutes. These images may be taken sequentially for as long as several hours and under certain circumstances may even be delayed up to 24 or 48 hours. Recently, techniques for obtaining tomographic scintigraphy (single-photon emission computed tomography [SPECT]) have considerably improved the anatomic information provided by radionuclide images. When evaluating renal function, small radiation detectors or gamma cameras placed directly over the kidneys can be used to generate time-radioactivity curves. This is known as a renogram.

Complications

There are no complications of nuclear medicine diagnostic procedures. The radiation doses involved are modest and often less than those for comparable conventional radiographic studies or CT.

Ultrasonography

Ultrasound can be used to image most parts of the GU system. It is a noninvasive study with no radiation exposure. Administration of contrast is not required, although newly developed ultrasound contrast agents often enhance the diagnostic yield of the examination. Characteristics of blood flow can be determined by US. The resolution of US imaging is limited in large and obese patients.

Technique

Two types of sonographic imaging are commonly used in the urinary tract: real-time gray-scale imaging and Doppler imaging. Real-time gray-scale imaging is used to depict the architecture and anatomy of the organ. Real-time imaging allows consistent modification of transducer position to obtain optimal projections. Doppler or flow imaging is used to assess the vascularity of the organ and masses and is usually combined with real-time gray-scale imaging.

Newer advances in ultrasound include advances in image presentation such as 3-D imaging and extended field-of-view imaging, so that data can be presented in a single image to facilitate the depiction of spatial relationships.

Complications

None known.

Indications

1. Kidney
    a) Evaluation of a renal mass. US can detect fluid-filled renal masses with more than 98% accuracy. Solid mass lesions larger than 1 cm in diameter are also routinely identified. The ultrasound appearance of cysts and solid masses is quite distinctive, although complex or complicated cysts may share certain imaging characteristics of solid lesions. The detection of neoplasms is aided by demonstrating flow within them by means of color-flow or power Doppler. US may also demonstrate IV and intracaval tumor extension in renal neoplasms. The ability to identify, characterize, and stage a renal mass is dependent on the depth of the lesion beneath the skin and the body habitus of the patient.
    b) Impaired renal function. In patients with renal insufficiency, US is helpful in assessing the size of the kidney and excluding urinary obstruction as a cause of the

renal failure. Dilated renal pelves and calyces usually indicated obstructive uropathy (Figure 3-12). Alteration in the normal echogenicity of the kidneys is seen in patients with medical renal disease. The kidneys may be smaller and more echogenic than normal.

c) As a guide to biopsy and other interventional procedures. By visualizing the kidney directly, entry into the kidney is facilitated for percutaneous renal biopsy or for entry into dilated renal collecting systems for antegrade pyelography preparatory to PCN.

d) Evaluate filling defects seen in the collecting system on an IVU or RPG. These are most commonly caused by nonopaque calculi, urothelial neoplasms, and blood clots. Renal calculi are markedly echogenic, produce acoustic shadowing, and are readily detectable by US (see Figure 3-12A). Clots and tumors may also be demonstrated but not necessarily easily differentiated by US.

e) Evaluation of perinephric collections. Fluid collections around the kidney may represent an abscess, urinoma, or hematoma. This situation is usually encountered with renal transplants. Determining the etiology of a fluid collection is usually not possible by US alone. A complex fluid mass is more likely an abscess or hematoma rather than a lymphocele or urinoma.

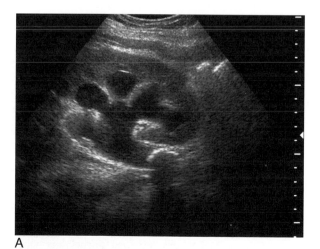

A

FIGURE 3-12. (Continued)

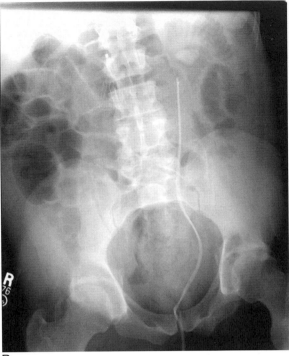

B

FIGURE 3-12. (Continued)

f) Renal surveillance. Kidneys at risk for the development of specific diseases can be periodically monitored by US (e.g., the contralateral kidney following
nephrectomy for Wilms' tumor and evaluation of
family members of patients with hereditary disorders
such as polycystic disease and tuberous sclerosis).
The status of existing diseases such as hydronephrosis
can also be monitored to determine whether the
process is static, improving, or worsening.

g) Renovascular problems. Gray-scale ultrasound contributes little to evaluation of RAS except for measurement
of renal size and demonstrating renal morphology. With
color-flow Doppler, arterial and venous lesions (e.g.,
occlusions, stenoses, aneurysms, fistulas, malformations)
of the extrarenal and intrarenal arteries and veins
can be demonstrated and flow velocities estimated.

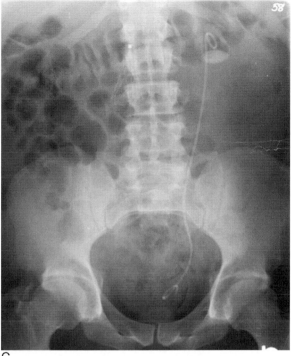

C

FIGURE 3-12. Hydronephrosis due to a proximal ureteral stone.
A. Renal ultrasound shows marked hydronephrosis proximal to a
shadowing echogenic calculus. **B.** Retrograde catheter was distal to
stone and did not drain left kidney. **C.** Double pigtail internalized
stent was then placed and patient underwent SWL.

The technique also allows for demonstration of bland and
tumor thrombus in the renal vein and inferior vena cava
in patients with renal tumors.

h) Renal transplant evaluation. The transplanted kidney,
because of its superficial position in the pelvis, is particularly well suited for US evaluation. The combination of Doppler and gray-scale sonography (duplex
Doppler) makes it possible to evaluate renal allografts
for such complications as rejection, RAS, and arterial
or venous thrombi. Surgical complications such as
hydronephrosis and lymphocele formation are also
easily assessed by US.

    i) Fetal renal ultrasound. The detection of fetal hydrone-phrosis alerts physicians to the need for additional urologic evaluation in the early neonatal period. The availability of fetal therapy is an exciting development and still in early stages.

2. Ureter. US has limited usefulness in most ureteral disorders but for a few instances. Dilated ureters may be seen, ureteroceles demonstrated within the bladder, and small calculi may be imaged, especially in the pelvic ureter. Color-flow demonstration of asymmetric jets of urine from the ureteral orifices in the bladder often indicates the presence of ureteral obstruction.

3. Bladder. Uses of US in urinary bladder evaluation include the measurement of residual urine after voiding, guidance for suprapubic aspiration, and evaluation of intravesical masses and diverticula.

4. Prostate and seminal vesicles. US of the prostate is useful to estimate prostatic size. Transrectal ultrasound (TRUS) is widely used to localize a suspicious prostate lesion for transrectal biopsy. TRUS and pelvic US are also useful in the evaluation of a pelvic mass and for aspiration of cystic lesions such as seminal vesicle cysts.

    TRUS should not be used as a routine screening modality in an asymptomatic population but is helpful in the presence of a palpable nodule or elevated prostatic specific antigen level to identify suspicious lesions as well as to direct transrectal biopsies of suspicious foci, in addition to routine sextant biopsies.

5. Scrotum and external genitalia
    a) US is the primary imaging modality to evaluate the scrotum and its contents. It can differentiate intratesticular from extratesticular masses as well as solid from cystic scrotal masses. US is also helpful when inflammation or neoplasm of the testis or epididymis is associated with a secondary hydrocele that prevents adequate palpation of the underlying lesion. Color-flow Doppler is very helpful in the scrotum and external genitalia. Perfusion patterns may help to differentiate inflammation from neoplasms and to substantiate a diagnosis of torsion or infarction.
    b) Undescended testicles can often be identified in the inguinal canal (but not within the abdomen) with US. To localize cryptorchid intra-abdominal testes, MRI or CT scan is usually used.
    c) In male sexual dysfunction, inadequacies of flow in the cavernosal arteries are readily identified, and this technique has become a standard part of the evaluation of the

impotent patient. Fibrous or calcified plaques in the tunica albuginea in Peyronie's disease can be easily identified. Retrograde filling of the urethra with saline during gray-scale scanning can identify strictures of the distal male urethra and assess the perurethral tissues for associated scarring. This technique, believed to allow for selection of the most appropriate treatment of urethral stricture, has not gained widespread acceptance. Standard contrast retrograde urethrography remains the most widely used study to evaluate the male urethra.

d) In the female, translabial or endoluminal (endourethral) US has been used to identify urethral diverticula but is not favored by most urologists and radiologists over voiding cystourethrography and MRI.

6. Intraoperative US. This technique is often used to assist in partial nephrectomy in patients with one or more small renal tumors and is particularly helpful in localizing small tumors that are intrarenal with little or no exophytic component.

Computed Tomography

Basic Principles

A narrowly collimated x-ray beam is rotated about the patient and a number of contiguous or slightly overlapping cross-sectional slices, each varying in thickness from 3 mm to 1 cm, are made through the anatomic areas of interest. Although many visceral structures can be recognized by their suggestive CT appearance, others have similar densities. To enhance structural differences, CM is frequently given. This is the same type as is used for urography and other urologic studies. Following administration of CM, multiple images are repeated. Many pathologic lesions can be recognized on the basis of their appearance before and after contrast administration. The advantage of CT over ordinary radiography is the greater contrast resolution of CT, which is approximately 10 times that possible with conventional radiography. The useful display of tomographic cross-sectional anatomy in CT, relatively unaffected by surrounding high x-ray absorbing tissues such as bone, is another distinct advantage. Complex computer algorithms allow reconstruction of CT data into many forms, including different planes, such as coronal and sagittal.

Technique

1. Preparation is the same as for any procedure in which CM is to be administered except that a dilute mixture

of barium or Gastrografin is administered orally before the CT study to identify the small and large bowels and thereby avoid confusion of fluid-filled bowel with abdominal masses or lymph nodes. In those patients being studied specifically for urinary tract calculi, oral contrast material is omitted.

2. After a series of non-contrast scans through the area of interest, sections are repeated following contrast administration. CM allows better characterization and delineation of renal masses, permits evaluation of renal vein and caval patency in renal neoplasm, compares blood flow to each kidney, and helps differentiate vascular structures from solid masses, such as retroperitoneal lymphadenopathy. The contrast is usually administered as a rapid bolus using a power injector.

Complications

The complications are limited to those described under CM. Contraindications are identical to those for IVU. Some unusually obese patients may not be candidates for CT because they cannot fit into the gantry or are too heavy for the table.

Indications

CT plays a major role in uroradiologic diagnosis. Indications have been broadening consistently as the efficacy and utility of CT are fully appreciated. Some of its more important uses are as follows:

1. Renal masses
   a) Diagnosis. CT is very accurate in detecting and characterizing renal masses, identifying renal pseudotumors, and differentiating simple as well as complex cystic masses from solid lesions of the kidney (Figure 3-13). Because fresh blood is recognizable on CT, hemorrhagic lesions and hematomas are easily recognizable. Renal parenchymal and urothelial neoplasms also have suggestive appearances on CT. With the increasing application of CT for all manner of abdominal symptoms, there is increasing serendipitous diagnosis of small renal masses ranging in size from 1 to 3 cm. The diagnosis of renal cancer is made when a lesion enhances after contrast administration and thus increases in density.

      As smaller renal masses are diagnosed and resected, it is becoming apparent that small benign tumors, particularly small lipid-poor angiomyolipomas, may

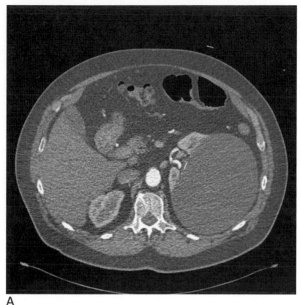

A

FIGURE 3-13. (Continued)

    be indistinguishable from renal cell cancers (RCCs) on imaging.

b) Staging of renal neoplasms. CT is superb at demonstrating perinephric extension, evidence of renal vein or IVC tumor thrombus, regional and abdominal lymphadenopathy, and the presence of liver or adrenal metastases. It is invaluable in the preoperative evaluation of neoplasms.

c) Postoperative. CT can detect local or distant intra-abdominal recurrence of neoplasm after partial or total nephrectomy for malignant disease.

d) Characterizing renal cysts. A cyst with homogenous low attenuation (<20 HU) and thin imperceptible walls represents a simple renal cyst (see Figure 3-13), whereas nodular enhancement of walls, thick irregular septations, and central enhancement are indicative of a malignancy. Cysts with characteristics that span these extremes are a diagnostic dilemma. Benign cysts complicated by hemorrhage and malignant cysts are the primary differential diagnostic possibilities that

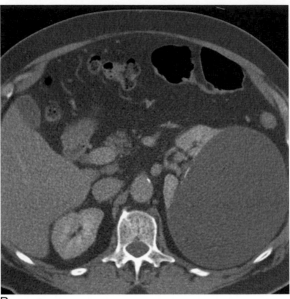

B

FIGURE 3-13. Left renal cyst. Arterial phase **(A)** and homogenous nephrographic phase **(B).** The large left renal cyst does not enhance, indicating it is benign.

have to be distinguished in such cases. MRI is often helpful in evaluation of such indeterminate lesions, as subtle enhancement of the lesion may be detectable on MRI but not on CT.

2. CT in patients with urolithiasis. The use of noncontrast CT for the evaluation of patients with acute renal colic is now accepted as the study of choice, with sensitivity and specificity for detection of renal calculi ranging between 97% and 100%. No oral or IV contrast is administered, and the diagnosis is available in a few minutes from the start of the scan. Definitive diagnosis requires identification of a stone in the ureter with proximal hydronephrosis. Perinephric fluid or stranding may also be seen.

Nearly all stones are dense on CT, with the notable exception being a drug calculus, as in patients on protease inhibitor therapy for human immunodeficiency virus (HIV) infection. As CT becomes more widely used, there are numerous reports of unsuspected renal and non-renal diagnoses that may masquerade clinically as renal colic. These include aortic aneurysms, spinal problems, renal vein thrombosis, diverticulitis, appendicitis, acute pyelonephritis, and so forth. The diagnosis of pyelonephritis and renal vein thrombosis may be difficult on non-contrast enhanced scans and may require the administration of IV contrast.

The increasing use of CT in the emergency room setting is raising concerns about the radiation exposure to patients with urolithiasis who have a chronic and recurrent disease and may present repeatedly with symptoms of colic. Vigilance on the part of the physicians and personnel taking care of such patients is recommended, so that patients receive no more radiation than absolutely necessary.

In pregnant patients with suspected stone disease in whom imaging confirmation is necessary, a non-contrast CT appears to be the best technique to establish the diagnosis and is preferable to a limited IVU, previously the standard imaging recommendation.

3. CTU. In the past several years, there has been increasing interest in using CT for a complete evaluation of the urinary tract, to include evaluation of the parenchyma for masses and the urothelium for pathology. The availability of newer multidetector scanners now makes feasible the imaging of the urinary tract in multiple phases. Unenhanced scans are first obtained through the abdomen and pelvis to evaluate for stones. Imaging is next performed approximately 100 seconds after the start of contrast administration to evaluate the renal parenchyma. Twelve minutes later, repeat imaging is performed through the abdomen and pelvis to evaluate the urothelium. Postprocessing is then performed and anteroposterior and coronal oblique images that simulate an IVU are created. Preliminary data are promising but there is no study to date that has directly compared the abilities of IVU and CTU in detecting urothelial abnormalities. CTU is a radiation heavy technique, with patients receiving approximately three times the radiation dose of an IVU.

   CT is also of help in staging transitional cell carcinoma of the renal collecting systems.

4. Renal inflammatory disease. Most patients with acute pyelonephritis do not require imaging for confirmation of the clinical diagnosis. However, because non-contrast CT is so widely used in the assessment of patients who present with acute flank pain and suspected renal colic, patients with clinically unsuspected

pyelonephritis will often have the diagnosis suggested on a CT scan. If a patient does not respond to appropriate antibiotic therapy, CT is useful in determining if complications have developed, such as a renal or perinephric abscess and assessing inflammatory perinephric extension.

5. Hydronephrosis. CT is superb for determining the level and etiology of hydronephrosis. The administration of oral and IV contrast is advisable in such patients to obtain as much information as possible.

6. Perinephric collections. Perinephric abscess, urinoma, and hematoma can be readily recognized and often differentiated by CT.

7. Trauma. CT is widely employed and very informative in assessing the extent of renal trauma and its possible complications, including vascular injury, extravasation from vascular system or urinary tract, urinoma formation, and impaired renal viability. When deep lacerations are identified at CT, imaging should be carried through into the excretory phase to determine if the collecting system is involved.

8. Retroperitoneal masses. CT and MRI are the best methods of evaluating most retroperitoneal masses including neoplasms (see Figure 3-6). With very large masses, the organ of origin may be difficult to determine on axial imaging alone. The addition of coronal and sagittal imaging is useful in such situations.

9. Retroperitoneal lymph nodes. CT and MRI are the most reliable methods currently available to evaluate for enlarged retroperitoneal lymph nodes. This is an important part of the staging of many urologic tumors including those arising in the testis, bladder, and prostate. In general, retroperitoneal and iliac lymph nodes are believed to be pathologically enlarged only when the short axis diameter is more than 1 cm.

10. Retroperitoneal fibrosis. In suspected cases of retroperitoneal fibrosis, CT can usually demonstrate the fibrous plaque, and CT and MRI are the two most important diagnostic modalities in evaluating for the disease.

11. Renal transplants. CT shares with MRI the ability to evaluate ailing renal transplants for hydronephrosis and perinephric fluid collections. Azotemia precludes the use of CM to evaluate vascular integrity.

12. Potential renal donors can be evaluated with cross-sectional and reconstructed CT images of renal parenchyma, vessels, collecting system, and ureters (CT, CT angiography, and CTU).

Urinary Bladder

CT is valuable in staging tumors confined to the urinary bladder when the perivesical fat planes are preserved. However, perivesical stranding could be attributable to inflammation or tumor, thereby limiting the staging value of CT. Obvious lymphadenopathy can be detected. MRI surpasses CT as the dominant imaging study in staging bladder cancer. Both techniques are limited, however, by their inability to detect small or microscopic metastases in normal-sized lymph nodes and minimal or microscopic tumor invasion of peripelvic fat and contiguous surfaces.

Prostate and Seminal Vesicles

With CT, congenital anomalies, cysts, and abscesses of the seminal vesicles can be well visualized and prostate abscesses detected. CT, however, has been replaced by MRI in assessing the prostate for most pathologies, including prostate cancer.

Adrenal Gland

Adrenal masses are a common finding on abdominal CT scans, and the vast majority represent benign adenomas, even in patients with a known underlying primary malignancy. An adrenal mass that measures less than 10 HU in density on unenhanced scans most likely represents an adrenal adenoma, and no further workup is necessary for such a mass. Masses that are greater than 10 HU on non-contrast CT are indeterminate in nature and can represent either lipid-poor adenomas or malignant lesions. The addition of delayed imaging at 15 minutes after contrast administration is helpful in such cases. Adrenal adenomas are vascular lesions from which contrast washes out quickly. If there is greater than 66% calculated washout of contrast from a lesion, it is most likely to represent an adenoma.

Adrenal myelolipoma is a benign lesion that may contain macroscopic fat (areas with density measurements less than −10 HU) (Figure 3-14). Adrenal carcinomas are usually large lesions at diagnosis.

Magnetic Resonance Imaging

MRI is a valuable adjunct and problem solver in imaging urinary tract pathology. The high contrast resolution of MRI makes it valuable in tissue characterization. Current

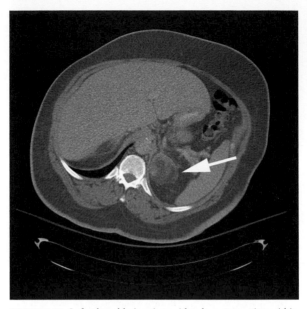

FIGURE 3-14. Left adrenal lesion *(arrow)* has low attenuation within it that represents fat, indicating that it is a myelolipoma.

indications for MR include the assessment of a renal mass that is not characterized on other imaging studies—small degrees of enhancement within a lesion not detectable on CT may be apparent on MRI, establishing the diagnosis of neoplasm. MR is also helpful in characterizing adrenal lesions. The use of endorectal and endovaginal coils allows high resolution imaging of the prostate gland, seminal vesicles, urinary bladder, and the urethra. Technical details of MRI cannot be addressed in this review.

INTERVENTIONAL URORADIOLOGY

This section discusses commonly performed nonvascular interventional procedures in the urinary tract.

Percutaneous Nephrostomy

Percutaneous nephrostomy (PCN) refers to the percutaneous placement of a drainage catheter or access sheath into the kidney, using radiologic guidance.

Indications for PCN

PCN is performed to relieve urinary obstruction, to gain access to the collecting system for therapeutic and diagnostic procedures, to divert urine to allow closure of a ureteral fistula or a dehiscent urinary tract anastomosis, and to allow assessment of residual recoverable function in a chronically obstructed kidney. These indications are elaborated on further later.

1. PCN to relieve urinary obstruction. PCN is most often requested in patients in whom imaging studies demonstrate hydroureteronephrosis; these studies may indicate the etiology as well as the anatomic level of the obstruction. Calculus disease is responsible for obstruction in approximately a third of patients with urinary obstruction who undergo PCN and malignancy in the rest, with carcinoma of the bladder, cervix, and colon being the most common primary tumors to cause urinary obstruction. When ureteral obstruction results in renal impairment, non-contrast computed tomography (NCCT) appears to be the best imaging modality to identify calculous causes of obstruction, whereas magnetic resonance urography (MRU) is superior for identifying non-calculous causes of obstruction. In patients with normal renal function, contrast-enhanced CT can identify the presence and cause of hydronephrosis in nearly all cases. MRU is particularly helpful in delineating the anatomy in patients with urinary diversion to bowel conduits.

   It is important to attempt, or at least to consider, the perurethral retrograde approach for renal drainage (ureteral intubation with cystoscopic guidance) in a patient with urinary obstruction before resorting to a PCN. Percutaneous drainage should ideally be reserved for patients in whom retrograde attempts are either unsuccessful or not feasible.

   In patients with obstruction, accompanied by signs or symptoms of urosepsis, PCN drainage provides rapid decompression of the obstructed collecting system and defervescence of the urosepsis. However, when obstruction and infection are due to renal or ureteral calculi, retrograde ureteral drainage is as effective in draining the collecting system as is PCN. In these cases, the decision to perform PCN or retrograde ureteral catheter drainage should be made by assessing what the best therapy for the stone would be. For instance, patients who have large renal calculi that would be best managed by percutaneous methods should have a PCN performed, whereas patients with smaller ureteral calculi that would be amenable to SWL should be drained by a ureteral catheter placed by a retrograde perurethral approach with cystoscopic guidance (see Figure 3-12).

PCN drainage can help to preserve or improve renal function until the cause of obstruction can be relieved in patients in whom the obstruction is expected to respond to treatment, such as chemotherapy, radiation therapy, or surgery. In patients with terminal malignancies and bilateral obstruction in whom ureteral stents cannot be placed, unilateral PCN drainage is usually preferred to bilateral drainage, to avoid the inconvenience of two externally draining nephrostomy bags. Unilateral drainage suffices in most patients to maintain renal function at an acceptable level and the less affected kidney (as judged by less hydronephrotic changes or parenchymal atrophy on imaging studies) is chosen for drainage (Figure 3-15).

2. PCN to gain access to the collecting system. PCN is often just the first step in performing a variety of other

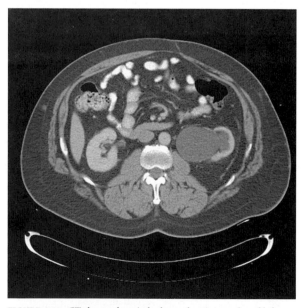

FIGURE 3-15. CT shows chronic hydronephrotic atrophy of left kidney due to colon cancer. Patient developed right hydronephrosis a few months later, necessitating a right nephrostomy.

interventional procedures in the kidney and ureter. Some examples of procedures that can be performed through a PCN track include the treatment of renal or ureteral calculi (stone fragmentation, removal, or chemolysis), ureteral interventions such as stricture dilation or stent placement, retrieval of foreign bodies such as fractured stent fragments, nephroscopic surgery such as endopyelotomy for UPJ obstruction, and brush biopsy or percutaneous therapy of urothelial tumors. Interventions can often be done at the same sitting as the PCN if the procedure is not complicated by excessive bleeding and if there is no infection.

3. PCN to divert urine. PCN is often performed to divert the urine to allow closure of a ureteral fistula, ureteral leak, or a dehiscent urinary tract anastomosis. PCN drainage alone is rarely successful in totally diverting the urine; the addition of ureteral stenting is usually required to bridge leaking ureteral segments or dehiscent anastomoses, and ureteral occlusion is usually necessary in patients with intractable fistulas, most commonly vesicovaginal fistulas. Urine diversion by PCN alone has been used with some success to treat patients with intractable hemorrhagic cystitis.

4. PCN to assess residual renal function. Renal drainage by PCN may allow assessment of residual recoverable function in a chronically obstructed kidney that appears to be either non-functioning or poorly functioning. The presence of renal parenchymal atrophy on CT or renal US does not necessarily predict a poor potential for functional recovery after drainage with a PCN, although a kidney that is reduced to a hydronephrotic shell is unlikely to recover function significantly.

Preprocedural Evaluation Prior to PCN

Preprocedural evaluation in patients being considered for PCN includes a clinical history to identify a potential bleeder as well as routine laboratory tests of coagulation and renal function. This is discussed further in the section on contraindications to the procedure.

Prophylactic antibiotics are beneficial in decreasing the development of sepsis in both high-risk patients (e.g., those with struvite stones, diabetes, urinary tract obstruction, indwelling catheters, previous manipulation, or instrumentation of the urinary tract) and patients with a low risk for developing sepsis. Antibiotics should be administered in such a way that maximum blood levels are attained during the procedure, that is immediately prior to or less than 2 hours before the procedure, and should be continued after the procedure for 24 to 48 hours in low-risk groups and for 48 to 72 hours in high-risk groups. In patients with urinary obstruction, antibiotic therapy should be continued until satisfactory renal drainage is ensured to avoid postprocedural bacteremia.

The risk of periprocedural sepsis is increased in the elderly, in diabetics, and in patients with indwelling catheters, stones, ureterointestinal anastomosis, or the clinical presence of infection; septic shock can occur in as many as 7% of patients with pyonephrosis. The organisms that commonly infect the GU tract are gram-negative rods and include *Escherichia coli, Proteus, Klebsiella,* and enterococcus. Antibiotic prophylaxis should ideally be based on culture results. In patients with obstruction and overt clinical infection in whom a specific organism has not yet been identified, broad-spectrum antibiotic therapy active against the common urinary pathogens is prudent.

Contraindications to PCN

The only absolute contraindication to PCN is the presence of an uncorrectable bleeding disorder; however, if the bleeding diathesis is due to a coagulopathy caused by urosepsis, urinary drainage will be necessary before the bleeding abnormality can be corrected. If there is severe hyperkalemia because of the obstructive uropathy, with serum potassium levels above 7 mEq/L, emergency hemodialysis and/or ion exchange therapy should be considered before PCN to rapidly correct the electrolyte abnormalities.

Correction of abnormal coagulation is needed if international normalized ratios (INR) and activated partial thromboplastin time (PTT) are greater than 1.5 times above the normal range. Fresh frozen plasma (FFP) will correct congenital factor deficiency and acquired coagulopathy. The corrective effect lasts only 6 hours, so the procedure has to be appropriately timed with the FFP infusion. If patients are on heparin, discontinuing the infusion and waiting 2–3 hours to perform the procedure is often sufficient because heparin has a half-life of 60 minutes (longer in patients with liver disease). Activated coagulation time can be checked if there is clinical concern. Abnormalities related to warfarin can be corrected with vitamin K_1 or FFP administration.

If the patient is taking aspirin or other drugs known to interfere with platelet function (examples include nonsteroidal anti-inflammatory drugs and newer beta-lactam antibiotics), a planned elective procedure can either be postponed for 3 to 10 days after the last dose of aspirin, or the bleeding time can be used as a guide with the procedure being delayed if the bleeding time exceeds the upper range of normal. Platelet transfusion will correct drug-induced prolongation of the bleeding time, if needed. Platelet counts greater than 50,000/dL are a safe value for most patients.

PCNs are often performed as an inpatient procedure but may be performed on an outpatient basis. Patients who may not be suitable candidates for outpatient PCN include those with hypertension, untreated urinary tract infection, coagulopathy, and staghorn calculi as these patients may be more likely to have complications such as procedure-related sepsis or bleeding.

Technique

1. Monitoring of patients—Continuous electrocardiogram monitoring during the procedure is advisable. Large-bore and secure IV access should be routinely established before the procedure so that IV sedation and analgesia can be administered during the procedure and IV access is readily available if other medications need to be administered. IV sedation combined with local anesthesia is sufficient to keep most patients comfortable; such patients require transcutaneous oximetry.

2. Localization of collecting system—The renal collecting system is localized by US if it is hydronephrotic. In a moderately or severely dilated collecting system, US guidance is successful in aiding entry into the collecting system in 85–95% of patients; conversely, in mildly dilated collecting systems, the success rate may be as low as 50%.

   Fluoroscopic guidance is used for the procedure if there is a radio-opaque stone that can serve as a target for puncture or if the collecting system can be opacified with contrast. If renal function is normal (as in a patient with a urinary fistula), the collecting system can be opacified with contrast excreted after IV administration. Opacification of the collecting system by injecting through a retrograde catheter is helpful in patients with nonopaque calculi, for planned percutaneous endopyelotomy, and in patients with nondilated collecting systems and urinary stones. Blind punctures of the kidney using anatomic landmarks are apt to require multiple punctures for optimal entry and should be measures of last resort; ultrasound guidance can facilitate appropriate and safe puncture of the collecting system with the fewest number of sticks.

3. The patients are positioned in either a prone or a prone oblique position with the ipsilateral side elevated 20–30 degrees; however, if the patient cannot lie prone, the procedure can be performed in a supine oblique position— CT guidance is particularly helpful in this case. Initial puncture can be performed with CT guidance and the subsequent manipulations for catheter placement are performed with fluoroscopic guidance. Preprocedural CT or MR scanning is necessary and highly recommended in patients with aberrant anatomy (e.g., severe scoliosis, congenital abnormalities) so that the relationship of the kidney to the liver, spleen, colon, gallbladder, and pleural space can be determined.

4. The flank is cleansed, and a subcostal skin entry site in the posterior axillary line is anesthetized. A needle is advanced into the collecting system from the flank, urine aspirated, contrast material injected, and a guidewire inserted through the needle into the kidney. The procedure is monitored fluoroscopically.

5. The needle is removed and the nephrocutaneous track enlarged by passing fascial dilators over the guidewire.

6. A drainage catheter, usually an 8-F "pigtail" catheter with a self-retaining mechanism, is passed over the guidewire and positioned in the renal pelvis. The guidewire is removed and the catheter is secured to the skin and attached to a closed gravity drainage bag.

Results

1. A PCN catheter can be successfully placed in 98–99% of patients with obstructed kidneys and dilated collecting systems.

2. Nondilated collecting systems or complex stone cases are technically challenging; reported success rates of catheter placement are 85–90%.

3. When obstruction is complicated by urosepsis or azotemia, the response to renal decompression is marked and often immediate, with fever and flank pain improving in 24–48 hours after PCN drainage. As mentioned earlier, when obstruction and infection are due to ureteral calculi, retrograde ureteral catheterization and PCN are equally effective in relieving the obstruction and infection; neither technique is superior to the other in promoting rapid drainage or clinical defervescence.

4. In patients with azotemia secondary to obstruction, PCN returns renal function to normal or near normal levels in 7–14 days and can improve renal function enough to obviate dialysis in 28–30%. In patients with malignancies, the ureters can be obstructed by contiguous involvement or extrinsic compression. The need for external nephrostomy drainage is often permanent in such patients as ureteral stents often fail in adequately draining patients with extrinsic obstruction. The physical and financial burdens posed by the presence of a drainage catheter have to be weighed against the benefit of extending life for a few months. Long-term survival after palliative diversion for malignant ureteral obstruction is poor, with only 25% of patients alive at 1 year. Our approach in patients with bilateral obstruction due to malignancies is to initially drain the symptomatic side, if there is one, or drain the kidney that appears to have more preserved renal parenchyma as gauged by cross-sectional imaging. The contralateral kidney is drained only if there is suspected infection or if unilateral drainage does not improve renal function enough to administer the necessary chemotherapy.

Complications

1. The overall serious complication rate of PCN is low, with a mortality of 0.2% compared to a surgical mortality of 6.0%. Major complications include hemorrhage and sepsis.
2. Hemorrhage requiring transfusion or other therapy is a complication in 1–2.4% of patients and is related to renal arterial pseudoaneurysms or arteriovenous fistulas due to laceration of lobar arteries. Most hemorrhage associated with nephrostomy placement is transient and self-limited; it is not uncommon to have pink or slightly bloody urine drainage for several days after a nephrostomy, and this is not considered a complication. If the urine is grossly bloody or large clots are seen on the nephrostogram, repeated irrigation with cold saline and/or placement of a slightly larger catheter, at least 2-F larger, to tamponade the bleeding vessel are usually effective in controlling the bleeding. Serious vascular trauma is suspected if the urine continues to be grossly bloody after 3 to 5 days, if new intrapelvic clots are observed on nephrostograms, or if there is a significant drop in the hematocrit. If the drop in the hematocrit is out of proportion to the urine blood loss, a retroperitoneal hematoma should be suspected and a CT scan obtained. Angiography and possible arterial embolization should be considered in patients

who have significant continuous or recurrent bleeding for longer than 4 to 5 days after PCN placement.

3. Sepsis after nephrostomy tube placement can occur, particularly in patients with stone disease. Patients with pyonephrosis are more prone to this complication and may develop postprocedure fever or even septic shock, despite the use of aminoglycoside prophylaxis. Forceful opacification of the collecting system to visualize the site and cause of obstruction should be deferred in all patients with urinary obstruction until the collecting system has been adequately decompressed for 24 to 48 hours and the patient is afebrile.

4. Inadvertent injury of adjacent organs is uncommon. The colon may lie posterior or posterolateral to the kidney and can be entered during a PCN. Retrorenal position of the colon is more common in patients who are thin and have little retrorenal fat, who have colonic dilation, or who have abnormal anatomy such as marked kyphosis or scoliosis. When there is doubt about safe access, pre-procedure CT to delineate the anatomy is prudent.

   The complication can often be managed conservatively, with drainage of both the kidney and the colon by separate catheters until the nephrocolic fistula heals.

5. An intercostal approach (often required for access to the upper poles of the kidneys) causes more thoracic complications than a subcostal puncture. In expiration, a posterior intercostal approach between the 11th and 12th ribs poses little risk of injury to the spleen and liver, but the lungs remain vulnerable to puncture in many patients. Other thoracic complications include pleural effusion, pneumonia, atelectasis, hydrothorax, and pneumothorax.

6. Minor complications that may occur are catheter dislodgment and urine extravasation. Dislodgement is more common in obese patients and in disoriented patients and can be minimized by using self-retaining drainage catheters routinely exchanged every few months. Dislodgement in the first week after placement often necessitates a fresh track. Renal pelvic perforation is unusual in a routine PCN performed for drainage of an obstructed collecting system and is more likely to occur in patients with large staghorn stones. It is usually a self-limiting complication.

PCN for Nonobstructive Indications

Management of upper urinary tract calculi. Percutaneous management of urinary tract calculi is currently limited to patients who are not candidates for SWL or ureteroscopy.

Percutaneous techniques are also used to salvage SWL or ureteroscopic failures. The widespread worldwide availability of SWL, its efficacy, and its relative noninvasiveness compared to percutaneous nephrostolithotomy (PCNL) make it the treatment of choice for most renal and ureteral calculi. Lately, the role of ureteroscopy in stone treatment is also being reassessed due to the introduction of second- and third-generation SWL machines that appear to be less effective in stone fragmentation than the original unmodified Dornier HM-3 SWL machine. The newer machines have a smaller focal zone that in theory should hit the stone harder while sparing the renal tissues from trauma. In reality, newer machines have been disappointingly less effective in breaking up stones while causing more side effects such as perinephric hematomas. Recently, a success rate of only 61% has been reported for impacted upper ureteral stones as compared to 91% for ureteroscopy. PCNL has a reported 100% success rate for removal of large (>1.5 cm) impacted upper ureteral stones, although it is more invasive than SWL and may have a higher complication rate than ureteroscopy. Stone-free success is greatly influenced by the stone size, with stones that are 1 cm or less in size representing the ideal for SWL. Stone-free rates of 85–87% have been reported for stones that are 1–2 cm in size.

The availability of the many different treatment options has resulted in some controversy and confusion over the indications for each of the management options. The American Urological Association has published suggested guidelines for the treatment of stones. There are many situations in which percutaneous stone removal is the primary procedure of choice. Table 3-1 lists the current indications in which percutaneous techniques are considered to be the first line of treatment for renal calculi. In all of these clinical situations, SWL suffers from certain disadvantages and is less effective than PCNL in complete stone removal. These indications are discussed further later. Distal ureteral calculi are managed by retrograde ureteroscopy or, in select cases, ESWL.

Stone size. In patients with large calculi, SWL has a poor chance of complete success, a high probability of requiring adjunctive therapy, and a significant incidence of complications. As the size of stones increases to more than 2–3 cm, the fragmentation efficiency with SWL decreases, necessitating multiple SWL attempts before complete breakup occurs. The number of ancillary procedures required to aid the passage of calculus particles increases. Some calculi that are 3 cm or larger but are of low radiographic density (e.g., stones composed of struvite or apatite) may respond to

Table 3-1: Indications for Percutaneous Therapy for Stone Disease*

1. Size
   a. Large stones (>2–2.5 cm)
   b. Most staghorn calculi
2. Composition: cystine calculi
3. Anatomic considerations
   a. Compromised urine drainage (includes UPJ obstruction, ureteral strictures, stones in dependent calices, and stones in caliceal diverticula)
   b. Abnormal body habitus, for example, scoliosis, myelomeningocele
   c. Congenital abnormalities such as horseshoe kidneys, fusion anomalies
   d. Postoperative states: urinary diversion, renal transplant
4. Miscellaneous indications
   a. Removal of all stone material essential (see text for details)
   b. Stones for which other treatment modalities have failed

*These clinical scenarios could also be considered to be contraindications for shockwave lithotripsy (SWL).
UPJ, ureteropelvic junction.

multiple SWL treatments, but for most large stones, including staghorn calculi, SWL is not the treatment of choice. With stones larger than 2.5–3.0 cm, only 30–35% of patients may be stone-free with SWL, compared to 70–90% of those treated with PCNL. It is important, however, to recognize that a single stone larger than 25–30 mm is of a different significance than several stones that are each 5 mm in diameter; the former is initially better managed with percutaneous techniques, whereas SWL is better for multiple smaller stones that are scattered throughout the collecting system and therefore less accessible to percutaneous techniques. Although each stone may easily be targeted for SWL, the presence of multiple stones does decrease the efficiency of SWL and the stone-free rate as compared to a single small stone.

Staghorn stones. The primary approach to these stones should be by PCNL. Branched staghorn stones that fill the majority of the collecting system pose special problems because stones may be located deep in infundibula and calices that may be difficult to reach from the initial percutaneous tract. PCNL is initially used to rapidly remove large volumes of easily accessible stone with ultrasonic or electrohydraulic lithotripsy ("debulking"). If infundibulocaliceal fragments are inaccessible from the nephrostomy tract using the usual endourologic techniques, SWL is used to break up the small volumes of remaining stones, followed by PCNL to remove the residual fragments.

Urinary obstruction, compromised urinary drainage. Urinary stasis can predispose to calculus formation. The most common examples of stones in association with obstruction are in UPJ obstruction, caliceal diverticula, malrotated kidneys, ectopic kidneys, horseshoe kidneys, and obstruction due to renal cysts or other renal masses. Although SWL can successfully break up the symptomatic calculi in these situations, the fragments are unlikely to be able to successfully pass even if the stone debris is adequately fragmented. In these cases, percutaneous stone therapy is combined with endourologic treatment for the underlying obstructive process, such as endopyelotomy for UPJ stenosis, balloon dilation for infundibular or ureteral strictures, and so forth.

Stone composition. The composition of a calculus is critical to decide on the best method of management. Certain calculi, for example, cystine calculi, are readily fragmented by ultrasonic lithotripsy but are refractory to SWL, making PCNL the treatment of choice. On the other hand, uric acid calculi respond well to SWL but not to ultrasonic lithotripsy. Rough, spiculated cystine stones that have recently formed respond better to SWL than do homogenous, smooth, long-standing stones. High-power machines such as the original HM-3 also appear to be more effective. For stones larger than 2 cm, proceeding directly to PCNL is the best option. All stone material must be removed at the time of the percutanous procedure to ensure that the patient will remain stone-free. Medical treatment (acetyl cysteine) has been unreliable in removing residual fragments, but its efficacy may be improved by infusing the drugs through percutaneously placed catheters.

Stones composed of calcium oxalate dihydrate and struvite break up well with SWL or any other form of power lithotripsy, whereas stones composed either partially or completely of calcium oxalate monohydrate do not respond well to SWL. With these stones, the volume of the stone is the main determinant of the most desirable mode of therapy.

Stones that do not adequately fragment with SWL or are inaccessible by ureteroscopy require a PCN for percutaneous ultrasonic lithotripsy. PCNL is also indicated in patients in whom certain removal of all stone material is important (such as airline pilots). Residual stone fragments persist in a significant percentage of patients following SWL. As the passage of such fragments can cause renal colic, airline pilots may not be allowed to fly as long as stone fragments are present in the urinary tract.

Technique for PCNL

Two primary components in the percutaneous therapy of upper urinary tract calculi are the establishment of an access tract and the actual stone removal itself. Accurate access is the essential underpinning of a successful PCNL as a poorly placed track may make it impossible to remove even the most accessible of calculi. Fluoroscopic control is usually preferred for the procedure, especially if the calculi are radiopaque. CT is useful in preprocedural planning in patients with aberrant anatomy, so that the liver, spleen, colon, and pleural space can be avoided by the proposed track. If the calculi are faintly opaque or the collecting system is not dilated, placement of a retrograde catheter prior to the puncture is invaluable and allows both opacification and distention of the collecting system. Local anesthesia and IV sedation are generally sufficient for establishing the track. Subsequently, track dilation and stone extraction are performed in the operating room—experience has proven that tracts can be dilated acutely to 24–30 F with no adverse effects. After the procedure, the collecting system is inspected to ensure a stone-free state. It is standard practice to leave in a large-bore nephrostomy tube after the procedure to provide reliable drainage of urine, tamponade the track and allow the renal puncture to heal, and permit access to the collecting system if additional procedures are required. The nephrostomy catheter is removed in 48 hours to 1 week, after a nephrostogram demonstrates no leaks from the collecting system or residual stones. The routine placement of nephrostomy tubes after an uncomplicated PCNL with complete calculus clearance is being questioned, due to the discomfort associated with the presence of a large-bore nephrostomy tube. There are many reports in the literature about either placing small tubes after the procedure in conjunction with a double-J stent or performing a totally tubeless PCNL.

When the calculus is located in a calix or diverticulum, access should be obtained through that particular calix or diverticulum.

Contraindications

An uncorrected bleeding abnormality is the only absolute contraindication. The procedure should not be performed if a stone-bearing kidney is uninfected and nonfunctioning. A relative contraindication is the inability to establish a safe access track.

Complications

1. Bleeding. Significant arterial bleeding occurs in 0.5–1.5% of patients. Vascular injury during the placement of the access track or track dilation can lead to pseudoaneurysms, arteriovenous fistulas, perinephric hematomas, and loss of functional parenchyma. Initial puncture into a calix rather than an infundibulum or the renal pelvis is the least likely to cause major vascular injury and is the preferable site of puncture. If excessive bleeding occurs during or after PCNL, the nephrostomy tube can be clamped, to tamponade the track and the collecting system. If that fails, a larger nephrostomy catheter can be placed, which will tamponade the track better and also allow blood clots as well as residual calculus fragments to pass. Selective angiography and embolization should be considered if the previous measures fail.

2. Injury to adjacent organs. The colon can be nicked if it is positioned posterior to the kidney. The colonic injury may not be obvious until the postprocedure nephrostogram demonstrates colonic filling with contrast. If the nick is small, the injuries can be managed conservatively by draining the kidneys with a double-pigtail ureteral stent placed from below, pulling the nephrostomy tube into the colon, and leaving it to drainage to act as a colostomy tube. The track usually seals in a few days. If a more serious injury occurs, open repair may be required.

   Injury to the duodenum, liver, and spleen is uncommon. Pleural and lung injuries may occur with supracostal punctures.

3. Sepsis. PCNL is considered to be a clean-contaminated procedure in patients with sterile urine preoperatively but a rise in temperature is common after stone removal. Postoperative bacteremia can occur and some of the factors affecting the development of postoperative fever are the duration of surgery and the amount of irrigant fluid.

4. Perforation. During the process of stone removal, the renal pelvis can be perforated by a sharp fragment of stone or by one of the instruments (such as the ultrasound probe) in as many as 10% of cases. Most such perforations heal within 12–24 hours as long as good urine drainage is maintained. Serial nephrostograms will show that even sizable renal pelvic and ureteral lacerations heal in a few days without stricture formation.

A calculus can extrude through a urothelial tear—renal pelvic extrusions should be treated with nephrostomy drainage, whereas ureteral tears should be treated with stenting for a few weeks. In the absence of infection, extrusion of calculus material into the perinephric and periureteral tissues appears to be of no clinical consequence.

Treatment of Ureteral Calculi

SWL is the treatment of choice for upper ureteral calculi and has higher success rates if the stone can be pushed back into the kidney. These calculi can also be approached in a percutaneous, antegrade fashion. In the midureter, most authorities favor ureteroscopic extraction of calculi or retrograde displacement of the calculus into the kidney followed by SWL. For distal ureteral stones, ureteroscopic extraction is probably the technique of choice because of its high initial success rate, the rare need for secondary treatments and postureteroscopic interventions, and the low complication rate of ureteroscopy in the distal ureter. However, the treatment of choice for distal ureteral calculi is not settled, and there are many institutional and individual variations.

Ureterolithotomy for stone removal is unusual and performed on the rare occasion for stones that are impacted or embedded in the ureter and require open surgical removal.

Other Procedures Performed Through a PCN Access Track

In patients with **UPJ obstruction,** PCNL is often combined with an endopyelotomy. Briefly, incisions are made along the posterior and lateral margins of the UPJ, with the incisions extending through the ureteral wall into the periureteric fat. Such an approach avoids the vascular structures that are usually located anteriorly and medially. After the procedure, the ureter is stented for 6–8 weeks with a large-bore stent. The reported success for relief of obstruction varies from 64 to 86%. When an endopyelotomy is planned, PCNL access through a posterior interpolar calix or upper polar calix provides the most direct and straight access to the UPJ.

The percutaneous route is also well suited to the **removal of foreign bodies** (e.g., broken stents, guidewire fragments, internal ureteral stents, fungus balls) (Figure 3-16) from the renal pelvis and/or ureter. Stents that have not been changed in the recommended period may encrust, become brittle, and fracture—fractures are best approached with a combined percutaneous-endoscopic technique. Although the

stent fragments can be removed percutaneously, the fragments tend to be brittle and refracture into smaller pieces
when they are grasped with forceps or baskets. Therefore,
removal under endoscopic guidance is most likely to result

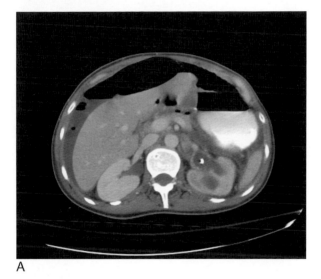

A

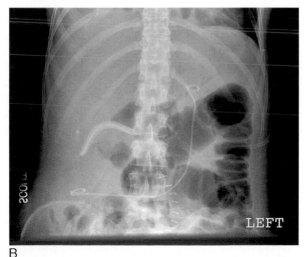

B

FIGURE 3-16. (Continued)

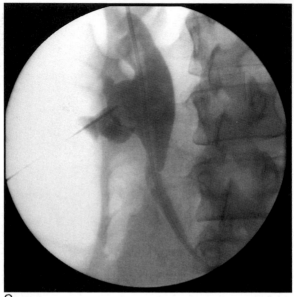

C

FIGURE 3-16. (Continued)

in complete extraction. Minimally encrusted stents may be removed without event but more severe encrustation can be complicated to treat and often requires ESWL in combination with endoscopic techniques.

URETERAL STENTING

Principles

1. Percutaneous ureteral stenting provides urinary diversion without the need for an external collection device when retrograde insertion of a ureteral stent is not possible or practical.
2. Most patients find a ureteral stent catheter more acceptable and convenient than a nephrostomy catheter.

Indications

1. Long-term stenting (months to years) is most frequently performed to bypass a ureteral obstruction.
2. Short-term stenting (weeks to months):

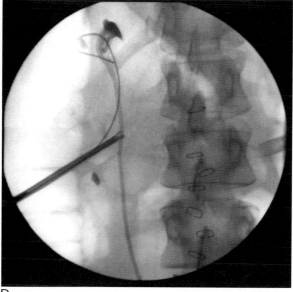

D

FIGURE 3-16. Percutaneous nephrostomy in patient with continent urinary diversion and occluded internalized stent. **A.** CT shows left-sided obstruction with delayed nephrogram. **B.** Abdominal film demonstrates an internalized stent in the continent pouch. Patient was febrile with urinary tract infection. The distal end of the stent could not be found even with pouch-endoscopy in the operating room. **C.** Percutaneous nephrostomy of the hydronephrotic left kidney. Patient was allowed to defervesce for a few days. Grossly purulent urine was aspirated. **D.** When patient was afebrile, the left ureteral stent was removed through the nephrostomy track.

    a) Facilitates healing of postoperative or traumatic pyeloureteral leaks or ureteral fistulas by diverting the urinary stream.

    b) Prevents stricture formation as ureteral injuries or implantations (native or allograft ureters) heal by providing a mold around which ureteral epithelialization is facilitated.

    c) Maintains ureteral caliber following balloon dilation or incision of benign ureteral strictures.

3. Catheters percutaneously placed into the ureters facilitate intraoperative ureteral identification during difficult surgical dissections (e.g., revision of an obstructed ureteroileal diversion).

4. Ureteral stents are often used in conjunction with non-operative treatment of renal and ureteral calculi. Prior to SWL, stents are used:
   a) To manipulate mid or upper ureteral calculi into the kidney or, if this is not possible, bypass them.
   b) To prevent stones from migrating back into the ureter prior to therapy.
   c) To facilitate localization of renal and ureteral stones during SWL.
   d) To allow for antegrade urinary drainage while stone fragments pass into the bladder. Stents are ideally inserted cystoscopically. Improperly positioned stents may require readjustment using fluoroscopy in the radiology department.
5. Antegrade insertion of ureteral stents prior to percutaneous therapy for renal calculi ensure that stone fragments created during ultrasonic lithotripsy do not inadvertently migrate into the ureter.

Contraindications

1. The presence of active renal infection.
2. Markedly diseased bladders that would be intolerant of a stent (e.g., radiation cystitis, bladder invasion by adjacent neoplasm).
3. Bladder fistulas.

Technique

1. Following PCN, a guidewire and catheter are manipulated through the abnormal (often stenotic) ureteral segment into the urinary bladder, bowel conduit, or urinary reservoir.
2. The catheter is replaced with a ureteral stent in which multiple side holes have been created where the stent will eventually be positioned in the renal pelvis. Kidney urine enters the stent through these side holes, travels through the catheter, and exits from its distal pigtail segment. Depending on ureteral caliber, urine may also flow around the stent. The proximal end of the stent protrudes from the skin and is obturated externally. This is an external ureteral stent catheter.
3. An external ureteral stent can be periodically changed from the flank over a guidewire.
4. Urinary drainage can be totally internalized by placing an internal ureteral stent with a pigtail configuration at both ends. The proximal pigtail is positioned in the renal pelvis and the distal pigtail in the bladder. Double pigtail

stents must be periodically changed (at least every 6 months) cystoscopically.

5. Patients who require ureteral stenting following ureteral diversion to a bowel conduit should have an external ureteral stent inserted in combined anterograde/retrograde fashion. A guidewire and catheter are first manipulated beyond the abnormal ureteral segment, through the bowel conduit, and out the stoma rather than into the bladder. The catheter is removed and a single pigtail drainage catheter passed retrograde into the renal pelvis. The distal end of this catheter protrudes through the stoma to drain into the urostomy collection bag. Internal ureteral stents should not be used in patients with ureteroenterostomies or continent urinary diversion reservoirs.

6. Catheters for intraoperative ureteral identification are percutaneously passed down the ureter to the point of ureteral obstruction. A PCN is also required to drain the kidney until surgical correction of the obstructed ureter has been accomplished.

7. Ureteral stents used as an adjunct to PCNL are passed into the pelvic ureter in conjunction with creation of a nephrocutaneous track through which endoscopes are inserted into the kidney.

8. If retrograde endoscopic attempts to pass catheters beyond ureteral obstructions and fistulas are unsuccessful, fluoroscopically guided retrograde perurethral catheter manipulations are often successful in the radiology department. This approach employs standard interventional equipment (e.g., catheters, guidewires, sheaths) passed through or over partially inserted ureteral catheters.

Results

1. Both internal and external ureteral stents allow patients to lead as active a life as their underlying condition will permit.

2. Ureteral obstructions can often be negotiated in antegrade (percutaneous) fashion even if retrograde cystoscopic catheterization is not possible (e.g., neoplastic obstruction of a ureteral orifice, distal ureteral angulation secondary to prostatic enlargement, spread of prostatic malignancy, ureteral reimplantation, tight ureteral stenoses, or urethral stricture).

3. Approximately 85–90% of ureteral obstructions and fistulas can be stented percutaneously. Very tightly obstructed ureters and ureters that are both tortuous and encased by tumor or fibrosis are the most frequent causes of failure of antegrade stent placement.

4. Internal ureteral stents may not drain kidneys as well as a PCN, especially when ureteral obstruction is caused by extrinsic compression or if intravesical pressure is elevated at rest or during micturition.

Complications

1. Improperly positioned stents will not provide optimal urinary drainage. This problem can be rectified with percutaneous, cystoscopic, or ureteroscopic techniques. Proximal stent migration can lead to perforation of the renal pelvis or calices, which can result in a urinoma or even catastrophic exsanguination due to erosion of the stent tip into a renal vessel. Stents that have migrated up into the kidney above a lower ureteral stricture or anastomosis can be extracted through a nephrostomy track under fluoroscopic guidance. A second approach is to use ureteroscopy to reposition the caudal end of the stent within the bladder. A stent that is positioned too far cephalad (so that the distal end is no longer within the urinary bladder) is usually related to placement of too short a stent rather than to cephalad migration.

2. Symptoms attributable to the intravesical coil of the stent (even when properly positioned) occur commonly, including microscopic hematuria, pyuria, lower abdominal pain, dysuria, urinary frequency, nocturia, and flank pain on voiding (due to renal reflux of bladder urine).

3. Fatigue fractures and encrustation of ureteral stents may occur if stents are not periodically replaced. This should be carried out at least every 6 months and more often in patients who form stones.

PERCUTANEOUS URETERAL OCCLUSION

Principles

1. Patients with advanced and often incurable pelvic or retroperitoneal malignancies may develop fistulas from the ureters, bladder, or urethra to the skin, vagina, or bowel. These fistulas are often accompanied by dysuria, incontinence, and skin maceration.

2. Most of these patients have previously undergone many surgical procedures, chemotherapy, and/or radiotherapy to palliate local cancer recurrence, are quite ill, and are usually not candidates for surgical urinary diversion.

3. Bladder drainage is usually either impractical or ineffective.
4. In the absence of complete ureteral obstruction, PCN alone does not satisfactorily divert urine, although it may decrease the amount of leakage at the fistula site.
5. Addition of external ureteral stents may further diminish leakage but often aggravates bladder symptoms.

Techniques

1. A variety of techniques may be used to occlude the ureter—all require concomitant percutaneous renal drainage. The techniques include the following: (1) ureteral obturation by percutaneously wedging a large catheter in the ureter proximal to a urinary leak; (2) other mechanical blocking devices, such as tissue adhesives, balloons, plugs, and coils; (3) percutaneous retroperitoneal ureteral clipping; and (4) endoscopic ureteral fulguration.
2. Renal embolization can obliterate renal function on the side of a ureteral leak. PCN drainage is obviated.

Results

1. All of these approaches may be effective for variable periods of time but, with the exception of embolization, require permanent PCN drainage, as these fistulas rarely heal.
2. These techniques do, however, improve the quality of life for patients with short life expectancies.

DILATION OF URETERAL AND URETHRAL STENOSES

Principles

1. Chronic ureteral stenting is not the optimal therapy for benign postoperative ureteral strictures, although it may be appropriate for malignant ureteral obstructions.
2. Many benign ureteral strictures are amenable to balloon catheter dilation or endourologic incision.
3. These procedures, if successful, can spare patients the nuisance of chronic indwelling stents or the risks of additional surgery.

Indications

1. An attempt at balloon catheter dilation of all benign ureteral strictures should be made before relegating patients

to additional surgery or to chronic PCN or indwelling ureteral stent drainage.

2. Endoscopic incision, employed alone or in combination with balloon dilation and ureteral stenting, can relieve certain UPJ obstructions (both congenital and acquired) as well as postoperative ureteroenteral anastomotic strictures.

3. Balloon dilation of ureters encircled by sutures sometimes results in disruption of the offending ligature, thus saving the patient an operation.

4. Balloon dilation of vesicourethral anastomotic strictures that develop after radical prostatectomy is a non-operative alternative to endoscopic incision and appears to be less likely to cause urinary incontinence.

Contraindications

1. Ureteral strictures caused by malignant disease, either primary or recurrent.

2. Inflammatory or traumatic urethral strictures appear to be more amenable to optical internal urethrotomy than to balloon dilation.

Technique

1. The strictured ureter is cannulated as described previously.

2. Biopsies and/or other imaging studies are obtained to confirm that the stricture is of benign etiology.

3. A catheter with an inflatable balloon capable of withstanding high pressure (15 to 17 atmospheres of pressure) and inflated diameter of 6–10 mm is used. Ureteral stenoses are generally inflated to 6–8 mm, and urethral stenoses are dilated with 8- to 10-mm balloons. The catheter is advanced across the stricture and the balloon inflated with diluted contrast material. A waist or narrowing is seen initially in the inflated balloon at the stricture site, which should disappear with continued or repeated inflations if the balloon dilation is technically correct.

4. Following dilation, a ureteral stent is placed, which remains in situ for 6 to 8 weeks to maintain luminal patency while the ureteral musculature heals. Stenting is accomplished with the largest catheter that can be comfortably accommodated. This is generally 10 F if the stent traverses the intramural ureter but may be larger if a ureteroenterostomy stricture is dilated and stented.

5. After 6 to 8 weeks, the stent is exchanged for a PCN and the efficacy of the dilation is assessed by nephrostograms and urodynamic studies prior to catheter removal.

6. If the ureteral stricture has been dilated and stented in a retrograde fashion per urethra with an internalized double pigtail catheter (usually 7–8 F), assessment of efficacy of balloon dilation is performed with an IVU obtained at 1, 6, and 12 months after stent removal.
7. Similar techniques have been adapted to treat congenital UPJ obstructions by balloon dilation, endoscopic incision, and stenting.

Results

1. Approximately 58% of all benign ureteral strictures can be successfully dilated with balloon catheters, usually with one attempt.
2. If there is poor response to the first attempt at balloon dilation, a second attempt at balloon dilation is worthwhile as some strictures will respond favorably to a second similar procedure.
3. The etiology and age of the stricture seem to influence the outcome of dilation therapy. Strictures not associated with ischemia or dense fibrosis may be successfully dilated (including those that occur in renal allograft recipients). Those associated with radiotherapy or surgical devascularization have a much lower rate of success. Strictures that have been present for less than 3 months respond much better to dilation therapy than do those that are more chronic in nature.
4. Endoscopic incision followed by balloon dilation and ureteral stenting is more effective than balloon catheter dilation alone for ureteroenteral anastomotic strictures and UPJ strictures.
5. Unsuccessful balloon dilation does not adversely affect other therapeutic options, including chronic indwelling ureteral stenting, surgical revision, or insertion of a metallic expandable ureteral stent (Wallstent or similar device). Although favorable short-term results have been reported with metallic ureteral stents, the long-term efficacy of metallic stents has not yet been established and remains an area of study.

Complications

1. No known permanent sequelae have resulted from unsuccessful dilation therapy. Laceration of ureteral mucosa or wall may occur with balloon dilation. These perforations heal uneventfully if the ureter is adequately stented and probably do not affect the outcome of dilation therapy.

PERCUTANEOUS DRAINAGE OF RENAL AND RELATED RETROPERITONEAL FLUID COLLECTIONS

Principles

1. Percutaneous drainage of renal and related retroperitoneal abscesses almost always obviates the need for surgical drainage. Cross-sectional imaging is used for guidance for the drainage.

Indications

Renal abscess or infected renal cyst that fails to improve with broad-spectrum antibiotics or a large infected renal or retroperitoneal fluid collection that requires drainage.

Contraindications

1. Absence of a safe percutaneous drainage route.
2. Small renal abscesses (less than 3 cm in diameter) can often be effectively treated with a course of IV antibiotics and may not require drainage.
3. Abnormal coagulation parameters.

Technique

1. The anatomic relationship of the fluid collection to its surrounding structures is assessed by cross-sectional imaging (CT or, less commonly, US). A safe, extraperitoneal route that avoids puncture of viscera, pleura, and major vessels is planned for diagnostic needle aspiration and catheter placement.
2. Diagnostic aspiration is performed with a 20- or 21-gauge needle to confirm the diagnosis.
3. If diagnostic aspiration yields infected material, a catheter is introduced into the collection under fluoroscopic control, the abscess drained completely, and the catheter securely sutured in place to provide continuous drainage. Injection of contrast medium (to evaluate the size and appearance of the abscess and assess whether it communicates with the collecting system) is minimized at the time of the drainage, to reduce the chances of inciting bacteremia or septic shock.
4. Septa within an abscess can usually be perforated with catheters and guidewires so that locules intercommunicate. Even so, multiloculated abscesses may require more than one catheter for complete drainage.

5. Multiple drainage catheters may be needed for renal abscesses that have spread retroperitoneally (one catheter for each component). Abscesses associated with ureteral obstruction require a PCN catheter in addition to the abscess drainage catheter.

6. Abscesses related to the urinary tract have less viscous contents than those that originate from the pancreas or gastrointestinal tract. Gravity drainage with 10- to 14-F pigtail or Malecot catheters is effective in draining most urinary tract abscess. If the abscess contents are very viscous, large sump catheters placed to suction and periodic irrigation with saline may be required.

7. When there is clinical defervescence with the percutaneous drainage, patients can be switched to oral antibiotics from parenteral therapy, discharged from the hospital with their drainage catheters in place, and followed as outpatients. Periodic follow-up catheter studies and CT scans are usually obtained at 1- to 2-week intervals to ensure that the catheter remains patent. Follow-up CT scans also demonstrate if there are undrained locules.

8. If a patient fails to improve on antibiotics and catheter drainage, a CT scan is obtained to detect undrained locules, enteric communications, or misplaced catheters.

9. Indications for catheter removal include the following:
   a) A satisfactory clinical response with defervescence of clinical signs of infection.
   b) Return of white blood cell count to normal.
   c) Cessation of drainage.
   d) Obliteration of the abscess cavity.

10. Drainage catheters usually need to remain in place for an average of 2–4 weeks for most urinary abscesses. Renal abscesses usually resolve in less time than do those that have spread extrarenally. The track will close following catheter removal if all infected material has been evacuated. Perinephric abscesses are often associated with an underlying abnormality such as stones or strictures that have to be treated after the abscess has resolved.

Results

Percutaneous abscess drainage can be expected to cure approximately 72% of renal and related retroperitoneal abscesses. This is a significant improvement compared to the results of surgical drainage and is due to the use of cross-sectional imaging techniques for evaluation, which allows the diagnosis of abscesses earlier in their development; needle aspiration to confirm the nature of a fluid collection; and also the efficacy of percutaneous drainage techniques.

Complications

1. Many patients develop transient bacteremia, febrile episodes, and even septic shock after percutaneous abscess drainage. These complications can be minimized by limiting catheter manipulation, lavage of the cavity, and/or contrast opacification of the abscess at the time of drainage. Definitive study of the abscess cavity should be deferred until the abscess has been effectively drained for several days.
2. Unsatisfactory clinical response may be due to partial drainage of septated collections or premature catheter removal.
3. An infected, obstructed calyceal diverticulum may be mistaken for a renal parenchymal abscess and continue to drain urine after the infection has cleared. Specific measures must then be directed toward dilating or occluding the neck of the diverticulum to prevent recurrence.

Percutaneous Drainage of Lymphoceles

1. Lymphoceles that occur after renal transplantation or pelvic surgery can be drained percutaneously but usually recur if only simple drainage is performed.
2. Sclerotherapy of the lymphocele cavity appears to be more effective in preventing fluid reaccumulation than simple catheter drainage alone. Agents used for sclerotherapy include tetracycline, povidone-iodine (Betadine), or absolute alcohol in combination with povidone-iodine.

Percutaneous Drainage of Urinomas

1. Urinomas are urine collections that result from extravasation of urine due to obstruction of the renal collecting system, surgery, or trauma and are often contained within a fibrous pseudocapsule.
2. Urinomas may cause secondary ureteral obstruction.
3. Large urinomas can be aspirated or drained in conjunction with management of the cause of the urine leak with PCN and ureteral stenting. However, not all urinomas require drainage as small (and occasionally large) urinomas will usually resorb spontaneously if the urinary obstruction is relieved.

RENAL CYST ASPIRATION AND ABLATION

Indications

1. Renal cyst aspiration is no longer used to discriminate between simple and complex cystic lesions when imaging studies are inconclusive. The use of high resolution renal CT and MRI allows characterization of most cystic lesions.
2. Primary indication for this procedure is to decompress and/or obliterate a symptomatic benign simple renal cyst.
3. Percutaneous ablation of a renal cyst is indicated if the lesion is producing pain, obstructive hydronephrosis, or segmental compression of portions of the collecting system with stasis of urine resulting in stone formation. Pain is the most common indication to perform renal cyst ablation.

Contraindications

1. An uncorrected bleeding diathesis.
2. Aspiration and ablation of cysts in autosomal dominant polycystic kidney disease are rarely performed because of the difficulty in localizing a specific cyst or locule that may be causing the symptoms. Here again, the most common indication is flank pain.

Technique

1. Renal cysts are aspirated with a 20-gauge needle, using CT, or most often, US guidance.
2. If the cyst is being punctured to ascertain whether it is responsible for the patient's flank or back pain, as much fluid as possible is aspirated from the lesion for a therapeutic trial. Ablation is deferred for a few weeks to see if the patient's flank pain responds to the cyst decompression, and if it recurs when fluid reaccumulates within the cyst.
3. For cyst ablation, a small catheter or sheath is placed in the lesion, the majority of the cyst fluid is aspirated, and a sclerosing agent then instilled into the cyst. The agent is left in for approximately a half-hour and then aspirated before the catheter is removed.
4. Many sclerosing agents can obliterate renal cysts. Absolute alcohol is most often used currently as it appears to be the most consistent in its action.

Results

1. Most renal cysts reaccumulate after diagnostic aspiration, even if the cyst is drained completely.

2. The majority of renal cysts can be permanently obliterated, thereby relieving the symptoms that prompted the intervention.

Complications

1. Improper needle placement may cause perinephric hemorrhage, inadvertent puncture of adjacent organs (e.g., lung, gastrointestinal tract), infection, arteriovenous fistula, and urinoma formation.
2. Extravasation of sclerosing agents into the perinephric tissues can cause fat necrosis, soft tissue fibrosis, or a febrile reaction.

URINARY TRACT BIOPSY TECHNIQUES

1. Soft tissue and visceral lesions related to the urinary tract, as well as suspicious nodes can readily be sampled for cytologic or histologic analysis when necessary for patient management. Prostate needle biopsy is considered elsewhere in this book.
2. Biopsies can be obtained with needles percutaneously placed into lesions (to biopsy renal masses, retroperitoneal masses, or nodes). Biopsy of urothelial lesions can be performed through percutaneously placed catheters or through retrograde catheters placed with cystoscopic guidance.

Indications

1. Evaluation of renal and adrenal masses in patients with a history of malignancy.
2. A significant number, approximately 20%, of small renal masses may be benign but indistinguishable from RCC by imaging criteria. There is increasing interest in biopsying these masses for management decisions.
3. Evaluation of urothelial irregularity or filling defects in patients with past history of bladder or upper tract urothelial cancer or with hematuria.

Contraindications

1. Contraindications to needle aspiration biopsy include the following:
   a) Hemorrhagic diathesis.
   b) Suspicion of an AVM in the area to be biopsied.
2. There are no contraindications to transcatheter brush biopsy.

Technique

1. Needle biopsy
   a) Most percutaneous biopsies are guided by CT or US, some by MRI, with operator preference, lesion size and location, and machine availability all factors that determine the modality used for guidance.
   b) Biopsies performed with small (21–22 gauge), thin-walled needles yield samples for cytologic evaluation. Larger needles (14–20 gauge), often used in conjunction with automated, spring-loaded biopsy devices, yield specimens for histologic evaluation.
   c) Aspiration biopsies are obtained and evaluated immediately by a cytopathologist to ascertain the adequacy of tissue sampling. Additional biopsies are performed until diagnostic material is obtained.
   d) Large needles provide tissue cores of sufficient size for conventional histopathologic examination.
2. Transcatheter biopsy
   a) This approach is most frequently used to obtain a brush biopsy of a pyelocalyceal or ureteral lesion suggestive of transitional cell carcinoma on noninvasive imaging studies.
   b) An open-ended catheter is passed cystoscopically into the ureter or kidney. A guidewire on which a nylon brush is mounted is then passed through the catheter and the suspicious abnormality "brushed" under fluoroscopy. Exfoliated cells retrieved by the brush are subjected to cytologic analysis. A variety of brush configurations are available for approaching lesions through the collecting system and ureter. Other biopsy instruments, including forceps and snares, can be passed through larger catheters or sheaths inserted into the upper urinary tract.

Results

1. Transcatheter and percutaneous brush biopsies yield true-positive results in more than 90% of cases. False-positive results are very infrequent.
2. Cytologic demonstration of malignant cells generally alters patient management by obviating the need for more invasive diagnostic techniques (including ureteroscopy), surgical biopsy, or staging procedures.
3. Negative findings do not exclude the presence of malignancy, as they may represent sampling error. Therefore,

thin-needle aspiration or transcatheter brush biopsy is of value only when positive results arc obtained.
4. Tissue core biopsies analyzed histologically may have fewer false-negative results.

Complications

1. Complications include the following:
   a) Blood vessel injury with bleeding, pseudoaneurysm, or arteriovenous fistula formation.
   b) Peritonitis due to bowel leak.
   c) Pneumothorax.
   d) Seeding of the needle track with malignant cells. This may be a more theoretical than actual risk. Only a handful of cases of spread of renal malignancy following aspiration biopsy have been reported. Nonetheless, because of the propensity for urothelial (but not parenchymal) tumors to spread along epithelial surfaces, suspected urothelial malignancies should not be biopsied percutaneously.
2. Brush biopsy is rarely associated with complications.
   a) Patient discomfort and hematuria are related to catheter manipulation and vigorous "brushing" of friable lesions. Therefore, it is best to perform these biopsies with conscious sedation to keep the patient comfortable.
   b) Collecting system or ureteral perforation with catheters or guidewires can occur but is innocuous if adequate urinary drainage is maintained for a day or two after the procedure, usually with a retrograde ureteral catheter.

TRANSCATHETER EMBOLIZATION

Principles

1. Renal abnormalities and varicoceles are the most common indications for transcatheter embolization in the most urinary tract.
2. A variety of embolic materials can be introduced through angiographic catheters. Particulate agents such as Gelfoam provide temporary vascular occlusion (hours to weeks). Mechanical, polymerizing, or sclerosing agents produce permanent occlusion.

Indications

1. Decrease blood flow through vascular renal or retroperitoneal tumors prior to surgery to facilitate surgical removal and minimize blood loss.

2. Control intractable bleeding from an incurable renal cell carcinoma, provide relief for tumor-related pain and paraneoplastic syndromes, and temporarily halt tumor growth (months to years).
3. Control renal hemorrhage secondary to traumatic aneurysms or AVMs.
4. Ablate renal function by infarcting all renal tissue as an alternative to bilateral surgical nephrectomy in patients with the following:
   a) End-stage renal disease and nephrotic syndrome with severe renal protein loss or uncontrollable hypertension.
   b) Ureterocutaneous fistulas usually secondary to irradiated pelvic malignancies.
5. Control post-traumatic pelvic hemorrhage.
6. Control intractable vesical hemorrhage associated with radiation cystitis when conservative urologic management is not effective or is contraindicated.
7. Occlude the internal spermatic vein in patients with testicular varicocele.

Technique

1. An angiographic catheter is selectively introduced into the vessel(s) supplying the tumor, malformation, organ, or other area to be devascularized and the selected embolic agent is introduced. These include particulate materials (autologous clot, Gelfoam, polyvinyl alcohol [Ivalon]), mechanical agents (e.g., stainless steel coils, detachable balloons), polymerizing fluids (e.g., isobutyl 2-cyano acrylate [bucrylate]), and other agents (e.g., absolute alcohol).
2. A renal artery occlusion balloon catheter helps prevent systemic reflux of embolic agents.
3. A post-embolization arteriogram is obtained to assess the effectiveness of embolotherapy.

Results

1. The efficacy of embolotherapy is judged on the post-embolization angiogram. Complete vascular occlusion may require the use of several embolic agents. For localized renal abnormalities (e.g., aneurysms, vascular malformations), segmental vessel embolization maximizes preservation of functioning renal tissue.
2. Internal spermatic veins supplying varicoceles may be occluded in 85–90% of cases with increase in sperm counts and motility in as many as 75% of infertile men.

Complications

1. Post-embolization syndrome. Most patients experience pain in the area of the embolized vessel, nausea, vomiting, and/or fever lasting 24 to 48 hours. Some may develop an ileus. These symptoms are related to tissue ischemia and infarction.
2. Undesired migration of embolic material. The most serious complication of renal artery embolization is reflux of embolic material and undesired migration to vessels supplying other organs such as spinal cord, bowel infarction, contralateral renal artery, and peripheral vessels.

IMAGE GUIDED ABLATION OF RENAL TUMORS

Percutaneous tumor ablation is becoming a viable option for patients with RCC in whom nephron-sparing surgery is contraindicated due to significant comorbidities. The role of percutaneous ablation therapy in patients without surgical contraindications is still unclear. The two techniques in current use are radiofrequency ablation (RFA) and cryotherapy.

Radiofrequency Ablation

RFA is the most widely used and studied tumor ablation technique. Electrodes are placed percutaneously in the tumor with CT guidance, and a high-frequency alternating current is applied to heat the tumor to 50°C, which coagulates the tissues. Tumors that can be successfully ablated are usually less than 5 cm in diameter and located in the periphery of the kidney. Centrally located tumors are more resistant to RFA than peripheral tumors, as the large vessels in the renal hilus disperse the heat, resulting in incomplete ablation. Ablation of centrally located tumors is also associated with a higher risk of injury to the collecting system. Anteriorly located tumors are often in proximity to the colon, and special maneuvers are necessary to prevent thermal injury to the colon. Tumor ablation is assessed by lack of enhancement of the lesion on follow-up contrast enhanced studies, and foci of enhancing tissue indicate the presence of viable tumor.

Cryoablation

Cryoablation has been used primarily with open conventional surgery but there is increasing interest in using this technique percutaneously. Cell death is produced by producing extracellular and intracellular ice crystal formation. The critical temperature required to produce complete necrosis is between -20 to $-50°C$. Experience with cryoablation of renal tumors is still very limited.

Other techniques that are also being investigated for renal tumor ablation include high-intensity focused ultrasound, microwave therapy, and renal ablation.

SELF-ASSESSMENT QUESTIONS

1. What is the best way to evaluate a patient presenting with acute flank pain?
2. What is the role of imaging in a patient with suspected acute pyelonephritis?
3. How should a patient with mild renal insufficiency and suspected transitional cell carcinoma be managed?
4. How should a patient with a primary neoplasm, such as a lung cancer, and an adrenal lesion be managed?
5. What factors influence the management of a patient with urinary tract calculi?

SUGGESTED READINGS

1. Dunnick NR, Sandler CM, Amis ES, Newhouse JH: *Essentials of Uroradiology,* 3rd ed. Williams and Wilkins, Baltimore, 2001.
2. Pollack HM, McClennan BL, eds: *Clinical Urography,* 2nd ed. Saunders, Philadelphia, 2000.
3. Morcos SK, Cohan RH, eds: *New Techniques in Uroradiology.* Taylor and Francis, New York, 2006.
4. Banner MP, ed: *Radiologic Interventions: Uroradiology.* Williams and Wilkins, Baltimore, 1998.

CHAPTER 4

Lower Urinary Tract Infections in Women and Pyelonephritis

Philip M. Hanno, MD, MPH

LOWER URINARY TRACT INFECTION

Definition

The urine is normally free of bacteria. *Bacteriuria* indicates the presence of bacteria in the urine. Bacteriuria can be symptomatic or asymptomatic. *Pyuria* is the presence of white blood cells in the urine and when seen in conjunction with bacteriuria is indicative of a true infection. *Asymptomatic bacteriuria* (ASB) is defined as the isolation of bacteria from the urine in significant quantities consistent with infection but without the local or systemic genitourinary signs or symptoms. The presence of ASB in the absence of symptoms or pyuria is often referred to as *colonization*. *Cystitis* refers to the symptoms of dysuria, urgency, frequency, and/or suprapubic pain. Infection (*bacterial cystitis*) is only one of many causes of this symptomatology, but one that is generally easy to prove or disprove with a simple urine culture. The differential diagnosis includes, but is not limited to, painful bladder syndrome/interstitial cystitis, radiation cystitis, bladder calculi, overactive bladder, and bladder cancer.

Other important definitions include the following:

1. Prophylactic antimicrobial therapy: prevention of infection in a sterile urinary tract by administration of antimicrobial medications.
2. Suppressive antimicrobial therapy: prevention of a clinically symptomatic infection in an asymptomatic patient whose urinary tract is colonized with bacteria.
3. Nosocomial urinary tract infection (UTI): those that occur in hospitalized or institutionalized patients.

Classification Schema

UTIs can be classified as to their *site of origin*. Cystitis refers to the nonspecific clinical syndrome of dysuria, urinary frequency, urgency, and suprapubic pressure. Fever, chills, and flank pain can indicate the presence of pyelonephritis, an interstitial inflammation caused by bacterial infection of the renal parenchyma. Surprisingly, based on symptoms, it can be remarkably difficult to differentiate infection involving the upper tracts from bacteriuria confined to the bladder. Many patients with pure lower tract symptoms will have positive cultures of renal pelvic and ureteral urine if catheterization of the upper tracts is performed. Conversely, some patients with flank pain will be found to have only cystitis on differential urine cultures. Fortunately, from a practical standpoint, it is not generally an important distinction, and localizing the site of infection in clinically uncomplicated infections is unnecessary.

UTIs can also be classified in terms of the *anatomic or functional status of the urinary tract* and the overall health of the patient. An uncomplicated infection indicates it is occurring in an otherwise normal urinary tract in a healthy individual. A complicated infection is one occurring in a functionally or structurally abnormal urinary tract or in a host with a compromised immune system or an infection with bacteria of increased virulence or antimicrobial resistance (i.e., nosocomial UTI).

Perhaps the most useful classification of UTI for the primary care provider is that devised by Tom Stamey of Stanford and is based on the relationship of UTI episodes with each other. *First infections* refer to isolated or remotely occurring bacterial cystitis. These are the most common infections in women, occurring in 25–30% of women between the ages of 30 and 40 years. *Unresolved bacteriuria* occurs when the urine cannot be sterilized despite antibiotic treatment. Common causes include pre-existing or acquired bacterial resistance, inadequate coverage of a second organism, rapid reinfection with a new organism during therapy, azotemia preventing access of the antibiotic to the urinary tract, and noncompliance with treatment. *Recurrent infection* is an infection diagnosed after successful treatment of an antecedent infection. This category represents 95% of recurrent UTIs in women. The other 5% may be caused by *bacterial persistence*. In this category, sterilization of the urine is short-lived, and within weeks, a relapse with the identical organism occurs. Such infections indicate a site of persistent infection within the urinary tract that could be a manifestation of an infected staghorn calculus, enterovesical fistula, or infected anatomic anomaly such as a diverticulum in the urinary tract.

Epidemiology

UTIs are considered to be the most common bacterial infection. They are generally associated with minimal morbidity except among specific subpopulations. Eleven percent of women report having had a UTI during any given year, and more than half of all women have had at least one UTI in their lifetime. One in three women has a UTI before the age of 24 years. This contrasts with men, in whom infection is uncommon until after the age of 50 when the problem of an enlarged prostate and outlet obstruction may occur. Between 3.5 and 7 million office visits a year are the result of UTI, and direct costs exceed $1.6 billion. It is difficult to assess the true incidence of UTI, as urine cultures are not often done in the outpatient setting, and symptoms are variable.

Catheter-associated UTI is the most common nosocomial infection. The risk of bacterial colonization increases with the duration of catheterization, approaching 100% at 30 days. UTI accounts for 25% of infections in the noninstitutionalized elderly. Thankfully, for such a common problem, UTI in the nonobstructed, nonpregnant female adult acts as a benign illness with no long-term sequelae. This is not true in other populations as noted in Table 4-1.

Symptomatic UTI is especially common among sexually active women. Modifiable behavioral risk factors include the use of a diaphragm and spermicides for contraception and frequency of sexual intercourse among premenopausal women. Estrogen deficiency is another risk factor, as is antimicrobial use itself. In women with a first UTI, 24% will have a second episode within 6 months, and up to half of women will have a second infection within a year. The risk

---

Table 4-1: Subpopulations at Increased Risk from Urinary Tract Infection (UTI)

Infants
Pregnant women
Elderly
Spinal cord injury
Indwelling catheters
Diabetes
Multiple sclerosis
Acquired immunodeficiency disease
Underlying urologic abnormalities

of recurrent uncomplicated bacterial cystitis remains unchanged whether the initial episode is left untreated to clear spontaneously or treated with short-term, long-term, or prophylactic antimicrobial therapy. Symptomatic episodes in the healthy population are more of a nuisance than a threat to health. No association between recurrent infections and renal scarring, hypertension, or renal failure has been established in patients with uncomplicated, simple recurrent UTI.

ASB is present in 3% of women in their early 20s, rising from 1% with the onset of intercourse in the late teenage years. It increases 1% per decade. The incidence of ASB in the pregnant population is similar to the nonpregnant population, but the implications are more concerning. The risk during pregnancy for pyelonephritis is increased substantially in those harboring bacteria in the urinary tract, especially during the end of the second and beginning of the third trimester. Studies suggest a 20–40% incidence of pyelonephritis if ASB is untreated in this population.

Diabetes increases the risk of UTI and bacteriuria among female but not male patients. UTIs in ambulatory patients with diabetes are considered complicated, with a heightened risk for pyelonephritis and severe complications if left untreated. UTI is more common in the multiple sclerosis population and can herald acute exacerbations and progression of the disease. Approximately 11–25% of elderly, noncatheterized patients can develop transient ASB, and persistent colonization in the elderly may affect up to 50% of geriatric women and be extremely difficult to eradicate.

Pathophysiology

The paradigm of uncomplicated UTIs is that bacterial virulence appears to be crucial for overcoming normal host defenses. With complicated UTI the paradigm is reversed, in that bacterial virulence is much less important, and host factors tend to be critical.

The bacteria responsible for UTIs are normally present in the bowel. *Escherichia coli* is the most common, accounting for 85% of community-acquired infections and up to 50% of nosocomial infections. Other common organisms include *Proteus* sp., *Klebsiella* sp., *Enterococcus faecalis*, and *Staphylococcus saprophyticus*. The female urethra is short, and bacteria generally enter the bladder in an ascending fashion.

Vaginal mucosal introital colonization generally precedes infection and is determined by bacterial adherence, the receptive characteristics of the epithelial surface, and the fluid that bathes both surfaces. Estrogens and pH affect attachment and colonization of the vaginal mucosa. Host defense mechanisms include the antiadherence properties of the vaginal and bladder mucosa, the hydrokinetic clearance of bacteria through voiding, and changes in urine pH and composition that may inhibit bacterial growth. Women with recurrent UTIs demonstrate increased adherence of bacteria in vitro to uroepithelial cells when compared to findings in women who have never had an infection. Studies suggest that this may be genetically determined.

Kunin has found strong statistical evidence that the female urethra has a powerful antimicrobial defense mechanism, which appears to differ in women with and without recurrent UTI. The female urethra is lined by cells identical to those of the vagina that respond readily to estrogens. The normally functioning urethra may help to protect the bladder from cystitis through the shedding of uropathogens bound to exfoliating urethral cells; trapping of bacteria by mucus secreted by the paraurethral glands; intermittent washout by urine; local production of immunoglobulins, cytokines, and defensins; and mobilization of leukocytes.

It is generally believed that some failure with the host defense mechanism allows for colonization of the introitus and vaginal mucosa in women subject to recurrent bacterial infection from reinfection outside the urinary tract. While colonized, these women can experience repeated infections for 6–12 months or more, each readily treated with antibiotics, but recurring within weeks or months. This introital colonization is of limited duration, and may resolve after 1 or 2 years and leave the patient asymptomatic until the next episode of colonization when subsequent bouts of infection begin.

Recent research by Gregory Anderson, Scott Hultgren, and colleagues at Washington University in Saint Louis has demonstrated a new and possibly important mechanism by which *E. coli* can seed the bladder urine in the absence of introital colonization. They have shown in animal models that bacteria can subvert the innate host defense responses by invasion into the bladder superficial cells. Intracellular bacteria mature into biofilms, creating pod-like bulges on the bladder surface. Pods contain bacteria encased in a polysaccharide-rich matrix surrounded by a protective shell of uroplakin. This can provide an internal reservoir of bacteria capable of causing clinical bacterial cystitis.

S. saprophyticus and enterobacterial species adhere to uroepithelial cells through different adhesive mechanisms than *E. coli.* After attachment, *Proteus* spp., *K. pneumoniae,* and *S. saprophyticus* each produce urease, which catalyzes the hydrolysis of urea in urine and causes the release of ammonia and CO_2. This elevates the urinary pH and can lead to the formation of bladder or kidney stones.

Risk factors for UTI include sexual intercourse, use of a diaphragm or cervical cap, and spermicidal jelly, which can alter the normal vaginal flora. The ABO blood group nonsecretor phenotype is at increased risk for vaginal colonization with uropathogenic bacteria. Urologic instrumentation, diabetes, and age-related changes in the elderly patient are also risk factors. Low estrogen levels allow vaginal pH to rise, resulting in a higher likelihood of vaginal colonization with *E. coli.* The use of oral contraceptive agents is unrelated. Personal hygiene habits are not generally related to recurrent UTI, and it is wise to assure patients that this represents a biologic phenomenon rather than a result of poor cleanliness.

Diagnosis: Signs and Symptoms, Diagnostic Studies

The history is a critical component in the diagnosis of UTI. The diagnosis is often made on history alone. The probability of bacterial cystitis in a woman with dysuria, urinary frequency, or gross hematuria is about 50% in the primary care setting. Urethritis and vaginitis can also cause acute dysuria in women. Cystitis is usually caused by enteric gram-negative bacilli or *S. saprophyticus.* Urethritis is caused by *Chlamydia trachomatis, Neisseria gonorrhoeae,* or herpes simplex virus. Vaginitis is caused by candidal species or *Trichomonas vaginalis.* Pyuria is rare in vaginitis but common in urethritis and cystitis. A positive urine culture is usually present in bacterial cystitis. Symptoms of cystitis are usually severe and more acute than those in urethritis, which can be mild, gradual in onset, and include vaginal discharge.

Symptoms suggesting vaginitis such as vaginal irritation or discharge reduce the likelihood of a diagnosis of cystitis by 20%. Dysuria and frequency in the absence of vaginal discharge raise the probability of acute UTI to 90%. If the woman has a history of culture-documented bacterial cystitis and experiences similar symptoms, the chance of a true infection approaches 90%.

Urologic investigation is not routinely indicated in women with isolated episodes of acute urinary frequency, dysuria, and urgency suggestive of lower UTI. Diagnosis is often empiric; however, a urinalysis and/or culture can provide helpful documentation of the true diagnosis and responsible organism (Table 4-2). Examination of urine sediment after centrifugation will show microscopic bacteriuria in more than 90% of infections with 10^5 colony forming units (cfu)/mL. Pyuria will be seen in 80–95% of infections, and microhematuria in about 50%. False-positive urinalyses are commonly caused by normal vaginal flora appearing to be gram-negative bacteria on urinalysis and pyuria that can be the result of a variety of other inflammatory conditions of the urinary tract. Alternatively, a false-negative urinalysis is commonly the result of urinary dilution from a high fluid intake in the symptomatic patient and frequent voiding, which prevents the bacteria in the bladder from multiplying to the high counts commonly associated with UTI.

If a urine culture is performed, it should be a carefully collected, midstream specimen to decrease the likelihood of any vaginal contamination. Approximately one third of women with acute symptomatic cystitis caused by *E. coli, S. saprophyticus,* or *Proteus* sp. have colony counts of

Table 4-2:   Diagnosis of Urinary Tract Infection (UTI)

Test	Sensitivity	Specificity
Pyuria	95%	71%
Bacteriuria	40–70%	85–95%
Dipstick	75%	82%
Nitrite + or		
leukocyte esterase +		
Midstream clean-catch		
pure culture		
>100,000 bacteria/mL	50%	80%
>1000 bacteria/mL	70–90%	High if dysuria

A positive dipstick (nitrite or leukocyte esterase positive) indicates that the likelihood of infection is 25% higher than the pretest probability. A negative test indicates that it is 25% lower. A positive dipstick in the setting of consistent symptoms suggests treatment can be instituted without urine culture provided there is an absence of factors associated with upper tract or complicated infection. A negative dipstick does not rule out infection when the pretest likelihood is high, and a urine culture in necessary in this situation. Culture is also critical in patients who do not respond to standard or initial therapy for UTI. Adapted from Fihn SD: Acute uncomplicated urinary tract infection in women. *N Engl J Med* 349:259–266, 2003.

midstream urine specimens ranging from 10^2 to 10^4 cfu/mL. Thus, a pure culture in the presence of symptoms must be considered significant, regardless of colony count.

Clues in the history that may suggest an increased risk of complicated UTI include childhood bladder or kidney infections, previous urologic surgery or instrumentation, an unusual causative organism, urolithiasis, or the presence of diabetes. If hematuria is noted, the physician is obligated to be sure that it is no longer present after treatment of infection. If it persists, a urologic imaging study and cystoscopy are necessary to rule out other urologic pathology. If a complicated UTI is suspected by history, a similar evaluation may be required.

Imaging studies should be considered in the following situations:

1. Women with febrile infections.
2. Men.
3. If urinary tract obstruction is suspected—History of:
   a) Calculi.
   b) Ureteral tumor.
   c) Ureteral stricture.
   d) Congenital ureteropelvic junction obstruction.
   e) Previous urologic surgery or instrumentation.
   f) Diabetes.
4. Persistent symptoms despite several days of appropriate antibiotic therapy.
5. Rapid recurrence of infection after apparently successful treatment.

Ultrasonography is an excellent initial screening test when imaging is indicated. It is noninvasive, does not cause radiation exposure, does not risk contrast reaction, and is generally readily available. It can identify stones, obstruction of the upper tracts, abscess, and many congenital abnormalities. Computed tomography (CT) and magnetic resonance imaging (MRI) provide the best anatomic data on the site, cause, and extent of infection. The key point to remember is that in the vast majority of symptomatic lower UTIs, imaging does not have a role to play in diagnosis or treatment.

Therapy: General Considerations

The management of UTIs is complicated by the increasing prevalence of antibiotic-resistant strains of *E. coli* and other common uropathogens. In the past, antibiotic resistance had been a problem only in the management of complicated nosocomial urinary infections. This resistance has now spread to uncomplicated community-acquired UTIs. Resistance to beta-lactams has increased from a rate of 20–30% in 1992 to up to 34% 4 years later. Trimethoprim-sulfamethoxazole (TMP-SMX) resistance had jumped to 18% by 1996, and *E. coli* strains resistant to ciprofloxacin increased from less than 1% in 1995 to 2.5% in 2001.

Resistance development tends to follow usage patterns, and as of 2006 quinolones had surpassed sulfas as the most common class of antibiotics prescribed for isolated outpatient UTI in women. This growth of the use of a potentially life-saving broad-spectrum antibiotic for what is, in most patients, a "symptomatic nuisance," raises concerns about increases in resistance to this importance class of antimicrobials in the future. The question arises as to whether it is better to potentially undertreat 5–20% of patients with recurrent UTI from reinfection and subsequently change antibiotics after 2 or 3 days if there is no clinical response, than to overtreat the vast majority with a quinolone. This author would answer yes in the majority of patients with uncomplicated, recurrent UTI from reinfection from a site outside the urinary tract.

Resistance patterns tend to be very local. Therefore, it is helpful to know the patterns of microbial resistance in your city and even in your hospital and surrounding outpatient clinics. Because urine levels of antibiotic are much more important than serum levels in determining efficacy for treating UTI, many antibiotics that appear to be poor choices based on sensitivity data relating to serum levels may eradicate UTI when administered because of high urinary excretion rates.

Uncomplicated Isolated Cystitis

Treatment of isolated cystitis is often empirical and not based on culture data. A drug should be chosen based on the following criteria: (1) the relative likelihood that it will be active against enteric bacteria that commonly produce UTIs, (2) ability to achieve high concentrations in the urine, (3) tendency not to alter the bowel or vaginal flora or to select for resistant bacteria, (4) limited toxicity, and (5) availability at reasonable cost to the patient. Because organisms causing isolated UTI in the community are generally pansensitive to antibiotics, cost and convenience are major factors in drug selection. Urine levels of antimicrobial rather than serum levels are important for efficacy in eliminating bacteria. Care must be taken in interpreting antibiotic susceptibility tests, as they are often based on serum levels of drug. In the past, physicians prescribed treatment for

5–10 days. It is now apparent that 3 days of antibiotic will suffice to clear the vast majority of uncomplicated UTIs. Single-dose therapy is slightly less efficacious, and symptoms can persist even after the urine has become sterile, leading to patient requests for more antibiotic.

An inexpensive, generic, narrower spectrum antibiotic is often a good choice in this setting. One can always move to a more expensive, broad-spectrum antibiotic if symptoms are not relieved in 2 or 3 days, and a subsequent culture indicates a resistant organism. However, in the vast majority of cases, the choice of TMP-SMX or nitrofurantoin will prove to be adequate to treat the infection, will be much less expensive for the patient, and will result in less chance of community bacteria acquiring resistance to powerful alternative antibiotics that can be life-saving when used in appropriate situations.

Unresolved Bacteriuria

Persistent symptoms following treatment for UTI necessitate urine culture and sensitivity testing. Choice of antibiotic will depend on the results obtained, and a 7- to 10-day course would be reasonable. Repeat culture and bacterial identification following treatment for unresolved bacteriuria is important to later differentiate the problem from recurrent infection from a site within the urinary tract.

Recurrent Bacterial Cystitis

A detailed culture history is critical in differentiating reinfection from a site outside the urinary tract as the cause of recurrent cystitis from reinfection from a site of bacterial persistence within the urinary tract. The former accounts for more than 95% of cases of recurrent UTI, but the latter is important, as a full urologic evaluation is mandatory. Bacterial identification is essential, as recurrent infections that occur after successful antimicrobial eradication (negative culture) and that are subsequently caused by varying strains of Enterobacteriaceae are pathognomonic for reinfection. The only confounding factor that might cause a similar scenario is reinfection from an enterovesical fistula with different organisms. In this unusual case, often the urine can never be sterilized, and infections may be with multiple organisms, thus leading to suspicion of a fistula.

This author tends to be aggressive in evaluating patients with long histories of recurrent UTIs in order not to miss a treatable etiology. A renal and bladder ultrasound will demonstrate normal anatomy, absence of infection stones, and low bladder urinary residual volume and serve as a good initial screening test in this group of patients. Cystoscopy can be reserved for those patients in whom there is suspicion of a fistula, infected suture, or voiding dysfunction that may be related to functional or anatomic obstruction.

Once it is clear that the patient's problem represents recurrent cystitis from reinfection from a site outside the urinary tract, usually gram-negative introital colonization, one can discuss treatment strategies with the patient. The patient should be reassured that the problem is largely one of controlling the symptoms and is not a threat to her urologic health. It is a treatable nuisance that most patients can manage on their own without numerous visits to physicians' offices. Years ago, many patients were treated with long-term, low-dose antibiotic therapy. This might have been 50 mg nitrofurantoin every evening or half tablet of TMP-SMX every other night for 6 months. At that point, treatment would stop in the hope that the introital colonization with uropathogenic gram-negative organisms had resolved, which tends to happen over time. Two or three episodes of UTI over the next 6 months would trigger another course of prophylaxis.

In an effort to decrease overall antibiotic usage, equally effective strategies have emerged. "Self-start" therapy relies on the patient to make the clinical diagnosis of UTI, which is not difficult for these patients. It presumes that symptom episodes in the past have been confirmed to be infectious by culture. Patients are given a prescription for an appropriate urinary antibiotic (nitrofurantoins, TMP-SMX, cephalexin), which they take for 2 or 3 days at the first symptom of infection. Although some physicians encourage dip-slide culture before and after medication, the author believes that if the symptoms respond quickly to a short course of antibiotic, culture is not necessary. Only if the symptoms do not respond or reoccur within a few days is a visit to the health care provider for appropriate culture and sensitivity testing required. Certainly, systemic symptoms such as fever and flank pain or the presence of gross hematuria should trigger a visit to the physician. With appropriate patient education, self-treatment seems to work very well in properly diagnosed recurrent UTI from reinfection. Antibiotic therapy for 3 days is similar to prolonged therapy in achieving symptomatic cure for cystitis, although prolonged therapy is marginally more effective in obtaining bacteriologic cure.

Single-dose therapy is another option in this setting. Although this might clear the bacteria from the urinary tract, symptoms often persist for 48 hours, and the patient is left unsure as to whether more antibiotic or a different antibiotic is required. If infections seem to be exclusively related to intercourse, and frequency of intercourse is not too high, one can consider a prophylactic antibiotic just before sexual activity to prevent infection. Those having sex four or more times weekly might be better off treating only symptomatic infections with short-term courses of antibiotics, thus limiting overall use of antibiotic.

Choice of Antibiotic

There are a variety of excellent, inexpensive, first-line antimicrobials to consider for the treatment of uncomplicated lower UTIs in women. Nitrofurantoin, although not effective against *Pseudomonas* and *Proteus* species, does cover the vast majority of pathogens encountered, and development of resistance over the last 30 years has not been a problem. It has high urine levels, a short half-life in the blood, and minimal effect on resident fecal and vaginal flora. It seems ideal for short-term use. It should not be administered to patients with known glucose-6-phosphate dehydrogenase (G6PD) deficiency. A rare pulmonary toxicity limits its use for long-term, low-dose continuous prophylaxis.

Trimethoprim with or without sulfamethoxazole is another widely used and very effective treatment for UTI. Although resistance to TMP-SMX has increased in the last decade, in many locales this is not a problem, and treatment can be changed if symptoms prove unresponsive or cultures show bacterial resistance. Alone or in combination these drugs will not eradicate *Enterococcus* and *Pseudomonas* species. They are inexpensive and can clear the vaginal flora of gram-negative uropathogens, although the clinical significance of this is questionable. Skin rashes and gastrointestinal side effects prove the main drawbacks.

Cephalosporins, as a group, have poor activity against *Enterococcus*. First-generation drugs are reasonable to treat uncomplicated UTI, but the second- and third-generation members of this group would best be reserved for culture-documented infections requiring their broader coverage. Ampicillin and amoxicillin, traditionally regarded as inexpensive first-line therapy, have generally fallen out of favor due to their interference with the fecal flora and the resultant emergence of resistant strains such that these drugs are now ineffective against as many as 30% of common urinary isolates.

Although the fluoroquinolones have a very broad spectrum of activity against most urinary pathogens including *Pseudomonas aeruginosa,* their routine use for treatment of uncomplicated UTI is to be avoided. Gram-positive activity is limited and efficacy against *Enterococcus* is poor. These are expensive, powerful oral agents. The fear that overuse may lead to the development of resistance and the fact that for most uncomplicated UTIs less expensive drugs are just as effective have tended to limit their use. Alarming reports of community-acquired UTIs caused by fluoroquinolones-resistant *E. coli* strains in some parts of the world suggest that we will see an evolution of resistance to these agents just as we have with sulfonamides, ampicillin, oral cephalosporins, and TMP-SMX unless a much more aggressive approach to the control of antimicrobial resistance is taken. The fluoroquinolones remain a valuable class of antibiotic, best restricted to complicated UTIs, pseudomonal infections, or treatment of resistant organisms.

Long-term use of antibiotics can lead to resistance, so methenamine salts (methenamine or hexamine hippurate) are often used. These are termed "urinary antiseptics." They are absorbed from the gut and pass into the urine where they release the chemical formaldehyde if the urine is acidic. To ensure urinary acidity, they are administered (1 gm twice daily) with vitamin C. Formaldehyde causes the breakdown of proteins essential to the bacteria, which ultimately results in their death. The Cochrane Review found that there is not enough evidence about whether methenamine hippurate can prevent UTIs, although it might work and more research is needed. This is unlikely to occur, as the methenamine salts are old, generic drugs that no company is likely to invest in to study. Adverse effects are minor and uncommon. This author likes to use methenamine hippurate in patients with recurrent UTI who harbor residual urine that allows the medication to release formaldehyde and keep bladder urine colony counts low, thus decreasing incidence of symptomatic infection. It is an ideal drug for patients on intermittent catheterization who present with recurrent symptomatic UTI. It is best to sterilize the urine with an appropriate antibiotic before initiating therapy.

Special Situations

Indwelling urinary catheters are used frequently in older populations. For either short- or long-term catheters, the infection rate is about 5% per day. During the initial 4 days of catheterization, concomitant antimicrobial therapy is associated with a decreased rate of infection. After 4 days, the infection rate is similar, whether or not antimicrobials are continued, but more resistant organisms are isolated from patients receiving antimicrobials. UTI follows formation of a biofilm on both the internal and external catheter surface. The biofilm is protective against antibacterials and also against the host immune response. Antimicrobial treatment of *asymptomatic catheter-acquired infection* (colonization) should be discouraged, because treatment in the presence of an indwelling catheter is unlikely to sterilize the urinary tract and acts to promote emergence of more resistant organisms, complicating management when subsequent symptomatic infection occurs. Treatment should be reserved for symptomatic infections only.

The prevalence of bacteriuria in the elderly patient is surprisingly high. Up to 20% of women and 10% of men older than 65 years have bacteriuria. The figures are even higher for nursing home residents. The need for treatment of *asymptomatic bacteriuria (ASB) in the elderly* is controversial. It is not uncommon for courses of antibiotics to be unsuccessful in long-term management of bacteriuria in this group of patients. Studies suggest that noncatheterized male and female residents with bacteriuria living in nursing homes have no higher frequency of courses of antimicrobial treatment, infections, or hospitalizations than those without persistent bacteriuria. As a result, screening for ASB in the elderly should be limited to those undergoing invasive urologic procedures and surgical procedures with implant material. Pyuria accompanying ASB is not an indication for antimicrobial treatment. In patients about to undergo surgery for implantation of foreign material, or any urologic surgery, the ASB should be treated and the urine sterilized if possible. Clearly, symptomatic UTIs in the elderly patient should be appropriately treated. In addition, it would seem prudent to treat any bacteriuria due to urea-splitting bacteria such as *Proteus mirabilis* to prevent stone formation. Otherwise, the routine treatment of ASB in the elderly appears unjustified and is often ineffective.

Pregnancy merits particular attention with regard to screening for bacteriuria and treatment of UTI. The prevalence of bacteriuria identified by screening is no higher in pregnant females than nonpregnant females of the same age. However, pregnancy results in physiologic changes that have important implications with regard to ASB and progression of infection. With pregnancy comes an increase in renal size, augmented renal function, hydroureteronephrosis, and anterosuperior displacement of the bladder. The frequency of acute pyelonephritis in pregnant women is significantly higher than that in their nonpregnant counterparts. Studies suggest a 20–40% incidence of pyelonephritis if ASB is untreated in this population. In addition, bacterial pyelonephritis in pregnancy has been associated with infant prematurity and perinatal mortality. These factors make it prudent to screen for ASB in pregnancy, treat it aggressively, and obtain follow-up cultures. An initial negative screening urine culture need not be repeated, as these patients are unlikely to develop bacteriuria later in pregnancy.

PYELONEPHRITIS

Infection of the upper urinary tract including the renal pelvis and kidney parenchyma is referred to as *pyelonephritis*. Acute pyelonephritis is characterized by acute suppuration accompanied by fever, flank pain, bacteriuria, and pyuria. Repeated attacks of acute pyelonephritis may result in chronic pyelonephritis, characterized by progressive renal scarring that can be asymmetric and involve both the cortex and pelvocalyceal system.

There are several potential routes of upper tract infection: (1) Ascending: Bacteria that reach the renal pelvis gain entry through the collecting ducts at the papillary tips and make their ascent through the collecting tubules. The presence of reflux of urine from the bladder or increased intrapelvic pressures from lower tract obstruction can facilitate upper tract infection, especially in the presence of intrarenal reflux. (2) Hematogenous: This is uncommon but can be a result of *Staphylococcus aureus* septicemia or *Candida* in the bloodstream. (3) Lymphatic: Very unusual form of extension to the renal parenchyma from an intraperitoneal infectious process (i.e., abscess).

Clinical Presentation

The classic clinical scenario is the acute onset of fever, chills, and flank pain in a patient with an obviously infected urine on urinalysis, subsequently proven on urine culture. One must keep in mind that some patients with flank pain and UTI do not have upper tract infection and that patients can have pyelonephritis in the absence of local or systemic symptoms. A high index of suspicion is required in a patient

Table 4-3: Potential Risk Factors for Pyelonephritis

Vesicoureteral reflux

Obstruction of the urinary tract (congenital ureteropelvic junction obstruction, stone disease, pregnancy)

Genitourinary tract instrumentation

Diabetes mellitus

Voiding dysfunction

Age (renal scarring rarely begins in adulthood but is generally related to intrarenal reflux in children)

Female gender

with one of the known risk factors for pyelonephritis (Table 4-3).

Additional symptoms of acute pyelonephritis may include systemic malaise, nausea, and vomiting. Lower tract symptoms including dysuria and urinary frequency are commonly present. Pyelonephritis can result in sepsis, hypotension, and death, especially in the scenario of infection behind an unrecognized upper tract obstruction.

On physical examination flank tenderness may be a prominent finding. An infected urine with the presence of large amounts of granular or leukocyte cases in the sediment is also suggestive of the diagnosis. *E. coli* possesses special virulence factors and accounts for 80% of cases of acute pyelonephritis. *Pseudomonas, Serratia, Enterobacter,* and *Citrobacter* are sometimes identified as causative microorganisms in complex cases with a history of urinary tract instrumentation, nosocomial infection, indwelling catheters, and/or ureteral stents.

Suspect *Proteus* or *Klebsiella* in patients with stone disease. *P. mirabilis* and some strains of *Klebsiella* contain the enzyme urease, which is capable of splitting urea with the production of ammonia and an alkaline environment. The latter is favorable for precipitation of the salt struvite (magnesium ammonium phosphate). Struvite may form branched calculi that harbor bacteria in the interstices of the stone. These so-called staghorn calculi can cause chronic renal infection, abscess, or chronic lower tract infection. The infection is difficult to cure unless the stone itself is removed.

The intravenous urogram may be normal or can show renal enlargement secondary to edema. Focal enlargement must be distinguished from a renal mass or abscess. Inflammation may cause a diminished nephrogram or delayed appearance of the pyelogram on the affected side. One of the most important aspects of any imaging study is to rule out the presence of urolithiasis and/or obstruction, which can lead to a life-threatening situation if not appreciated and relieved. Ultrasound can demonstrate many of the previously mentioned findings and help to rule out an obstructive process. CT is also useful in some cases, and may show patchy decreased enhancement suggesting focal renal involvement (Figures 4-1 and 4-2).

Complications

1. **Xanthogranulomatous pyelonephritis (XGP)** is an unusual, often severe, chronic renal infection that destroys the kidney. It is generally unilateral, associated with obstructing calculi, and results in an enlarged, nonfunctioning kidney that must be differentiated from malignancy. Perirenal fat may be involved with adjacent subcapsular inflammatory response. *Proteus* and *E. coli* are the primary microbes responsible for initiating the inflammatory process. Pathologically, the kidneys consist of yellow-white nodules, pyonephrosis, and hemorrhage. Granulomatous inflammation with lipid-laden macrophages known as xanthoma cells is seen histologically. Suspect XGP in the patient with persistent bacteriuria

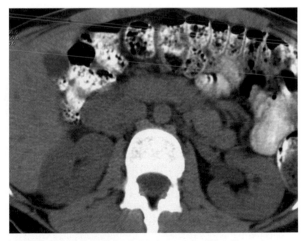

FIGURE 4-1. Acute pyelonephritis in 26-year-old woman. Precontrast CT is unhelpful in making diagnosis. (Courtesy of Parvi Ramchandami.)

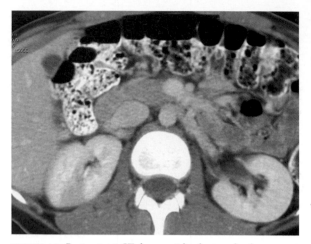

FIGURE 4-2. Postcontrast CT shows patchy decreased enhancement in right kidney. (Courtesy of Parvi Ramchandami.)

accompanied by flank pain, fever, and chills in the presence of an enlarged, nonfunctioning kidney with a stone or solid mass lesion. CT and ultrasound aid in diagnosis. Treatment is generally nephrectomy, removing the entire inflammatory mass.

2. **Chronic pyelonephritis** is rare in the absence of underlying functional or structural abnormalities of the urinary tract. The symptoms are those of the chronic renal failure it produces, and a history of recurrent acute pyelonephritis may be elicited. Urine cultures may be negative. A localized scar over a deformed calyx is a classic presentation on imaging studies. Pathologically, the kidneys are often diffusely contracted, scarred, and pitted. Histologically, periglomerular fibrosis is common in conjunction with atrophied tubules.

3. **Renal insufficiency** is a rare complication of acute pyelonephritis.

4. **Hypertension** is noted in more than 50% of patients with chronic pyelonephritis. This may be due to fibrosis of the renal parenchyma with resulting ischemia and secondary activation of the renin-angiotensin system. Although hypertension can accelerate progressive renal failure, the fact that nephrectomy cures hypertension in selected patients suggests that the reverse is also true.

5. **Renal abscess**, a collection of purulent material confined to the renal parenchyma, may follow insufficient

treatment of focal bacterial nephritis (lobar nephronia). Diagnosis is with CT and ultrasound. Needle aspiration and drainage of the abscess and prolonged antibiotic treatment often preclude the need for surgical drainage.

6. **Infected hydronephrosis** denotes the bacterial infection of a hydronephrotic kidney. When associated with suppurative destruction of renal parenchyma, the term *pyonephrosis* is used. Ultrasound and CT can usually make the diagnosis, and emergent drainage is required, usually by ureteral catheter or percutaneous catheter placement, until definitive relief of the obstruction is attempted.

7. **Perinephric abscess** can result from rupture of a cortical abscess or hematogenous seeding from another infected site. The primary treatment is drainage.

8. **Emphysematous pyelonephritis** is an acute necrotizing parenchymal and perirenal infection caused by gas-forming uropathogens. Diabetic patients are at increased risk. Complicating factors can include urinary tract obstruction secondary to calculi or sloughed necrotic papillae. Women are affected more commonly than men. Fever, vomiting, and flank pain constitute the classic triad of symptoms. The diagnosis is established by the finding on plain x-ray, CT, or ultrasound of intrarenal parenchymal gas. The disease can be fatal, and aggressive percutaneous renal and perirenal drainage or immediate nephrectomy, in combination with appropriate antibiotics, is critical. Most cases are associated with *E. coli*, though *Proteus, Klebsiella,* and *Candida albicans* can be responsible pathogens.

Management (Figure 4-3)

Acute pyelonephritis can be managed on an outpatient basis with oral antibiotics in the patient who is not septic and does not suffer from nausea and vomiting. TMP-SMX or a fluoroquinolone is a good choice pending culture results.

Dehydration, vomiting, or sepsis may require hospitalization and parenteral administration of antibiotics (Table 4-4). TMP-SMX, fluoroquinolone, or a combination of ampicillin and gentamicin are reasonable choices of antibiotic and should be administered parenterally until the patient is afebrile. They can then be switched to oral therapy. In the pregnant patient, ceftriaxone, aztreonam, or a combination of ampicillin and gentamicin can be administered

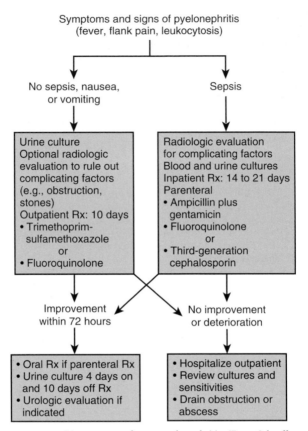

FIGURE 4-3. Management of acute pyelonephritis. (From Schaeffer AJ, Schaeffer EM: Infections of the urinary tract. In Wein AJ, Kavoussi LR, Novick AC, et al, eds: *Campbell-Walsh Urology,* 9th ed. Elsevier, New York [in press], with permission.)

with conversion to an oral cephalosporin when the patient is afebrile.

Therapy for uncomplicated pyelonephritis is generally recommended for 10 days, and a full 2-week course is recommended for those who present with sepsis. Complicated infection associated with hospitalization, catheterization, urologic surgery, or urinary tract abnormalities may require 3 weeks of antibiotic therapy along with associated urologic procedures to relieve obstruction that may be responsible for life-threatening sepsis.

Table 4-4: Guidelines for Parenteral Treatment of Pyelonephritis
Clinical severity of infection, suspected urosepsis
Presence of underlying anatomic urinary tract abnormality
Inadequate access to follow-up care
Renal failure
Presence of urinary tract obstruction (infection behind an obstruction can be a lethal combination)
Immunocompromised and/or elderly host
Failed outpatient management on oral antimicrobials

SELF-ASSESSMENT QUESTIONS

1. How is colonization different than infection?
2. In what situations should asymptomatic bacteriuria be aggressively treated?
3. How can recurrent urinary tract infections from bacterial reservoirs outside the urinary tract be managed?
4. The patient with persistent bacteriuria accompanied by flank pain, fever, and chills in the presence of an enlarged, nonfunctioning kidney with a stone or solid mass lesion should be suspected of having what disorder?
5. What important, potentially life-threatening condition must be ruled out in a patient with upper tract urologic infection?

SUGGESTED READINGS

1. Anderson GG, Palermo JJ, Schilling JD, et al: Intracellular bacterial biofilm-like pods in urinary tract infections. *Science* 301:105–107, 2003.
2. Fihn SD: Acute uncomplicated urinary tract infection in women. *N Engl J Med* 349:259–266, 2003.
3. Kass EH: Asymptomatic infections of the urinary tract. *J Urol* 168:420–424, 2002.
4. Katchman EA, Milo G, Paul M, et al: Three day vs longer duration of antibiotic treatment for cystitis in women: systematic review and meta-analysis. *Am J Med* 118:1196–1207, 2005.
5. Krieger JN: Urinary tract infections: what's new? *J Urol* 168:2351–2358, 2002.

6. Kunin CM, Evans C, Bartholomew D, Bates DG: The antimicrobial defense mechanism of the female urethra: a reassessment. *J Urol* 168:413–419, 2002.

7. Nicolle LE: Catheter-related urinary tract infection. *Drugs Aging* 22:627–639, 2005.

8. Schaeffer AJ, Schaeffer EM: Infections of the urinary tract. In Wein AJ, Kavoussi LR, Novick AC, et al, eds: *Campbell-Walsh Urology,* 9th ed. Elsevier, New York (in press).

9. Stamm WE, Schaeffer AJ: The state of the art in the management of urinary tract infections. *Am J Med* 113 (suppl 1A)1s–84s, 2002.

10. Wagenlehner FME, Naber KG, Weidner W: Asymptomatic bacteriuria in elderly patients. *Drugs Aging* 10:801–807, 2005.

Prostatitis and Lower Urinary Tract Infections in Men

Steve Lebovitch, MD and
Michel A. Pontari, MD

I. URINARY TRACT INFECTIONS

A. Incidence and Risk Factors

Urinary tract infections (UTIs) are the most common nosocomial bacterial infections in the United States and account for more than 7 million visits to physicians annually. The majority of infections are in women, with 20–50% of women developing a UTI during their lifetime and an incidence of infection 30 times higher in adult women than adult men. However, UTIs are more common in male infants than female infants, perhaps due to the higher incidence of congenital genitourinary disorders in males, and uncircumcised infants have more UTIs than those who are circumcised. The incidence of UTIs is similar for men and women older than the age of 50 years. The increased prevalence in men older than this age is secondary to prostatic enlargement with resultant bladder outlet obstruction and residual urine, urinary tract instrumentation, immobility or decreased activity, and decreased prostatic secretions. Asymptomatic bacteriuria may range from 15–35% in institutionalized elderly men and is frequently polymicrobial. A mortality rate as high as 3% is seen in the elderly population that goes on to develop upper tract infections and sepsis (Table 5-1).

B. Other Risk Factors

Other risk factors for UTIs include urethral stricture disease, neurogenic bladder, calculi, iatrogenic instrumentation, urethral catheters (5% per single catheterization and 5% increase per day of catheterization), external collecting devices, enteric fistulas, urachal cysts or sinuses, renal impairment, neutropenia, insertive anal intercourse, intercourse with an infected female partner, and lack of circumcision with inadequate meatal care. Diabetes mellitus can cause a neurogenic bladder with a large capacity and infrequent voiding. Elevated urinary

Table 5-1: Prevalence of Bacteriuria in Males		
Age Group	**Percent**	**Most Likely Cause**
Infants	2	Anatomic, noncircumcised
Young boys	0.1–0.5	
Young adults	<0.01–0.03	
Adults (30–65 years)	0.1	Sexual activity
Elderly (>65 years)	5–15	Anatomic and instrumentation

glucose impairs phagocytosis. Medications, such as steroids, lead to depression of the immune system, potentially increasing the prevalence of UTIs. Individuals with spinal cord injuries requiring tailored drainage regimens due to spastic or flaccid bladders are greatly at risk.

C. Pathogenesis

1. Routes of infection. The majority of uropathogens in men are introduced via the ascending route (through the urethra), as opposed to a hematogenous or lymphatic route, or direct extension.
2. Pathogens. Gram-negative enteric bacteria, particularly *Escherichia coli*, cause about 80% of UTIs in men. A smaller percentage are caused by *Klebsiella, Enterobacter,* and *Proteus.* Gram-positive organisms, such as enterococci and staphylococci, cause about one fifth of infections. Two or more organisms may be the cause of infection in bacterial prostatitis, urinary fistulas, and chronic diseases such as diabetes mellitus or those resulting from foreign bodies or calculi.
3. Host resistance
   a) *Washout of bacteria during micturition.* A lower inoculum size is required when urine flow is obstructed.
   b) *Bacterial antiadherence factors.* These include the mucopolysaccharide coating of the bladder epithelium and possibly urinary constituents including the normal flora of the urethra, Tamm-Horsfall mucoprotein, and immunoglobulins IgA and IgG.
   c) *Prostatic antibacterial factor.* This is secreted by the prostate and has important antimicrobial activity.

Spermine has some activity against gram-positive bacteria. Zinc is also believed to be antibacterial.

d) *Long male urethral length.* Long length inhibits retrograde ascent of bacteria. Furthermore, the male meatus, which is not located on the perineum, is less likely to come into contact with enteric bacteria compared to the female.

e) *Low pH of urine.* Urea and organic acids lower pH to less than 5.5 making it difficult for bacteria to thrive.

D. Diagnosis

Localization of Lower UTI

The Meares-Stamey four-glass urine test differentiates bacterial cystitis from chronic bacterial prostatitis.

1. Technique (Figure 5-1). The uncircumcised male must retract his foreskin prior to voiding and wipe the glans with an antiseptic swab. The first 10 mL of urine is collected in a sterile specimen container (voided bladder 1 [VB1]). After voiding 200 mL, a midstream specimen is collected in a separate container (VB2). The patient then stops voiding and prostatic massage is performed. The expressed prostatic secretion (EPS) is gently milked by proximal to distal pressure on the bulbar urethra and is collected in a fresh container. The next 10 mL of voided urine is collected immediately following prostatic massage (VB3). A modified Nickel's two-glass test evaluates for leukocytes and bacterial counts in the preprostatic

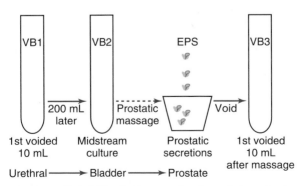

FIGURE 5-1. Bacterial localization procedure for male lower tract infection.

and postprostatic massage urine sample allowing for a simple screening tool in prostatitis.
2. Interpretation of culture results
   a. VB1 identifies the urethral flora. With urethral colonization or urethritis only, the VB1 is greatest.
   b. VB2-positive culture can result from bladder, prostatic, or urethral bacteria. If the VB2 culture is positive, the patient should be treated with an antibiotic that will sterilize the bladder and urethra but will not diffuse into the prostate (e.g., nitrofurantoin, for 3 days). After treatment, the localization cultures should be repeated.
   c. EPS/VB3. Cultures with substantially higher colony counts (tenfold) than VB1 indicate prostatic infection when VB2 culture is negative.

II. BACTERIAL CYSTITIS

A. Signs and Symptoms

Urinary frequency, urgency, hesitancy, dysuria, nocturia, suprapubic discomfort, low back pain, and hematuria or terminally blood-tinged urine may be present. Systemic symptoms such as fever, chills, and rigors are absent. Elderly people may be asymptomatic or may have gastrointestinal symptoms, such as nausea and vomiting.

B. Diagnosis

1. Urinalysis. On a clean-catch voided specimen, a positive leukocyte esterase and nitrite tests on dipstick suggest bacterial infection. On microscopic examination of a centrifuged specimen, greater than 10 white blood cells per high power field (WBC/HPF) indicates pyuria. Red blood cells may be seen. Gram stain is performed to look for bacteria. Casts are not seen.
2. Urine culture. Greater than or equal to 10^5 colony forming units (cfu)/mL of urine indicates true bacterial infection in men as opposed to contamination from periurethral bacteria. Polymicrobial growth without a predominant organism strongly suggests contamination.
3. Diagnostic imaging and cystoscopy. An intravenous urogram with renal ultrasound or computed tomography (CT) scan should be obtained after the first UTI to search for a possible urinary tract abnormality. Bladder ultrasound can evaluate the postvoid residual urine volume. Cystoscopy should be performed after urine sterilization in men

beyond middle age. Young adults to middle-aged men having a first uncomplicated UTI who are sexually active and respond to antibiotic treatment may not require a complete imaging and cystoscopic evaluation.

C. Screening

Infectious Diseases Society of America (ISDA) guidelines recommend screening for asymptomatic bacteriuria prior to any prostatic instrumentation or any case in which mucosal bleeding may be involved to allow for initiation of antimicrobial therapy prior to the procedure. Any antimicrobial therapy should be discontinued immediately postprocedure unless an indwelling catheter remains in place.

D. Treatment

1. *Bacterial cystitis.* Culture-appropriate antibiotics should be used for symptomatic men and asymptomatic men younger than age 60 years for 7 to 10 days. Asymptomatic bacteriuria in elderly men need only be treated in the face of detrimental organisms (e.g., urea-splitting bacteria), abnormal urinary tracts, or urinary tract instrumentation. Men with UTIs can generally be managed as outpatients with trimethoprim-sulfamethoxazole (TMP-SMX) (Bactrim, Septra), one double-strength tablet twice daily, or with a quinolone (ciprofloxacin 500 mg twice daily, or levofloxacin 250 mg once daily), for a period of 7–10 days.
2. *Candidal cystitis.* This may be seen in catheterized patients or those with diabetes mellitus, with immunosuppression, or on systemic antibiotics. The indwelling catheter should be removed, if possible, or changed. Any unnecessary steroid or antibiotic should be stopped. Continuous bladder irrigation with amphotericin B (50 mg/L sterile water every 24 hours) for 5 days may be used. Oral fluconazole 50–100 mg/day for 7 days is useful in treating *Candida albicans.*

III. PROSTATITIS AND CHRONIC PELVIC PAIN SYNDROME

A. Epidemiology

Prostatitis accounts for approximately one fourth of all male office visits for genitourinary tract symptoms. Half of all men will suffer from prostatitis symptoms sometime in their lives. Prostatitis accounts for approximately 2 million office visits to physicians in the United States annually.

B. Classification

Classification of the prostatitis syndromes is based on the presence of prostatic inflammation and bacterial infection. Only 10% of men with prostatitis syndromes have bacterial prostatitis. Classically, the four groups have been as follows: acute bacterial prostatitis, chronic bacterial prostatitis, non-bacterial prostatitis, and prostatodynia. In 1995, the Chronic Prostatitis Workshop of the National Institute of Diabetes, Digestive and Kidney Diseases reclassified the syndromes. Acute bacterial prostatitis is class I. Chronic bacterial prostatitis is class II. Nonbacterial prostatitis and prostatodynia are class III, called chronic abacterial prostatitis-chronic pelvic pain syndrome (CPPS), and are subcategorized depending on the presence or absence of leukocytes in the EPS and/or semen. Class IV describes patients without symptoms but with the presence of inflammation in the EPS, semen, or prostate tissue on biopsy or resection. Class IV patients require no treatment as they are asymptomatic.

C. Acute Bacterial Prostatitis—Category I Prostatitis

1. *Signs and symptoms.* Possible prodrome of vague pelvic and systemic symptoms. Acute onset of dysuria, urgency, frequency, nocturia, perineal and low back pain, difficulty voiding, fever, chills, and malaise. Prostate is enlarged, boggy, and tender on rectal examination, although examination should be minimized to avoid bacteremia.
2. *Laboratory results.* Elevated WBC. Pyuria and bacteriuria on urinalysis. Urine culture most commonly grows *E. coli. Klebsiella, Proteus mirabilis, Enterobacter,* and *Staphylococcus aureus* are also common; *Salmonella* is rare. Granulomatous prostatitis may result from miliary tuberculosis or systemic mycosis.
3. *Treatment.* Bed rest, antipyretics, analgesics, hydration, suprapubic cystotomy for urinary retention, and stool softeners. Acutely ill patients may require hospitalization for hydration and broad-spectrum parenteral antibiotics (ampicillin and gentamicin) until culture and sensitivity results are available. These antibiotics are able to penetrate the generally impermeable prostatic epithelium due to alterations in the epithelial barrier during intense

inflammation. Once afebrile, patients should be managed as outpatients with TMP-SMX or a fluoroquinolone for 3 to 4 weeks. Treatment is important to attempt to prevent the development of chronic prostatitis. *Salmonella* is treated with cotrimoxazole or chloramphenicol. Tuberculous and mycotic prostatitis are treated with antitubercular or antifungal therapies, respectively.

4. *Complications.* Prostatic abscess should be suspected in diabetic patients or in the presence of continued spiking fevers despite adequate antibiotics and a fluctuant prostate. Computer tomography or transrectal ultrasound (TRUS) can diagnose a prostatic abscess. It can be drained by transurethral incision or TRUS-guided transperineal percutaneous drainage. Chronic prostatitis is a possible sequela of acute prostatitis.

D. Chronic Bacterial Prostatitis—Category II Prostatitis

1. *Signs and symptoms.* Pelvic, perineal, or low back discomfort; dysuria and irritative voiding; clear discharge; recurrent UTI; and pain during or after ejaculation. Patients are asymptomatic between episodes. Physical examination is normal.

2. *Laboratory results.* Recurrent bacteriuria between courses of antibiotics is common. *E. coli* is present in 80% of cases. Klebsiella, Pseudomonas aeruginosa, *and* Proteus *are less common. The role of gram-positive organisms, including* Staphylococcus epidermitis *and* Staphylococcus saprophyticus, is debated as such organisms normally colonize the anterior urethra and contamination of prostatitic secretions cannot be avoided. Localization studies for these organisms usually are not reproducible, do not produce an immune response in prostatic secretions, and do not lead to relapsing and recurrent UTI in untreated patients, as do gram-negative prostatic infections. Little evidence has been found that *Mycoplasma,* fungi, obligate anaerobic bacteria, trichomonads, or viruses cause prostatitis. *Ureaplasma urealyticum* and *Chlamydia trachomatis* have been localized to the prostate in a small percentage of patients.

3. *Treatment.* Antibiotics are used either to eradicate the prostatic bacteria or to suppress bacteriuria and relieve symptoms. Curative antibiotics, such as TMP-SMX and the fluoroquinolones, are lipid soluble to penetrate the lipid membrane of the prostate and are concentrated within the prostate. TMP (160 mg) and SMX (800 mg)

twice daily or a fluoroquinolone in standard doses for 4 to 6 weeks are curative in 33–50% of patients. Treatment can be extended up to 12 weeks if cure is not obtained. A suppressive dose of one fluoroquinolone or TMP-SMX can be continued. Zinc and other vitamin supplements have not proven useful. Transurethral resection of the prostate should only be used in the presence of prostatic calculi or bladder outlet obstruction. Prostatic massage is of questionable benefit.

E. Chronic Nonbacterial Prostatitis—Category III/Chronic Pelvic Pain Syndrome (CPPS)

1. *Signs and symptoms.* Very similar to chronic bacterial prostatitis. May be intermittent in nature. The use of The National Institutes of Health Chronic Prostatitis Symptom Index (NIH-CPSI, Figure 5-2) is very useful in gauging patients' symptoms at baseline and to track any changes with treatment.

2. *Etiology.* Several etiologies have been proposed in the pathogenesis of chronic prostatitis/chronic pelvic pain syndrome (CP/CPPS). Proposed is a cascade of events that begins with a primary event which leads to immunologic stimulation, followed by an inflammatory response with a persistent immunologic stimulation, ultimately leading to neuropathic damage and NIH III prostatitis. Other mechanisms may result from an interactivity of endocrine, immunologic, neurologic, and psychologic factors. Bacterial pathogens have been analyzed in CP/CPPS, yet to date no specific infectious agent has been implicated as the one pathogen. Structural alterations of the lower urinary system may lead to obstruction and development of symptoms. Urine reflux into the prostate has been implicated causing irritation and inflammation.

3. *Evaluation.* Patients should be evaluated to rule out reversible causes of pelvic pain such as malignancy, stone, or true infection. One should send a urine culture. Patients with severe irritative voiding symptoms and/or hematuria should have a urine cytology. Up to 2% may have underlying bladder malignancy. Patients with symptoms of bladder outlet obstruction should have a video-urodynamic study to rule out bladder neck dysfunction.

4. *Treatment.* Antimicrobials may be started on a 4- to 6-week course despite negative urine culture. Nonsteroidal anti-inflammatory agents, hot sitz baths, tricyclic antidepressants for chronic neuropathic pain, anticholinergics, repeated prostate massage, and 5-alpha-reductase inhibitors can be

---

NIH-Chronic Prostatitis Symptom Index (NIH-CPSI)

Pain or Discomfort

1. In the last week, have you experienced any pain or discomfort in the following areas?

	Yes	No
a. Area between rectum and testicles (perineum)	$\square_1$	$\square_0$
b. Testicles	$\square_1$	$\square_0$
c. Tip of the penis (not related to urination)	$\square_1$	$\square_0$
d. Below your waist, in your pubic or bladder area	$\square_1$	$\square_0$

2. In the last week, have you experienced:

	Yes	No
a. Pain or burning during urination	$\square_1$	$\square_0$
b. Pain or discomfort during or after sexual climax (ejaculation)?	$\square_1$	$\square_0$

3. How often have you had pain or discomfort in any of these areas over the last week?

$\square_0$ Never
$\square_1$ Rarely
$\square_2$ Sometimes
$\square_3$ Often
$\square_4$ Usually
$\square_5$ Always

4. Which number best describes your AVERAGE pain or discomfort on the days that you had it, over the last week?

$\square$ $\square$ $\square$ $\square$ $\square$ $\square$ $\square$ $\square$ $\square$ $\square$ $\square$
0 1 2 3 4 5 6 7 8 9 10
NO PAIN   PAIN AS BAD AS YOU CAN IMAGINE

Urination

5. How often have you had a sensation of not emptying your bladder completely after you finished urinating, over the last week?

$\square_0$ Not at all
$\square_1$ Less than 1 time in 5
$\square_2$ Less than half the time
$\square_3$ About half the time
$\square_4$ More than half the time
$\square_5$ Almost always

6. How often have you had to urinate again less than two hours after you finished urinating, over the last week?

$\square_0$ Not at all
$\square_1$ Less than 1 time in 5
$\square_2$ Less than half the time
$\square_3$ About half the time
$\square_4$ More than half the time
$\square_5$ Almost always

Impact of Symptoms

7. How much have your symptoms kept you from doing the kinds of things you would usually do, over the last week?

$\square_0$ None
$\square_1$ Only a little
$\square_2$ Some
$\square_3$ A lot

8. How much did you think about your symptoms, over the last week?

$\square_0$ None
$\square_1$ Only a little
$\square_2$ Some
$\square_3$ A lot

Quality of Life

9. If you were to spend the rest of your life with your symptoms just the way they have been during the last week, how would you feel about that?

$\square_0$ Delighted
$\square_1$ Pleased
$\square_2$ Mostly satisfied
$\square_3$ Mixed (about equally satisfied and dissatisfied)
$\square_4$ Mostly dissatisfied
$\square_5$ Unhappy
$\square_6$ Terrible

Scoring the NIH-Chronic Prostatitis Symptoms Index Domains

Pain: Total of items 1a, 1b, 1c, 1d, 2a, 2b, 3, and 4 =_____
Urinary Symptoms: Total of items 5 and 6 =_____
Quality of Life Impact: Total of items 7, 8, and 9 =_____

FIGURE 5-2. NIH-Chronic Prostatitis Symptom Index (NIH-CPSI).

tried. Alpha-adrenergic blockers, muscle relaxants (diazepam), or even transurethral incision of the bladder neck or microwave thermotherapy can be used in patients with bladder neck/external sphincter spasms. Patients with refractory pain may even undergo sacral neuromodulations. See the basic algorithm for diagnosis of lower UTI in males (Figure 5-3).

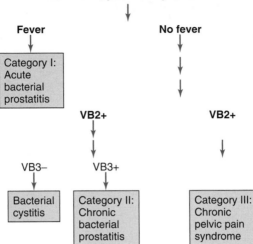

FIGURE 5-3. Basic algorithm for diagnosis of lower UTI in males. Symptoms of dysuria, frequency, suprapubic discomfort, and pain with ejaculation.

IV. INFECTION OF THE SEMINAL VESICLES

This is rarely diagnosed in the absence of chronic bacterial prostatitis or epididymitis and may be suspected by the palpation of a hard, swollen mass above the prostate on rectal examination.

V. EPIDIDYMITIS

A. Etiology

1. *Retrograde ascent* of urethral pathogen through the ejaculatory duct and vas deferens to the epididymis.

   a) Sexual transmission is responsible for most cases in men younger than age 35 years. *C. trachomatis* is most common, followed by *Neisseria gonorrhoeae.* Enteric organisms may be causative in males performing insertive anal intercourse.

   b) Nonsexual transmission is responsible for most cases in men older than age 35 years. The bacteria may be carried through the urethra by climbing an indwelling catheter as a scaffold.

2. *Antegrade descent* may occur when a bladder infection is present and is due to bladder outlet obstruction. The patient may have recently undergone urinary tract instrumentation or operation (transurethral resection of prostate may lead to reflux of urine down vas deferens). A prostatic infection may rarely be the source of bacteria. An ectopic ureter emptying into a seminal vesicle is an uncommon cause of recurrent epididymitis.

3. *Hematogenous* spread of bacteria from a distant source may occur and can result in infection with organisms such as *Haemophilus influenzae, Cryptococcus, Brucella,* or *Mycobacterium tuberculosis.*

4. *Amiodarone* is selectively concentrated in the epididymis and can cause inflammation of the head of the epididymis. Dose reduction leads to resolution.

B. Signs and Symptoms

The epididymis may be swollen up to 10 times its normal size. It is exquisitely tender. When the testicle is involved (epididymo-orchitis), the epididymis may not be palpable as a separate structure. A reactive hydrocele and scrotal wall erythema are common. Elevation of the testicle when the patient is recumbent may relieve the pain. Fever, chills, and irritative voiding symptoms are frequent. Urethral discharge is occasionally present.

C. Evaluation

One should perform urinalysis and urine culture. Gram stain of urethral specimen should be obtained when sexually transmitted disease is suspected. Scrotal ultrasound with Doppler flow should be performed. This shows increased blood flow to the inflamed epididymis and helps differentiate from testicular torsion.

D. Differential Diagnosis

Testicular torsion, torsion of appendix testis, testicular abscess, testis tumor, mumps orchitis, and tuberculosis (TB).

E. Treatment

Bed rest, scrotal elevation and support, ice packs, and pain relief with nonsteroidal anti-inflammatory agents are standard. Men requiring urinary drainage should undergo placement of a suprapubic catheter if a transurethral catheter does not pass easily. Surgical drainage of a scrotal abscess or testicular infarct may be necessary. Antibiotic therapy consists of treatment with a fluoroquinolone or TMP-SMX for 10 days for an infection from a source in the bladder. If the infection is chlamydial, treat with doxycycline 200 mg initially, followed by 100 mg twice daily for 10 days. Ceftriaxone 250 mg intramuscularly, ciprofloxacin 500 mg orally, or ofloxacin 400 mg orally, in a single dose, will treat gonorrhea and should be administered when treating for *Chlamydia*.

SELF-ASSESSMENT QUESTIONS

1. What are the most common organisms that cause lower urinary tract infections in men?
2. When the VB2 culture is positive, what must be done to determine whether the patient has bacterial cystitis or bacterial prostatitis?
3. Under which circumstances should a positive urine culture from an elderly man (older than 65 years) be treated?
4. What is the most common type of prostatitis? How is it treated?
5. What type of catheter should be placed in a patient with acute bacterial prostatitis or epididymitis when urinary drainage is required?

SUGGESTED READINGS

1. Centers for Disease Control and Prevention: Sexually transmitted diseases treatment guidelines. Available at http://www.cdc.gov/STD/treatment/TOC2002TG.htm.
2. Meares EM, Jr, Stamey TA: Bacteriologic localization patterns in bacterial prostatitis and urethritis. *Invest Urol* 5:492, 1968.
3. Nicolle LE, Bradley S, Colgan R, et al: Infectious Diseases Society of America guidelines for the diagnosis and treatment of asymptomatic bacteriuria in adults. *Clin Infect Dis* 40:643–654, 2005.
4. Nickel JC: Prostatitis and related conditions. In Walsh PC, Retik AB, Vaughan ED Jr, Wein AJ, eds: *Campbell's Urology,* 8th ed. Saunders, Philadelphia, 2002, pp. 603–630.
5. Nickel JC, Moon T: Chronic bacterial prostatitis: an evolving clinical enigma. *Urology* 66:2–8, 2005.
6. Schaeffer AJ: Infections of the urinary tract. In Walsh PC, Retik AB, Vaughan ED Jr, Wein AJ, eds: *Campbell's Urology,* 8th ed. Saunders, Philadelphia, 2002, pp. 515–602.

CHAPTER 6

Specific Infections of the Genitourinary Tract

Ricardo E. Dent, MD and
Ashok K. Batra, MD, FACS

I. GENITOURINARY TUBERCULOSIS

A. General Considerations

1. Tuberculosis (TB) has been known to occur in humans for more than 7000 years. In 18th century Europe, the disease reached epidemic proportions and wiped out nearly one fourth of the population of England. The cause of this disease remained a mystery until the 19th century, when Robert Koch published his first article outlining the pathogenesis of the disease in 1882. In 1926, Edgar Medlar was the first to describe TB renal involvement. He demonstrated that microscopic renal lesions were typically bilateral and almost always found in the renal cortex. *Mycobacterium tuberculosis* and *Mycobacterium bovis* are the two most common infectious human pathogens.

2. The World Health Organization estimates that 2 billion people are infected with TB (one third of the world population). In 2004, 1.7 million deaths resulted from TB. This makes TB the number one infectious disease killer worldwide. Once infected with TB, 5–10% will develop active disease over their lifetime. Centers for Disease Control and Prevention (CDC) data from 2004 indicate that the incidence of TB declined to 4.9 cases per 100,000 in the United States. This signifies a 2.3% decrease from the previous year and a 46% decrease from 1992. The case rate among US-born persons was 2.6 per 100,000 and 22.8 for foreign-born persons. A resurgence of TB has been seen in areas with a high prevalence of acquired immunodeficiency syndrome. The disease is the most common opportunistic infection of this population worldwide.

3. Involvement of the genitourinary (GU) system is seen in 4–8% of people with TB. Approximately 9% of patients with pulmonary TB and 26% of those with miliary disease

have associated infection of the kidneys, ureters, or genital organs.

4. The GU tract is the leading secondary site of involvement among extrapulmonary organs, primarily involving young adults. Male cases predominate over female cases in a ratio of 3:1.

5. Bacille Calmette-Guérin (BCG) is highly effective in protecting children from meningitis and miliary TB. Its efficacy against pulmonary TB in adults is variable. Countries with low disease prevalence generally prefer withholding vaccination to maintain the diagnostic value of purified protein derivative (PPD) skin testing.

B. Pathogenesis

1. Almost all TB infections are acquired by inhalation of aerosolized droplets of bacteria. TB bacilli spread to the kidneys hematogenously and proceed to lodge in periglomerular capillaries and create abscesses. Once infected, the immunocompetent host has a lifetime risk of 5–10% for developing active disease. Although TB elicits both a cellular and humoral immune response, it is only the cellular response that determines the outcome of an infection.

2. Involved sites may be dormant for many years, and given favorable conditions, they reactivate and spread by caseation and cavitation. TB is strictly aerobic and has a doubling time of 15–20 hours (*Escherichia coli* has a doubling time of just over an hour).

3. Conditions that favor reactivation include debilitating disease, trauma, steroid therapy, diabetes, anemia, immunosuppression, and acquired immunodeficiency syndrome (AIDS). Tumor necrosis factor inhibitors such as infliximab have also been linked to reactivation of latent TB.

4. The characteristic granulomatous lesion is known as a *tubercle.* It consists of a central giant cell of Langhans surrounded by lymphocytes and fibroblasts. Tubercles in the glomeruli may either heal or spill into the nephrons where they are caught in the narrow loop of Henle and form more tubercles.

5. Tubercles caseate and slough into the calyceal fornix. Bacilli that spill down the ureters have the potential to create extensive tissue fibrosis that may result in ureteral stricture formation, bladder inflammation, and contracture. The calyceal stem and pelviureteral junction are the areas most frequently affected.

6. Approximately 4% of initial tubercles result in destructive TB. When caseation is progressive, the disease may involve the entire renal pelvis leading to a calcified mass of caseous material called a "putty kidney." Severely damaged kidneys have reduced renal blood flow that may result in secondary hypertension.

7. If early renal lesions do not heal (the response of each kidney is independent of the other), passage of infected urine through the urogenital tract can lead to involvement of the ureters, bladder, prostate, seminal vesicles, vas deferens, epididymis, and testis. Rarely, the primary hematogenous lesion in the urinary tract may settle in the prostate.

8. BCG therapy is commonly employed for the treatment of superficial bladder cancer. Sometimes, this results in TB infection of the bladder, prostate, and, occasionally, the kidneys. Even miliary TB has been reported after BCG treatment.

C. Clinical Features and Diagnosis

1. Renal involvement is generally silent (Table 6-1). It frequently presents with vague urinary symptoms. Therefore, a high index of suspicion along with careful history taking are essential for the diagnosis. The interview should specifically cover a history of "contact" and/or a previous history of pulmonary TB and a history of recurrent urinary tract infections unresponsive to standard antibiotics. In the male, the earliest indication may be tuberculous epididymitis or cystitis. Epididymitis is frequently the only symptom. Infections of the testis are almost always secondary to infection of the epididymis. Females may present with

---

Table 6-1:   Clinical Findings in Genitourinary Tuberculosis (TB)

Sterile pyuria
Nocturnal painless frequency of micturition
History of present or past TB elsewhere in the body
Unexplained hematuria
Chronic cystitis unresponsive to antibiotics
Chronic epididymitis with epididymal nodularity and/or
  thickened or beaded vas deferens
Nodularity of prostate, shrunken "bean bag" prostate
Induration of seminal vesicles
Dull flank pain and renal colic
Chronic draining scrotal sinus
Hematospermia (rare)

bladder pain and dysuria. Back pain and hematuria are not uncommon. Recurrent *E. coli* infections may serve as a warning sign for the urologist.

2. Bladder biopsy is contraindicated in active tuberculous cystitis.

3. The severity of symptoms does not correlate with the degree of urinary tract involvement.

4. The diagnosis is made by finding *M. tuberculosis* in the urine or semen.

   a) Three to five consecutive early morning urines are cultured: repeat if results are negative. Although the urine is frequently sterile, 50% of patients have microscopic hematuria. Sterile pyuria is a classic finding.

   b) Acid-fast stains on concentrated urinary sediment from 24-hour specimen may be positive in 50–60% of cases, but culture corroboration is essential. If cultures are positive, antibiotic sensitivities are performed. Polymerase chain reaction (PCR) of urine has sensitivity and specificity of more than 95% and 98%, respectively. DNA probes allow clinicians to differentiate between various mycobacterial species and strains. Adenosine deaminase levels of pleural fluid have proven useful in the diagnosis of pulmonary TB. Sputum diagnosis of TB requires 10^4 mycobacteria per mL.

   c) A negative tuberculin skin test makes the diagnosis unlikely, but a conversion of a previously negative test to positive should raise the index of suspicion.

   d) Radiographs alone are not sufficient for diagnosis. Plain radiographs may show calcification, and intravenous urogram (IVU) is standard practice. IVU reveals various features of TB and helps rule out obstruction and nonfunctioning units.

   e) Drug-sensitivity testing is essential. However, due to the slow growth of TB, results may not be available for more than 8 weeks.

5. Differential diagnosis.

   a) Chronic nonspecific cystitis or pyelonephritis.

   b) Acute or chronic nonspecific epididymitis.

   c) "Urethral syndrome," interstitial cystitis.

   d) Necrotizing papillitis of one or both kidneys.

   e) Schistosomiasis.

D. Therapy

1. General considerations (Table 6-2).

   a) The aim of antituberculous therapy is to treat the active disease promptly and render the patient noninfective in the shortest period of time.

Table 6-2:	Common Antituberculous Chemotherapeutic Agents		
Drug	Doses	Side Effects	Remarks
First Line			
Isoniazid (INH)	5–10 mg/kg per day, to max 300 mg/day	Peripheral neuritis, hepatitis	Bactericidal, pyridoxine for neuritis
Rifampin	10–20 mg/kg per day, to max 600 mg/day	Hepatotoxicity, hypersensitivity, transient leukopenia or thrombocytopenia	Bactericidal, orange discoloration of urine
Ethambutol	15 mg/kg per day	Retrobulbar neuritis, color vision changes	Tuberculostatic, baseline visual acuity tests
Streptomycin	750–1000 mg/day IM for 1 month, then 95 mg/kg IM twice per week	Nephrotoxicity, ototoxicity	Bactericidal
Pyrazinamide	15–30 mg/kg to max 2000 mg/day	Hepatotoxicity, elevates serum uric acid	Monitor liver function and serum uric acid
Second Line			
Amikacin/kanamycin	15 mg/kg/day to max 1000 mg	Auditory and renal toxicity, hypokalemia, hypomagnesemia	Only available parenterally

(Continued)

Table 6-2.—Cont'd			
Drug	**Doses**	**Side Effects**	**Remarks**
Aminosalicylic acid	150 mg/kg to max 12 g/day	Hypersensitivity, GI irritation, hepatotoxicity	Tuberculostatic
Capreomycin	500–1000 mg/day once per day for 3 months, then twice per week	Nephrotoxicity, ototoxicity	Use with caution in elderly
Ciprofloxacin	750–1500 mg per day	Abdominal cramps, GI irritation, interactions with warfarin and theophylline	Antacids containing aluminum, magnesium, or calcium reduce absorption
Cycloserine	10–20 mg/kg per day to max 500 mg/day	Psychosis	Contraindicated in epileptics
Ethionamide/ protionamide	500–1000 mg per day	GI irritation, hepatotoxicity, hypothyroidism, metallic taste	Antacids/antiemetics may help tolerance
Rifabutin	5 mg/kg per day to max 300 mg	Rash, hepatitis, fever, neutropenia, thrombocytopenia	Drug of choice in HIV, orange discoloration of secretions

GI, gastrointestinal; HIV, human immunodeficiency virus; IM, intramuscular.

b) The quantity of the bacillary population is related to the extent of the disease.

c) Multiple drugs work synergistically against resistant organisms in early treatment.

d) Close follow-up of the GU tract is essential during therapy, as asymptomatic ureteral strictures (especially in the lower third) may occur during the healing phase. Tuberculous strictures lend themselves to percutaneous or transurethral dilation techniques. Steroids may be beneficial.

e) Surgical intervention may play an increasing role with trends toward shorter duration of chemotherapy.

2. Primary agents are rifampin, isoniazid, pyrazinamide, and either ethambutol or streptomycin. Pyridoxine (25–50 mg daily) should be added to regimens that include isoniazid to prevent neuropathy. After 2 months of therapy (for a susceptible isolate) only the rifampin and isoniazid are continued for an additional 4–6 months. Popular combination regimens include rifampin 600 mg daily, isoniazid 300 mg daily, pyrazinamide 25 mg/kg daily, and ethambutol 25 mg/kg daily for 2 months followed by rifampin 600 mg and isoniazid 300 mg daily for 4–6 more months.

3. Second-line agents include rifabutin (preferred over rifampin for patients taking protease inhibitors and nonnucleoside reverse transcriptase inhibitors), aminoglycosides (kanamycin/amikacin), fluoroquinolones (ciprofloxacin/levofloxacin/ofloxacin), capreomycin, cycloserine, aminosalicylic acid, ethionamide, and protionamide (see Table 6-2 for doses and side effects). Worldwide mycobacteria are becoming increasingly resistant to commonly used drugs (Table 6-3 includes mechanisms of action and antibiotic resistance information).

4. Surgical therapy.

a) Emergent surgical procedures are undertaken to drain perinephric abscesses, remove nonfunctioning renal tissue, and bypass ureteral strictures.

b) Elective surgery, when indicated, is performed 4–6 weeks after chemotherapy has begun and the inflammatory process has stabilized. This decreases the incidence of postoperative strictures.

c) Partial nephrectomy is sometimes attempted for calcified polar lesions increasing in size. Reconstructive ureteral surgery is performed as necessary. Severely contracted, nonfunctional bladders are managed by augmentation procedures.

Table 6-3:   Mechanism of Action and Recognized Mutational Resistance of Commonly Used Antituberculous Agents

Drug	Mechanism of Action	Site of Mutational Resistance
Isoniazid	Inhibits mycolic acid synthesis Catalase-peroxidase enzyme	*inhA* (regulatory region, mycolic acid gene) and *katG* (catalase-peroxidase gene)
Rifampin	Inhibits RNA polymerization	β-Subunit *rpoB* (RNA polymerase gene)
Pyrazinamide	Inhibits fatty acid synthesis	*pncA* (pyrazinamidase gene)
Ethambutol	Inhibits cell wall synthesis (blocks arabinosyl transferase)	*embB* (gene for arabinosyl transferase enzyme)
Streptomycin	Inhibits protein synthesis	*rpsL* (gene for ribosomal S12 protein); 16-S ribosomal RNA gene
Amikacin	Inhibits protein synthesis	16-S ribosomal RNA gene
Quinolones	Inhibits DNA structure	*GyrA* (gyrase A gene)

From Walsh PC, Retik AB, Darracott EV, Wein AJ, eds: *Campbell's Urology*, 8th ed. Philadelphia, Saunders, 2002.

    d) Nephrectomy is performed for a grossly diseased nonfunctioning kidney or diseased kidney with severe secondary hypertension.

E. Follow-up

1. Patients should be re-evaluated 3, 6, and 12 months after completion of therapy and their urine cultured for acid-fast bacillus (AFB). They may be discharged following a year of disease-free follow-up.

2. Imaging studies such as kidney, ureter, and bladder (KUB) x-rays, computed tomography (CT), and intravenous urography are required to follow the status of calyceal deformities and renal calcifications.

II. GENITOURINARY SCHISTOSOMIASIS

A. General Considerations

1. Caused by a blood fluke (parasitic trematode worm), this disease was first recognized by Egyptian physicians of the 12th dynasty (1900 ac). In 1851, Theodor Bilharz first described the worms in the human mesenteric venous plexus and linked them to the disease.
2. Approximately 200 million humans are infested with schistosomes, namely *Schistosoma mansoni, Schistosoma japonicum,* and *Schistosoma haematobium.* In the United States, there are more than 400,000 people living with the disease. Incidence of urinary involvement is 40–60%.
3. GU schistosomiasis is primarily caused by *S. haematobium.* It is endemic in Africa and certain areas of the Middle East such as Southern Iraq.
4. *S. mansoni* and *S. japonicum* cause intestinal tract and liver disease.
5. Urogenital infection by *S. haematobium* may cause infertility, ectopic pregnancies, and anemia due to chronic blood loss. The syndrome is known as female genital schistosomiasis. The cervix and bladder may develop "sandy patches" that are characteristic of the disease. On x-ray, the "calcified bladder" is a thick, circumferential sandy patch that contains a multitude of schistosome eggs.

B. Etiology and Life Cycle

1. Adult schistosomes are delicate cylindrical worms, 1–2 cm in length. They have adapted for existence in venules and have a mean life span of 3.4 years. A single pair spawns from 250,000–600,000 eggs in their lifetime.
2. Humans are infected through contact with infested fresh water in small canals, ditches, or drains. The infective larval stage, free swimming cercariae, penetrates the skin or mucous membranes.
3. Cercariae (shed by the snails in fresh water sources) penetrate through unbroken human skin and reach the general circulation and are pumped by the heart throughout the body. Only worms that reach the portal circulation survive.

4. Adult worms reaching their definitive destinations in the venous plexi mature and mate. Females lay eggs (200–500 per day) in the submucosa of the involved tissues: the bladder, lower ureters, and seminal vesicles in the case of GU schistosomiasis. Eggs are extremely antigenic and produce an intense inflammatory reaction in the tissues where they are deposited. About 20% erode through the viscera of deposition (intestine, bladder) and are eliminated.

5. Ova are eliminated in human feces and urine. If they reach fresh water, they start their asexual cycle (snail) resulting in the production of sporocyst. They hatch, and the contained larvae, ciliated miracidia, find a specific freshwater snail that they penetrate. There, they form sporocysts that ultimately form the cercariae that leave the snail and pass into the freshwater to begin their sexual cycle after reaching their human host.

C. Pathogenesis and Clinical Features

1. Stage 1: Generalization or incubation period.
   a) Young schistosomes rapidly acquire host-derived antigenic materials on their body surface and become immunologically camouflaged.
   b) Secretions and excretions of the worms may engender hypersensitivity and general manifestations of illness.
   c) Allergic skin reactions, cough, fever, malaise, body and bone aches, and gastrointestinal (GI) symptoms may be present.
2. Stage 2: Deposition of ova by mature worms in the target area.
   a) Because female worms may lay eggs for years, the disease is slowly progressive.
   b) Toxic and antigenic products of a viable miracidium pass through the shell of the egg and elicit a granulomatous inflammatory response around the egg, forming pseudotubercles.
   c) General symptoms include "swimmers itch" and Katayama syndrome (fever, lethargy, and myalgia). Acute symptoms generally occur 3–9 weeks after infection.
   d) GU symptoms include painful terminal hematuria, dysuria and pyuria, hematospermia, and vesical irritability.
3. Stage 3: Late complications.
   a) End result of repeated, chronic infections.
   b) Infection of urinary tract—usually coliform organisms (*E. coli, Klebsiella, Pseudomonas*). Definitive association

with *Salmonella typhi* and *Salmonella paratyphi* infections.

c) Schistosomal bladder polyps, secondary infection, stones, urinary tract calcification.

d) Fibrosis is the ultimate result of infection and may involve the bladder, urethra, and ureters, leading to hydronephrotic renal atrophy and bladder contraction. Schistosomal "contracted bladder" syndrome occurs late in the course of the disease and presents as constant, deep lower abdominal and pelvic pain, urgency, both diurnal and nocturnal frequency, and incontinence.

e) Bilharzial bladder cancer syndrome has an early onset (40–50 years of age) and results in squamous cell carcinoma (60–90%) and adenocarcinoma (5–15%). More than 40% of squamous cell carcinomas are exophytic and carry a good prognosis.

D. Diagnosis

1. Diagnosis of infection.

   a) Urine sediment reveals elliptical terminally spined eggs of *S. haematobium*. The highest yield may be obtained at mid-day. Sending the patient on a short walk before urine collection may facilitate shedding of eggs from the bladder mucosa. Number of eggs per 10 mL of urine has the best sensitivity and specificity of all estimates of intensity for current infection.

   b) Rectal or bladder mucosal biopsy may also be performed to look for eggs.

   c) Serologic tests such as enzyme linked immunosorbent assay (ELISA) and immunoblot are very sensitive and specific. However, positive results do not always correlate with the worm burden and do not help distinguish between previous exposure and current infection or reinfections.

2. Diagnosis of sequelae and complications.

   a) Plain x-ray of abdomen classically reveals bladder calcification. Seminal vesicle, urethral, and distal ureteral calcifications may be seen.

   b) IVU is essential to look for obstructive uropathy. CT scanning and ultrasound may be employed for the detection of obstructive and destructive lesions.

   c) Cystoscopy may be used to obtain mucosal biopsies for original diagnosis and is also utilized to assess for complications such as bladder cancer.

E. Therapy

1. Medical management.
   a) *S. haematobium* is sensitive to two oral drugs: praziquantel (Biltricide) and oxamniquine.
   b) Praziquantel, a heterocycline prazinoisoquinoline, is the drug of choice for treatment of all species. Dosage for *S. haematobium* is 20 mg/kg by mouth every 6–8 hours times 3 doses, given with food. It reliably cures 60–90% of patients and substantially decreases the worm burden in those that are not cured. The drug causes titanic contractions and tegumental vacuoles that cause the worms to detach and die.
   c) Oxamniquine is no longer available in the United States.
   d) Re-examination of urine or feces 1 month after treatment is recommended to assess efficacy.
2. Surgical management.
   a) Surgical procedures are reserved for complications of infection such as ureteral stenosis, bladder fibrosis, and bladder carcinoma. Procedures include ureteral dilation, ureteral reimplantation, partial cystectomy, bladder augmentation, and cystectomy with urinary diversion.

III. GENITAL FILARIASIS (BANCROFTIAN FILARIASIS)

A. General Considerations

1. Currently, no form of human filariasis is endemic in the United States. In 2004, more than 250 million people in more than 39 countries were treated for the disease.
2. The World Health Organization has identified lymphatic filariasis as the second leading cause of permanent disability in the world after leprosy.
3. Filarial infection is widespread in tropical and subtropical countries. Although numerous filarial species cause human disease, urologic problems are most common with *Wuchereria bancrofti* (90%). *Onchocerca volvulus,* the agent of African river blindness, can also cause scrotal elephantiasis, also known as hanging groin. *Brugia malayi* infections are rare in this country.
4. *W. bancrofti* is a human parasite without a known animal reservoir and with a cycle that proceeds from human to mosquito and back to human. Mosquito bites transmit the filarial larvae into the human host.

5. Periodic bancroftian filariasis is found throughout tropical Africa, North Africa, tropical coastal borders of Asia, southern parts of Indian subcontinent, Queensland, the West Indies, Puerto Rico, and northern South America.

B. Etiology and Life Cycle

1. Adult filarial *W. bancrofti* are 4- to 10-cm worms approximately 0.2 mm in diameter; they reside in the lymphatic system and live for decades.
2. The female worm is viviparous, producing microfilariae that can be found in the peripheral blood at night (nocturnal periodicity) and in the lungs during the day. Microfilariae live from 3–6 months.
3. If ingested by suitable mosquitoes, microfilariae develop in the thoracic muscles of the insect and move to the mouth parts after 2 weeks.
4. They enter the skin of human hosts through puncture wounds of a mosquito bite and move to the lymphatics where males and females meet, mate, and mature. One year later, microfilariae begin to appear in the blood.

C. Pathogenesis and Clinical Features

1. Host response to microfilariae differs from the immune response to adult worms. Various features of occult and overt infections have been described. The clinician will see a range of pathology from circulating eosinophilia to eosinophilic granulomas in the lymph nodes and spleen.
2. Severity of lesions is related to load of adult worms, site of infection, and host susceptibility.
3. Maturing adults in the lymphatics cause fibrotic and inflammatory changes that can eventually lead to lymphatic obstruction.
4. The syndrome of "filarial fever" resembles malaria and involves headache, malaise, fever, lymphadenopathy, and urticarial rash.
    a) It occurs in the acute phase and is typically afilaremic.
    b) Often, no history of this can be obtained. The fever persists for 3–5 days and may be low or high grade. Bancroftian filariasis tends to initially center in the epididymis and spreads centrifugally with repeated infections, whereas brugian filariasis initially begins in distal lymphatics.
5. In the chronic phase, 10–15 years after the onset of the first acute attack, lymphatics of inguinal region, upper

arm, and spermatic cord are affected. Funiculoepididymitis and orchitis are known to occur. Common findings include the following:

a) Chronic lymphadenopathy.

b) Retrograde lymphangitis with bacteria and mycotic superinfection.

c) Lymphatic obstruction with resulting edema, especially in lower limbs (elephantiasis) and scrotum (hydrocele formation).

d) Renal lymphaticourinary fistula formation resulting in chyluria.

6. Tropical pulmonary eosinophilia.

a) This is due to hyperergic reaction to filariae.

b) It is characterized by peripheral eosinophilia, lymphadenopathy, and pulmonary infiltrates. There is very little to no urologic involvement.

D. Diagnosis

1. In early stages, microfilariae are usually present in smears of blood obtained at night. The nocturnal microfilariae may be provoked before drawing blood with a single daytime dose of 1–2 mg/kg of diethylcarbamazine.

2. In long-standing, chronic disease, blood smears are usually negative.

a) Peripheral eosinophilia may be present.

b) Microfilariae may sometimes be found in hydrocele fluid or chylous urine.

c) Filarial complement fixation tests are useful for the detection of disease. Currently, specific serodiagnostic tests for *W. bancrofti* are available. ELISA test for IgG antibody against recombinant filarial antigen is also useful. IgE and IgG4 may be observed in patients with active filarial disease.

3. Differential diagnosis includes nonfilarial congenital lymphatic defects and obstructions, tuberculous inguinal lymphadenitis, schistosomiasis, and lymphatic obstruction from malignancy.

E. Therapy

1. Even though chemotherapy is effective in eliminating *W. bancrofti,* structural changes may not be reversible. The primary goal of treatment is to eliminate as many adult worms and microfilariae as possible.

2. Diethylcarbamazine (Hetrazan or DEC).

a) Mainstay of the treatment. It is known to be effective against adult worms and microfilariae.

b) Dose: 6 mg/kg per os (PO) once (similar effect as multiple doses). Alternatively, give orally over 14 days. Day 1, 50 mg PO once; day 2, 50 mg PO three times a day; day 3, 100 mg PO three times a day; days 4–14, 2 mg/kg PO three times a day. Repeat at 3- to 6-month intervals.

c) Toxicity (anorexia, nausea, vomiting, pruritus) may be due to dying microfilariae. Concurrent administration of corticosteroids may decrease the allergic manifestations.

d) In countries like Africa with a high incidence of onchocerciasis (river blindness) and Loa loa, the drug is not commonly used due to a high incidence of severe adverse reactions.

e) Mechanism of action is unknown, but is thought to involve sensitizing microfilariae to phagocytosis.

3. Doxycycline.
   a) Often given along with DEC to decrease the number of adult worms and microfilaria.
   b) Dose: 100–200 mg/day for 4–6 weeks.

4. Ivermectin (Mectizan).
   a) It is effective against microfilariae but has no effect on the adult worms. Sometimes used in combination with DEC.
   b) Given as single dose of 150–200 µg/kg PO. It is usually well-tolerated with few side effects. Like DEC, it needs to be repeated to prevent recurrent filaremia. It is often used in combination with albendazole.
   c) Paralyzes the parasites, acting as a γ-aminobutyric acid (GABA) receptor agonist by potentiating the inhibitory signals sent to motor neurons.

5. Suramin (Antrypol, Moranyl).
   a) A complex derivative of urea that is effective against adult worms but has many side effects.
   b) Standard dose is 66.7 mg/kg/day intravenous (IV) in 6 weekly doses.

6. Mebendazole (Vermox, Banworm).
   a) Causes worm death by blocking uptake of glucose and other nutrients in susceptible adult worms.
   b) 100 mg PO twice a day for 3 days, repeat if not cured in 3 weeks.

7. Albendazole (Albenza, Eskazole, Zentel).
   a) Broad-spectrum antihelminthic. Inhibits ATP production in worms, resulting in immobilization and death. Sometimes used in combination with DEC.
   b) 400 mg PO single dose.

IV. RARE PARASITIC GENITOURINARY INFECTIONS

A. Hydatid Disease (Echinococcosis)

1. *Echinococcus granulosus,* a small taeniid-type tapeworm, is endemic in the sheep-herding regions of the world (e.g., Australia, Argentina, Spain, Middle East, Greece, Turkey, and parts of Asia). Although rare in the United States, cases have been reported in several western states, including California, Arizona, New Mexico, and Utah. Renal hydatids may occur in up to 3% of cases.

2. Incubation occurs over a long period of time and symptoms depend on the size and location of the lesions. Common urologic symptoms include a chronic dull flank pain and lower back discomfort presumably caused by cystic pressure. Occasionally, cysts become large enough to rupture, giving rise to urinary and systemic symptoms. Cysts frequently involute and become calcified.

3. Indirect hemagglutination and ELISA are the most commonly used methods to test for *Echinococcus* antibodies. Casoni's test is a valuable skin test for diagnosis. In most cases, eosinophilia is limited or absent.

4. Plain radiographs, CT scans, and magnetic resonance imagings (MRIs) are useful in identification of the disease. Ultrasound can be an extremely useful tool. A floating membrane or "water lily" sign is pathognomonic (described in multiple imaging modalities). Septated cysts with a honeycomb pattern are likely to be echinococcal.

5. Due to the extremely antigenic nature of *Echinococcus,* it is important to differentiate between echinococcal and amebic abscesses before surgical excision. Praziquantel has been recommended preoperatively or in the case of operative spillage of cyst contents. Rupture of cysts can lead to anaphylaxis and significant metastatic seeding of the disease.

6. Surgical treatment ranges from simple excision to various emergency surgical procedures for obstruction and abscess formation, including nephrectomy.

7. Medical therapy primarily involves albendazole and mebendazole. When cysts are accessible, meta-analysis supports percutaneous aspiration-injection-reaspiration (PAIR) + albendazole. Before and after drainage: albendazole, > 60 kg 400 mg PO twice a day or < 60 kg, 15 mg/kg/day with meals for 28 days. Afterwards, puncture (P) and aspiration (A), then instillation (I) of isotonic

saline before reaspiration (R). This allows a cure rate of more than 95%, whereas surgical excision has a cure rate close to 90%. The albendazole cycle may be repeated 3 times.
8. Mebendazole is believed to be less effective. Dose: 50 mg/kg/day PO for at least 3 months.

B. Amebiasis

1. This disease is quite prevalent in the developing countries with poor sanitary conditions.
2. Amebic infections uncommonly affect the kidneys.
3. The right kidney is more frequently involved, usually in association with liver abscess.
4. Amebic involvement of urethra and bladder is occasionally seen in association with fulminant amebic sepsis and multiorgan involvement.
5. Symptoms include fever, renal pain, and hematuria (sometimes seen in association with renal vein thrombosis).
6. Diagnosis may sometimes be established only on biopsy. A stool antigen test has a sensitivity of 87% and specificity of 90%. Serum antigen and PCR tests are also highly sensitive and specific.
7. Liver abscesses will appear hypoechoic and homogenous. CT of liver may show fluid levels and a low-attenuation lesion with an enhancing rim.
8. Drugs used to treat amebiasis include metronidazole, tinidazole, paromycin, ornidazole, chloroquine, and iodoquinol. For severe infections, use metronidazole (750 mg IV to PO three times a day for 10 days) or tinidazole (2 gm daily for 5 days) followed by paromycin 500 mg PO three times a day for 7 days.
9. Surgery should be delayed until reasonable control of the infection has been achieved.

V. GENITOURINARY FUNGAL INFECTIONS

A. General Considerations

1. Fungal infections have been documented since the days of Hippocrates. Schmorl first described renal involvement with *Candida* in 1890. Rafin described bladder involvement with *Candida* in 1927.
2. With the increasing number of immunocompromised patients (especially transplant, human immunodeficiency virus [HIV], and elderly), systemic fungal infections are

becoming increasingly prevalent. Fungi are the fourth most common cause of nosocomial bloodstream infections and cause more than 9% of all nosocomial infections. With disseminated infections, the mortality rate is close to 50%. European studies indicate that fungi are responsible for 17% of all nosocomial infections in the intensive care unit.

3. There are two types of fungal infections:
   a) Primary fungal infections (blastomycosis, coccidioidomycosis, and histoplasmosis).
   b) Opportunistic fungal infections (candidiasis, aspergillosis, cryptococcosis, and mucormycosis). *Candida albicans, Candida tropicalis, Candida parapsilosis,* and *Candida glabrata* account for the majority of opportunistic fungal infections. *Candida* is the most prevalent of the fungi and accounts for almost 90% of all the fungal infections affecting the GU tract. *C. albicans* is the most common among the *Candida* species. Candidiasis is described in detail.
4. Diagnosis of most fungal infections is achieved through tissue culture. Enzyme immunoassay and radioimmunoassay can also be extremely helpful.
5. Treatment typically consists of surgical debridement when necessary, accompanied with systemic antifungal therapy.

B. Primary Fungal Infections

1. Blastomycosis
   a) Endemic in the mid-western and south-central regions of the United States. Incidence is 1–2 cases per 100,000 in areas with endemic disease.
   b) Clinical manifestations range from asymptomatic infection; flu-like syndromes; pneumonia with fever, lobar infiltrates, and cough; chronic respiratory illness; or fulminant infection with high fever, diffuse infiltrates, and respiratory failure.
   c) GU infection is reported to occur in 20–30% of patients with systemic disease. Prostatitis and epididymitis are the most common urologic manifestations.
   d) Medical therapy consists of amphotericin B for disseminated infection. Long-term itraconazole or fluconazole is used for focal uncomplicated disease.
2. Coccidioidomycosis
   a) Endemic in the hot and dry climates of the western United States. Incidence is approximately 15 cases per 100,000 in areas with endemic disease.

b) Symptomatic infection (approximately 40% of cases) presents as a flu-like illness with fever, cough, headache, rash, and myalgias. Urologic symptoms include voiding dysfunction with or without scrotal swelling.

c) GU infection occurs in 30–46% of patients with systemic disease. Renal involvement is manifest with microabscesses or granulomas. Bladder infection may present with hematuria or pneumaturia.

d) Medical therapy consists of amphotericin B. Itraconazole or fluconazole is given for long-term outpatient therapy.

3. Histoplasmosis

a) Endemic in temperate climates throughout the world and in the United States in the Ohio, Missouri, and Mississippi River valleys. Approximately 80% of the population in endemic areas is skin-test positive for the organism. Approximately 250,000 individuals are infected annually, with clinical manifestations developing in less than 5%. Disseminated disease develops in 4–27% of immunocompromised patients that are infected.

b) The organism, *Histoplasma capsulatum,* is commonly found in bird and bat guano. Clinical disease frequently mimics TB but rarely affects the kidneys. Superficial penile ulcers may develop in disseminated disease.

c) Symptomatic infection presents as a flu-like illness with fever, cough, headache, and myalgias. A sepsis syndrome may develop in patients with HIV. GU infection should be considered a manifestation of systemic disease in which kidney, bladder, prostate, and epididymis may be seeded.

d) Medical therapy consists of amphotericin B followed by long-term itraconazole.

C. Opportunistic Fungal Infections

1. Aspergillosis

a) Organism may grow in decomposing vegetation, potted plants, spices, and marijuana. Yearly incidence is approximately 1–2 per 100,000.

b) In immunosuppressed patients, invasive pulmonary disease presents with fever, cough, and chest pain. The infection may then spread to sinuses, brain, skin, bone, and GU system.

c) GU infection is a manifestation of systemic disease. Kidneys may be affected by obstruction caused by bezoars or focal infiltrating disease manifested by abscesses or pseudotumors. Prostate infection presents with frequency, dysuria, or bladder outflow obstruction.

d) Medical therapy consists of voriconazole or amphotericin B. Combination voriconazole with caspofungin is preferred in immunosuppressed patients.

2. Cryptococcosis

   a) Incidence is only 0.4–1.3 cases per 100,000 in the general population. Among patients with AIDS, the annual incidence is 2–7 cases per 1000.

   b) Initial pulmonary infection is usually asymptomatic. When the disease spreads systemically, meningoencephalitis can be a serious concern.

   c) Renal cryptococcus infection manifests as pyelonephritis or focal abscess. The lower GU tract may develop bladder outflow obstruction or prostatitis.

   d) Medical therapy consists of amphotericin B originally followed by either fluconazole or itraconazole.

3. Mucormycosis

   a) The disease is extremely rare and clinical manifestations are typically rhinocerebral.

   b) Desferrioxamine therapy has been associated with the disease.

   c) Urologic manifestations present with fever and flank pain in patients with underlying immunosuppression.

   d) Treatment consists of extensive surgical debridement and amphotericin B. Azoles and caspofungin are usually not helpful.

D. Candidiasis (Opportunistic Fungal Pathogen)

1. Pathogenesis and clinical manifestations

   a) *Candida* species normally inhabit mucocutaneous body surfaces. Alterations in host defenses allow the organism to invade body tissues while in the mycelial phase, which is more resistant to cellular defenses than the yeast phase.

   b) Risk factors include use of broad-spectrum antibiotics, diabetes mellitus, corticosteroids, indwelling catheters, granulocytopenia, bone marrow transplant, solid organ transplant, burns, severe trauma, recent surgery, GI surgery, and antineoplastic drugs.

   c) Bladder involvement may be asymptomatic or present with urgency, hematuria, frequency, nocturia, severe dysuria, and suprapubic pain.

    d) Upper tract involvement may be asymptomatic or present with signs and symptoms of pyelonephritis, perinephric abscess, or obstruction from fungus balls.

    e) Systemic candidiasis generally involves the lungs or kidneys and presents with fever, chills, hypotension, lethargy, petechiae, and embolic phenomena.

2. Diagnosis

    a) Blood and urine cultures must be evaluated in the context of the clinical setting, as candidemia and candiduria may occur as a transient phenomenon.

    b) Diagnosis of fungal cystitis is based on clinical presentation of irritative bladder symptoms, history of predisposing factors, positive urinary fungal cultures (greater than 10^4 colony forming units [CFU]/mL; however, in the presence of an indwelling catheter, these counts cannot be used to differentiate colonization from true infections), negative bacterial and acid-fast cultures, cystoscopy, bladder biopsy (to rule out tumor), and tissue cultures.

    c) Blood cultures, ophthalmologic examination, and PCR may help diagnose systemic involvement.

    d) IVU may show calyceal defects and ureteral obstruction due to fungal masses or bezoars.

3. Treatment

    a) Asymptomatic candiduria implies colonization without tissue invasion and generally resolves when predisposing factors (antibiotics and indwelling catheters) are removed. Urinary alkalinization with sodium bicarbonate to a pH of 7.5 may be helpful.

    b) Symptomatic or intractable vesical candidiasis (greater than 15,000/CFU) should be treated with systemic and/or intravesicular antifungal agents. Various intravesical irrigation agents have been used with success such as amphotericin B (50 mg/1000 mL of 5% dextrose water solution per 24 hours as a continuous infusion) and miconazole (50 mg/1000 mL normal saline per day). Local therapy is undertaken once obstructive disease is corrected and invasive disease has been excluded.

    c) First-line medical therapy for candidemia in stable patients includes: fluconazole (6 mg/kg/day or 400 mg daily [qd] IV or PO for 7 days, then PO for 14 days after last positive blood culture) or caspofungin (70 mg IV on day 1 followed by 50 mg IV qd); or amphotericin B (0.6 mg/kg/day IV, total dose 5–7 mg/kg). Alternatively, voriconazole (loading dose 6 mg/kg q 12 hours × 1 day IV, then 3 mg/kg every 12 hours IV).

d) Unstable patients require: amphotericin B (0.8–1 mg/kg/day ± flucytosine 37.5 mg/kg q 6 hours PO) or fluconazole (>6 mg/kg/day or 400–800 mg qd IV).

e) Surgical therapy. Ureteroscopy, percutaneous nephrostomy along with irrigation and removal of fungal bezoars, and placement of drains and stents may be required to clear the fungus. This is generally followed by medical therapy with or without continuous irrigation with antifungal agents.

VI. FOURNIER'S GANGRENE

A. General Considerations

1. In 1883, a French venereologist named Jean-Alfred Fournier described a rapid, fulminating gangrene of the genitalia in young male patients. Currently, the eponym Fournier's gangrene is applied to any large fulminating penoscrotal and perineal gangrenous processes, also known as necrotizing fasciitis.

2. There is no predilection for race. This condition has been described in all ages, although the mean age tends to be between 20 to 50 years. Male to female ratio is 10:1.

3. Clinical presentation begins with irritation, itching, and erythema of the scrotum, which progresses to groin necrosis within a matter of hours. Crepitance may be felt with clostridial infections. Systemic symptoms include fever, malaise, chills, and sweats. Usually, genital discomfort is out of proportion with the physical findings.

4. Diabetes is the most commonly associated medical condition. There may be a GU history of urethral stricture or fistula or a GI history of an anorectal process such as fistula, fissure, or abscess. Other associated risk factors include alcoholism, chronic steroid use, cirrhosis, morbid obesity, malignancies, HIV, local trauma, paraphimosis, and periurethral urinary extravasation. In many cases, no etiologic source is found.

B. Pathogenesis

1. The source of infection is either the GU or GI tract. Once the local inflammatory response becomes activated, decreasing oxygen tension in the tissues promotes the growth of anaerobic and facultative anaerobic organisms.

2. The infection is typically polymicrobial. Common organisms include: gram-positive cocci (*Streptococcus* and *Staphylococcus*), gram-negative rods (Enterobacteriaceae), and anaerobic organisms (*Bacteroides, Clostridia, Streptococcus*).

C. Clinical Features and Diagnosis

1. A high index of suspicion is critical. A young diabetic patient with scrotal discomfort and systemic toxicity out of proportion to the physical signs of rapidly advancing erythema, edema, bronzing of skin, bleb formation, or a foul-smelling discharge should warn the urologist of a fulminant and rapidly progressive process. In advanced presentation, the patient may be septic and hemodynamically unstable. Pain may subside as the tissue becomes progressively necrotic.

2. Common presenting signs include scrotal swelling (94%), fever (70%), acute urinary retention (19%), spontaneously drained abscess (11%), and dysuria or urethral discharge (5–8%).

3. Urine, tissue, and blood cultures are standard. Serum creatinine, blood urea nitrogen (BUN), electrolytes, hematologic and coagulation studies, and arterial blood gas analysis are recommended.

4. A KUB is recommended and, if indicated, retrograde urethrogram, cystoscopy, and proctoscopic examinations are done. CT scans may detect smaller amounts of soft tissue gas than plain radiographs. Ultrasound can be useful if testicular torsion is considered in the early differential diagnosis. MR is generally not feasible due to the aggressiveness of the disease and the logistical challenges of critical illness.

D. Therapy

1. Prompt and aggressive therapy is required. This includes rapid assessment and stabilization of the patient along with administration of broad-spectrum antibiotics.

2. Antibiotics. Triple antibiotic therapy that includes an aminoglycoside and anaerobic coverage is recommended. Imipenem or meropenem are very useful as single-agent therapy for polymicrobial infections.

   a) Gentamicin (3–5 mg/kg per day) for gram-negative organisms.

   b) Clindamycin (600 mg every 4 hours) for adequate anaerobic coverage. Metronidazole can be used alternatively.

    c) A third-generation cephalosporin such as ceftriaxone should be used. Penicillin G (3–5 million U every 6 hours) for *Clostridia* is frequently recommended. An infectious disease consult is also practical.

3. Surgical therapy. Wide excision and debridement of all devitalized tissues are recommended. A suprapubic catheter is needed for urinary diversion. The patient should be monitored carefully postoperatively and further debridements performed as necessary. This frequently leaves large denuded areas between the lower abdomen and upper thighs that may require the testicles to be placed in upper medial thigh pouches. Some studies have demonstrated that postoperative hyperbaric oxygen therapy enhances wound healing. A wide variety of scrotal reconstruction techniques can be performed once the patient is stable and the wound is healing. Despite the current advances, mortality is high and approaches 25%.

SELF-ASSESSMENT QUESTIONS

1. How does TB spread to the kidneys?
2. What is the most common presenting symptom of genitourinary TB?
3. What combination of drugs is commonly used to treat TB?
4. Which schistosome species is responsible for GU involvement?
5. What is the drug of choice for all species of schistosomes?
6. Which organism is most commonly involved with GU filariasis?
7. What is most common cause of opportunistic GU fungal infections?
8. What are the drugs of choice for *Candida* and *Aspergillus* infections?
9. What are the common risk factors for developing opportunistic GU fungal infections?
10. What are the common presenting signs of Fournier's gangrene?

DISCLAIMER

The views expressed in this chapter are those of the authors and do not represent the policies of the United States Food and Drug Administration.

SUGGESTED READINGS

1. Centers for Disease Control and Prevention home page: Available at http://www.cdc.gov/az.do.

2. Centers for Disease Control and Prevention home page: Division of Bacterial and Mycotic Diseases: aspergillosis, Blastomycosis, Candidiasis, Coccidioidomycosis, and Cryptococcosis. Accessed Apr 15, 2006. Available at http://www.cdc.gov/ncidod/dbmd/diseaseinfo/.

3. Centers for Disease Control and Prevention home page: Division of Bacterial and Mycotic Diseases: histoplasmosis. Oct 12, 2005. Apr 15, 2006. Available at http://www.cdc.gov/ncidod/dbmd/diseaseinfo/histoplasmosis_t.htm.

4. Centers for Disease Control and Prevention home page: Division of Tuberculosis Elimination: treatment of Tuberculosis. Jun 4, 2003. Apr 15, 2006. Available at http://www.cdc.gov/mmwr/preview/mmwrhtml/rr5211a1.htm.

5. Centers for Disease Control and Prevention home page: Division of Tuberculosis Elimination: trends in Tuberculosis. Mar 23, 2006. Apr 15, 2006. Available at http://www.cdc.gov/mmwr/preview/mmwrhtml/mm5511a3.htm.

6. Centers for Disease Control and Prevention home page: Parasites and health: amebiasis. Jan 21, 2004. Apr 15, 2006. Available at http://www.dpd.cdc.gov/dpdx/HTML/Amebiasis.htm.

7. Centers for Disease Control and Prevention home page: Parasites and health: echinococcosis and lymphatic filariasis. Nov 22, 2004. Apr 15, 2006. Available at http://www.dpd.cdc.gov/dpdx/.

8. Centers for Disease Control and Prevention home page: Parasites and health: schistosomiasis. Aug 30, 2004. Apr 15, 2006. Available at http://www.dpd.cdc.gov/dpdx/HTML/Schistosomiasis.htm.

9. Dreyer G, Noroes J, Figueredo-Silva J, et al: Pathogenesis of lymphatic disease in bancroftian filariasis: a clinical perspective. *Parasitol Today* 16:544–548, 2000.

10. Emedicine from WebMD home page: Available at http://www.emedicine.com.

11. Fry DE: Editorial comment: the story of hyperbaric oxygen continues. *Am J Surg* 189:467–468, 2005.

12. Gilbert DN, Moellering RC, Eliopoulos GM, Sande MA: *The Sanford Guide to Antimicrobial Therapy 2005.* Antimicrobial Therapy Inc., Hyde Park, 2005.

13. The Global Alliance to Eliminate Lymphatic Filariasis home page: Dec 30, 2005. Apr 15, 2006. Available at http://www.filariasis.org/index.

14. Golden MP, Vikran HR: Extrapulmonary tuberculosis: an overview. *Am Fam Physician* 72:1761–1768, 2005.

15. Grayson DE, Abbott RM, Levy AD, et al: Emphysematous infections of the abdomen and pelvis: a pictorial review. *Radiographics* 22:543–561, 2002.

16. Hoerauf A, Mand S, Volkmann L, et al: Doxycycline in the treatment of human onchocerciasis: kinetics of Wolbachia endobacteria reduction and of inhibition of embryogenesis in female Onchocerca worms. *Microbes Infect* 5:261–273, 2003.

17. Keane J, Gershon S: Tuberculosis associated with infliximab, a tumor necrosis factor a-neutralizing agent. *N Engl J Med* 345:1098–1104, 2001.

18. Lenk S, Schroeder J: Genitourinary tuberculosis. *Curr Opin Urol* 11:93–96, 2001.

19. Madeb R, Marshall J, et al: Epididymal tuberculosis: case report and review of the literature. *Urology* 65:798.e22–798.e24, 2005.

20. Matos MJ, Bacelar MT, Pinto P, et al: Genitourinary tuberculosis. *Eur J Radiol* 55:181–187, 2005.

21. Mawhorter SD, Curley GV: Prostatic and central nervous system histoplasmosis in an immunocompetent host: Case report and review of the prostatic histoplasmosis literature. *Clin Infect Dis* 30:595–598, 2000.

22. Merino E, Boix V, et al: Fournier's gangrene in HIV-infected patients. *Eur J Clin Microbiol Infect Dis* 20:910–913, 2001.

23. Morpurgo E, Galandiuk S: Fournier's gangrene. *Surg Clin North Am* 82:1213–1224, 2002.

24. Neal P: Schistosomiasis: an unusual cause of ureteral obstruction, a case history and perspective. *Clin Med Res* 2:216–227, 2004.

25. Pedrosa I, Saiz A, Arrazola J, et al: Hydatid disease: radiologic and pathologic features and complications. *RadioGraphics* 20:795–817, 2000.

26. Poggensee G, Feldmeier H: Female genital schistosomiasis: Facts and hypotheses. *Acta Tropica* 79:193–210, 2001.

27. Ross AG, Bartley PB: Current concepts: schistosomiasis. *N Engl J Med* 346:1212–1220, 2002.

28. *The Sanford Guide to Antimicrobial Therapy 2005.* Antimicrobial Therapy Inc., Hyde Park, 2005.

29. Seo R, Oyasu R, Schaeffer A, et al: Blastomycosis of the epididymis and prostate. *Urology* 50:980–982, 1997.

30. The U.S. National Library of Medicine, Levy D, ed: MedlinePlus: mucormycosis. Jul 14, 2004. Apr 15, 2006. Available at http://www.nlm.nih.gov/medlineplus/ency/article/000649.htm.

31. Walsh PC, Retik AB, Darracott EV, Wein AJ: *Campbell's Urology,* 8th ed. Philadelphia, WB Saunders, 2002.

32. Wikipedia: Available at en.wikipedia.org/wiki/Main_Page.

33. Wise GJ, Marella VK: Genitourinary manifestations of tuberculosis. *Urol Clin North Am* 30:111–121, 2003.

34. Wise GJ, Talluri GS, et al: Fungal infections of the genitourinary system: manifestations, diagnosis, and treatment. *Urol Clin North Am* 26:701–718, 1999.

35. Wise GJ: Genitourinary fungal infections: a therapeutic conundrum. *Expert Opin Pharmacother* 2:1211–1226, 2001.

36. The World Health Organization home page: Available at www.who.int/en/.

37. World Health Organization home page: Tuberculosis. Mar 2006. Apr 15, 2006. Available at http://www.who.int/tb/en/.

C H A P T E R 7

Painful Bladder Syndrome (Interstitial Cystitis)

Philip M. Hanno, MD, MPH

Painful bladder syndrome (PBS), formerly referred to as interstitial cystitis (IC), is a condition diagnosed primarily on the basis of clinical symptomatology. It requires a high index of suspicion on the part of the health care provider. It should be considered in the differential diagnosis of the patient presenting with chronic pelvic pain, often exacerbated by bladder filling and associated with urinary frequency. **The *sine qua non* of the diagnosis is the presence of pain associated with the bladder.** The older term IC was not at all descriptive of the clinical syndrome and not accurate with regard to the pathologic findings. The reader should realize that the older term is still in use and common in the literature but gradually becoming less so.

Originally considered a bladder disease, it is now positioned in the medical spectrum as a chronic pain syndrome that may begin as a pathologic process in the bladder in most, but not all, patients. In a small percentage of patients it can progress into a disorder that even cystectomy may not benefit!

PBS encompasses a major portion of the "painful bladder" disease complex, which includes a large group of patients with bladder and/or urethral and/or pelvic pain, irritative voiding symptoms (urgency, frequency, nocturia, dysuria), and sterile urine cultures. Painful bladder conditions with well-understood and established etiologies include radiation cystitis, cystitis caused by micro-organisms that are not detected by routine culture methodologies, and systemic disorders that affect the bladder (Table 7-1). **PBS is a diagnosis of exclusion.** It may have multiple causes and represent a final common reaction of the bladder to different types of insults. Essentially, one must be confident that the patient with PBS is not actually suffering from any known cause of bladder pain before making the diagnosis.

Table 7-1:   Causes of Frequency and Urgency

Interstitial cystitis
Upper motor neuron lesion
Habit
Large fluid intake
Pregnancy
Bladder calculus
Urethral caruncle
Radiation cystitis
Large postvoid residual
Genital condyloma
Diabetes mellitus
Cervicitis
Periurethral gland infection
Atrophic urethral changes
Vulvodynia
Urinary tract infection
Chemical irritants: contraceptive foams, douches, diaphragm,
    obsessive washing
Overactive bladder
Vulvar carcinoma
Diuretic therapy
Bladder cancer
Urethral diverticulum
Pelvic mass
Chemotherapy
Bacterial urethritis
Renal impairment
Diabetes insipidus

DEFINITION

The International Continence Society (ICS) defines PBS as "the complaint of suprapubic pain related to bladder filling, accompanied by other symptoms such as increased daytime and night-time frequency, in the absence of proven urinary infection or other obvious pathology." The term IC has classically been used to describe the clinical syndrome of urgency/frequency and pain in the bladder and/or pelvis that is unrelated to any defined urologic pathology. When considering PBS/IC, the symptom of pain should be broadened to include "pressure" and "discomfort." The ICS considers IC to be a subset of the broader PBS syndrome and reserves the "interstitial cystitis" designation to patients with PBS and "typical cystoscopic and histologic features," without further specifying what these features are. In the absence of clear criteria for IC, this chapter refers to PBS/IC and IC interchangeably, as all but the recent literature terms the syndrome IC.

Urgency is left out of the definition of PBS/IC, as it would tend to obfuscate the borders of overactive bladder (OAB) and PBS/IC and proves to be unnecessary for definition purposes. One can often separate out those patients with the urgency of PBS/IC from those with the urgency of OAB by doing a cystometrogram. The OAB patient will generally have uninhibited bladder contractions, whereas the PBS/IC patient will have a stable bladder with hypersensitivity during bladder filling. A simple question will often suffice to differentiate between the two conditions. "Is your urgency to find a restroom because you are afraid you will wet yourself or is it because you are in increasing pain and discomfort?" The former strongly suggests OAB, and the latter is most consistent with PBS/IC. OAB is more than 10 times more common in the population than PBS/IC, and the treatment algorithm is very different, making the differential diagnosis critical (Figures 7-1, 7-2, and 7-3).

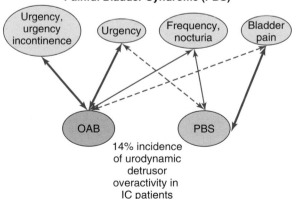

FIGURE 7-1. Relationship of overactive bladder and painful bladder syndrome. (From Abrams P, Hanno P, Wein A: Overactive bladder and painful bladder syndrome: there need not be confusion. *Neurourol Urodyn* 24:149, 2005.)

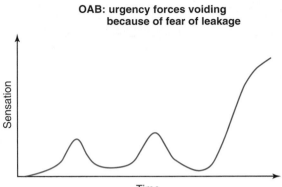

FIGURE 7-2. Undulating onset of urgency typical of overactive bladder.

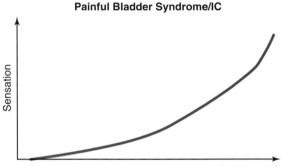

FIGURE 7-3. Gradually increasing pain and resulting urgency typical of painful bladder syndrome.

EPIDEMIOLOGY

Epidemiology studies of PBS/IC suffer from the lack of a universally accepted definition, the absence of a validated diagnostic marker or clinical test that ensures the diagnosis is made in a uniform manner by different clinicians in different geographic areas, and the lack of a pathognomonic finding on histologic biopsy of bladder tissue. There is considerable variability in studies on incidence and prevalence not only within the United States but around the world. The first population-based study included patients with IC in Helsinki,

Finland. The prevalence was 18.1 per 100,000 women and 10.6 per 100,000 population. The annual incidence of new female cases was 1.2 per 100,000. Severe cases accounted for 10% of the total. Only 10% of cases were in men.

Another early population study from the United States in 1987 first demonstrated the potential extent of what had been considered a very rare disorder. It concluded that, although there were 43,500–90,000 diagnosed cases of IC in the United States (twice the prevalence in Finland), up to half a million people had symptoms of painful bladder and sterile urine, considerably expanding the population of potentially affected individuals. The median age at onset was 40 years and there was a 50% remission rate not clearly related to therapy that lasted a mean of 9 months.

More recent epidemiologic studies using different operational definitions have yielded wildly disparate data, from 35–24,000 per 100,000 in the United States, to 1.2 per 100,000 in Japan and 7 per 100,000 in the Netherlands. Most studies show a female to male preponderance of 5:1 or greater. In the absence of a validated marker, it may be difficult to differentiate chronic pelvic pain syndrome (CPPS) in men ("nonbacterial prostatitis") from PBS. **In males who have chronic pelvic and perineal pain in the presence of urinary frequency and no history of urinary infection, PBS/IC should be considered high in the differential diagnosis.** Men with primarily pain complaints in the absence of any voiding dysfunction fit the more classic description of type 3 CPPS rather than PBS/IC. Only 5–10% of patients with PBS/IC in most series have true bladder ulceration (Hunner's ulcer). Men with PBS/IC tend to be diagnosed at an older age than women and have a higher incidence of Hunner's ulcer.

All patients with presumed PBS/IC with microhematuria should undergo cystoscopy, urine cytology, and bladder biopsy of any suspicious lesion to be sure that a bladder carcinoma is not masquerading as PBS/IC. It would seem that in the absence of microhematuria, and with a negative cytology, the risk of missing a cancer is negligible but not zero. **There is no evidence that PBS/IC itself is associated with a higher risk of bladder cancer or transitions to cancer over time.**

ETIOLOGY

It is likely that PBS/IC has a multifactorial etiology (Figure 7-4). A "leaky epithelium," mast cell activation, neurogenic inflammation, primary pelvic floor dysfunction, and

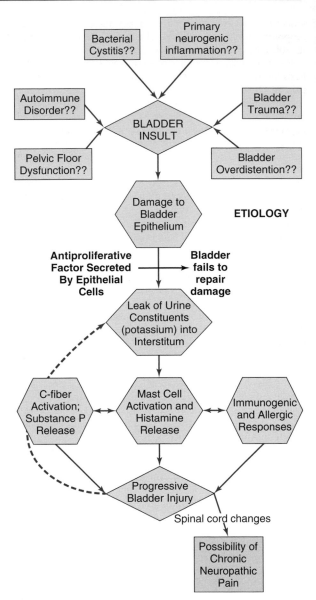

FIGURE 7-4. Synthesis of PBS/IC etiologic theories.

sequelae of bladder infection or pelvic surgery have all been proposed at one time or another. There are little data to support the role of an active infectious etiology, but it is conceivable that a viral or bacterial cystitis could begin the cascade that ultimately leads to a self-perpetuating process resulting in chronic bladder pain and voiding dysfunction.

The discovery of *antiproliferative factor* (APF) by Susan Keay and her group at the University of Maryland represents a potential major advance in the search for the etiology of PBS/IC and perhaps even in the quest for a more rational treatment approach. It remains to be confirmed by other laboratories around the world. Dr. Keay observed that cells from the bladder lining of normal control subjects grow significantly more rapidly in culture than cells from PBS/IC patients. Normal bladder cells were cultured in the presence of urine from patients with PBS/IC, asymptomatic controls, patients with bacterial cystitis, and patients with vulvovaginitis. Only urine from PBS/IC patients inhibited bladder cell proliferation. The presence of APF was found to be a sensitive and specific biomarker for PBS/IC. It was found in bladder urine but not in renal pelvic urine of PBS/IC patients, indicating production by the bladder urothelial cells. Subsequent studies indicated that APF is associated with decreased production of heparin binding epidermal growth factor-like growth factor (HB-EGF). APF activity was related to increased production of EGF, insulin-like growth factor-1, and insulin-like growth factor binding protein-3 by the bladder cells from IC patients but not by the cells from healthy bladders. Studies of PBS/IC patients and asymptomatic controls showed urine levels of APF, HB-EGF, and EGF to reliably differentiate PBS/IC from controls.

APF may prove to be an accurate marker of PBS/IC if confirmed by other centers. It appears to have the highest sensitivity and specificity of the variety of possible markers tested and fits nicely into the etiologic schema portrayed in Figure 7-4. It has been shown to differentiate men with bladder-associated pain and irritative voiding symptoms from those with pelvic/perineal pain alone and other non-specific findings compatible with the chronic pelvic pain syndrome in men (CPPS III), previously categorized as non-bacterial prostatitis.

It has been hypothesized by Keay and colleagues that PBS/IC may result from an inhibition of bladder epithelial cell proliferation caused by the APF, which is mediated by its regulation of growth factor production from bladder cells. Conceivably, any of a variety of injuries to the bladder from a traumatic or infectious process **in a susceptible individual** may result in PBS/IC if APF is present and suppresses production of HB-EGF. Theoretically, if production of APF could be "turned off" by genetic techniques, or its effects were nullified by exogenous HB-EGF, the clinical syndrome might be prevented.

DIAGNOSIS

The diagnosis of PBS/IC is the diagnosis of chronic pain, pressure, and/or discomfort associated with the bladder, usually accompanied by urinary frequency in the absence of any identifiable cause. A high index of suspicion is required on the part of the clinician, as many patients suffer for years in the absence of the correct diagnosis. **Pelvic pain and urinary frequency lasting more than 3 months and unrelated to urinary infection establish a working diagnosis.** Some patients will not complain of pain, but if the clinician asks them why they void so often, they will admit to a "pressure" or "discomfort" that is relieved, at least momentarily, by emptying the bladder.

An intravesical potassium chloride challenge (KCl test) has been proposed for diagnosis. It compares the sensory nerve provocative ability of sodium versus potassium using a 0.4M potassium chloride solution. Pain and provocation of symptoms by potassium constitute a positive test. The test is very nonspecific, failing to diagnosis at least 25% of PBS/IC patients presenting with classic symptoms and overdiagnosing much of the population with OAB, urinary infection, and nonspecific pelvic pain as having PBS/IC. **Prospective and retrospective studies looking at the KCl test for diagnosis in patients presenting with symptoms of PBS/IC have found no benefit of the potassium test in comparison with standard techniques of diagnosis.**

A variety of IC symptom scales have been developed. They are designed to evaluate the **severity** of symptomatology and monitor disease progression or regression with or without treatment. They have not been validated as diagnostic instruments.

As PBS/IC is a diagnosis of exclusion, one must rule out infection and less common conditions including, but not limited to, carcinoma, eosinophilic cystitis, malakoplakia, schistosomiasis, scleroderma, and detrusor endometriosis. In men younger than the age of 50, videourodynamics are useful to eliminate other treatable causes of voiding dysfunction. Many drugs including cyclophosphamide, aspirin, nonsteroidal anti-inflammatory agents, and allopurinol have caused a nonbacterial cystitis that resolves with drug withdrawal.

In the presence of microhematuria, local cystoscopy is essential to rule out bladder cancer or other lesions. Cystoscopy under anesthesia with bladder distention can identify the typical mucosal "cracking and bleeding" that one sees with Hunner's ulcer (Figure 7-5), present in about 10% of patients with PBS/IC. However, this procedure is not mandatory to diagnose the syndrome, and it is certainly justifiable to begin conservative therapy for PBS/IC without bladder distention having been performed. **Bladder biopsy is indicated only if necessary to rule out other disorders that might be suggested by the cystoscopic appearance.** Glomerulations (petechial bleeding points) (Figures 7-6 and 7-7) are not specific for PBS/IC, and only when seen in conjunction with the clinical criteria of bladder pain and frequency can the finding of glomerulations be viewed as significant. They are commonly seen after radiation therapy, in patients with bladder carcinoma, and after exposure to toxic chemicals or chemotherapeutic agents. They are often identified in patients on dialysis, patients with gravity

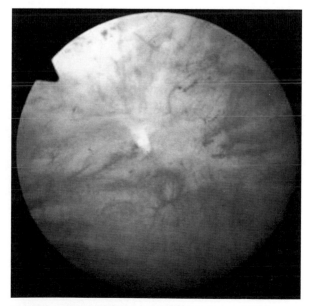

FIGURE 7-5. Typical appearance of Hunner's ulcer on initial endoscopy and prior to distention, mucosal tearing, and bleeding.

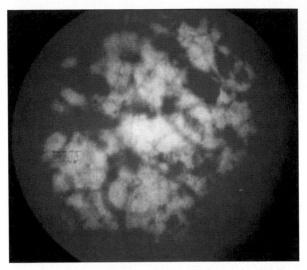

FIGURE 7-6. Typical appearance of glomerulations and mucosal hemorrhage after bladder distention under anesthesia.

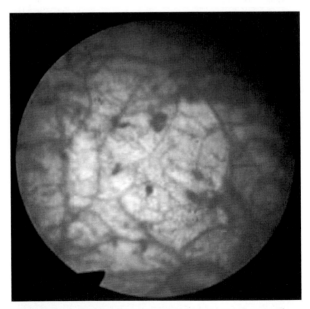

FIGURE 7-7. Typical appearance of glomerulations and mucosal hemorrhage after bladder distention under anesthesia.

incontinence, or after urinary diversion—all conditions in which the bladder has not filled for prolonged periods. They are absent in many patients with PBS/IC.

INITIAL MANAGEMENT

After diagnosis, the first decision the practitioner faces is whether to institute therapy. If the patient has not had an empiric course of antibiotics for his or her symptoms, such a trial with one course of treatment is not unreasonable. Doxycycline is a good choice. Generally, patients diagnosed with PBS/IC have already been on several courses of antibiotics by the time the diagnosis is even entertained.

If the patient's symptoms are mild to moderate, the withholding of immediate treatment is worth considering. Someone who awakens once or twice a night and voids at 2- to 3-hour intervals with minimal pain symptoms is someone active treatment would be unlikely to benefit. **Data that early intervention affects the natural history or course of the disease are lacking and an argument for the early institution of therapy cannot be supported on the basis of epidemiologic data or clinical trials.** Patient education and empowerment are important initial steps in therapy. Reassuring the patient that this is not a life-threatening disease; others have similar problems and have learned to live with them; there is a spontaneous remission rate; and symptoms do not invariably progress does much to alleviate the stress that accompanies the diagnosis. The Interstitial Cystitis Association is an important resource for information and support for patients (www.icahelp.org).

Timed voiding and behavioral modification can be useful in the short term, especially in patients in whom frequency rather than pain predominates. Many clinicians believe that stress reduction, exercise, warm tub baths, and efforts by the patients to maintain a normal life style all contribute to quality of life. Biofeedback, soft tissue massage, and other physical therapies may aid in pelvic floor muscle relaxation and alleviate pain and frequency. Although elaborate dietary restrictions and an "IC diet" are unsupported by any peer-reviewed literature, many patients do find their symptoms are adversely affected by specific foods and would do well to avoid them. Often these include caffeine, alcohol, and beverages that might acidify the urine such as cranberry juice.

Education and conservative therapy help many patients but often more active intervention is required.

ORAL THERAPY

Although many oral medications have been tried for the treatment of PBS/IC, amitriptyline, sodium pentosanpoly-sulfate, and hydroxyzine are the only commonly used medications outside of research trials.

Amitriptyline has become one of the most popular oral agents for the treatment of PBS/IC. It is a tricyclic antidepressant and is an old, inexpensive drug available only in its generic form. This class of medication has at least three main pharmacologic actions: (1) central and peripheral anticholinergic activity, (2) blockage of the active transport system in the presynaptic nerve ending responsible for the reuptake of serotonin and norepinephrine, and (3) sedation that may be central or related to antihistaminic properties. It is believed that amitriptyline has analgesic properties and potentiates the body's own endorphins. It may help to stabilize the mast cells in the bladder and also increase bladder capacity through its effect on the beta-adrenergic receptors in the bladder body. Finally, the sedative effects can help the patient sleep.

The physician prescribing amitriptyline should be very familiar with the drug, as it has many significant side effects. These commonly include daytime sedation, constipation, increased appetite, and dry mouth. It should not be prescribed for potentially suicidal patients or for those with cardiac problems or arrhythmias. The patient with PBS/IC should be started on a dose of 10 mg before bed. The dose is gradually increased by 10 mg each week to a maximum dose of 50 mg at bedtime at the start of the fifth week. If tolerated, this dose is maintained.

Parson's suggestion that a defect in the epithelial permeability barrier, the glycosaminoglycan layer, contributes to the pathogenesis of PBS/IC has lead to an attempt to correct such a defect with the synthetic sulfated polysaccharide sodium pentosanpolysulfate (PPS). This is a heparin analogue (trade name Elmiron) that is sold in an oral formulation. Three to 6% of each dose is excreted into the urine. Two placebo-controlled multicenter trials in the United States served as the pivotal studies for Food and Drug Administration approval for the pain of IC. In the initial study, overall improvement of greater than 25% was reported by 28% of the PPS-treated group versus 13% in the placebo group. In the follow-up study, the respective figures were 32% on PPS versus 16% on placebo. Average voided volume on PPS increased by 20 mL. No other objective improvements were documented. A recent NIDDK study looking at both PPS and hydroxyzine (see later) alone and in combination compared to placebo failed to show a statistically significant response to either medication. **Elmiron appears to have a beneficial effect in a minority of patients who take it for 3–6 months**. There are no convincing data that a longer trial is worthwhile in nonresponders. The dose is 100 mg three times daily. Side effects include a 6% incidence of reversible hair loss, gastrointestinal upset, and skin rash. It is generally well tolerated, although not highly efficacious.

Antihistamines have been used for their properties against mast cell activation. Hydroxyzine, an H1 antagonist, was studied in 40 patients treated with 25 mg before bedtime, increasing to 50 mg at night and 25 mg in the morning in those for whom sedation from the medicine was not a problem. The vast majority of patients had symptom improvement, but these good results have not been confirmed in placebo-controlled trials. Cimetidine, an H2 antagonist, has been reported effective in a British trial, but confirmatory studies are lacking and the mechanism of action is unexplained. It is not commonly used in PBS therapy.

Improvement with systemic steroids was first described in 1953. They have fallen out of favor due to the risk of chronic administration. Recently it has been reported that prednisone at a dose of 25 mg daily for 1–2 months and then tapered as tolerated may be effective in patients with otherwise unresponsive ulcerative disease.

Although the exact role of autoimmunity in the etiology of PBS/IC remains controversial, recent Finnish studies suggest good results with low-dose cyclosporine, an antirejection medication used in organ transplantation. In a direct comparison with PPS, cyclosporine-treated patients had a 75% response rate compared to a 19% response rate with Elmiron. Suplatast tosilate, an antiallergy compound marketed in Japan, has shown efficacy in a small, uncontrolled PBS study in which improvements in symptoms and bladder capacity were correlated with changes in autoimmune parameters. These findings provide clues for future research.

INTRAVESICAL THERAPY

Dimethylsulfoxide (DMSO) is the only Food and Drug Administration (FDA)-approved medication for intravesical instillation for the treatment of PBS/IC. It is a product of the wood pulp industry and a derivative of lignin. It has exceptional solvent properties and is freely miscible with water, lipids, and organic agents. Pharmacologic properties include membrane penetration, enhanced drug absorption, anti-inflammatory, analgesic, collagen dissolution, muscle relaxant, and mast cell histamine release. Intravesical delivery by urethral catheter of 50 mL of a 50% solution (Rimso-50) allowed to remain in the bladder for 15 minutes and repeated at weekly intervals for 6 weeks is effective in ameliorating symptoms in about 60% of patients for a period of several months to over a year. Some patients who respond to an initial 6-week course are treated monthly for 6 months. Patients emit a garlic-like odor for several hours after treatment and may experience a short-term symptom exacerbation. It is often administered as part of a "cocktail" including 10 mg triamcinolone (Kenalog), 44 mEq sodium bicarbonate, and 40,000 units heparin.

Heparin, an exogenous glycosaminoglycan, can be administered intravesically in sterile water as a single agent. Forty thousand units in 20 mL of sterile water self-administered via catheter by the patients daily and held for 30–60 minutes has been reported beneficial, but no placebo-controlled studies have confirmed efficacy.

In a large multicenter randomized trial, intravesical bacille Calmette-Guérin (BCG) failed to show a statistically significant benefit compared to placebo. Capsaicin and resiniferatoxin, agents that desensitize C fiber afferent neurons, have failed to gain acceptance for intravesical therapy. The possible therapeutic value of intradetrusor injection of botulinum toxin type A is currently being determined in clinical trials. Older intravesical treatments such as chlorpactin, a derivative of bleach originally used to treat bladder tuberculosis, and silver nitrate are rarely used today for treatment of PBS/IC.

HYDRODISTENTION

Hydrodistention under anesthesia is often the first therapeutic modality employed as part of the diagnostic evaluation. There is no one correct way to do this procedure. Our method is to perform a cystoscopic examination (which is often unremarkable), obtain urine for cytology, and distend the bladder for 1–2 minutes at a pressure of 80 cm H_2O. The bladder is emptied and then refilled to look for glomerulations or ulceration (see Figures 7-5 to 7-7). A therapeutic hydraulic distention follows for another 8 minutes. Biopsy, if indicated, is performed after the second distention with the bladder contracted. Little is to be gained by distending the bladder to more than 1 L volume, even if the pressure of 80 cm H_2O has not been reached, and the risk of temporary retention seems to increase as the volume infused increases. Although more than 50% of patients may experience some symptom relief after distention, this is often transitory and rarely lasts longer than 6 months. In those in whom relief is prolonged, it is worth considering a repeat distention in the future for therapy. A finding of a bladder capacity of less than 200 mL under anesthesia does not bode well for the success of nonsurgical therapeutic efforts.

NEUROMODULATION

Direct sacral nerve stimulation with the Interstim device from Medtronics has recently been explored in the treatment of PBS/IC and urgency/frequency. **Patients who do best with this treatment modality are those who have identifiable pain and dysfunction in the pelvic muscles.** Early studies suggest that about half of patients with PBS may derive benefit from neuromodulation, and several new devices are currently in testing for this application.

SURGICAL THERAPY

The surgical therapy of PBS/IC is an option after all trials of conservative treatment have failed. PBS, although a cause of significant morbidity, is a nonmalignant process. **Surgery should be reserved for the motivated and well-informed patient who falls into the category of extremely severe, unresponsive disease, a group that comprises fewer than 10% of patients.** Surgical intervention is aimed at increasing the functional capacity of the bladder or diverting the urine stream. Augmentation (substitution) cystoplasty and urinary diversion with or without cystectomy have been used as a last resort with good results in selected patients.

PHILOSOPHY OF MANAGEMENT

A reasonable management algorithm developed by an international committee for the International Consultation on Continence 2004 meeting is presented in Figure 7-8. Although there are many differences of approach to the treatment of PBS/IC, this author believes that it is best to progress through a variety of treatments. Whereas the shotgun approach of initial multimodal therapy has many adherents, employing or adding one treatment at a time makes the undulating natural history of the disease itself an ally in the treatment process. One should

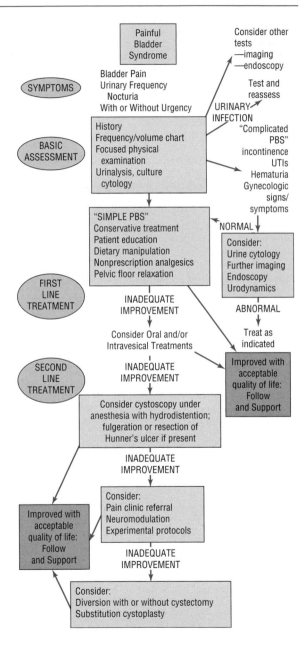

FIGURE 7-8. Suggested management algorithm. (From Hanno P, Baranowski A, Fall M, et al: Painful bladder syndrome [including interstitial cystitis]. In Abrams PH, Wein AJ, Cardozo L [eds]: *Incontinence*, 3rd ed. Paris, Health Publications Limited, 2005, vol 2, Chapter 23, pp 1456–1520.)

encourage patients to maximize their activity and live as normal a life as possible, not becoming a prisoner of the condition. Although some activities or foods may aggravate symptoms, nothing has been shown to negatively affect the disease process itself. Therefore, patients should feel free to experiment and judge for themselves how to modify their life style without the guilt that comes from feeling they have harmed themselves if symptoms flare. Dogmatic restriction and diet are to be avoided unless they are shown to improve symptoms in a particular patient.

SELF-ASSESSMENT QUESTIONS

1. What symptoms are characteristic of painful bladder syndrome/interstitial cystitis (PBS/IC)?
2. What disorders need to be considered in the differential diagnosis of PBS/IC?
3. How can the physician differentiate overactive bladder from PBS/IC?
4. Discuss the most promising diagnostic test for PBS/IC.
5. Consider the arguments for the different treatment approaches used in patients with this disorder.

SUGGESTED READINGS

1. Abrams P, Hanno P, Wein A: Overactive bladder and painful bladder syndrome: there need not be confusion. *Neurourol Urodyn* 24:149, 2005.
2. Hand JR: Interstitial cystitis: report of 223 cases (204 women and 19 men). *J Urol* 61:291, 1949.
3. Hanno P, Baranowski A, Fall M, et al: Painful bladder syndrome (including interstitial cystitis). In Abrams PH, Wein AJ, Cardozo L (eds): *Incontinence*, 3rd ed. Health Publications Limited, Paris, 2005, vol 2, Chapter 23, pp 1456-1520.
4. Hanno P, Keay S, Moldwin R, van Ophoven A: International Consultation on IC—Rome, September 2004/Forging an International Consensus: Progress in painful bladder syndrome/interstitial cystitis. Report and abstracts. *Int Urogynecol J Pelvic Floor Dysfunct* 16(suppl 1)S2, 2005.

5. Keay SK, Szekely Z, Conrads TP, et al: An antiproliferative factor from interstitial cystitis patients is a frizzled 8
   protein-related sialoglycopeptide. *Proc Natl Acad Sci
   U S A* 101:11803, 2004.
6. Nordling J, Anjum FH, Bade JJ, et al: Primary evaluation
   of patients suspected of having interstitial cystitis (IC).
   Eur Urol 45:662, 2004.
7. van Ophoven A, Pokupic S, Heinecke A, Hertle L: A prospective, randomized, placebo controlled, double-blind
   study of amitriptyline for the treatment of interstitial
   cystitis. *J Urol* 172:533, 2004.
8. Waxman JA, Sulak PJ, Kuehl TJ: Cystoscopic findings
   consistent with interstitial cystitis in normal women
   undergoing tubal ligation. *J Urol* 160:1663, 1998.

CHAPTER 8

Nephrolithiasis

John J. Pahira, MD and
Millie Pevzner, MD

I. EPIDEMIOLOGY

1. The annual incidence of nephrolithiasis in the United States is 12 cases per 10,000 persons.
2. The prevalence of nephrolithiasis in the United States is 5% in males and 3% in females.
3. Nephrolithiasis accounts for 7–10 of every 1000 hospital admissions.
4. Males have a threefold increased risk of developing stones over females (high urinary citrate concentrations in women) with peak age at onset of 20–40 years.
5. With no treatment, 10% of all first-time stone formers will have recurrent disease within 1 year and 50% within 5 years.
6. Uric acid and calcium stones are more frequent in males, whereas infectious stones are more common in females.
7. The incidence of kidney stones has increased in industrialized countries due to high dietary protein intake. Bladder stones are more common in underdeveloped countries.

II. COMPOSITION OF RENAL STONES

1. Calcium oxalate: 36–70%.
2. Calcium phosphate (hydroxyapatite): 6–20%.
3. Mixed calcium oxalate and calcium phosphate: 11–31%.
4. Magnesium ammonium phosphate (struvite): 6–20%.
5. Uric acid: 6–17%.
6. Cystine: 0.5–3%.
7. Miscellaneous: xanthine, silicates, and drug metabolites, 1–4%. Indinavir (most common protease inhibitor) causes stones in up to 6% of patients. These stones are radiolucent on x-ray and on a computed tomography (CT) scan.

III. PATHOGENESIS AND PHYSIOCHEMICAL PROPERTIES

A. Factors Influencing Stone Formation

1. Genetics

a) Idiopathic hypercalciuria is inherited as an autosomal dominant trait.

b) Cystinuria is an autosomal recessive defect on chromosome 2.

c) Primary hyperoxaluria, type 1 and 2, is inherited as an autosomal recessive defect.

d) Lesch-Nyhan syndrome is an X-linked disease causing hyperuricemia.

e) Familial renal tubular acidosis (RTA), Ehlers-Danlos syndrome, Marfan's syndrome, Wilson's disease.

2. Environmental

a) Dietary factors:
   i) High animal protein and sodium intake increase the risk of calcium stones. There is a new trend toward low carbohydrate diets with increased animal protein.
   ii) High purine diets lower urinary pH and cause hyperuricosuria.
   iii) Vitamin B_6 (pyridoxine) deficiency results in increased formation and excretion of oxalate.
   iv) Dehydration, inadequate fluid intake, vitamin C excess, calcium supplements, calcium-containing antacids contribute to stone formation.

b) Geographical factors:
   i) Higher during summer months.
   ii) Higher in Southeast United States and lower in Mid-Atlantic and Northwest regions.

B. Physical and Biochemical Parameters

1. Supersaturation is not dependent solely on the solute concentration but also on ionic strength, complexation, urine volume, and urine pH. Ionic strength is determined by the presence of monovalent ions in the urine. Its increase will allow more crystals to be in solution without supersaturation. The presence of certain substances in the urine, such as citrate and pyrophosphate, that naturally complex with any potential solute reduces the free ion activity.

2. Urinary organic (e.g., glycosaminoglycans, nephrocalcin, Tamm-Horsfall protein, uropontin) and inorganic inhibitors (e.g., citrate, magnesium, and sulfates) inhibit various phases of stone formation.

3. Epitaxy is overgrowth of one type of crystal on the surface of a preexisting one that is of different type. This process of heterogenous nucleation is seen with amorphous calcium phosphate and uric acid facilitating the crystallization of calcium oxalate salt.

4. Crystal retention can occur due to the interaction between renal epithelial cells and salt crystal, which results in their internalization and submucosal plaque formation (Randall's plaques). These crystals aggregate and erode toward the papillary surface to form a nidus for further stone growth. Reduced urine output and stasis due to anatomic abnormalities of the genitourinary tract can facilitate stone formation. A horseshoe kidney, calyx or bladder diverticula, obstructive disorders, and medullary sponge kidney can all predispose to increase crystal retention.

C. Etiologic Factors of Specific Stone Types

1. Calcium Stones

Calcium oxalate develops in acidic urine (pH less than 6.0). Calcium phosphate develops in alkaline urine (pH greater than 7.5). With calcium phosphate stones, rule out urinary tract infection (UTI), RTA, and hyperparathyroidism. Promoters of calcium stones include hypercalciuria, hypocitraturia, hyperuricosuria, hyperoxaluria, dietary factors, and absence of inhibitors (Table 8-1).

a) Hypercalciuria. **Normocalcemic hypercalciuria** (idiopathic hypercalciuria) occurs in 30–60% of calcium oxalate stone formers and in 5–10% of nonstone formers. Diagnosis is made with normal serum calcium and

Table 8-1: Normal Values of Urinary Excretion of Substances Affecting Stone Formation

Substance	Men (mg/day)	Women (mg/day)
Urinary calcium	<300	<250
Urinary uric acid	<800	<750
Urinary citrate	450–600	650–800
Urinary oxalate	<45	<45

elevated urinary calcium on a random diet. The upper level of normal is 250 mg/day for women and 300 mg/day for men. **Absorptive hypercalciuria** (AH) is characterized by jejunal hyperabsorption of calcium possibly due to increased serum calcitrol (1,25 dihydroxy vitamin D_3) and increased sensitivity of vitamin D receptors. Increased serum calcium causes suppression of parathyroid hormone (PTH) function and increases the filtered load of calcium. Suppression of PTH decreases renal tubular reabsorption of calcium leading to excess urinary calcium loss. Serum calcium is normal. AH is of three distinctive types:

i) AH Type I will not be controlled by diet. Urinary calcium remains elevated even on a restricted diet.

ii) AH Type II is dietary dependent. Urinary calcium will normalize on a low calcium diet.

iii) AH Type III is secondary to a renal leak of phosphate. Decreased serum phosphate stimulates increased vitamin D_3, leading to increased small bowel absorption of phosphate and calcium and an increased renal excretion of calcium. (Rare.)

Renal hypercalciuria (renal leak) is characterized by impaired proximal tubular reabsorption of calcium, thus there is wasting of calcium. This results in increased serum PTH, with subsequent increase in the synthesis of $1,25(OH)_2D_3$. In this way, serum calcium homeostasis is maintained. Hypercalciuria occurs even during a restricted calcium diet.

Resorptive hypercalciuria (subtle hyperparathyroidism) is characterized by increased bone resorption due to underlying primary hyperparathyroidism with excessive PTH. Hyperparathyroidism indirectly enhances intestinal calcium absorption by stimulating vitamin D_3 production. Increased urinary calcium exceeds the tubular absorption capability. These patients present with high normal serum calcium, elevated urinary calcium, and a mild elevation in PTH. Treatment with thiazides will cause serum calcium to rise and confirm the diagnosis.

Hypercalcemic hypercalciuric states are seen in the following:

i) Primary hyperparathyroidism; 50% will present with nephrolithiasis, but this accounts for only 1–5% of all patients with urinary stones. It is caused by adenoma in 85% and diffuse multigland hyperplasia in 15% of patients. Elevated PTH stimulates bone resorption and increased intestinal absorption of calcium, increased renal calcium tubular reabsorption, and increased tubular excretion of phosphorus. This results in increased calcium phosphate product in blood and deposition of calcium salts in kidney (nephrocalcinosis). Stones are primarily calcium phosphate. Fasting urinary calcium is elevated (Table 8-2).

ii) Sarcoidosis is associated with an increased production of $1,25(OH)_2D_3$ by the macrophage within the sarcoid granuloma. Stones are primarily calcium oxalate. PTH levels are low or immeasurable.

iii) Other etiologies include hyperthyroidism, hypervitaminosis D, milk alkali syndrome, immobilization, Paget's disease, multiple myeloma, and other malignancies (lung, breast, renal cell, head and neck cancers).

b) Hypocitraturia. Seen as a sole abnormality in 5–10% of patients with stones and in 50% of patients who have other associated metabolic disturbances. Citrate forms a soluble salt with calcium and inhibits the formation of calcium oxalate or calcium phosphate crystals. Acidosis is the most important etiologic factor. It reduces urinary citrate by enhancing tubular citrate reabsorption and metabolism to bicarbonate. Causes of hypocitraturic calcium stones include:

Table 8-2: Summary of Laboratory Findings

	PHPT	AHI	AHII	AHIII	RH	HUCN
Serum Ca	↑	N	N	N	N	N
Serum PO	↓/N	N	N	↓	N	N
Serum PTH	↑	N/↓	N/↓	N/↓	↑	N
Urine Ca	↑/N	↑	↑	↑/N	↑	N
Urine Ca (fasting)	↑/N	N	N	N	↑	N
Urine Ca (1 gm Ca load)	↑/N	↑	↑	↑	↑/N	N
Urine uric acid	N/↑	N/↑	N/↑	N	N/↑	↑
Bone density	N/↓	N	N	N	N/↓	N

PHPT, Primary hyperparathyroidism; AHI, absorptive hypercalciuria, type I; AHII, absorptive hypercalciuria, type II; AHIII, absorptive hypercalciuria, type III; RH, renal hypercalciuria; HUCN, hyperuricosuric calcium oxalate nephrolithiasis.

    i) Chronic diarrheal syndromes associated with enteric hyperoxaluria.

    ii) Distal RTA (type I RTA).

    iii) Idiopathic.

    iv) A diet high in salt and animal protein.

    v) Hypokalemia.

    vi) UTI with bacteria degrading citrate.

    vii) Thiazides.

c) Hyperuricosuria. Ten to 20% of patients with hyperuricosuria have calcium oxalate stones. Uric acid crystals may act as a nidus facilitating the nucleation of calcium oxalate crystal and may also decrease the activities of some urinary inhibitors. At a urinary pH of less than 5.5, the dissociated form of uric acid predominates and the urine will be saturated with monosodium urate, which can induce heterogenous nucleation of calcium oxalate. It can also enhance calcium oxalate crystallization by complexing with urinary inhibitors. Causes of hyperuricosuria include:

    i) Excessive dietary purine intake.

    ii) Increased endogenous uric acid production as in patients with myeloproliferative disorders, acute tumor lysis syndrome after radiation or chemotherapy.

    iii) Chronic diarrheal diseases (regional enteritis, short gut syndrome, and inflammatory bowel diseases).

d) Hyperoxaluria. Oxalate forms insoluble complexes with calcium in the gastrointestinal tract and in the urine. The activity of stone disease correlates better with the urinary oxalate level rather than urinary calcium.

    i) Mild metabolic hyperoxaluria (MMH). Increased urinary oxalate may be due to MMH, which causes increased urinary oxalate excretion, or it may be due to diet. High dietary content of oxalates or vitamin C may increase urinary oxalate to 50–60 mg/day. A low calcium diet (less than 500 mg/day) increases urinary oxalate excretion. Reducing oxalate in diet helps treat this condition.

    ii) Enteric hyperoxaluria. Seen in small bowel malabsorption of variable etiology, this includes inflammatory bowel disease, bowel resection, and jejunoileal bypass. There is an increase of intestinal bile salts and fatty acids, which bind to calcium salt and form calcium soaps. As there is less calcium available to bind with luminal oxalate, there is increased oxalate available for absorption. Colonic mucosal permeability to free oxalate is also increased. Both factors contribute to significant gut absorption of oxalate. These patients tend to have low urinary citrate and magnesium as a result of chronic metabolic acidosis and hypokalemia due to ongoing diarrhea. Treatments include lowering dietary oxalate and fat, combined with oral calcium, citrate, and magnesium supplements. Cholestyramine helps to bind fatty acids and bile salts in the gut.

iii) **Primary hyperoxaluria (PH).** PH Type I is an autosomal recessive trait in which the conversion of glyoxalate to glycine is diminished due to a defect in the liver enzyme alanine-glyoxylate aminotransferase activity. This results in increased conversion of glyoxalate to oxalate. There is increased oxalate production and excretion early in childhood. These patients present with early stone formation, nephrocalcinosis, tubulointerstitial nephritis, and subsequent renal failure. PH Type II is a rare deficiency of D-glycerate dehydrogenase and glyoxalate reductase. This leads to increased urinary oxalate excretion. Only 21 cases have been reported.

2. Uric Acid Stones

Uric acid is an end product of purine metabolism of endogenous or exogenous sources. It is a weak acid with pK of 5.35 at physiologic pH. At a urine pH of less than 5.5, the majority of uric acid exists in its insoluble undissociated form, which is the major constituent of uric acid stone. As the urine pH increases to higher than 5.5, more soluble dissociated monosodium urate crystals are formed, favoring calcium oxalate and calcium phosphate stone formation. Stones are usually round, smooth, yellow-orange, and radiolucent. The main risk factor for crystallization of uric acid is the high concentration of urate, which is attributable either to a high excretion of urate or to a low urine volume and a low urinary pH. Although most patients with uric acid nephrolithiasis excrete more than 750 mg/day of uric acid, idiopathic uric acid stone disease can occur without hyperuricosuria. Patients may increase risk for stones with excessive purine intake, hyperuricemia secondary to gout, myeloproliferative disorders, and treatment with cytotoxic drugs.

3. Struvite Stones (Triple Phosphate, Infected Stone)

True struvite stones are composed of a combination of magnesium ammonium phosphate ($MgNH_4PO_4 \cdot 6H2O$) and carbonate apatite ($Ca_{10}(PO_4)_6 \cdot CO_3$). Fifty percent of struvite stones may contain a nidus of another stone composition. These stones can grow to encompass the entire collecting system. This is known as a staghorn calculus. A urine pH equal to or greater than 7.2 and the presence of ammonia in the urine are essential for the crystallization of ammonia in the urine. Struvite stones form only when urease producing organisms split urea into ammonia, bicarbonate, and carbonate ion. The most common organism associated with struvite calculi is *Proteus mirabilis.* Others include *Haemophilus influenzae, Staphylococcus aureus, Yersinia enterocolitica,* and to a lesser extent *Ureaplasma urealyticum, Klebsiella pneumoniae, Pseudomonas* species, and enterococci with the exception of *Escherichia coli.* Because of increased susceptibility of women to UTIs, struvite stones are more common in females than men with a ratio of 2:1. However, struvite stones formed in the bladder are more frequent in men. Factors that predispose to UTIs increase the likelihood of struvite stone formation. These include congenital or acquired anatomic abnormalities, neurologic disorders, and indwelling foreign bodies. In patients with spinal cord lesions, 8% will form renal calculi, with 98% of the stones composed of struvite.

4. Cystine Stones

Cystinuria is an autosomal recessive disorder due to the mutation in the SLC3A1 amino acid transporter gene on chromosome 2. This causes impaired transtubular reabsorption of filtered dibasic amino acids (cystine, ornithine, arginine, and lysine) and results in excessive urinary excretion. Cystine precipitates in hexagonal crystals due to its low solubility within normal urinary pH. Heterozygotes (asymptomatic) excrete more than 400 mg of cystine per day, whereas homozygote stone formers excrete more than 600 mg/day. Positive urine cyanide-nitroprusside colorimetric reaction is a qualitative screen.

IV. CLINICAL MANIFESTATIONS OF NEPHROLITHIASIS

1. Asymptomatic nephrolithiasis may be discovered during the course of radiographic studies undertaken for unrelated reasons.
2. **Pain is the most common symptom,** varying from mild ache to severe intense pain requiring hospitalization and parenteral analgesic medications. Renal colic occurs when stones produce obstruction of the urine flow. Typically, it

begins suddenly in the early morning hours and intensifies over a period of 15–30 minutes into a steady pain that causes nausea and vomiting. The pain develops in paroxysms that are related to movement of stone in the ureter and associated ureteral spasm. Paroxysms usually last 20–60 minutes. Obstruction can occur at one of four sites along the course of the ureter: the ureteropelvic junction (UPJ); midureter at the level of iliac vessels; the posterior aspect of the pelvis in women, where the ureter is crossed anteriorly by pelvic blood vessels and the broad ligament; and the ureterovesical junction. The site of obstruction determines the location of pain. An upper ureteral or renal pelvic obstruction leads to flank pain, with costovertebral angle tenderness that may radiate laterally around the flank and into the abdomen. Pain may also be felt in the testis, because the nerve supply to the kidney and testis is the same. Midureteral calculi will produce more abdominal discomfort in the mid and lower abdomen. A lower ureteral obstruction causes pain that can radiate to the groin, bladder, scrotum, or labia. Renal colic can also be due to the passage of blood clots or sloughed renal papillae.

3. **Microscopic or gross hematuria occurs in 95% of patients.** Hematuria may be absent if the stone is causing complete obstruction.
4. **Nausea and vomiting** are frequently associated with renal colic.
5. Frequency, urgency, and dysuria can result from stone impaction at the ureterovesical junction and/or associated UTI.
6. There may be a low-grade fever without associated infection.
7. Staghorn calculi do not produce symptoms unless small pieces break off and pass into the ureter. Long-term, bilateral disease can result in chronic renal failure.

V. EVALUATION OF PATIENTS WITH NEPHROLITHIASIS

The National Institutes of Health (NIH) consensus conference on prevention and treatment of kidney stones suggested that all patients, even those with a single stone, should have a basic workup (history and physical, labs, urinalysis and culture, imaging, stone analysis) to rule out systemic causes of nephrolithiasis. More comprehensive evaluation needs to be done in the following:

1. All children
2. African Americans (stone disease is much less common in this demographic)
3. Patients with growing, bilateral, or recurrent stones (metabolically active disease)
4. Patients with a strong family history of stones
5. Patients with systemic disease or underlying metabolic disorders that predispose to stone formation
6. When the recovered stone is not composed predominantly of calcium oxalate
7. Solitary kidney

A detailed evaluation (a basic evaluation plus 24-hour urine collection) should be undertaken 3–4 weeks after the last episode of renal colic and as the patients resume the normal fluid and dietary intakes.

A. Medical History

The following questions should be considered to identify specific risk factors:

1. Chronology of stone events: age at first stone passage, number and size of stones passed, the particular kidney involved with each event, spontaneous passage versus need for active intervention, associated UTIs, and the symptoms noted with each episode.
2. The presence of systemic diseases or underlying metabolic disorders that enhance stone formation (e.g., Crohn's disease, colectomy, sarcoidosis, hyperparathyroidism, hyperthyroidism, RTA, and gout).
3. The presence of a family history of stones.
4. Intake of medication that can increase the risk of stone formation (e.g., acetazolamide, ascorbic acid, corticosteroids, calcium-containing antacids, triamterene, acyclovir, and indinavir).
5. Occupation and life style. Professionals have a greater tendency to stone formation than manual laborers. High protein and sodium dietary intake increases the risk of stone formation. Habitual tea drinking may lead to oxaluria.
6. The analysis of previous stones.

B. Physical Exam

May provide clues to underlying systemic causes (e.g., tophi secondary to gout, enterocutaneous fistulas with Crohn's disease).

C. Laboratory Tests

1. Urinalysis. High specific gravity can indicate inadequate hydration. Low urine pH (less than 5.5) is seen with uric acid stones, whereas high urine pH (at or about 7.2) is seen in patients with RTA and struvite stones. Microscopic or gross hematuria is often seen. The presence of white blood cells in the urine may be seen in the absence of infection. Crystalluria can help in defining stone type (hexagonal cystine crystal, coffin lid phosphate crystal, rhomboidal uric acid crystal). Bacteriuria must be further evaluated with urine culture.

2. Urine culture. Early detection of UTIs is important. Determine the presence of urease-producing bacteria.

3. Cystine screening. Addition of sodium nitroprusside to urine with cystine concentration higher than 75 mg/L alters the urine color to purple-red.

4. Blood tests. Complete blood count (CBC) may show mild peripheral leukocytosis. White blood count (WBC) higher than $15,000/mm^3$ may suggest an active infection. Serum chemistry includes calcium, phosphate, uric acid, sodium, potassium, chloride, bicarbonate, albumin, and creatinine. If calcium level is elevated, an intact PTH should be checked.

5. Twenty-four hour urine collection. Urine is collected in a container with boric acid as a preservative, which may falsely lower urinary pH. Collection is done to determine total urine volume, pH, calcium, citrate, magnesium, oxalate, phosphate, sodium uric acid (cystine, if screening test is positive), and creatinine.

6. Stone analysis. Analysis with x-ray crystallography or infrared spectrography.

7. Urinary acidification test. With oral ammonium chloride load (0.1 gm/kg body weight) given over 30 minutes for the diagnosis of distal type I RTA. Urine pH fails to drop below 5.3.

D. Radiologic Evaluation

1. Plain film of the kidneys, ureters, and bladder (KUB). This is 90% sensitive in detecting urinary calculi. Determining the size, number, and location of the stones allows for a rational planning of stone removal. Ninety-two percent of stones, with the exception of pure uric acid, cystine, indinavir, and xanthine stones, are at least partially radio-opaque and can be detected by a KUB. KUB has the advantage of being quick, inexpensive, and easily obtainable and provides an accurate measure of

stone size. Its limitations include the inability to detect nonopaque calculi and those that are less than 2 mm. It is difficult to differentiate renal from extrarenal calcification on a supine film. The study cannot be used in pregnant patients.

2. Intravenous pyelogram (IVP). This is the diagnostic procedure of choice to best define intrarenal and ureteral anatomy. It has a high sensitivity and specificity for determining stone location and the degree of obstruction. IVP can detect radiolucent stones and define anatomic abnormality contributing to stone formation. Patients are requested to strain their urine if they have to void during the procedure in response to intravenous contrast that induces diuresis.

3. Ultrasonography (US). Procedure of choice in patients known to have allergy to contrast, pregnant females, and children. Sensitivity of US to renal calculi is less than radiography. False negatives occur in the presence of small renal calculi or in obese patients. Calculi in the ureter between the level of the iliac crest and the ureterovesical junction cannot be evaluated satisfactorily. US will detect radiolucent calculi and urinary tract obstruction if present. It is also used to follow the size of existing stones and formation of new ones. US is also used to rule out other etiology in patients presenting with acute flank pain.

4. CT scans. A noncontrast-enhanced CT scan is the most rapid and cost-effective method for rapidly diagnosing nephrolithiasis and obstruction in patients with acute flank pain. It has a sensitivity of 97% and specificity of 96%. It is more sensitive than radiography, sonography, or both combined in detecting all types of stones. Helical or spiral CT scanning is superior to nonhelical CT, as it requires less cooperation from the patient.

VI. MANAGEMENT OF NEPHROLITHIASIS

A. Treating Patients with Acute Renal Colic

1. Aggressive intravenous fluid hydration is usually not necessary unless the patient is dehydrated and unable to take fluid orally. It may actually aggravate the degree of obstruction and increase patient discomfort.

2. Parenteral analgesia.
   a) Parenteral analgesics may be needed if pain is severe and associated nausea and vomiting render patients unable to tolerate medication via the oral route.

    b) The parenteral nonsteroidal anti-inflammatory drugs (NSAIDs) such as ketorolac (Toradol) are as effective in alleviating renal colic, if not more, than standard narcotic analgesics.

    c) The risk of NSAID-related renal dysfunction due to their hemodynamic effects or direct tubulointerstitial diseases can be increased in states of dehydration or the concomitant administration of radiocontrast materials.

    d) NSAIDs (ketorolac) should be avoided in older patients; patients with renal failure, volume depletion, or bilateral ureteral obstruction; and pregnant patients.

    e) NSAIDs are appropriate for patients with renal colic who have a known addiction to narcotics or in those who need to immediately return to a setting where they cannot be under the influence of narcotics.

    f) Epidural analgesia can be used for a pregnant patient with symptomatic calculi.

3. There is no benefit from using smooth muscle relaxants.
4. Referral to the urologist should be made if the following occur:

    a) Persistent pain.

    b) Patient unable to pass the stone due to size (larger than 8 mm).

    c) Urinary extravasation detected on IVP study.

    d) High-grade obstruction with a large stone.

    e) Patients with a solitary kidney.

    f) Failure of outpatient conservative measures to induce passage of the stone.

    g) The presence of urinary infection, especially when there is obstruction.

    h) Early referral of pregnant patients.

B. Medical Treatment of Nephrolithiasis

1. General Conservative Measures

a) Nonpharmacologic intervention may reduce the 5-year incidence of stone recurrence by approximately 60%.

b) **High fluid intake** of at least 8–10 glasses (10 oz.) per day, with a goal of keeping urine volume more than 2 L/day. Patients are instructed to drink enough fluids to keep their urine clear.

c) Relatively low animal protein diet (0.8–1.0 gm/kg/day) helps to reduce stone formation. Patients are instructed to eat 8 oz. of meat, chicken, or fish per day and to have one vegetarian day per week.

d) A low-sodium diet (2–3 gm/day or 80–100 mEq/day) is effective in reducing calcium excretion in hypercalciuric patients. Patients are instructed to avoid salty food and the salt shaker.

e) The role of dietary calcium restriction is controversial because extreme dietary calcium restriction can reduce bone density and cause a negative calcium balance. In recent studies, high calcium intake actually reduced the incidence of oxalate stones, presumably by increasing intestinal binding of calcium to oxalate. We advise patients to have one serving of dairy with each meal and to avoid dietary calcium at night.

f) Avoid stone-provoking drugs. (e.g., calcitrol, calcium supplements, loop diuretics, probenecid).

g) Avoidance of oxalate-rich foods helps to reduce stone formation. Patients are encouraged to monitor intake of tea, spinach, chocolate, nuts, fruit juices, and so forth.

2. Specific Medical Therapy of Different Stone Types

a) Calcium Stones

i) Absorptive hypercalciuria type I. Thiazide diuretics decrease urinary calcium by as much as 150 mg/day by (1) inducing mild volume depletion, which results in compensatory rise in the proximal tubular reabsorption of sodium and calcium, and (2) directly enhancing distal tubular calcium reabsorption. Chlorthalidone 25–50 mg daily or indapamide 1.25–2.5 mg/day; hydrochlorothiazide (HCTZ) 25–50 mg twice a day can be used. Continued sodium restriction is stressed (evaluated by 24-hour urinary sodium of less than 100 mEq/day).

Hypokalemia secondary to diuretic use may reduce citrate excretion; thus, supplementation with potassium citrate is necessary. Potassium supplementation includes:

1. Polycitra K syrup 15–30 mL twice daily.
2. Polycitra K crystals 1 packet twice daily.
3. Urocit K 10–20 mEq twice daily.

A potassium-sparing diuretic such as amiloride can be added at a dose of 5–10 mg/day. Potassium supplements should not be given with amiloride, because the combination can lead to severe hyperkalemia. Avoid triamterene because of its propensity to stone formation.

Sodium cellulose phosphate is a nonabsorbable calcium and magnesium binding resin. As it binds to intestinal calcium, more oxalate is unbound and available for absorption. Thus, dietary oxalate should be restricted. Dosage is 2.5–5 gm given with each meal. Long-term use can induce negative calcium balance and mandate monitoring bone density. Thus, this drug should be avoided in patients with osteoporosis. Magnesium supplement may be necessary.

ii) Absorptive hypercalcemia type II. Dietary calcium restrictions include a moderate restriction of 600 mg/day or one to two servings of dairy with meals. Dietary sodium restriction is essential to decrease hypercalciuria. Thiazide and potassium citrate supplements are offered when the previously discussed conservative measures are not effective.

iii) Absorptive hypercalciuria type III. Orthophosphate (Neutra-Phos-K) reduces serum $1,25(OH)_2D_3$ levels and increases urinary inhibitory activity. Recommended dosage is 250–500 mg three to four times daily.

iv) Renal hypercalciuria. Thiazides enhance tubular calcium reabsorption. This normalizes serum calcium and suppresses PTH. HCTZ 50 mg twice daily or indapamide 1.25–2.5 mg/day can be given. Dietary sodium is restricted to 2 gm/day, and urinary sodium kept to less than 100 mEq.

v) Hyperuricosuric calcium oxalate nephrolithiasis. Increase fluid intake and decrease dietary purine intake, especially red meat, fish, and poultry. Alkalinize urine with potassium citrate to keep pH higher than 6.5 but less than 7.5. Urinary pH greater than 7.5 may facilitate precipitation of calcium phosphate crystals.

Xanthine oxidase inhibitor (allopurinol) may reduce stone formation by 80%. It is given when serum uric acid is higher than 8 mg/dL or urinary uric acid is greater than 800 mg/24 hours. The recommended dose of allopurinol is 100–300 mg daily.

vi) Hypocitraturia. Potassium citrate increases intracellular pH and therefore citrate production. Polycitra K or Urocit K can be used, with a goal to keep urinary citrate above 400 mg. Ingestion of 4 oz. of lemon juice a day mixed with water as lemonade for a total volume of 2 L may increase urinary citrate by twofold.

vii) Enteric hyperoxaluria.
  1. Phase I.
    a. Treat underlying disease (regional enteritis, blind loop syndrome, biliary tract disease, etc.).
    b. Increase fluid intake.
    c. Low dietary fat (50 gm/day) and oxalate.

    d. Calcium supplementation, 2–3 tablets (500 mg each) with each meal. Use calcium citrate (better than calcium carbonate).

    e. Cholestyramine, 1–4 gm four times daily with meals and at bedtime.

  2. Phase II (add if phase I is unsuccessful).

    a. Pyridoxine (vitamin B_6) 25–50 mg two to four times daily.

    b. Potassium citrate to increase urinary citrate as an inhibitor.

    c. Magnesium supplement with magnesium gluconate 0.5–1 gm three times daily.

    d. Allopurinol should be added if the stones contain uric acid.

viii) Primary hyperoxaluria. Pyridoxine can decrease endogenous production of oxalate. The dose is 100–800 mg/day. Oral orthophosphate (2 gm, of elemental phosphorus per day) can be given in four divided doses. Also oral magnesium, potassium citrate supplements, and increased fluid intake can be used. A combined liver/kidney transplant may be necessary in pyridoxine-resistant patients.

b) Uric Acid Stones

i) Increase fluid intake especially at night to increase urine volume to 2 L/day.

ii) Decrease dietary animal protein (8–10 oz. of animal protein/day) to decrease sulfur content. A vegetarian day once weekly with no animal protein is recommended.

iii) Urinary alkalinization with potassium citrate to keep urine pH above 6.5. Patients can check their urine pH using nitrazine papers and adjust the dose accordingly. If urine pH remains at or below 6.0, check patient compliance to low protein diet and medication intake.

iv) Acetazolamide (Diamox) is given at a dosage of 250–500 mg at bedtime to maintain an acceptable urine pH at night.

v) Allopurinol is given if urinary uric acid remains at or above 800 mg/day despite good dietary compliance and urine pH equal to or above 6.5.

c) Cystine Stones

i) Patients should increase fluid intake to maintain urine output more than 3 L/day to allow maximal dissolution of cystine stones. Urinary alkalinization with potassium citrate is used to keep urine pH 7.0–7.5. This increases cystine solubility by threefold.

ii) If urine cystine is above 500 mg/L or the previous measures are ineffective, D-penicillamine is used. It forms a soluble disulfide with cysteine, thereby decreasing the availability of free cysteine to form cystine. Each 250-mg dose decreases cystine concentration by 75–100 mg/day. This therapy has many side effects and should be discontinued once stone dissolution occurs. Thiola (mercaptopropionylglycine) has been shown to be as effective as D-penicillamine but with a better safety profile. Thiola is now used more widely than D-penicillamine. Captopril contains sulfhydryl groups that bind cysteine and thus decreases urinary cystine excretion. It is better tolerated than other medications and is a good choice when thiols are not tolerated.

C. Surgical Management of Nephrolithiasis

1. General

a) On presentation, 66–75% of stones are located in the ureter, 80% of which are 4 mm or less.

b) Seventy-five to 80% of stones pass spontaneously.

c) Indications for surgical intervention include persistent renal colic refractory to oral pain medications, the presence of obstructive uropathy secondary to stones, refractory hematuria, urinary infections, struvite stones, and the size and composition of the stone.

D. Therapeutic Modalities

1. Extracorporeal Shock Wave Lithotripsy (ESWL)

a) The first commercially available kidney stone lithotriptor, the Dornier Human Model 3 (HM3), was introduced in 1983.

b) The first patient treated in the United States with ESWL was at the Methodist Hospital of Indiana in February 1984.

c) Principle: Shock waves are high-energy focused pressure waves that can travel in air or water. When passing through two different mediums of different acoustic impedence, energy is released, which results in the fragmentation of stones. Shock waves travel harmlessly through substances of the same acoustic density. Because water and body tissues have the same density, shock waves can travel safely through skin and internal tissues. The stone is a different acoustic density and when the shock waves hit it, they shatter and pulverize it. Urinary stones are thus fragmented, facilitating in their spontaneous passage.

d) Lithotripsy devices all share four main features.

   i) Energy source (electrohydraulic, piezoelectric, electromagnetic).

   ii) Coupling mechanism (water bath or water cushion and gel).

   iii) Focusing device (ellipsoid, spherical disc, acoustic lens).

   iv) Stone localization (fluoroscopy, ultrasound).

e) The Dornier HM3 device used an ellipsoid reflector and fluoroscopy guidance to localize the stone. One third of the energy is unreflected and unfocused leaving the ellipsoid slightly ahead of the focused waves. These unfocused waves, called precursorial shock waves, are painful when they strike the skin. Newer devices now eliminate the water bath of the HM3 and deliver shock wave energy across a soft membrane that couples to the patient with gel (Figure 8-1).

f) Indications for ESWL. Renal and ureteral calculi at all locations that require surgical treatment can be treated with ESWL. The overall success for stones less than 2 cm is 80–90%. Stones in a lower pole calyceal location and impacted ureteral calculi have a 60–70% chance of successful fragmentation. It may be difficult for a patient to clear stone fragments from a lower pole calyx. Postprocedure positioning exercises may help stone fragments clear. Impacted ureteral calculi may benefit from pre-ESWL manipulation into a nonobstructing upper tract position. A ureteral stent is usually placed at the time of manipulation to help fragments clear. In general, patients require some type of anesthesia to control pain during ESWL procedures. Intravenous sedation may be adequate with some types of ESWL technology, but general anesthesia with control of respiratory movement of the kidney has been shown to facilitate stone fragmentation with ESWL.

g) Contraindications of ESWL.

   i) Absolute: pregnancy, bleeding diathesis, and obstruction below the level of the stone.

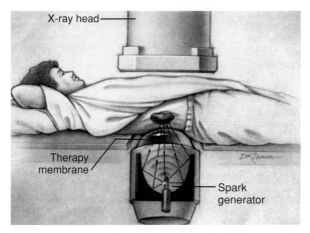

FIGURE 8-1. Basic design of extracorporeal shock wave lithotriptor. Using fluoroscopy the urinary stone is localized at the second focus point.

    ii) Relative: calcified arteries and/or aneurysms and cardiac pacemaker (pacemaker should be reprogrammed).
  h) Complications of ESWL.
    i) Failure to fragment the stone or inadequate fragmentation occurs in 10–20% of treatments. Multiple or large fragments may cause an obstruction of the ureter and pain. Additional treatment will be required, such as repeat ESWL or ureteroscopy and stone fragment manipulation.
    ii) Complications related to shock wave include skin bruising, subscapular and perinephric hemorrhage, pancreatitis, hearing loss, and urosepsis.
  i) Adjunctive modalities. Stents are used with stone burdens greater than 1.5 cm to decrease the risks of obstruction and sepsis. Stents are used to increase the treatment success with upper or midureteral calculi by pushing the stone into the renal pelvis or simply by-passing the stone. Used only when patients are symptomatic preop.
  j) Combined therapy. Large stone burdens or staghorn calculi often require initial debulking with percutaneous procedures followed by ESWL for residual stones.

2. Percutaneous Nephrolithotomy (PCNL)

a) Indications.
   i) Staghorn calculi. The American Urological Association (AUA), in 1994, published recommendations targeting the treatment of staghorn calculi. Their guidelines recommend PCNL as the first-line treatment followed by ESWL or repeat PCNL as needed.
   ii) Large renal stone burden. Primary PCNL for calculi greater than 3 cm carries a success rate approaching 100%, with a lower rate of ancillary procedures (8%).
   iii) Large lower pole renal calculi. There is a much lower success rate with ESWL due to the impedance of gravity-assisted drainage. PCNL is more cost-effective than ESWL for lower pole calculi greater than 1 cm.
   iv) Cystine calculi. Although cystine calculi are ductile (firm) and resistant to ESWL, they are actually softer than other calculi types in terms of microhardness. This feature makes them suitable for ultrasonic lithotripsy or laser fragmentation.
   v) Abnormalities of renal and upper tract anatomy. Percutaneous approach is favorable in patients with UPJ obstruction, caliceal diverticula and obstructed infundibula (hydrocalyx), ureteral obstruction, malformed kidneys (e.g., horseshoe and pelvic), and obstructive or large adjacent renal cysts.
   vi) Abnormalities of patient anatomy. Occasionally, obesity or musculoskeletal deformity may prevent the use of ESWL. In contrast, the effectiveness of PCNL is generally not affected by obesity, although modification of the technique is necessary.
   vii) Shock wave lithotripsy and ureteroscopy failures.
   viii) Nephrolithiasis in transplanted kidneys. With the kidney located superficially in the iliac fossa, ultrasound can localize the site of the calculi with precision, then appropriate access for PCNL is obtained.
b) Contraindications of PCNL include uncontrolled bleeding diathesis, untreated UTI, and inability to obtain optimal access for PCNL due to obesity, splenomegaly, or interposition of colon.
c) The technique is establishment of access at a lower pole calyx, dilation of the tract with a balloon dilator or Amplatz dilators under fluoroscopy, and stone removal with graspers or its fragmentation using electrohydraulic, ultrasonic, or laser lithotripsy. A nephrostomy tube is left

for drainage or a ureteral stent. An antegrade nephrostogram is performed in 24–48 hours to ensure adequate
drainage. If the kidney is adequately draining with no
residual stones, the nephrostomy tube is removed.

d) Complications of PCNL include hemorrhage (5–12%),
perforation, and extravasation (5.4–26%); damage to
adjacent organs (1%); ureteral obstruction (1.7–4.9%);
and infection/urosepsis (3%).

e) PCNL has a success rate of 98% for renal stones and
90% for ureteral stones (Figure 8-2).

3. Rigid and Flexible Ureteroscopy (URS)

a) This remains the gold standard for treatment of middle
and distal ureteral calculi.

b) Rigid ureteroscopes are easier for stone manipulation
because of better flow and visibility.

c) Flexible ureteroscopes are available for diagnostic and
therapeutic uses. Because of their deflection capabilities,
they can access the entire upper urinary tract.

d) The stones are removed using the stone basket or graspers. Alternatively, endoscopic lithotripsy devices are
used for stone fragmentation (electrohydraulic, ultrasonic, or laser lithotripsy).

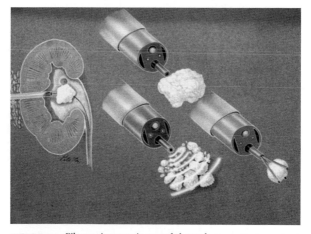

FIGURE 8-2. Fiberoptic scope is passed through a percutaneous tract
and an ultrasonic probe fragments the stone, which can be removed
by suction or with grasping forceps. (Courtesy of David Klemm,
Medical Illustration Department—Georgetown University.)

e) Efficacy of URS includes success rates of 98–99% for distal ureteral calculi, 51–97% for midureteral calculi, and 58–88% for upper ureteral calculi.

f) Complications of URS include failure to retrieve the stone, mucosal abrasions, false passages, and ureteral perforation; complete ureteral avulsion; ureteral stricture (3–11%); and urosepsis.

4. Open Surgery

a) Since the era of ESWL, advanced PCNL, and ureteroscopic techniques, its role has diminished to less than 1%.

b) It is still indicated for large complete staghorn calculi and large stone burden in conjunction with UPJ obstruction.

5. Factors Influencing Therapeutic Choice

a) Stone burden (size and number). ESWL treatment of large stones (greater than 2 cm) creates a large quantity of fragments called "Steinstrasse" (street of stone), which may accumulate in the ureter and cause obstruction. Stones larger than 2 cm in diameter are best treated with PCNL due to higher stone-free rates and lower retreatment rates. Multiple smaller stones may be easily targeted by ESWL. Most complete staghorn calculi are best managed initially by percutaneous debulking followed by ESWL of residual fragments.

b) Stone location. Renal and upper ureteral stones are best managed with ESWL or PCNL. Lower ureteral stones are best managed with ureteroscopy using basket extraction or in situ lithotripsy with a Holmium laser or electrohydraulic lithotripsy. Lower pole calyceal stones are more accessible with PCNL than those in the upper pole. Narrowed calyceal infundibulum or UPJ decreases the stone free rate after ESWL and stones are best managed percutaneously.

c) Stone composition. If stone analysis is not available, composition is suggested by history and radiographic appearance. Pure calcium phosphate and calcium oxalate monohydrate stones may be refractory to ESWL. Calcium oxalate dihydrate stones fragment easily with ESWL. Cystine calculi are resistant to fragmentation with ESWL but may be degraded by ultrasonic/laser energy. Uric acid calculi are easily fragmented by ESWL.

d) Extraurinary factors. The presence of retroperitoneal masses, bony abnormalities such as scoliosis, coagulation abnormalities, pregnancy, cardiac pacemakers, and extrarenal vascular calcifications may influence the choice of therapy.

e) Bladder calculi can be managed with laser lithotripsy or electrohydraulic lithotripsy or a combination of both. In some cases, stones may be removed by opening the bladder at the time of a suprapubic or retropubic prostatectomy.

SELF-ASSESSMENT QUESTIONS

1. A 31-year-old man presents to the emergency room with colicky left flank pain radiating to his groin. He is afebrile, has no significant past medical history, and has never had a kidney stone. A CT scan reveals a 4-mm distal left ureteral stone. How would you manage this patient?

2. A 42-year-old morbidly obese woman presents to your office with a history of recurrent renal calculi requiring surgical intervention. A stone analysis reveals that her stone is composed of calcium oxalate. She wants to know how she can reduce her rate of stone recurrence. How would you counsel her?

3. What is the differential diagnosis for a pure calcium phosphate stone?

4. A 35-year-old man with a long history of cystine stones has been poorly compliant with his medications. He currently has bilateral staghorn calculi. What are the treatment options for this patient, both immediate and long term?

5. What dietary factors can contribute to the development of calculi?

SUGGESTED READINGS

1. Borghi L, Schianchi T, Meschi T, et al: Comparison of two diets for the prevention of recurrent stones in idiopathic hypercalciuria. *N Engl J Med* 346:77–84, 2002.
2. Coe FL, Evan A, Worcester E: Kidney stone disease. *J Clin Invest* 115:2598–2608, 2005.
3. Evan AP, Coe FL, Lingeman JE, Worcester E: Insights on the pathology of kidney stone formation. *Urol Res* 33: 383–389, 2005.
4. Lingeman JE, Kim SC, Kuo RL, et al: Shockwave lithotripsy: anecdotes and insights. *J Endourol* 17:687–693, 2003.
5. Parks JH, Worcester EM, O'Connor RC, Coe FL: Urine stone risk factors in nephrolithiasis patients with and without bowel disease. *Kidney Int* 63:255–265, 2003.

C H A P T E R 9

Urologic Emergencies

Jeffrey P. Weiss, MD, FACS and
Ira J. Kohn, MD

I. INTRODUCTION

This chapter is designed to aid the urologist when called to
the emergency room (ER) or to a hospitalized inpatient
for matters worthy of immediate attention. Urinary trauma,
stones, sepsis, and sexually transmitted diseases are the
topics of specific chapters covered in detail elsewhere in this
manual. Apart from the four immediately aforementioned
issues, the following is an outline of reasons a urologist will
make an unscheduled trip to evaluate and treat a hospital
inpatient or outpatient:

- Gross hematuria
- Urinary retention
  - Noncatheterized patient
  - Catheterized patient
- Flank pain
  - Ureteral obstruction
    - Stone
    - Clot
    - Malignancy
      - Extrinsic
      - Intrinsic
    - Surgical complication
  - Renal vascular occlusion
    - Arterial
    - Venous
  - Renal hemorrhage
- Scrotal pain
  - Torsion of testis
  - Epididymitis
  - Torsion of appendages
  - Tumor
- Fractured penis
- Anuria
- Priapism
  - Low flow
  - High flow

- Genital skin problems
  - Phimosis
  - Paraphimosis
  - Balanoposthitis
  - Fournier's gangrene
  - Zipper injuries

II. GROSS HEMATURIA

When called to see a patient with gross hematuria the urologist should see to it that a cart containing equipment to satisfactorily place a new catheter is at the ready. The cart will have a wide assortment of Foley catheters including coude tip, as well as filiforms and followers, sounds, and a catheter guide or stylet. It is likely that a standard 16-F Foley catheter is in place, as passage of this type of catheter is generally a reflex response to gross hematuria on the part of nonurologic medical personnel. Often the catheter tip has not quite made its way into the urinary bladder (e.g., is held up in the prostatic urethra). If the urine is densely bloody, an attempt to ascertain position of the catheter should be made by means of gentle irrigation with a catheter-tip syringe, at first using only a small amount of irrigant. If possible, a urologic history should be sought, because patients with known urethral stricture disease or small, noncompliant bladders (e.g., due to prior pelvic radiation therapy) will cause special difficulty in catheter placement even by the experienced urologist. In the case of satisfactory catheter placement in which irrigant immediately exits around the catheter, a small rigid bladder should be suspect and confirmed with cystography. Perforation is an increased risk for such bladders, in which irrigant will flush in easily but is not easily withdrawn. The flexible cystoscope is ideally a standard device available on the hospital "GU cart" to aid in anatomic diagnosis of the source of hematuria as well as to be an invaluable aid to management of Foley catheter placement. Once the catheter is ascertained to be in good position and the bladder of normal capacity and compliance, clot irrigation may follow through a large-bore catheter. Generally more than one 60-mL syringeful of irrigant will have to be instilled to aspirate clot. Suction on the syringe barrel will remove clot after which time the remaining irrigant is allowed to drain by gravity so as not to insidiously overdistend the bladder. The procedure is then repeated as many times as necessary to clear all clot. When the procedure is deemed too painful by the medical staff or patient, clot removal should be done under general anesthesia, even if it is considered risky. Patients with heart disease are often safer asleep in the hands of an anesthesiologist than when writhing in pain on a hospital floor at the mercy of an insensitive staff urologist. Aggressive irrigation should not be done blindly at the bedside when either catheter position or bladder integrity is in doubt. Once clots are entirely removed, continuous bladder irrigation (CBI) with physiologic saline solution is recommended for lower urinary tract bleeding. If bleeding comes from an upper tract lesion such as renal tumor, clots entering the bladder will be already formed, and CBI will be useless. In this case, intermittent hand irrigation is preferable, followed by efforts to stop bleeding from the upper tract source.

Once catheter management has been optimized, the urologist should go through an algorithm to assess the cause of hematuria and, when possible, institute therapy to control it. Thus, check the chart to see if the patient's initial (uninstrumented) urinalysis (UA) was normal. If so, the hematuria is often simply the result of complicated Foley catheter insertion. If there was pyuria to any degree, infection should be suspected and treated. If the patient has a coagulopathy, its etiology should be sought and reversed if indicated. If coagulation defects are intentionally induced (e.g., warfarin or platelet inhibitors), discussion with the medical staff as to its degree of necessity should be promptly initiated. Cessation of such anticoagulation will usually result in correction of hematuria, although it may be necessary to continue anticoagulation despite hematuria if the underlying condition necessitating its use is critical. Ideally computed tomographic urography and cystoscopy should be done at a safe and convenient time after the emergent treatment of hematuria for completeness, even when mundane local causes such as Foley catheter trauma or infection are suspected.

III. URINARY RETENTION

A. Noncatheterized Patient

Whenever possible it is useful to try to obtain a history of prior difficulties with passage of a Foley catheter owing to urethral stricture, bladder neck contracture, or small capacity fibrotic/end-stage bladder. In men, a coude catheter will usually overcome obstruction caused by trilobar/median lobe hyperplasia. When this fails, gentle passage of a van Buren sound will allow for determination of the site of obstruction, which may simply be scarring of the bladder neck in which case a catheter guide will successfully result in Foley placement. If urethral stricture is suspected on the basis of sound passage, it is far less traumatic to utilize filiforms and followers to dilate the stricture than sounds. If a flexible cystoscope is available, it should be used for the same purpose; passage of a flexible guidewire may then facilitate passage of a Councill-tip catheter (one containing a center lumen with end-hole). The latter will more likely pass when a 5-F open-ended ureteral catheter is first passed over the wire to establish a stiffer tract over which to pass the Councill catheter. Interventional radiologists are helpful in diagnosing the etiology of infravesical obstruction and subsequent passage of urethral drainage catheters using guidewire exchange techniques under radiologic guidance.

Pitfalls in placement of drainage catheters in patients in retention include sepsis and postobstructive diuresis. The former may be prevented by checking a UA prior to instrumentation with appropriate antimicrobial prophylaxis when the UA is abnormal. The latter will occur when obstruction is long-standing and associated with hydronephrosis, hypertension, volume overload, and renal insufficiency.

B. Catheterized Patient

Urinary retention in a patient with a Foley catheter installed may be due to obstruction of the drainage lumen by clot, stone, tissue, or debris. Gentle irrigation may suffice to clear the obstructing agent. Obtaining a history of the circumstances surrounding placement of the catheter as well as inspection of catheter position may lead to clues as to the etiology of obstruction. Thus, for example, if a catheter appears to be inserted only a short way into the urethra, the tip may not be seated well into the bladder. The most common scenario would be difficult catheter insertion followed by inflation of the balloon in the prostatic fossa. Bladders with very small capacity may cause confusion as to adequate placement, and irrigation may be of little help as irrigant may rapidly exit around the catheter. Replacement of the catheter should be done as described in the "Gross Hematuria" section. Cystography may additionally be invaluable to confirm catheter position and, at times, as an aid to catheter placement. When placement of a urethral catheter proves too difficult or impossible, percutaneous placement of a suprapubic drainage catheter may be done either as a bedside procedure using a Stamey-type of catheter in case of a palpable bladder, or one guided by x-ray or ultrasound when the status of bladder filling is indeterminate.

IV. FLANK PAIN

A. Ureteral Obstruction

1. Stone

The mainstay for current diagnosis of obstructing ureteral calculus is noncontrast computed tomography (CT) scanning. All stones are visible on CT with the exception of indinavir stones. Matrix calculi are difficult to detect by CT, but careful inspection with the help of computer-generated tools such as bright and contrast adjustment may reveal such low-density material in the urinary tract. Further discrimination of the type of stone may be discerned through analysis of Hounsfield unit density. Calcium oxalate stones, for example, have a Hounsfield density range of 650 units as compared with uric acid calculi whose Hounsfield density is in the range of 350 units. Ultrasound is unfortunately nonspecific in that the presence of hydronephrosis correlates only poorly with the diagnosis of acute urolithiasis. However, stones keep company with other stones so that, if the clinical history and UA are consistent with stone and ultrasound discloses the presence of nephrolithiasis, a presumptive diagnosis may be made. Ultrasound has its greatest application during pregnancy owing to the lack of ionizing radiation, as well as in follow-up of patients suspected of having passed calculi. However, sonographic resolution of hydronephrosis noted during the acute episode is suggestive, but not assurance, of interim stone passage.

2. Intrinsic Noncalculous Ureteric Obstruction

All that is acute ureteral colic is not stone. Blood clot owing to urinary tract infection, stone, coagulopathy, or upper tract malignancy may cause acute ureteral obstruction. Fungus balls should be suspected in the milieu of a history of chronic obstructive uropathy combined with frequent or prolonged antibiotic therapy for bacterial urinary infection. Diabetics and immunocompromised patients (e.g., those with acquired immunodeficiency syndrome [AIDS], transplant immunosuppressive therapy, or cancer treated by chemotherapy) are particularly at risk for development of fungus balls, which may derive from a variety of micro-organisms such as *Monilia* and *Aspergillus*. Fungus balls may be detected as low-density structures in the urinary tract. Removal by means of endoscopic procedures using percutaneous and ureteroscopic approaches may be necessary adjunctive treatment to antifungal therapy in these patients. Cholesteatoma, keratinizing desquamative squamous metaplasia of the upper urinary tract, is a rare cause of ureteral obstruction and flank pain and is a reactive phenomenon associated with chronic urinary tract infection whose exact pathophysiology is indeterminate. Management may employ minimally invasive techniques such as ureteronephroscopy although advanced cases may result in nephrectomy.

3. Extrinsic

Cancer arising in organs adjacent to the urinary tract may gradually occlude the ureters unilaterally or bilaterally. However, there is usually a point at which such obstruction becomes acutely symptomatic due to associated urinary infection or renal failure when both kidneys are involved or in cases of solitary functioning kidney. In this case, emergency evaluation and treatment are warranted. Cancer of the uterus, bowel, and pancreas and lymphoma are the most common causes of ureteral obstruction owing to nonurinary malignancies. Treatment is generally with double pigtail ureteral stent placement or percutaneous nephrostomy. Women with cervical cancer having undergone high-dose pelvic radiation are at risk for development of hematuria and vesicovaginal fistula when treated with chronic indwelling ureteral stents; these patients are sometimes best served with simple nephrostomy.

4. Intrinsic

Cancer of the prostate, bladder, renal pelvis, and ureter constitute the usual gamut of intrinsic urinary tract malignancies causing acute symptomatic obstruction and emergency management. Radiographic imaging with CT and retrograde urography as well as endoscopic techniques to diagnose the primary tumor are carried out along with establishment of acute drainage using similar management strategies as those outlined previously. Retroperitoneal fibrosis may cause acute unilateral or bilateral obstruction. Etiologies include idiopathic as well as aneurysm of adjacent great vessels. Ureteral stent placement is usually easy and effective as initial management.

5. Surgical Complication

Ureters are sometimes inadvertently occluded or partially resected during surgical procedures such as hysterectomy and bowel resection. Intraoperative recognition of this complication will greatly mitigate the degree of difficulty of restoration of intrinsic urinary tract drainage. The urologist can count on the occasional instance in which he or she is called emergently to the operating room to evaluate a ureteral injury. Ureteral trauma will be explored further in the formal Urinary and Genital Trauma chapter elsewhere in this manual. Unfortunately, recognition of iatrogenic acute ureteral injury is often delayed by days, weeks, or months. Diagnostic and management strategies involve the usual armamentarium of various forms of urography and drainage using endoscopic or percutaneous techniques.

B. Renal Vascular Occlusion

1. Arterial

Occlusive arterial disease, whether intrinsic (renal arterial stenosis) or extrinsic (embolic phenomena), can result in acute renal ischemia and accompanying renal pain mimicking ureteral obstruction. In this situation, the urologist will be called to evaluate a patient with flank pain and microscopic or gross hematuria who will have no evidence for urolithiasis on noncontrast CT scanning. A history of atrial fibrillation should be sought as well as whether the patient has had prior open heart surgical placement of valvular prostheses. Intracardiac thrombus owing to acute myocardial infarction as well as vegetations associated with endocarditis may result in emboli to the renal arterial vasculature. Diagnosis of renal ischemia/infarction is most easily made during the arterial phase of the contrast CT scan, which demonstrates a characteristic wedge-shaped area of hypoperfused renal parenchyma. Nuclear renal scanning, although useful as a determinate of vascular perfusion, is nonspecific in diagnosis of acute renal infarction whether segmental or total. Once diagnosed, acute renal vascular occlusion may be treated with systemic anticoagulation in case of thromboembolic disease and endovascular stent reconstitution of arterial blood flow when technically possible.

2. Venous

Renal vein thrombosis is a rare cause for acute flank pain and is associated with dehydration, hypercoagulable states, extrinsic renal vein narrowing occasioned by retroperitoneal tumor or fibrosis, and glomerulonephritis. Diagnosis once again is usually suspected based on the ubiquitous CT scan, which reveals an enlarged, congested kidney that has reduced or absent function after administration of intravenous contrast media. Anticoagulation with heparin or clot-dissolving agents can result in restoration of renal function.

C. Renal Hemorrhage

Nontraumatic renal hemorrhage is due to bleeding from pre-existing renal tumors of any size. These may be benign (angiomyolipoma, more likely to bleed when >5 cm in diameter) or malignant (renal cell carcinoma). Arteriovenous malformations as well as renal artery aneurysms may be sources of acute renal hemorrhage causing acute flank pain with or without hematuria. Patients taking anticoagulants, particularly warfarin, are at added risk for renal hemorrhage due to underlying renal pathology even when the latter is minor. Treatment utilizes angiographic ablative techniques with or without surgical intervention and reversal of coagulopathy.

V. SCROTAL PAIN

First and foremost, a call to see the patient with acute scrotal pain should lead to prompt response owing to the possibility that the underlying condition may be a surgical emergency, namely, testicular torsion. Every other cause for scrotal pain is less urgent outside the realm of trauma.

A. Torsion of Testis

Sudden onset of unilateral persistent scrotal pain in males from approximately age 8 to any age should be evaluated by personnel with expertise in the diagnosis of torsion. Fever, flank pain, and lower urinary tract symptoms are absent in the typical symptom complex, although nausea may be present. Physical exam usually makes the diagnosis: high riding testis with absent cremasteric reflex and lack of relief of pain with caudal scrotal support (Prehn's sign) are the key to physical diagnosis of torsion. Color Doppler ultrasound is helpful to confirm the impression of the lack of torsion. However, a normal color Doppler study should never be substituted for the history and physical exam, which alone will justify operation (unilateral detorsion and bilateral scrotal orchiopexy with nonabsorbable suture) when they are strongly suggestive or torsion. The authors suggest using CV5 Gore-Tex suture, which lays flat and allows tissue ingrowth minimizing the chance for subsequent failure. Manual detorsion may be attempted in the emergency department although it is rarely successful in convincingly resolving torsion. Intraoperative decision as to whether to perform orchiectomy is based on time of onset of pain (less than 8 hours is best; many surgeons will hold out hope for a favorable outcome if pain developed within the prior 24 hours) and appearance at surgery. A blue testis that visibly "pinks up" on the operating table is reasonable for orchiopexy even after more than 8 hours of pain. A necrotic testis should be removed. Strong consideration for orchiopexy on the asymptomatic side should be given in that the "bell clapper deformity" of the twisted testis is usually bilateral putting the remaining testis at risk for future torsion.

B. Epididymitis

Acute scrotal pain is most often due to epididymitis. In boys and young men the etiology is usually inflammatory and in older men the cause is more likely lower genitourinary (GU) infection. UA and culture are mandatory after physical exam, which reveals a swollen, reddened scrotum and epididymal tenderness with relatively less testicular tenderness; testis should be anterior to the epididymis and with a vertical lie. Scrotal ultrasonography will reveal symmetric blood flow to the testes and a swollen hypervascular epididymis. When infection is not suspect, nonsteroidal anti-inflammatory drugs (NSAIDs) and a brief period of rest (3–5 days) usually suffices for treatment. Antibiotics (7–10 days of fluoroquinolone) are reserved for those suspected of having GU infection. Those with fever and leukocytosis may require intravenous antibiotics along with NSAIDs.

C. Torsion of Appendages

The appendix testis is a mullerian remnant, whereas the appendix epididymis is a wolffian remnant. Either may twist on its blood supply and cause an acute pain syndrome often discernible by a focal tender paratesticular mass called a "blue dot sign." Although history and physical accompanied by a competent ultrasound may secure the diagnosis, many such male patients will undergo exploration through an inguinal incision owing to the difficulty in distinguishing torsion of the appendages from neoplasm. In cases in which the diagnosis is clear cut in the emergency department or office setting, the patient may be treated with 72 hours of NSAID and close follow-up.

D. Tumor

Testis pain or palpable mass should be evaluated with sonography, which is sensitive for germ cell tumor. In cases of testis mass, alpha-fetoprotein and beta-human chorionic gonadotropin (HCG) should be sent and inguinal exploration of the testis should be done without delay to institute prompt diagnosis and treatment of testicular cancer or stromal tumor.

VI. FRACTURED PENIS

Rupture of the corpora cavernosa may occur during vigorous sexual intercourse involving turgid erections, which therefore place this condition in the younger male. The usual story is that the erect penis became disengaged from the vagina and hit some impervious part of the female anatomy causing an acute bend in the penis accompanied by the feeling or even "sound" of a snap and followed by acute penile pain of varying degree, loss of erection, and subsequent penile ecchymosis. The ecchymosis takes the distribution of limiting genital fascial barriers along the lines of those involved with trauma to the urethra: If the Buck's fascia is intact, the injury is limited to the space below this fascial level causing mostly penile swelling. If Buck's fascia is disrupted, urinoma/hematoma spreads along the lines of the Colles' fascia to the scrotum, perineum, or anterior abdominal wall, limited at the thigh level owing to the insertion of the Colles' fascia into the fascia lata. Diagnosis is often delayed by the patient who is invariably mortified at the idea of disclosing the circumstances of the injury to emergency medical personnel. The urethra may rupture along with the corpora cavernosa, a problem that can be diagnosed either with retrograde urethrography when suspected preoperatively or during careful urethral dissection and inspection at exploration. Although the diagnosis is always made clinically, magnetic resonance imaging (MRI) may be a useful imaging modality albeit impractical as it is both slow and not always promptly available. Surgical treatment is best carried out promptly on recognition of the injury and may be done either through a circumcising subglanular incision or corporal extroversion through a penoscrotal incision. Suture of the ruptured corpora involves straightforward approximation of tunical edges by absorbable suture such as PDS. Ruptured urethra should be repaired over a urethral catheter with absorbable suture approximating both mucosa and spongiosum.

VII. OLIGURIA AND ANURIA

Urologists are often requested to evaluate an oligo/anuric patient owing to the possibility that upper or lower urinary tract obstruction may contribute to renal failure. A systematic evaluation should allow for prompt identification and treatment of anatomic or functional urinary obstruction.

A. Definition

Anuria: urine output <50 mL/24 hours
Oliguria: urine output <500 mL/24 hours

B. Differential Diagnosis

1. Prerenal Azotemia

a) Volume depletion (dehydration, hemorrhage)
b) Low cardiac output
c) Renal artery stenosis
d) Systemic vasodilation (septic shock, anaphylaxis, drug overdose)

2. Intrinsic Renal Parenchymal Disease

a) Acute tubular necrosis
b) Acute glomerulonephritis
c) Acute interstitial nephritis
d) Chronic glomerular nephritis

3. Postrenal Azotemia

a) Upper urinary tract obstruction
  i) Calculus
  ii) Tumor
  iii) Papillary necrosis
  iv) Ureteral stricture
b) Lower urinary tract obstruction
  i) Atonic detrusor/detrusor areflexia
    Neurogenic

Spinal cord injury
Cerebral vascular accident
Multiple sclerosis
Peripheral denervation (abdominoperineal resection)
Non-neurogenic
Chronic voiding dysfunction
Obtunded/drug overdose
   ii) Bladder outlet obstruction
      Benign prostatic hypertrophy (BPH)
      Urethral stricture
      Bladder/urethral calculus
      Phimosis

C. Evaluation

1. History

a) Voiding difficulty
b) Urinary tract stones
c) Diabetes
d) Congestive heart failure

2. Physical Examination

a) Signs of dehydration (skin turgor, sunken eyeballs, etc.)
b) Abdominal/flank distention, tenderness, or mass
c) Palpably distended bladder
d) Obstructing phimosis/balanitis xerotical obliterans (BXO)
e) Peripheral edema
f) "Uremic skin frost"

3. Laboratory Studies

a) Blood urea nitrogen (BUN)/creatinine (Cr), electrolyte profile
b) Complete blood count (CBC) (especially regarding anemia)
c) UA (regarding pyuria, hematuria, proteinuria)

4. Urinary Tract Imaging

a) Ultrasound or CT scan
   Hydroureteronephrosis
   Unilateral
   Bilateral
   Renal atrophy/scarring
   Echogenic renal parenchyma
b) Bladder: Postvoid residual urinary volume

D. Management

1. Circumvent Lower Urinary Tract Obstruction

Foley catheter
Suprapubic tube

2. Circumvent Upper Urinary Tract Obstruction

Ureteral stents
Percutaneous nephrostomy

3. Monitor Urine Output

4. Serial BUN/Cr Measurement

5. Correct Electrolyte Profile

6. Nephrology Evaluation

VIII. PRIAPISM

A. Definition

The term priapism is derived from Priapus, the Greek god of fertility and protector of horticulture often depicted with a wooden sickle in his hand and his phallus proudly erect. Priapism refers to a pathologic condition of prolonged penile erection unrelated to sexual stimulation or failing to subside following orgasm. Oftentimes priapism is associated with penile pain although the onset of pain may be delayed until 6–8 hours have elapsed. Priapism has been observed in males of all ages, including infants. The age-related peak incidence of priapism follows a bimodal distribution with the highest incidence occurring between the ages of 5–10 and 20–50 years. The vast majority of causes in the younger age group is secondary to neoplasm or sickle cell anemia (trait).

B. Classification

1. Ischemic

Ischemic, venous, or low-flow priapism refers to a condition of failure of venous outflow with resultant cessation of arterial inflow creating an acidotic and hypoxic environment within the corpora cavernosum. The net effect creates increased intracorporeal pressure similar to a compartment syndrome and acidosis resulting in painful engorgement and eventual smooth muscle necrosis, fibrosis, and permanent erectile dysfunction if not expediently reversed.

2. Nonischemic

Significantly less prevalent than ischemic priapism, nonischemic, arterial, or high-flow priapism is a result of unregulated increased arterial inflow causing prolonged penile tumescence. Perineal or direct penile trauma is the underlying event causing arterial rupture leading to increased intracorporeal arterial inflow. The erection in nonischemic priapism is oftentimes painless and less than fully rigid.

C. Etiology/Pathophysiology

1. Approximately 50% of all episodes of priapism are thought to be idiopathic.
2. Pharmacotherapy.
   a) In adults, inappropriate dosing of intracavernous therapy for erectile dysfunction with vasoactive agents such as alprostadil, papaverine, phentolamine, and combinations thereof are thought to be the most common cause of ischemic priapism. Intraurethral alprostadil suppositories and oral phosphodiesterase inhibitors have a much lower incidence of priapism.
   b) Antidepressants such as trazodone.
   c) Antipsychotics such as chlorpromazine, phenothiazine, and clozapine.
   d) Antihypertensives such as hydralazine, prazosin, and guanethidine.
   e) The high fat content of total parenteral nutrition.
   f) Cessation of anticoagulation with heparin or coumadin may result in a rebound hypercoagulable state.
   g) Recreational drugs such as cocaine or alcohol.
3. Hematologic diseases.
   a) Sickle cell anemia. The oxygen tension in the corpora cavernosa predisposes to erythrocyte sickling leading to venous stasis and obstruction resulting in priapism.
   b) Leukemia.
   c) Hb Olmsted.
   d) Thrombophilia.
4. Neurologic conditions.
   a) Lumbar spinal stenosis.
   b) Cerebrovascular disease.
   c) Seizure disorders.
5. Neoplasm. Bladder and prostate cancer have been implicated in metastatic infiltration of the corpora resulting venous outflow obstruction. This type of

priapism is usually treated with chemotherapy or radiation therapy.
6. Nonischemic priapism usually results from direct trauma to the penis, perineum, or pelvis. The cavernosal artery has been identified as the most commonly injured vessel in nonischemic priapism.

D. Evaluation

1. History.
   a) Duration and quality of erection.
   b) Pain or no pain.
   c) Medication or recreational drug use.
   d) History of sickle trait or hypercoagulable states.
2. Physical examination.
   a) Penile exam will reveal a rigid, painful erection with a softer glans penis with ischemic priapism, whereas a semierect painless penis is often noted with nonischemic priapism.
   b) Signs of genital/perineal trauma.
   c) Regional lymphadenopathy.
3. Laboratory tests.
   a) Aspiration of corporeal blood for blood gas measurement.
      Ischemic: Dark venous blood.
      pH <7.25, PO_2 <30 mm Hg, PCO_2 >60 mm Hg.
      Nonischemic: Bright red arterial blood.
      pH >7.30, PO_2 >50 mm Hg, PCO_2 <40 mm Hg.
   b) Complete blood count (CBC) may suggest underlying leukemia. Sickle prep if appropriate.
4. Doppler ultrasound reveals no cavernosal arterial flow with ischemic priapism, whereas a ruptured cavernosal artery with unregulated blood flow and blood pooling are characteristic of nonischemic priapism.

E. Treatment of Priapism

The ultimate goal of treatment is to cause detumescence that will relieve pain and hopefully decrease the risk for intracorporeal fibrosis that may result in permanent erectile dysfunction in at least 25% of affected patients. Emergency treatment on patient presentation is advised as a time-dependent window of opportunity exists in terms of successful resolution of the priapic episode and maintenance of normal erectile function. Treatment generally follows a stepwise approach based on etiology of priapism.

1. *Ischemic Priapism*

a) The first line of treatment is analgesics or a dorsal penile
nerve block for pain control in combination with intracorporeal irrigation and evacuation of old blood from
the corpora cavernosa utilizing a 19- to 21-gauge butterfly (scalp) needle. If this is unsuccessful, then injection of
an alpha agonist into the corporeal space to cause vasoconstriction is advised. Epinephrine, norepinephrine,
and phenylephrine have all been utilized. Phenylephrine,
a pure alpha-1 adrenergic agonist with minimal cardiac
side effects, has become the agent of choice. Phenylephrine solution is made by mixing 1 mL of phenylephrine 10
mg/mL with 19 mL of normal saline resulting in a final
phenylephrine solution of 500 μg/mL. Phenylephrine
solution is then instilled in aliquots of 500 μg every 5
minutes until detumescence occurs or for a series of
10–12 injections before deemed unsuccessful. Constant
cardiac monitoring of blood pressure and heart rate is
advised during treatment with these sympathomimetic
agents. Lower concentrations should be used in children
and patients with severe cardiovascular disease.

b) Second-line treatments involve the creation of various
surgical fistulas between the engorged corpus cavernosum and the glans penis, corpus spongiosum, and dorsal
or saphenous vein. It is the hope that these fistulas will
spontaneously close sometime after detumescence.

Glans-cavernosal shunts: The **Winter's shunt** is created
by inserting a Tru-Cut biopsy needle through the glans
penis into the corpora cavernosum under local anesthesia. Removal of several cores of tunica albuginea separating the glans and corpora is advised. The *Ebbehoj
procedure* is performed by inserting a number 10 or 15
scalpel blade vertically through the glans penis into the
corpora cavernosa, then rotating the blade 90 degrees
and removing it horizontally. The skin of the glans penis
may then be approximated with an absorbable suture.

Open surgical procedures: An **Al-Ghorab shunt** is created by dorsal dissection at the level of the coronal sulcus
down to the distal tips of the corporeal bodies where
5-mm elliptical incisions are made bilaterally and dark
old blood is evacuated until detumescence ensues. The
incisions are then closed with absorbable sutures. The
Quackels Cavernoso-Spongiosal shunt is created with
the patient in the dorsal lithotomy position through a
perineal incision with dissection carried down to the
bulb of the corpus spongiosum where incisions are made

in the adjacent corpus spongiosum and corpus cavernosum. The corpus cavernosum in then drained of old blood and the two structures sutured together either unilaterally or bilaterally. In the *Grayhack procedure*, the saphenous vein is transected several centimeters inferior to the inguinal ligament at the saphenofemoral junction and mobilized and tunneled subcutaneously to a second incision at the lateral base of the penis where a tension free end-to-side anastomosis is made with the corpora cavernosa. Similarly the deep and superficial dorsal veins of the penis have also been used for cavernoso-dorsal venous shunts.

2. Sickle Cell Associated Priapism

Initial treatment of sickle cell associated priapism should include corporeal aspiration of old blood and, if unsuccessful, injection of a vasoactive agent. Adjunctive treatments that may have some additional benefit in the sickle cell population include hydration, analgesia, oxygenation, and exchange transfusion.

3. Nonischemic Priapism

The initial management of nonischemic priapism is reassurance and watchful waiting. These patients can be observed safely for several months for spontaneous closure of the fistula with no increased incidence of erectile dysfunction. Ice packing may cause vasospasm and thrombosis aiding early spontaneous closure. Definitive treatment of persistent nonischemic priapism requires selective internal pudendal arteriography to identify the fistulous site, followed by selective angiographic embolization, and open surgical ligation reserved for instances of failed repeat embolization.

IX. FORESKIN EMERGENCIES

A. Phimosis

Phimosis is the inability to retract the foreskin over the glans penis due to narrowing, constriction, and/or adhesions. Congenital neonatal foreskin adhesions usually spontaneously lyse during the first several years of life. Forceful retraction of the phimotic foreskin during infancy is ill advised and may result in fissures and eventual scarring of the distal foreskin. Poor genital hygiene may result in chronic infection causing adhesions between the inner foreskin and underlying glans penis as well as fibrosis resulting inability to retract the foreskin. Complications of phimosis include balanitis, posthitis, paraphimosis, voiding dysfunction, and penile carcinoma.

Patients may present with complaints of erythema, itching, discharge, or pain with sexual intercourse. Minor phimosis can be managed with improved genital hygiene and sometimes topical application of a corticosteroid cream. Phimosis preventing emergency catheter placement can oftentimes be circumvented by use of a coude catheter, catheter guide, nasal speculum to visualize the meatus, or flexible cystoscope and guidewire placement. Mild balanoposthitis can be treated with broad-spectrum oral antibiotics. Severe balanitis may require emergency dorsal slit circumcision aided by local anesthesia. Elective formal circumcision should be considered for persistent symptoms or recurrent infection.

B. Paraphimosis

Paraphimosis refers to the retracted foreskin becoming trapped proximal to the glans penis resulting in edema, inflammation, and pain. Left untreated it can progress to ischemia of the glans penis and eventual gangrene. Treatment consists of initial firm compression to decrease edema followed by manual reduction often aided by placement of a lubricant at the level of the proximal glans penis. However, dry gloved hands are essential in gaining traction of the outer foreskin when pulling it back over the glans into the anatomic position. A local anesthetic block can be utilized for pain control during the procedure. In rare instances, direct incision of the constricting band may be necessary to allow manual retraction. Paraphimosis is frequently the result of a partially phimotic foreskin and elective circumcision may be indicated.

X. GENITAL SKIN INFECTIONS

A. Balanoposthitis

Balanitis refers to inflammation of the cutaneous layers of the glans penis, whereas posthitis is inflammation of the prepuce. These two conditions oftentimes occur simultaneously and are associated with phimosis. Meticulous genital hygiene is the cornerstone of prevention. Oral antibiotics (e.g., cephalexin) or antifungals (e.g., fluconazole) in combination with cleansing will often lead to resolution.

B. Scrotal Abscess

Scrotal/perineal abscesses usually result from infection of a local hair follicle (folliculitis) or sebaceous cyst. It is important rule out any associated process that may manifest as drainage of pus in the scrotal region such as an epididymal abscess or tracking perirectal abscess sometimes associated with diverticular disease. Therefore, in addition to physical examination, scrotal ultrasound or pelvic CT scan may be indicated. Management of local scrotal abscesses include treatment with skin coverage antibiotics (e.g., cephalexin) combined with incision and drainage of loculated collections if spontaneous drainage does not occur.

C. Fournier's Gangrene

1. General Characteristics

a) Fournier's gangrene is a fulminant necrotizing fasciitis of the male genitalia and perineum.
b) The greatest incidence is between ages 20 to 50 years with no predilection for race.
c) Mortality rates average 25% despite aggressive treatment.
d) Initiating events include urethral strictures, perianal abscess, fissures, urethrocutaneous fistulas, GU trauma, and instrumentation.
e) Predisposing immunocompromised states such as diabetes mellitus, human immunodeficiency virus (HIV), cancer, and chronic ethanol or intravenous drug abuse are often associated.

2. Pathogenesis

a) Microbiology: Infections are frequently polymicrobial. The most frequently cultured organisms include gram-negative rods from the Enterobacteriaceae family and gram-positive streptococci and staphylococci. Anaerobic bacteria including *Bacteroides fragilis,* streptococci, and *Clostridium* are often present.
b) Pathophysiology: The involved micro-organisms act synergistically causing obliterative endarteritis resulting in soft tissue necrosis and gangrene. Infection usually involves the skin and subcutaneous tissue sparing the underlying muscle. Spread of infection may be initially limited by fascial planes such as Buck's fascia for infections of urethral origin and Colles' fascia for infections of anorectal origin.

3. Diagnosis

A high index of suspicion is tantamount to diagnosis and emergency treatment. Patients typically present with a painful and/or erythematous, edematous, foul-smelling genital cellulitis oftentimes with areas of eschar or necrosis. Crepitus is a classic finding associated with anaerobic infection. CT scan will usually reveal subcutaneous air as well as any associated abnormalities such as diverticular disease or pelvic fluid collections. These patients are often febrile or frankly septic.

4. Treatment

a) Panculture and prompt initiating of treatment with triple antibiotic coverage (e.g., penicillin G 3–5 million units every 6 hours, gentamicin 3–5 mg/daily, and clindamycin 600–1200 mg/day). Adjustment of antibiotics when culture and susceptibility results are known.

b) Metabolic stabilization with vigorous intravenous hydration; correction of electrolyte imbalances and hyperglycemia.

c) Emergency surgery with wide excision and debridement of all devitalized tissue. Mere incision and drainage has been shown to substantially increase mortality rates.

d) Cystoscopy to assess for urethral stricture and suprapubic tube placement.

e) Proctosigmoidoscopy to assess for associated anorectal anomalies and possible bowel diversion.

f) Vigilant postoperative wound examination with repeat debridement if necessary for devitalized tissue. Frequent wound irrigation with hydrogen peroxide, bacitracin, and so forth, and wet to dry dressing changes employing 25% Dakin's solution.

g) Adjuvant hyperbaric oxygen therapy decreases the spread of necrotizing fasciitis especially with gas-forming anaerobic organisms and promotes wound healing.

h) Once a clean bed of granulation tissue is noted, closure by a variety of reconstructive techniques including skin grafting and local flaps may be undertaken.

XI. FOREIGN BODIES

A. Zipper Injuries

Zipper-associated genital lacerations should be treated conservatively with initial pressure to minimize bleeding, careful genital hygiene, and topical application of an antibiotic ointment (e.g., Polysporin) to prevent local irritation.

Zipper entrapment of the penile or scrotal skin requires emergency zipper disassembly. This is accomplished by using a wire cutter to sever the connective metallic assembly of the zipper allowing the teeth of the zipper to separate. A local anesthetic block may help to control pain during the procedure.

B. External Rings

Various types of constricting bands (rings, washers, bolts, pipes, etc.) oftentimes employed purportedly as "sexual aids" may result in local tissue edema secondary to compression making removal challenging. Left in place, tissue necrosis will ultimately ensue. If generous lubrication and compression of local edema do not allow for safe and easy removal, then a standard ring or bolt cutter will need to be utilized. Similarly, a variety of genital piercings, which have recently achieved significant popularity, may serve as a source of inflammation and/or infection necessitating immediate removal.

C. Intraurethral Foreign Bodies

Various foreign bodies placed in the urethra may become trapped. Pretreatment identification of the exact type of foreign body and proximal extent of migration is advised. Evaluate radiographically with CT scan or kidneys, ureters, and bladder (KUB) x-ray if the object is completely radio-opaque (screws, BBs, etc.). If feasible, attempt endoscopic extraction. Objects located proximal to the external sphincter or densely embedded/adherent to local tissue may require open exploration and removal. Irregularly shaped, sharp, or relatively large objects, especially in the posterior urethra, may be least traumatically extracted by endoscopic relocation to the bladder and suprapubic cystotomy. Place a Foley catheter postoperatively in an attempt to decrease risk for stricture formation in most instances.

POSTCIRCUMCISION COMPLICATIONS

1. Infection can usually be treated with an oral cephalosporin.
2. Incision separation if small will heal by secondary intent or absorbable suture skin approximation for larger defects.
3. Hematomas if large and painful can be evacuated by separation of skin edges and placement of a compressive but not glans ischemic dressing.

4. Bleeding is usually controlled by application of manual pressure for 10–15 minutes. Persistent bleeding may require topical cauterization with a silver nitrate applicator stick or placement of an absorbable suture. Brisk bleeding from the ventral surface is often indicative of laceration of the frenular artery and will require suture ligation for hemostasis.

SELF-ASSESSMENT QUESTIONS

1. Describe the various imaging modalities available to diagnose acute obstruction in cases of stone, intrinsic or extrinsic tumor, blood clot, or pregnancy.
2. What are the underlying medical conditions that predispose to acute renovascular occlusion (arterial, venous)?
3. Create an algorithm for treatment of acute ischemic priapism.
4. What is the single best test for diagnosis of testis torsion?
5. The disruption of which fascial layer determines the route of extravasation of urine and/or blood following penile fracture?

SUGGESTED READINGS

1. Edelstein CL, Alkunaizi A, Yaqoob MM, et al: Etiology, pathogenesis, and management of renal failure. In Walsh PC, Retik AB, Vaughan ED Jr, Wein AJ (eds): *Campbell's Urology,* 7th ed. WB Saunders, Philadelphia, pp 315–341.
2. Nakada SY, Hoff DG, Attai D: Determination of stone composition by noncontrast spiral computed tomography in the clinical setting. *Urology* 55:816–819, 2000.
3. Sadeghi-Nejad H, Seftel AD: The etiology, diagnosis and treatment of priapism: review of the American Foundation for Urologic Diseases consensus panel report. *Curr Urol Rep* 3:492, 2002.
4. Shingal R, Payne CK: Emergency room urology. In Hanno PM, Malkowicz SB, Wein AJ (eds): *Clinical Manual of Urology.* McGraw Hill, New York, 2001.
5. Siroky MD, Oates RD, Babayan RK (eds): *Handbook of Urology: Diagnosis & Therapy.* Lippincott Williams & Wilkins, Philadelphia, 2004.
6. Walsh PC, Retik AB, Vaughan ED, et al (eds): *Campbell's Urology,* 8th ed. Elsevier, London, 2002.
7. Vick R, Carson C III: Fournier's disease. *Urol Clin North Am* 26:841, 1999.

8. Zaman ZR, Kommu SS, Watkin NA: The management of penile fracture based on clinical and magnetic resonance imaging findings. *BJU Int* 96:1423–1424, 2005.

C H A P T E R 10

Urinary and Genital Trauma

Jonathan L. Wright, MD, MS and
Hunter Wessells, MD, FACS

INTRODUCTION

Trauma is the leading cause of death among young persons, and disability far exceeds mortality. At present, injuries are responsible for 11% of global mortality and 13% of global disability adjusted life years. By 2020, road traffic injuries are projected to become the sixth leading cause of death and the third leading cause of worldwide disability. Urologic injuries, although only accounting for a small percentage of all injuries, are responsible for both mortality and long-term morbidity. Whereas kidney injuries cause acute hemorrhage and can be immediately life threatening, lower urinary tract and genital trauma leads to lifelong disability and impaired quality of life.

KIDNEY INJURIES

Initial Evaluation

The kidneys are the most commonly injured genitourinary organ. Population based studies have determined the rate of renal injury to be 1.1–1.2% of all trauma patients. Evaluation of the kidneys for injury is required in the trauma patient presenting with microscopic or gross hematuria (Figure 10-1). However, the degree of hematuria correlates poorly with renal injury severity, and patients with renal artery thrombosis or pedicle avulsion may not have hematuria. A high degree of suspicion for renal trauma is required for patients who do not meet the hematuria criteria for imaging but who have experienced a fall from a height, have sustained a direct blow to the flank, or have other clinical indicators (e.g., persistent flank pain or severe associated injuries).

Hemodynamically stable patients with suspected renal trauma and indications for imaging should undergo computed tomography (CT) with a portal venous phase scan to identify active arterial bleeding and parenchymal lacerations, followed by 10-minute delayed images to identify urinary

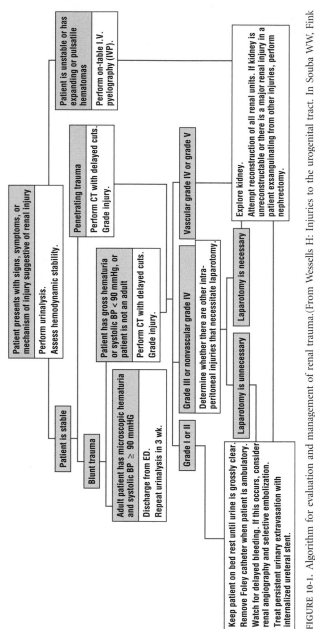

FIGURE 10-1. Algorithm for evaluation and management of renal trauma. (From Wessells H: Injuries to the urogenital tract. In Souba WW, Fink MP, Jurkovich GJ, et al. [eds]: *ACS Surgery.* WEBMD, New York, 2005.)

The following text appears within the flowchart:

Patient presents with signs, symptoms, or mechanism of injury suggestive of renal injury
Perform urinalysis.
Assess hemodynamic stability.

Patient is stable

Blunt trauma

Adult patient has microscopic hematuria and systolic BP ≥ 90 mmHG
Discharge from ED.
Repeat urinalysis in 3 wk.

Patient has gross hematuria or systolic BP < 90 mmHg, or patient is not an adult
Perform CT with delayed cuts.
Grade injury.

Penetrating trauma
Perform CT with delayed cuts.
Grade injury.

Patient is unstable or has expanding or pulsatile hematomas
Perform on-table I.V. pyelography (IVP).

Grade I or II

Grade III or nonvascular grade IV
Determine whether there are other intraperitoneal injuries that necessitate laparotomy.

Laparotomy is unnecessary
Keep patient on bed rest until urine is grossly clear. Remove Foley catheter when patient is ambulatory. Watch for delayed bleeding. If this occurs, consider renal angiography and selective embolization. Treat persistent urinary extravasation with internalized ureteral stent.

Laparotomy is necessary

Vascular grade IV or grade V
Explore kidney.
Attempt reconstruction of all renal units. If kidney is unreconstructable or there is a major renal injury in a patient exsanguinating from other injuries, perform nephrectomy.

contrast extravasation. Hemodynamically unstable patients should not undergo CT imaging until other measures have determined that emergent laparotomy is not required. Diagnostic peritoneal lavage (DPL) and ultrasonography have been used in this scenario. If the patient requires immediate laparotomy, on-table intravenous pyelography can provide useful information (see later).

Classification

The American Association for the Surgery of Trauma (AAST) Organ Injury Scale is used to classify blunt and penetrating renal injuries and corresponds closely to the appearance of the kidney on CT (Figure 10-2). A recent study from the National Trauma Data Bank (NTDB) found that the AAST scale for renal injuries predicted morbidity (nephrectomy, dialysis) in both blunt and penetrating injured patients and mortality in blunt trauma patients (Tables 10-1 and 10-2). This confirms earlier validation studies showing a relationship between injury severity and operative interventions on the kidney.

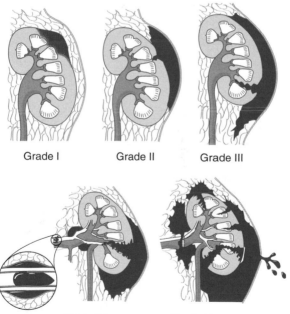

Grade I   Grade II   Grade III

Grade IV   Grade V

FIGURE 10-2. AAST organ injury scale for the kidney. (From McAninch JW, Santucci RA: Genitourinary trauma. In Walsh PC [ed]: *Campbell's Urology*, 8th ed. WB Saunders, St. Louis, 2002.)

Table 10-1:   Multivariate Predictors of Morbidity and Mortality for Blunt Renal Trauma*

	Nephrectomy (n = 289)	Dialysis (n = 33)	Death (n = 709)
AAST I	Ref	Ref	Ref
AAST II	2.5 (1.0–6.2)	1.5 (0.41–5.6)	0.95 (0.65–1.4)
AAST III	12 (5.6–25)	1.3 (0.45–4.6)	1.3 (0.90–2.0)
AAST IV	64 (34–120)	3.7 (1.2–11)	1.4 (0.97–2.0)
AAST V	127 (68–236)	4.7 (1.4–16)	1.9 (1.3–2.7)
Bowel surgery	2.3 (1.8–2.9)	3.9 (1.5–10)	
Spleen surgery	2.2 (1.8–2.8)		2.1 (1.4–3.0)
Liver surgery	1.5 (1.2–2.0)		
ISS > 15			2.8 (1.4–5.6)
ISS > 24			3.0 (2.0–4.4)
ISS > 47			1.7 (1.3–2.3)
SBP < 90			2.0 (1.5–2.6)
Abd AIS > 3		5.3 (1.9–15)	
Head AIS > 3			2.5 (1.9–3.4)
Age > 40 years	1.3 (1.0–1.5)	4.0 (2.2–7.3)	2.0 (1.6–2.4)

*Blank cells indicate the parameter was not an independent predictor for that particular outcome.
AAST, American Association for the Surgery of Trauma; AIS, Abbreviated Injury Scale; ISS, injury severity score; SBP, systolic blood pressure.

Management

Increasingly, renal trauma management is conservative with multiple series showing successful renal preservation despite high-grade injury. The indications for nephrectomy in renal trauma include persistent, life-threatening hemorrhage, pedicle avulsion, or an expanding, pulsatile or uncontained retroperitoneal hematoma. Complications that once required open surgery can be managed nonsurgically: Active arterial bleeding and arterial pseudoaneurysms are controlled with angioembolization, and perinephric abscesses and urinomas can be treated with percutaneous drainage and/or indwelling ureteral stents.

Currently, 20–50% of all penetrating renal injuries and fewer than 5% of blunt injuries are managed operatively. Grade I and II renal injuries should be managed with observation alone. Most grade III and IV injuries can be managed nonoperatively with close monitoring, serial

Table 10-2: Multivariate Predictors of Morbidity and Mortality for Penetrating Renal Trauma*			
	Nephrectomy (n = 333)	Dialysis (n = 6)	Death (n = 249)
AAST I	Ref		
AAST II	1.1 (0.3–3.7)		
AAST III	7.7 (3.2–18)		
AAST IV	25 (10–63)		
AAST V	31 (12–82)		
Firearm injury	25 (10–63)		
Bowel surgery	31 (12–82)		
Spleen surgery			0.42 (0.22–0.81)
Liver surgery			0.44 (0.23–0.87)
ISS > 24			4.6 (2.27–9.2)
SBP < 90			2.8 (1.6–4.9)

*Blank cells indicate the parameter was not an independent predictor for that particular outcome. There were too few patients with dialysis (n = 6) for a meaningful prediction model.
AAST, American Association for the Surgery of Trauma; ISS, injury severity score; SBP, systolic blood pressure.

hematocrit measurement, and repeat imaging in selected cases. Patients are kept on bed rest until the urine is grossly clear. Foley catheter drainage is necessary only until other injuries are stable and the patient can void spontaneously. Thrombosis of the renal artery or its branches is treated nonoperatively unless the contralateral kidney is absent or injured, in which case emergency revascularization is indicated.

Renal exploration often leads to nephrectomy, which may be the result of damage control in the exsanguinating patient or surgeon unfamiliarity with renal reconstructive techniques. Other predictors of nephrectomy include the AAST renal injury scale, the Injury Severity Score (ISS), transfusion requirements, and operations on other intra-abdominal organs.

Operative Management

A significant number of patients with a penetrating injury and a minority of those with blunt trauma require immediate laparotomy before radiographic evaluation. In these patients, if a major renal injury is suspected based on the size of the perinephric hematoma, an intraoperative intravenous pyelogram (IVP) (one-shot IVP) is recommended before renal exploration to confirm the presence of a contralateral functioning kidney and potentially to rule out major injury. A plain abdominal film is obtained 10 minutes after bolus injection of 2 mL/kg of iodinated contrast material. If the injured kidney is adequately imaged and found to be normal, exploration may be omitted. In the critically ill patient with multiple injuries, renal exploration is indicated only if a pulsatile or expanding hematoma is present, in which case a rapid nephrectomy is usually necessary. Less severe injuries can be managed with perinephric drains, embolization, and other adjunctive techniques described later (see the "Complications" section).

Operative management of grade III, IV, and V injuries consists of hemorrhage control first, followed by repair of the collecting system and parenchymal closure. A midline transabdominal incision permits exploration of the kidneys and provides optimal access to the renal hilum. Before opening Gerota's fascia, isolation of the renal artery and vein should be achieved by opening the posterior peritoneum medial to the inferior mesenteric vein or by reflecting the ipsilateral colon (provided that the perinephric hematoma is left undisturbed). Once the renal vessels are isolated, Gerota's fascia is opened. If massive bleeding occurs when the hematoma is entered, Rummel tourniquets or vascular clamps are applied to the renal artery. If bleeding persists, venous injury is likely and the renal vein should be occluded as well. Sharp and blunt dissection to completely expose the kidney facilitates identification of injury to the parenchyma, the renal pedicle, or the collecting system. The renal capsule should be preserved to facilitate subsequent repair.

The principles of renal reconstruction include sharp debridement of the devitalized tissue, achievement of hemostasis, collecting system closure, coverage of the defect, and drainage. Bleeding points must be controlled using figure of eight sutures of fine absorbable monofilament.

Once hemostasis is satisfactory, 2–3 mL of methylene blue is injected into the renal pelvis while occluding the ureter to identify injuries to the collecting system. The collecting system openings are closed with 4–0 absorbable sutures. The defect in the parenchyma can be filled with folded absorbable gelatin sponges as the capsule is closed over the bolsters. In the future, novel hemostatic sponges may provide hemostasis comparable to the classic reconstructive steps. If the renal capsule has been destroyed, coverage options include an omental or perinephric fat flap, a patch of polyglycolic acid or peritoneum, or an entire sac of polyglycolic acid wrapped around the kidney, with the parenchymal edges kept well apposed. Gerota's fascia is not reapproximated. Closed-suction drainage is recommended only after collecting system repair. Internalized stents are reserved for complex injuries (e.g., large lacerations of the renal pelvis or the ureteropelvic junction [UPJ]).

Complications

The most significant early complications are urinary leakage and delayed bleeding. For grade IV injuries with substantial extravasation (Figure 10-3), follow-up imaging 48–72 hours after the initial scan is recommended to evaluate the degree of ongoing urinary extravasation. If the amount of extravasation has not improved, double J ureteral stenting is indicated. The urinary bladder should be drained with a Foley catheter until extravasation resolves, which can take days to weeks. Ultrasonography is useful for following such collections and for reducing the patient's radiation exposure. If the perinephric fluid collection is large enough to compress the ureter or becomes infected, additional percutaneous drainage is required.

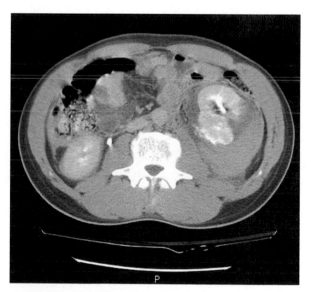

FIGURE 10-3. Grade IV renal laceration with urinary extravasation and perinephric hematoma.

Delayed bleeding is a rare but life-threatening complication of major lacerations. Pseudoaneurysm formation is the most common cause of delayed bleeding and usually occurs within the first 2 weeks post injury. Selective arterial embolization is an effective treatment that obviates the need for exploration in most instances.

Postinjury renal scintigraphy is recommended in patients with grade IV and V injuries to identify patients who are at risk for chronic renal insufficiency. The optimal timing of postoperative nuclear medicine imaging has not been determined, but by 3 months, the hematoma and inflammation related to the injury usually have resolved. Either mercaptoacetylglycine (MAG3), dimercaptosuccinic acid (DMSA), or diethylenetriamine penta-acetate (DTPA) scanning will assess the relative function of the injured kidney.

Hypertension is a rare late complication of renal injury that is renin mediated from an ischemic segment of parenchyma. Etiologies include renal artery injury leading to stenosis, extrinsic compression from urinary or blood extravasation (Page kidney), or arteriovenous fistula. Excision of the nonperfused segment or nephrectomy may be required.

URETERAL INJURIES

Initial Evaluation

Ureteral trauma is rare, accounting for approximately 1% of all genitourinary injuries. Ureteral injuries more commonly occur with penetrating trauma and patients usually have multiple associated abdominal injuries. Hematuria may be absent in 25–70% of patients, which contributes to a delay in diagnosis, especially in blunt trauma patients. A high index of suspicion is thus necessary to prevent a delay in diagnosis with resultant late consequences such as urinoma, sepsis, and nephrectomy. Stable patients with suspected ureteral injuries should undergo a CT with intravenous contrast and delayed images. Unstable patients taken to the operating room without imaging can be evaluated intraoperatively with a one-shot IVP (described previously). In one study, all penetrating ureteral injuries were found at ureteral exploration; indications for exploration include a retroperitoneal hematoma and a projectile trajectory that put the ureter at risk. Injection of indigo carmine into the collecting system identifies sites of laceration or avulsion. Ureteral injury at the UPJ or near the iliac vessels can occur after severe deceleration or ejection from a high-speed vehicle, particularly in children because the hyperextensibility of their spines leading to avulsion at the UPJ.

Management

Management depends on the segment of ureter injured (Figure 10-4) and the timing of diagnosis. Injuries recognized initially should be surgically repaired. If patients are unstable, ligation of the ureter and nephrostomy tube drainage or exteriorization of a ureteral stent allow elective repair either days later or months later. If there was a delay in diagnosis leading to abscess or urinoma formation,

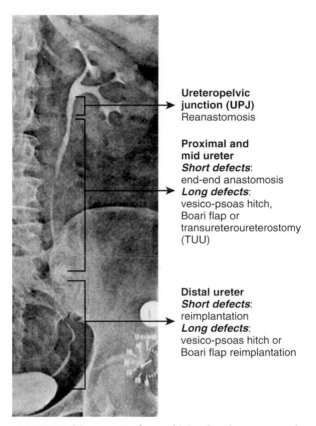

Ureteropelvic junction (UPJ)
Reanastomosis

Proximal and mid ureter
Short defects:
end-end anastomosis
Long defects:
vesico-psoas hitch,
Boari flap or
transureteroureterostomy
(TUU)

Distal ureter
Short defects:
reimplantation
Long defects:
vesico-psoas hitch or
Boari flap reimplantation

FIGURE 10-4. Management of ureteral injury based on segment of ureter injured. (From Kuan J, Routt ML, Wessells H: Genitourinary and pelvic trauma. In Mulholland, MW, Lillemoe KD, Doherty GM, et al. [eds]: *Greenfield's Surgery: Scientific Principles and Practice,* 4th ed. Lippincott, Williams & Wilkins, Philadelphia, 2006.)

percutaneous nephrostomy and ureteral stenting followed by a delayed definitive management as an operative approach at that point is likely to result in nephrectomy.

The principles of ureteral reconstruction include debridement of devitalized tissue, a spatulated tension-free anastomosis, watertight closure, stenting, coverage of the repair, and drainage. Gunshot ureteral injuries should be debrided proximal and distal to the injury until bleeding ureter is encountered, to decrease the risk of anastomosing an ischemic edge from the blast-induced microvascular damage. However, in all cases, mobilization of the ureter should be limited to ensure that the blood supply is not compromised. Partial transections may be closed primarily. All repairs should be performed with interrupted 5.0 or 6.0 absorbable sutures over an internalized or externalized stent. Closed-suction retroperitoneal drainage and Foley catheter decompression of the bladder are essential. Drains can be removed after 2–3 days unless output is consistent with a urine leak as determined by creatinine measurement. Bladder catheterization for 7 days is recommended after reimplantation. In combined bladder and ureteral reconstructions, contrast cystography is indicated before catheter removal. Ureteral stents are removed at 4–6 weeks. Contrast-enhanced CT or renal scintigraphy 3 months after stent removal should be performed to identify silent obstruction.

Upper Ureter

Disruption of the upper ureter or the UPJ is repaired with primary anastomosis of the ureter to the renal pelvis. In addition to a ureteral stent, a nephrostomy tube may be inserted intraoperatively.

Mid Ureter

Ureteral injuries above the pelvic brim that cannot be anastomosed to the renal pelvis are repaired with a ureteroureterostomy. The ureteral ends are spatulated on opposite sides for the anastomosis. In cases of associated colonic, duodenal, or pancreatic injuries, an omentum flap or retroperitoneal fat should be used, when possible, as an additional layer of coverage. In rare cases in which a large defect prohibits ureteroureterostomy, a transureteroureterostomy may be performed. In this case, the injured ureter is directed behind the mesocolon to the contralateral side and anastomosed to a 1- to 2-cm opening in the medial side of the uninjured ureter. A stent (5-French pediatric feeding tube or a single-J ureteral stent) should be placed across the anastomosis and be brought through the bladder.

Distal Ureter

Injuries below the pelvic brim are best managed with reimplantation into the bladder. The distal stump is ligated, and after the anterior bladder wall is opened, the spatulated end of the ureter is brought through a new hiatus on the back wall of the bladder. Larger defects can be bridged with a vesicopsoas hitch after mobilizing the contralateral bladder pedicle. In rare cases in which complex bladder or pelvic vascular injuries preclude extensive pelvic dissection, a transureteroureterostomy may be performed.

Complications

The most common complication of ureteral injury is fistula formation. This usually occurs due to distal obstruction or ureteral necrosis. Fistulas should be managed with antegrade or retrograde drainage of the collecting system with percutaneous or endoscopic techniques. Drainage of periureteral fluid collections is essential. If recognition of an injury or a complication is delayed, reconstruction should be deferred for at least 3–6 months until all inflammation has subsided.

INJURIES TO THE BLADDER

Initial Evaluation

Bladder injury occurs in approximately 1% of all trauma patients, and most are due to blunt injuries and associated with a pelvic fracture. Whereas 90% of bladder ruptures have an associated pelvic fracture, only 9% of pelvic fractures have an associated bladder rupture. However, even in the absence of overt genitourinary injury, there are increasing data to suggest that patients with pelvic fractures are at increased risk of urinary and sexual dysfunction.

Bladder rupture is best diagnosed with CT cystography (Figure 10-5), although plain film cystography is an acceptable alternative. Figure 10-6 illustrates an algorithm for evaluation and management of bladder trauma. The indications for cystography include blunt trauma with gross hematuria in the presence of free abdominal fluid on CT, blunt trauma with a pelvic fracture and any degree of hematuria (>3 red blood cells [RBCs] per high-power field [hpf]), stable penetrating trauma with any degree of hematuria, and an injury to the

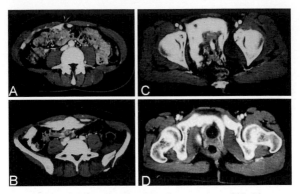

FIGURE 10-5. CT cystogram images of extraperitoneal bladder rupture. Note contrast tracking to the umbilicus (**A**); contrast tracking lateral to colon, not to be confused with contrast outlining loops of small intestine in an intraperitoneal injury (**B**); "molar tooth" configuration of contrast surrounding the bladder in the upper space of Retzius (**C**); contrast surrounding the lower bladder and bladder neck region (**D**).

pelvis. The sensitivity and specificity of CT cystography at one large trauma center were 95% and 100%, respectively. Recently, specific fractures patterns have been identified as predictors of bladder injury, namely pubic symphyseal diastasis >1 cm and obturator ring fracture with >1 cm displacement. Bladder injuries are classified as either extraperitoneal or intraperitoneal. The distinction can be made on CT or conventional cystography and the classification is important because of different management strategies.

Management

Extraperitoneal Injuries

Blunt, extraperitoneal bladder injuries are generally managed nonoperatively with 7–10 days of catheter drainage. Contraindications to a nonoperative approach include penetrating injuries, urinary infection, pelvic fractures requiring internal fixation of the pubis, the presence of bony fragments in the bladder, bladder neck injury, rectal injury, and female genital lacerations associated with pelvic fracture. Stable patients undergoing laparotomy for associated injuries who can tolerate additional procedures are also candidates for operative repair. In patients undergoing internal fixation of the pelvis, the bladder may be approached extraperitoneally through the incision used to expose the pubic symphysis.

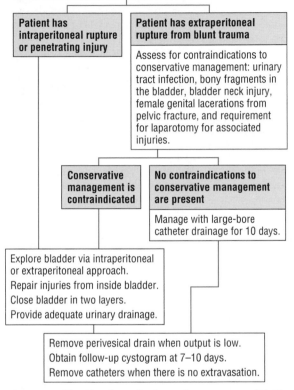

FIGURE 10-6. Algorithm for evaluation and management of bladder trauma. (From Wessells H: Injuries to the urogenital tract. In Souba WW, Fink MP, Jurkovich GJ, et al. [eds]: *ACS Surgery*. WEBMD, New York, 2005.)

Most extraperitoneal bladder injuries associated with pelvic fractures are anteriorly located, small in size, and easily managed without an extensive bladder exploration.

Prior to removing the catheter, CT cystography should be performed. If extravasation persists, the catheter should be left in place and cystography repeated at appropriate intervals until healing occurs.

Intraperitoneal Injuries

All intraperitoneal bladder ruptures require exploration and repair. The bladder is opened vertically at the site of rupture and a full intravesical examination performed to exclude a concomitant extraperitoneal injury, which can occur in 8% of cases. The ureteral orifices and bladder neck should be inspected. Additional lacerations found within the bladder are closed with 3–0 absorbable sutures, approximating the detrusor and mucosa in one layer and providing hemostasis. The primary laceration, usually at the dome, is closed with two layers of continuous 2–0 slowly absorbable sutures; a 20-French urethral catheter should be placed to maximize drainage. Suprapubic catheters are not indicated unless an unrepaired urethral injury is present or severe hematuria resulting from coagulopathy or extensive injuries necessitates additional drainage to allow for clot irrigation and additional bladder decompression. A closed-suction drain near the bladder closure is recommended and can be removed after 2–3 days unless the creatinine level in the drainage fluid indicates urinary leakage. Similar to extraperitoneal injuries, the catheter should be left in place for 7–10 days and cystography performed prior to removing the catheter.

Complications

Complications of bladder injury are primarily due to a delay in diagnosis leading to azotemia, ascites, and sepsis. Bladder neck injury, if not identified and repaired, may result in an incompetent proximal sphincteric mechanism and subsequent incontinence. Persistent leakage after repair is rare and usually responds to catheter drainage. Persistent extravasation suggests catheter obstruction, bony fragments, or ischemic complications of injury or embolization.

<u>URETHRAL INJURIES</u>

Urethral injuries associated with pelvic fracture occur in 3% of males and 6% of females. Only a minority of patients will have concomitant bladder injuries. Characteristics of typical patients with urethral injury include age younger than 40 years; multiple associated injuries to the head, abdomen, and chest; involvement in motor vehicle crashes; and high injury severity scores. Figure 10-7 illustrates an algorithm for the evaluation and management of urethral trauma.

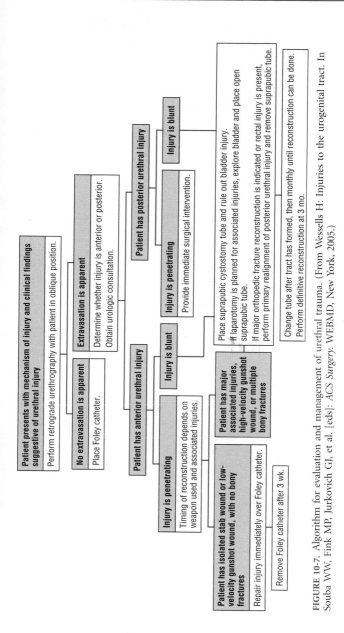

Patient presents with mechanism of injury and clinical findings suggestive of urethral injury

Perform retrograde urethrography with patient in oblique position.

No extravasation is apparent

Place Foley catheter.

Extravasation is apparent

Determine whether injury is anterior or posterior. Obtain urologic consultation.

Patient has anterior urethral injury

Injury is penetrating

Timing of reconstruction depends on weapon used and associated injuries.

Patient has isolated stab wound or low-velocity gunshot wound, with no bony fractures

Repair injury immediately over Foley catheter.

Remove Foley catheter after 3 wk.

Injury is blunt

Patient has major associated injuries, high-velocity gunshot wound, or multiple bony fractures

Place suprapubic cystostomy tube and rule out bladder injury.
If laparotomy is planned for associated injuries, explore bladder and place open suprapubic tube.
If major orthopedic fracture reconstruction is indicated or rectal injury is present, perform primary realignment of posterior urethral injury and remove suprapubic tube.

Change tube after tract has formed, then monthly until reconstruction can be done.
Perform definitive reconstruction at 3 mo.

Patient has posterior urethral injury

Injury is penetrating

Provide immediate surgical intervention.

Injury is blunt

FIGURE 10-7. Algorithm for evaluation and management of urethral trauma. (From Wessells H: Injuries to the urogenital tract. In Souba WW, Fink MP, Jurkovich GJ, et al. [eds]: *ACS Surgery*. WEBMD, New York, 2005.)

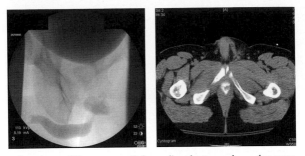

FIGURE 10-8. CT cystogram *(left panel)* and retrograde urethrogram *(right panel)* of urethral disruption demonstrating contrast extravasation.

Mechanisms

Pelvic fractures are the most common cause of posterior urethral injury in males. The classic injury is a distraction injury at the prostatomembranous junction. Variations occur including complete and partial disruption, and the tears can occur either above or below the urogenital diaphragm (Figure 10-8). Multivariable analysis of fracture patterns showed that displaced fractures of the pubis and medial one third of the inferior pubic ramus are independently associated with urethral injury in men.

The female urethra is rarely injured, but a recent review from our institution showed that urethral and bladder neck injuries were always associated with pelvic fracture. Longitudinal tears may originate in the bladder neck, whereas avulsion type injuries probably share similar mechanisms with male type distractions of the membranous urethra.

Anterior urethral (penile and bulbar urethral) injuries are commonly caused by straddle injury, in which the corpus spongiosum is crushed against the pubic symphysis. Other mechanisms include penile fracture, amputation, or penetrating injuries to the genitalia.

Initial Evaluation

Signs and symptoms of urethral injury are variable, and thus careful history, physical examination, and radiographic imaging are critical to determine the location, nature, and extent of injury. Inability to void and painful attempts to void suggest urethral injury. Blood at the urethral meatus, the classic sign of injury to the urethra, indicates that imaging should be performed immediately. Other signs include a palpable bladder, butterfly perineal hematoma, and high riding prostate. In female patients, many urethral and bladder neck injuries are missed and only detected at time of operative exploration. Therefore, the presence of vaginal bleeding should prompt urgent speculum examination and consideration for imaging or cystoscopy.

Imaging of the urethra with urethrography in males and cystography in females remains the recommended initial evaluation for suspected urethral injury. The sensitivity and specificity of urethrography are high in men. Conversely, cystography may miss some female urethral or bladder neck injuries. Thus, in cases of suspected injury not clearly defined on radiographic imaging, we advocate cystoscopy as an adjunctive diagnostic measure.

Management

Traumatic posterior urethral distraction injuries in men have traditionally been managed by means of suprapubic cystostomy, with reconstruction delayed for 3–6 months. Most urethral injuries, however, including female and male injuries, can undergo immediate realignment. Sutured repair is not recommended for male posterior urethral distraction defects but should be used for all female injuries.

Anterior urethral injuries in men are best treated with immediate repair. One exception is the patient with a straddle-type crush injury to the bulbar urethra, which should always be treated with urinary diversion and delayed repair. Another is a high velocity gunshot wound associated with extensive tissue destruction.

Posterior Urethra

Posterior urethral (prostatic and membranous urethral) realignment without sutured repair renders definitive reconstruction unnecessary in a significant percentage of men. Bladder neck injury and female urethral injury warrant early surgical intervention. Simultaneous rectal and vaginal injury may occur in this setting. Evacuation of the pelvic hematoma, irrigation, placement of drains, and primary realignment (men) or repair (women) of the urethra are strongly recommended. Another relative indication for realignment of posterior urethral injuries in men is open reduction and internal fixation of anterior pelvic ring fractures. Realignment allows early removal of suprapubic cystostomy tubes from the orthopedic field.

Primary realignment is usually performed through a lower midline abdominal incision, which allows antegrade passage of instruments through the bladder at the same time as retrograde passage of instruments from the urethral meatus. Flexible cystoscopes or magnetic-tipped catheters advanced under fluoroscopic guidance are used to place a wire into the bladder beyond the injury, and a Council-tip Foley catheter is then advanced over the wire. Neither mucosal approximation nor direct anastomosis is the goal. Suprapubic catheter drainage is not required, but a perivesical drain should be left in place for 48 hours.

Anterior Urethra

Immediate reconstruction is preferred for penetrating injuries of the bulbar and penile urethra and for urethral injuries associated with penile fracture. For these partial or complete transections without major tissue loss, primary repair is associated with a lower stricture rate than simple realignment. Wounds accompanied by major tissue loss and defects larger than 2 cm (e.g., grade V injuries) or complicating associated injuries are best treated with suprapubic tube urinary diversion (see later) and subsequent reconstruction at a tertiary referral center.

Suprapubic Cystostomy

Suprapubic cystostomy remains standard management of prostatomembranous urethral disruption and straddle injuries to the bulbar urethra. Percutaneous placement of the tube under fluoroscopic guidance when possible allows temporary urinary diversion for initial stabilization and evaluation of the patient. Cystography can be performed via the suprapubic tube to rule out bladder injury. Straddle injuries must be treated with diversion unless the disruption is only partial and allows safe passage of a guidewire or catheter under fluoroscopic guidance. Suprapubic cystostomy is recommended for penetrating trauma to the urethra if the injuries were caused by high-velocity weapons and are characterized by extensive tissue loss, if serious associated injuries are present, or if bony fractures prevent proper placement of the patient in the lithotomy position.

Postintervention Care

After primary realignment of urethral injuries, the urethral catheter is left in place for 6 weeks, at which time a pericatheter retrograde urethrogram is obtained, with the expectation that any extravasation will have resolved. The Foley catheter should remain in place for 3 weeks after immediate surgical repair of the anterior urethra, at which time contrast voiding cystoure-thrography is obtained.

If extravasation is present, continued catheter drainage for another 1–2 weeks is needed before repeating the study. If the patient initially underwent diversion with a suprapubic tube alone, the tube should be changed after a tract has formed (usually about 4 weeks after the procedure) and then monthly until reconstruction can be performed. Stricture formation or complete obliteration of the urethra may be the final result of this nonoperative approach. Subsequent radiographic studies will indicate whether secondary endoscopic or open procedures are needed.

GENITAL INJURIES

Genital injuries are significant because of their association with injuries to major pelvic and vascular organs and the chronic disability resulting from penile, scrotal, and vaginal trauma. As trauma is predominantly a disease of young persons, genital injuries affect health related quality of life and contribute to the burden of disease related to trauma. Injuries to the female genitalia have additional consequences when associated with sexual assault and interpersonal violence. A recent Consensus Group on Genitourinary Trauma provided an overview and reference point on the subject. This chapter reviews the mechanism, initial evaluation, and operative management of injuries to the male and female external genitalia.

Mechanisms

The male genitalia have a tremendous capacity to resist injury. The flaccidity of the penis limits the transfer of kinetic energy during trauma. In contrast, the fixed crura of the penis in relation to the pubic rami, and the female external genitalia in their similar relationships with these bony structures, are prone to blunt trauma from pelvic fracture or straddle injury. The erect penis becomes more prone to injury: Missed intromission or manual attempts at detumescence can cause penile fracture. Firearms and missiles have enough kinetic energy to overcome the protective mechanisms of flaccidity.

The looseness and laxity of genital skin generally have a protective role, allowing the skin to deform and slide away from a potential point of contact; however, in the case of machinery injury, rotating or suction devices can entrap a portion of the genital skin. The entire penile and scrotal skin can be trapped and avulsed.

Deep genital structures have multiple sources of arterial inflow including the dorsal, cavernosal, and bulbourethral arteries. Thus, ischemic loss of the penis is only seen with complete amputation or prolonged constriction injury. Likewise the testis derives blood supply from the cremasteric, testicular, and vasal arteries. Because burns start superficially and progressively spread their damage down into deeper tissues in the opposite fashion from Fournier's gangrene, preservation of some portion of the vascular integrity of the skin is likely in most chemical and thermal injury.

A rare cause of penile injury is amputation. When assault is the cause, appropriate police reporting is required. Other causes require special input from psychiatric and psychological experts. Penile amputation may be a manifestation of depressive and psychotic behavior, due to either schizophrenia or illicit drug abuse. Constriction rings can cause loss of superficial skin, deep urethral necrosis, or complete penile loss.

Lacerations and avulsions of the scrotum not involving the testis may occur due to blunt trauma, machinery accidents, stab wounds, and occasional firearm injury. Complete avulsion of the scrotal skin is rare and is usually the result of power takeoff, auger, or devastating motor vehicle crashes involving widespread skin loss or degloving. Evaluation of the testis for potential rupture is mandatory and involves physical examination, scrotal ultrasonography, or direct exploration.

Pelvic fractures with symphyseal or pubic ramus displacement can cause severe injury to the deep structures of the penis, including crural avulsion from its vascular and neural supply.

Presentation

Penetrating injuries to the external genitalia have a high likelihood of associated injuries to the spermatic cord and testis, urinary bladder and urethra, rectum, and vascular structures of the iliac and femoral region. Urethral injury occurs in 10–38% of penile fractures and up to 22% of penile gunshot wounds. Blood at the meatus implies injury, whereas its absence does not rule out significant urethral trauma.

A delay in presentation is common after penile fracture and constriction ring use, usually due to patient embarrassment. Missed intromission, acute bending, and a popping sound followed by immediate detumescence of the penis and acute pain are characteristic of penile fracture. Penile swelling is usually limited to the attachments of Buck's fascia and only the shaft of the penis will be ecchymotic; a localized hematoma has been termed as an "eggplant deformity." A perineal butterfly hematoma or scrotal bleeding can occur when the deep investing fascia of the penis has been ruptured by penetrating or blunt trauma. Entrapment of the genitalia by industrial machinery including augers, power takeoff from farm tractors, and suction devices can lead to avulsion of the genital skin. Genital and perineal burns are present in less than 5% of burn victims.

Initial Evaluation

The evaluation and initial management of genital injuries involve recognition of associated injuries, control of hemorrhage, and certain mechanism-specific interventions. Penetrating injuries to the penis have associated injuries in up to 83% of patients. In the absence of obvious signs of urethral injury, catheterization should be attempted. The catheter can help maintain orientation when structures are distorted by hematoma. Hematuria suggests the possibility of a bladder or upper urinary tract injury. Rectal injuries must be identified to avoid complications such as fistulas and Fournier's gangrene.

Bleeding from the penis can usually be controlled in the emergency department with gauze wraps to tamponade any bleeding. Excessively tight compressive dressings that compromise blood supply to the distal penis must be avoided. Burns should be covered with appropriate dressings depending on the mechanism; 1% silver sulfadiazine cream is appropriate. Chemical burns can be irrigated with saline; alkaline burns with dilute acetic acid; and for acid burns, sodium bicarbonate is recommended.

Bite injuries by animals or humans require appropriate antibiotic coverage for the species as well as tetanus toxoid administration. Empirical broad-spectrum antibiotics such as amoxicillin/clavulanic acid are appropriate for dog, rat, cat, bat, skunk, and raccoon bites as well as human bites. The possibility of rabies transmission must be considered. Dog and cat bites most commonly lead to pathogenic infection with *Pasteurella* organisms; anaerobic organisms may also be present. Human bites are more likely to cause complications than dog bite wounds. The predominant human oral bacterial organism is *Eikenella corrodens*; however, transmission of viral infection including hepatitis and human immunodeficiency virus (HIV) is possible.

After penile amputation or self-mutilation, urinary diversion should be established with a suprapubic cystostomy. Immediate management requires attention to two basic goals: resuscitation of the patient and preparation for surgical replantation. The stump is covered with sterile saline soaked gauze dressings. Transfusion may be required. The amputated penis is treated with a two-bag system. The amputated organ is wrapped in sterile saline gauze and placed in a first bag, which is then placed into a second bag containing ice. Appropriate transfer to tertiary centers can be accomplished with successful reimplantation more than 24 hours after injury.

Ancillary tests to detect penile fracture, such as cavernosography or magnetic resonance imaging (MRI), have limited sensitivity and specificity and are not clinically useful. If all penetrating and blunt ruptures of the tunica albuginea and superficial penile structures are explored and repaired, radiographic studies of the corpora cavernosa are not necessary.

Operative Management

The ultimate goal of reconstructive surgery is to have an organ with normal function and appearance. General wound care principles include irrigation, debridement, and closure of all wound layers. Most lacerations of the genital skin can be closed primarily due to the excellent blood supply.

Penile Trauma

Exposure of the deep cavernosum and tunica albuginea can be achieved through a circumferential subcoronal incision via degloving or for deeper wounds a penoscrotal, infrapubic, or even perineal incision. For penile fracture, the degloving incision allows complete inspection of the urethra and cavernosa. Primary closure can be achieved in virtually all cases. We close injuries of the tunica albuginea in a transverse fashion to prevent narrowing of the corpora. Penetrating defects in the tunica albuginea may be so large as to preclude primary closure. In such instances, which are rare in civilian practice, off the shelf fascia, pericardium, or other collagen matrix type products may be helpful. For severe disruptions of deep crural structures, plication maneuvers to exclude a proximal crus may be necessary. Given the high likelihood of arterial injury with both blunt and penetrating disruption of the crura, arterial insufficiency and erectile dysfunction may occur regardless of techniques to repair the tunica albuginea.

The tunica albuginea is closed with interrupted slowly absorbable sutures. Extensive irrigation, usually with a pulse lavage system and normal saline, is appropriate to remove any foreign body. In cases of penetrating impalement injuries or gunshot wounds, foreign material including clothing, missile fragments, or pieces of bone may enter the deep structures of the penis and urinary tract. These must be actively sought in such cases and removed.

Defects of glanular tissue do not preclude a good outcome: Debridement and trimming of skin edges to create a clean wound allow for closure of fairly large defects. Although the size of the glans may be reduced, its overall contour can usually be maintained.

Genital Bite Injuries

Simple uncontaminated bite injuries can be irrigated and closed primarily if appropriate antibiotics are administered, contamination is minimal, and the wound is closed within 6–12 hours. Grossly contaminated bite injuries should be left open and allowed to granulate. Most penetrating injuries to the penis and genitalia can be closed primarily as long as devitalized tissue is debrided, foreign material is removed, and appropriate antimicrobial coverage is given. Xeroform gauze and loosely wrapped gauze sponges complete the dressing. Local application of antibiotic ointments should be started once the dressings are taken down. Wound infections are uncommon after repair of penile injuries.

Burns

Management of burns, electrical injuries, and other skin injuries of the genitalia should be conservative. The rich vascular supply may allow a greater degree of skin preservation than would be expected in other areas of the genitalia. Skin grafting for such injuries is a rare event. Complete loss of genital skin usually implies a devastating burn from which patients may be unlikely to survive. In contrast, less than complete surface area burns of the genitalia have a remarkable capacity for recovery, and skin grafting is the exception rather than the rule.

Avulsion injuries of the male genitalia often present complex situations such as loss of the scrotum, perineum, urethra, and penis.

Penile Amputation

Penile amputation requires precise management of urethral, cavernosal, neurovascular, and skin transection in all but the most distal injuries. Simple urethral and tunica albugineal reapproximation of complete shaft amputation will usually lead to survival and function of the organ, although skin loss is unavoidable and sensation of the glans and accompanying ejaculatory function will be lost. Urethral stricture is also more common. Thus, whenever possible we advocate complete reattachment with microvascular and nerve reattachment. With a clean cut, virtually no preparation is required. However, if the penis has been avulsed or cut with a blunt instrument, or purposefully mutilated by the patient or the assailant, reattachment may be problematic.

Reapproximation starts with the tunica of the corpus spongiosum, the urethral epithelium over a catheter, followed by the ventral-most aspect of the tunica albuginea of the corpus cavernosum. Reanastomosis of the deep arteries of the cavernosum usually is not required or easy. We only perform dorsal arterial reanastomosis. Once the tunica albuginea of the corpus cavernosum has been reapproximated, the ends of the dorsal neurovascular structures are brought into proximity. Microvascular repair using an operating microscope and fine permanent suture allows reanastomosis of one or both dorsal arteries, the dorsal nerves, and the deep dorsal vein. Failure to reanastomose the deep dorsal vein may lead to glans hyperemia and venous congestion of the shaft skin, which can compromise the success of the reattachment. Postoperatively, venous congestion is a major problem even with microvascular reattachment. We have found that the use of medical leeches is very helpful in reducing swelling and hematoma related to venous congestion and postoperative bleeding.

Scrotal Trauma

Scrotal skin lacerations can be closed primarily in the absence of gross infection or heavy contamination. Meticulous hemostasis is required to avoid hematoma; the scrotum allows bleeding without tamponade. Layered closure of the dartos fascia and skin, with a drain brought out dependently, limits postoperative hematoma. Interrupted suturing reduces ischemia and allows further drainage between the sutures. Skin suture choice is usually absorbable monofilament. In complex wounds, nonabsorbable nylon sutures are preferable. Xeroform gauze or other antibacterial dressings and ointments should be placed on the incisions, and the scrotum should be surrounded with loose gauze.

Complete scrotal avulsion is a devastating injury (Figure 10-9). The avulsed skin is not usually suitable for

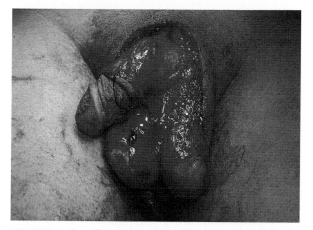

FIGURE 10-9. Scrotal and penile skin avulsion from machinery injury.

regrafting. Machinery injuries with rotating mechanisms may damage the intrinsic microvasculature of the skin. We do not advocate immediate grafting but instead recommend an interval of local care and dressing changes with saline soaked gauze. This allows the wound bed to granulate, after which very successful results can be obtained with split thickness skin grafts obtained from thigh donor sites. Testicular transplantation into subcutaneous thigh pouches can be a temporizing or permanent measure dependent on patient age, sexual function, and overall prioritization of trauma injuries.

INJURIES TO THE FEMALE GENITALIA

Mechanism

Female genital injuries involving severe pelvic fractures or sexual assault and interpersonal violence require specialized treatment. Although many vulvar lacerations are the result of sports-related straddle-type injuries, genital trauma is reported in 20–53% of sexual assault victims. If such history is elicited, appropriate support services and police involvement must be secured. Informed consent for the patient assessment should be obtained if a history of sexual assault has been verified. This assessment must include history, physical examination, and collection of laboratory and forensic specimens as outlined by the American College of Obstetrics and Gynecologists.

Female patients with external genital injuries should be suspected of having injury to the internal female organs as well as the lower urinary tract and urethra. Many female urethral injuries are associated with vaginal bleeding. Female genital injury in the setting of pelvic fracture or impalement injury should include cystourethrography, proctoscopy, and laparotomy as indicated. Unrecognized associated urinary tract and gastrointestinal (GI) injuries in the face of vaginal trauma may lead to abscess formation, sepsis, and death.

Management

Perineal and vulvar lacerations can usually be managed in the emergency department. Large hematomas should be incised and drained, with ligation of any bleeding vessels. As with the male genital skin, closure with interruptive absorbable sutures is standard. Drains can be used if there is a large cavity, if hemostasis is suboptimal, or if there is suspected contamination.

Internal lacerations to the vagina and cervix can be closed in the emergency department as long as there is not severe bleeding. Large lacerations associated with bleeding and hematoma require speculum examination under anesthesia to completely assess and repair the injuries. Vaginal lacerations are closed with continuous absorbable sutures, and vaginal packing is critical for hemostasis.

Complex vaginal and perineal lacerations, associated with pelvic fracture, rectal injury, or other adverse features, require a more systematic approach. Evaluation under anesthesia is mandatory including speculum examination, cystoscopy or cystography, and rigid proctoscopy. Diversion of the fecal stream is rarely indicated unless perineal injuries extensively involve the rectum, anus, or external sphincter. Bladder ruptures should be repaired if associated vaginal lacerations are present, to prevent deep pelvic infection, abscess, or formation of vesico-vaginal fistulas.

CONCLUSIONS

Urogenital trauma demands care and attention to prompt diagnosis, selection of management modality, integration of the multidisciplinary trauma team, and careful follow-up to monitor for long-term complications and disability.

SELF-ASSESSMENT QUESTIONS

1. What is the role of CT compared to intraoperative IVP (so-called one-shot IVP) in renal trauma?
2. List the key principles of renal reconstructive surgery for trauma and how do they differ from those used for partial nephrectomy in renal cell cancer.
3. How should one manage delayed bleeding after non-operative management of major laceration?
4. What are the indications for operative management of extraperitoneal bladder injuries?
5. What is the role of the urologist in the acute management of posterior urethral disruption associated with pelvic fracture?

SUGGESTED READINGS

1. Brandes S, Coburn M, Armekakas N, McAninch J: Diagnosis and management of ureteric injury: an evidence-based analysis. *BJU Int* 94:277–289, 2004.
2. Chapple C, Barbagli G, Jordan G, et al: Consensus statement on urethral trauma. *BJU Int* 93:1195–1202, 2004.
3. Gomez GG, Ceballos L, Coburn M, et al: Consensus statement on bladder injuries. *BJU Int* 94:27–32, 2004.
4. Kuan J, Wright JL, Rivara F, et al: American Association for the Surgery of Trauma Organ Injury Scale for kidney injuries predicts nephrectomy, dialysis, and death in patients with blunt injury and nephrectomy for penetrating injuries. *J Trauma* 60:351–356, 2006.
5. Morey AF, Metro MJ, Carney KJ, et al: Consensus on genitourinary trauma: external genitalia. *BJU Int* 94:507–515, 2004.
6. Santucci RA, Wessells H, Bartsch G, et al: Evaluation and management of renal injuries: consensus statement of the renal trauma subcommittee. *BJU Int* 93:937–954, 2004.
7. Wessells H: Injuries to the urogenital tract. In Souba WW, Fink MP, Jurkovich GJ, et al (eds): *ACS Surgery.* WEBMD, New York, 2005, pp 1262–1279.
8. Wessells H, Long L: Penile and genital injuries. *Urol Clin North Am* 33:117–126, 2006.
9. Wright JL, Kuan J, Nathens A, et al: Renal and extra-renal predictors of nephrectomy from the National Trauma Data Bank. *J Urol* 1753:1970–1975, 2006.
10. Wright JL, Nathens AB, Rivara FP, et al: Sexual and excretory dysfunction one year after pelvic fracture. *J Urol* 176:1540–1545, 2006.

Urethral Stricture Disease

Michael J. Metro, MD

I. DEFINITION

1. A urethral stricture is fibrotic tissue that renders the normally compliant urethral lumen inelastic. This results in the narrowing of the urethral lumen and the slowing of urine flow through it. Strictures occur as a result of inflammation or trauma from iatrogenic or external sources.
   a) The term urethral stricture is correctly used to describe lesions of the anterior urethra. In contrast, posterior urethral "strictures" are really urethral distraction defects that occur in the setting of pelvic fracture.
2. The anterior urethra begins at the urogenital diaphragm and includes the bulbar urethra, the penile or pendulous urethra, and the fossa navicularis and meatus.
3. The posterior urethra includes the prostatic and membranous urethra (Figure 11-1).

II. ETIOLOGY

A. Trauma

1. Anterior urethra.
   a) Straddle injuries can injure the bulbar urethra when the urethra is crushed against the undersurface of the pubic symphysis.
   b) Penetrating injuries can involve the penile urethra.
2. Posterior urethra.
   a) Urethral distraction defects as a result of pelvic fracture occur within the membranous urethra. This roughly 2-cm long segment is between two relatively fixed points (the prostatic apex and the proximal corpus spongiosum, which is fixed to the cavernous bodies).

B. Iatrogenic

1. Injuries result from traumatic catheterization, instrumentation during other urologic surgeries (transurethral

311

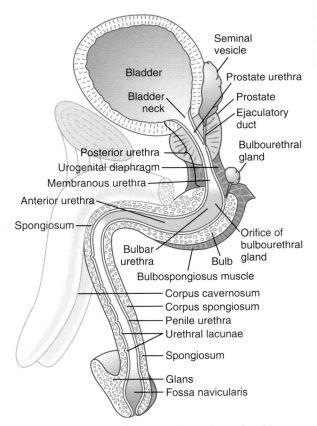

FIGURE 11-1. Anatomy of anterior and posterior urethra. (Courtesy of Jack W. McAninch, MD.)

resection of the prostate [TURP], ureteroscopy), or self-induced injury from traumatic Foley catheter removal.

C. Infection

1. Gonococcal urethritis classically causes anterior, mostly penile, urethra strictures.
2. Other sexually transmitted diseases such as *Chlamydia trachomatis* can also result is stricture disease.

III. CLINICAL PRESENTATION

A. Obstruction

1. The classic history is that of obstructive urinary symptoms, that is, slowing of urinary stream, decreased caliber of the stream, increase in voiding time, incomplete bladder emptying, and post-void dribble.
2. Meatal strictures can result in splaying or splitting of the urinary stream.

B. Secondary Complications

1. Infection.
   a) Obstruction of the flow of urine often leads to "upstream" infection such as prostatitis or epididymo-orchitis.

IV. DIAGNOSIS

Largely a clinical diagnosis based on history. Clinical suspicion can be supported by a flow rate and curve determination and/or assessment of post-void residual.

A. Urethroscopy

1. Can be used to confirm a clinical suspicion; accurate diagnosis of length and location of stricture should be performed radiographically.

B. Retrograde Urethrogram (RUG) and Voiding Cystourethrogram (VCUG)

1. Accurate assessment of length and location of a stricture is achieved by the correct performance of an RUG and a VCUG.
2. The patient should be placed obliquely at 45 degrees, with the bottom leg flexed 90 degrees at the knee and the top leg straight. This allows unobstructed lateral imaging of the urethra and limits imaging foreshortening, which occurs with anteroposterior projection.
3. A 12- or 14-F Foley catheter is then placed within the fossa navicularis and the balloon is inflated with 2 mL of saline to prevent dislodgement.
4. Contrast is then injected by way of the catheter to opacify the urethra and images are obtained.

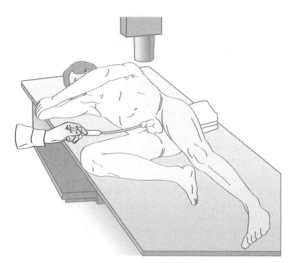

FIGURE 11-2. Positioning for performance of retrograde urethrogram (RUG). (Courtesy of Jack W. McAninch, MD.)

5. The bladder is then filled in a retrograde fashion via this catheter, or a small feeding tube (5 or 8 F) can be navigated through the stricture to allow for bladder filling. This component of the study can show what aspect of the urethral stricture is truly urodynamically significant as proximal dilation and distal diminution of urethral caliber will be seen (Figure 11-2).

V. ASSOCIATED CONDITIONS

1. Urethral carcinoma can present with a urethrocutaneous fistula secondary to urethral obstruction from stricture and must be ruled out with a biopsy in all patients presenting in this fashion.
2. Periurethral abscess proximal to distal obstruction from the urethral stricture.
3. A urethral diverticulum can form proximal to the site of obstruction and cause post-void dribbling or infections.

VI. TREATMENT

1. The first step in determining course of treatment needs to involve a discussion of goals of therapy with the patient.

Most treatments that involve dilation or incision can certainly treat the acute problems of urinary obstruction but do not have good long-term success rates (30–50%). Formal urethroplasty, utilizing a variety of techniques, can provide long-term success rates near 90% at the expense of a longer operation and longer immediate postoperative convalescence.

2. Algorithm for treatment.

3. **Urethral dilation** can be performed in the office with local anesthesia with lidocaine jelly and is still a mainstay of therapy for stricture disease. A well-performed dilation may be the least traumatic of all of the minimally invasive techniques. Urethral sounds or filiforms and followers can be employed to perform the dilation. Both techniques are not without risks, however. Urethral false passages and trauma can lead to development of longer and more complex strictures. Urethral dilation should be considered a palliative procedure as definitive successes are extremely rare.

4. A combination of flexible endoscopy and filiform placement can be a valuable tool to ensure correct luminal placement of the filiform. The filiform, placed in parallel next to the scope, is seen to traverse the stricture as opposed to a passage based on feel.

5. Soft dilation is a practice of the placement of a urethral catheter that is changed and increased in size over a period of days or weeks. This has not resulted in long-term success but can atraumatically extend the life of a dilation.

6. Direct vision incisional urethrotomy (DVIU).

   a) Incisional urethrotomy is performed endoscopically under sedation or general anesthesia and involves visualizing the stricture endoscopically and incising with a cold knife at the 12 o'clock position to open the stricture. A Foley catheter is then placed for 2–10 days. The goal of the incision is to allow for re-epithelialization of the urethral lumen, which will result in a lumen of normal caliber.

   b) Urethrotomies with a hot knife or a laser should be avoided secondary to the addition of thermal injury to the spongiosal tissue making recurrences longer and more severe.

   c) Results.

      i) The success rate of incisional urethrotomy depends on length and location of the stricture. Short-term (< 6 months) success rates are excellent but long-term success occurs in only 50% of cases. Subsequent urethrotomies have an even lower chance of long-term success with the second having a 20% chance of success and the third having virtually no chance of success. Incisions of pendulous strictures should be considered palliative as true long-term successes are rare.

ii) A regimen of urethral self-dilation after DVIU or dilation can extend the life of a urethrotomy and lengthen the time needed for subsequent incisions or dilations.

iii) Injections of steroids into strictures after incisions have been tried but have not resulted in improved results.

d) Conclusions.

i) Despite low long-term success rates, dilations and incisions of a urethral stricture are commonly repeatedly performed. Referral to a urologist with specific training in urethral reconstruction does not happen as often as it probably should. The open reconstructive procedures are technically difficult and are not a casual operation. Repeated incisions and dilations should be considered palliative and not therapeutic unless the only aim is to establish urethral continuity. Management guidelines generally recommend referral for urethroplasty in young individuals and those that have failed two, and possibly one, endoscopic attempt at treatment depending on the stricture characteristics.

VII. OPEN RECONSTRUCTION

1. The optimal choice of techniques for formal open reconstruction of a urethral stricture is dependent on length and location of the stricture as determined by retrograde urethrography.

2. Intraoperative sonourethrography can provide data at the time of surgery including exact length of stricture, degree of luminal narrowing, and location that may help in determining technique for reconstruction.

3. The sonourethrogram is performed by placing a 10- or 12-MHz small parts transducer in the perineum with the patient placed in a frog-leg position. Saline is injected via a catheter-tipped syringe to distend the urethra in a retrograde fashion. The bladder is filled and suprapubic pressure is applied to provide antegrade filling of the urethra. The stricture can then be measured and the degree

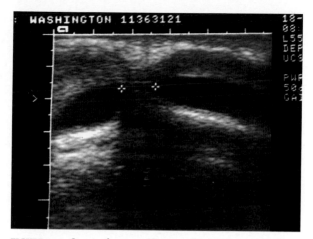

FIGURE 11-3. Sonourethrogram. (Courtesy of Jack W. McAninch, MD.)

of luminal narrowing can be determined, which aids in determining the width of a flap or graft that may be required (Figure 11-3).

A. Anastomotic Urethroplasty

1. Indications

a) Bulbar strictures less than 2 cm can reliably be treated with an anastomotic or end-to-end (ETE) urethroplasty.
b) Penile or pendulous strictures, unless exceedingly short or in an impotent man, cannot be managed by ETE due the resultant chordee that will be present postoperatively. The pendulous urethra lacks the elasticity of the bulbar urethra and its location on the penile shaft makes chordee with an erection unavoidable.

2. Procedure

a) The urethra is mobilized by dividing the fibromuscular septum, which attaches the urethra dorsally to the cavernosal bodies. Mobilization is performed until a tension-free anastomosis can be ensured. The strictured urethra is excised and a spatulated anastomosis is performed over a 16-F urethral catheter. The anastomosis is performed in one layer dorsally where the spongiosum is thin and in two layers ventrally where the spongiosum is robust.

b) Urethroscopy and cystoscopy should be performed after the urethra is opened to document absence of more proximal stricture or foreign bodies (stones) in the bladder.

3. Postoperative

a) The urethral catheter is maintained for 2 weeks.
b) A VCUG is done at the time of catheter removal to document the absence of extravasation and the presence of an adequate caliber urethra. The bladder is filled via the existing urethral catheter and is then removed. Fluoroscopic visualization of the subsequent void is performed.

4. Success Rate

a) Long-term success rates between 90% and 95% should be expected.
b) Success is defined by the presence of a normal flow rate, an unobstructed flow pattern, and the absence of the need for subsequent instrumentation such as dilation or incision.
c) Self-dilation/calibration after all open urethroplasty cases is not required and should be discouraged.

B. Substitution Urethroplasty

1. Substitution urethroplasty is performed for bulbar strictures > 2 cm and for most pendulous strictures. Grafts rely on the blood supply of surrounding tissues for support, whereas flaps bring their own pedicled blood supply for use in areas where blood supply is less robust or reliable.
2. The penile urethra circular fasciocutaneous flap, described by McAninch, has been a mainstay of reconstruction for strictures of the entire anterior urethra. More recently, with the popularity of the buccal mucosa graft, its use is reserved for pendulous strictures or for reoperations in the bulbar urethra where a free graft repair has failed.
3. The flap is raised by making two parallel circumferential incisions, usually 15–2.0 cm apart, under the coronal margin. The proximal incision is taken down above the superficial lamina of Buck's fascia and carried toward the base of the penis. The distal incision is carried below this layer of Buck's fascia and again taken down to the base of the penis. In this fashion a pedicled flap, usually of 15–18 cm in

length, and dependent on the superficial lamina of Buck's fascia for vascular support, can be raised.

4. The flap is utilized as a ventral onlay after the urethra has been opened ventrally through the stricture. 6–0 Maxon or PDS is used to perform a running anastomosis that incorporates the flap and the dorsal urethral plate over a 16-F catheter.

5. The catheter is left for 3 weeks at which time a VCUG confirms adequate healing.

6. Long-term success rates are between 85% and 90%.

7. **Buccal mucosa**—For substitution urethroplasty in the bulbar urethra, the buccal mucosa graft has achieved huge popularity and should be considered the gold standard.

   a) **Properties**—Buccal mucosa has a thick epithelium that makes it easy to handle, has a thin lamina propria that improves graft take, and is an epithelial surface that is accustomed to being wet leading to less inflammation.

   b) **Harvest**—Grafts can be harvested from the inner cheek, the lower lip, and even the lateral tongue.

   c) **Dorsal or ventral** grafts can be placed as dorsal or ventral onlays depending on surgeon preference. Advocates of the ventral approach point to the improved vascularity of the corpus spongiosum over the corporal bodies, which support the dorsal onlay, and the relative simplicity of the surgical technique. Those that favor the dorsal onlay (Table 11-1) point to a lesser incidence of graft sacculation due to improved mechanical support of the corporal bodies and the ability to place that graft in less vascularly robust areas of the urethra such as the pendulous urethra.

VIII. POSTERIOR URETHRA

Pelvic fracture urethral distraction defects (PFUDDs)— Strictures of the posterior urethra are more properly referred to as PFUDDs. The membranous urethra is short (2 cm) and is positioned between two relatively fixed points (prostatic apex and the proximal corpus spongiosum). Ten percent of all pelvic fractures result in posterior urethral disruptions that occur due to the shearing forces applied at the membranous urethra. Urethral disruptions are more common with anterior disruptions of the pelvic ring and with bilateral rami fractures.

Table 11-1: Algorithm for Diagnosis and Management of Urethral Strictures

Signs and Symptoms of Stricture

In Office
Flow Rate and Curve,
Post-Void Residual
Diagnostic Urethroscopy

Obliterative Stricture	Urethral Stricture	Meatal Stenosis	Bladder Neck Contracture (BNC)

Suprapubic Tube (SPT) — (Obliterative Stricture / Urethral Stricture)

Meatal Dilation
↓
Failure?
↓
Self Meatal Dilation Failure?
↓
Meatoplasty

Bladder Neck Dilation Failure?
↓
Bladder Neck Incision Failure?
↓
Transurethral Resection of Bladder Neck (TURBNC) Failure?

Retrograde urethrogram (RUG)
Voiding Cystourethrogram (VCUG)
↓
Determine Length and Location of Stricture

Bulbar < 1 cm	Bulbar < 2 cm	Bulbar > 2 cm	Pendulous	Membranous

DVIU
Failure?
↓
Repeat RUG/VCUG

Intraoperative Sonourethrogram

< 2 cm? → **End-to-End Urethroplasty**
> 2 cm? → **Buccal Mucosa Urethroplasty**

Anastomotic Repair
↓
Utilize 4 Step Urethral Mobilization

Aggressive TURBNC Failure?
↓
TURBNC +/- Urolume
↓
May Need Procedure for Incontinence

Fasciocutaneous Flap Urethroplasty or Dorsal Onlay Buccal Mucosa Urethroplasty

A. Diagnosis

The classic presentation of the posterior urethral disruption is blood at the urethral meatus, which occurs in up to 93% of cases. The diagnosis is also made when attempts at urethral catheter placement fail. A rectal exam may reveal a high-riding prostate, which is present due to the prostate being elevated out of the pelvis secondary to surrounding hematoma. Diagnosis is confirmed by RUG, which may reveal a complete or partial disruption or a contusion in which the lumen is compressed by surrounding hematoma but remains in continuity. A complete disruption is present when no injected contrast is found to enter the bladder while some contrast is able to enter the bladder when a partial disruption is present.

B. Initial Management

There exists some controversy in the initial management of a posterior urethral disruption. Some experts advocate only urinary diversion with a suprapubic catheter placement, whereas some recommend an attempt at urethral realignment when the clinical situation allows. Advocates for realignment point to a decreased stricture rate of 70% versus nearly 100% with simple diversion. Proponents of suprapubic diversion point to a minor increase in the incidence of impotence and incontinence with realignment.

1. **Anastomotic**—All repairs of PFUDDs are anastomotic or end-to-end repairs. The goal of the surgery is to mobilize the urethra enough to ensure an anastomosis that is tension free. A stepwise approach to this urethral mobilization has been outlined by George Webster and others. The four-step approach entails:
   a) **Division of dorsal attachments of the urethra to the corpus cavernosum**—This can be carried distally to the peno-scrotal junction with no risk of chordee.
   b) **Crural separation**—Separation of the corporal bodies for 3–4 cm forms a groove in which the urethra can lie to allow for a more direct route to the proximal urethra.
   c) **Inferior pubectomy**—Removal of a portion of the inferior pubis with a rongeur or osteotome also allows for a more direct route for the distal urethra to travel to reach the proximal urethrotomy.
   d) **Urethral rerouting**—Finally, urethral rerouting around a corporal body allows the urethra to lie in a more dorsal fashion thus shortening the distance between the two urethral ends.

C. Results

Success rates of 90% or more should be expected when performed by surgeons familiar with the technique. It is important to note that some degree of erectile dysfunction occurs in up to 70% of men with posterior urethral injuries.

A recovery of function is the rule in more than 60% of these patients after definitive urethroplasty and resolution of the pelvic hematoma. Incontinence is rare with only 6% of men reporting problems with stress incontinence.

IX. BLADDER NECK CONTRACTURES

Bladder neck or vesical neck contractures occur as a result of prostatic surgery and can be very difficult to treat as the recurrence rate is high. An incidence of 5–15% can be expected after radical retropubic prostatectomy and approximately 3% after TURP. Initial treatment usually is a bladder neck dilation, followed by incisions, and then finally resections of the vesical neck. The result of "fixing" a bladder neck contracture can be stress incontinence and patients must be made aware of this. Formal open reconstruction of the bladder neck often requires an abdominoperineal approach and is quite difficult. Continence is rare after such a procedure. The one remaining acceptable place for a Uro-Lume stent may be across the bladder neck in refractory cases of contracture. An artificial urinary sphincter is sometimes necessary to regain continence once a contracture is definitively treated.

X. SPECIFIC CONDITIONS CAUSING URETHRAL STRICTURE

1. Balanitis xerotica obliterans (BXO) is the term used to describe genital lichen sclerosis in the male. Histologically, it is characterized by hyperkeratosis and lymphocytic infiltration.
    a) Patients with BXO present most commonly with meatal stenosis and have findings of loss of elasticity of the glanular and preputial skin, loss of skin pigment, and induration of hyperkeratosis of the glans.
    b) Conservative treatment involves application of topical steroids (triamcinolone, betamethasone) and meatal dilation.
    c) Assessment must include retrograde urethrography as the disease can involve the more proximal urethra, or prior instrumentation may have induced stricture disease here.
    d) Formal reconstruction often involves substitution urethroplasty, often in two stages, as the penile skin, normally used to treat strictures here, is often histologically

abnormal in these patients and repairs based on flap of this tissue are bound to fail.

2. Fossa navicularis strictures are almost always caused by iatrogenic trauma from instrumentation when not caused by BXO.

a) Local flap urethroplasty is the mainstay of definitive treatment for strictures in this area.

3. The "hypospadias cripple" is a term used to describe the unfortunate man who has undergone prior failed hypospadias repair, usually multiple times. Strictures in these men are usually complex and require expert referral for formal reconstruction, which usually involves two-stage reconstruction with buccal mucosa grafting.

SELF-ASSESSMENT QUESTIONS

1. What is the anatomic landmark that separates the anterior from the posterior urethra?
2. What are the main causes of stricture disease?
3. What are the symptoms of stricture disease?
4. What are the noninvasive and invasive diagnostic tests used to diagnose urethral strictures?
5. What is the correct technique and patient positioning to perform a retrograde urethrogram (RUG)?

SUGGESTED READINGS

1. Anger JT, Raj GV, Delvecchio FC, Webster GD: Anastomotic contracture and incontinence after radical prostatectomy: a graded approach to management. *J Urol* 173:1143–1146, 2005.

2. Barbagli G, Palminteri E, Lazzeri M: Dorsal onlay techniques for urethroplasty. *Urol Clin North Am* 29:389–395, 2002.

3. Barbagli G, Palminteri E, Rizzo M: Dorsal onlay urethroplasty using penile skin or buccal mucosa in adult bulbourethral strictures. *J Urol* 160:1307–1309, 1998.

4. Flynn BJ, Delvecchio FC, Webster GD: Perineal repair of pelvic fracture urethral distraction defects: experience in 120 patients during the last 10 years. *J Urol* 170:1877–1880, 2003.

5. Greenwell TJ, Castle C, Andrich DE, et al: Repeat urethrotomy and dilation for the treatment of urethral stricture are neither clinically effective or cost-effective. *J Urol* 172:275–277, 2004.

6. Heyns CF, Steenkamp JW, De Kock MLS, Whitaker P: Treatment of male urethral strictures: is repeated dilation of internal urethrotomy useful? *J Urol* 160:356–358, 1998.

7. Jordan GH: Management of membranous urethral distraction injuries via the perineal approach. In McAninch JW, Carroll PR, Jordan GH (eds): *Traumatic and Reconstructive Urology*. Saunders, Philadelphia, 1996, pp 393–410.

8. McAninch JW: Fasciocutaneous penile flap in reconstruction of complex anterior urethral strictures. In McAninch JW, Carroll PR, Jordan GH (eds): Traumatic and Reconstructive Urology. Saunders, Philadelphia, 1996, pp 609–614.

9. Rosen MA, McAninch JW: Preoperative staging of the anterior urethral stricture. In McAninch JW, Carroll PR, Jordan GH (eds): *Traumatic and Reconstructive Urology*. Saunders, Philadelphia, 1996, pp 551–564.

10. Rosen MA, McAninch JW: Stricture excision and primary anastomosis for reconstruction of the anterior urethral stricture. In McAninch JW, Carroll PR, Jordan GH (eds): *Traumatic and Reconstructive Urology*. Saunders, Philadelphia, 1996, pp 565–570.

CHAPTER 12

Urinary Fistula

Eric S. Rovner, MD

A fistula represents an extra-anatomic communication between two or more epithelial or mesothelial lined body cavities or the skin surface. Although most fistulas in the industrialized world are iatrogenic, they may also occur as a result of congenital anomalies, malignancy, inflammation and infection, radiation therapy, iatrogenic (surgical) or external tissue trauma, ischemia, parturition, and a variety of other processes. The potential exists for fistula formation between a portion of the urinary tract (i.e., kidney, ureters, bladder, and urethra) and virtually any other body cavity including the chest (pleural cavity), gastrointestinal (GI) tract, lymphatics, vascular system, genitalia, skin, and reproductive organs. Classification is generally based on the organ of origin in the urinary tract and the termination point of the fistula (i.e., vagina, skin, GI tract). The presenting symptoms and signs are variable and depend to a large degree on the involved organs, the presence of underlying urinary obstruction or infection, the size of the fistula, and associated medical conditions such as malignancy.

Treatment of urinary fistula depends on several factors including its location, size, and etiology (malignant or benign). Prevention of urinary fistula is, of course, paramount; however, proper nutrition, infection, and malignancy are important considerations not only when assessing a patient for the risk of creation of a fistula during any given intervention but also during an evaluation for the repair of an existing urinary fistula.

I. VESICOVAGINAL FISTULA

A. General Considerations

Vesicovaginal fistula (VVF) is the most common acquired fistula of the urinary tract.

1. VVFs have been known about since ancient times; however, it was not until 1663 that Hendrik von Roonhuyse first described surgical repair. In 1852, James Marion Sims published his now famous surgical series describing

his method of surgical treatment of VVF using silver wire in a transvaginal approach. Of note, it was not until his 30th attempt at closure of VVF that he achieved success.

B. Etiology

The most common cause of VVF differs in various parts of the world.

1. In the industrialized world, the most common cause (75%) is injury to the bladder at the time of gynecologic surgery—usually abdominal hysterectomy. Obstetric trauma accounts for very few VVFs in the United States and other industrialized nations.
   a) Post-hysterectomy VVFs are thought to result most commonly from an incidental unrecognized iatrogenic cystotomy near the vaginal cuff.
      i) The operative approach to hysterectomy is an important factor as bladder injuries are at least three times more common during abdominal hysterectomy compared to vaginal hysterectomy.
   b) The incidence of fistula after hysterectomy is estimated to be approximately 0.1–0.2%.
   c) Other causes of VVF in the industrialized world include malignancy, pelvic radiation, and obstetrical trauma including forceps lacerations and uterine rupture.
2. In the developing world where routine perinatal obstetrical care may be limited, VVFs most commonly occur as a result of prolonged labor with resulting pressure necrosis to the anterior vaginal wall and underlying trigone of the bladder from the baby. In some instances, VVF may result from the use of forceps or other instrumentation during delivery.
   a) Obstetric fistulas tend to be larger, located distally in the vagina, and may involve the proximal urethra.
   b) The constellation of problems resulting from obstructed labor is not limited to VVF and has been termed the "obstructed labor injury complex" and includes varying degrees of each of the following: urethral loss, stress incontinence, hydroureteronephrosis, renal failure, rectovaginal fistula, rectal atresia, anal sphincter incompetence, cervical destruction, amenorrhea, pelvic inflammatory disease, secondary infertility, vaginal stenosis, osteitis pubis, and foot drop.

c) In sub-Saharan Africa the incidence rate of obstetric VVF has been estimated at 10.3 per 100,000 deliveries.

C. Presentation

1. The most common complaint is constant urinary drainage per vagina although small fistulas may present with intermittent wetness that is positional in nature.

   a) VVF must be distinguished from urinary incontinence due to other causes including stress (urethral) incontinence, urge (bladder) incontinence, and overflow incontinence.

   b) Patients may also complain of recurrent cystitis, perineal skin irritation due to constant wetness, vaginal fungal infections, or rarely pelvic pain. When a large VVF is present, patients may not void at all and simply have continuous leakage of urine into the vagina.

   c) VVF following hysterectomy or other surgical procedures may present on removal of the urethral catheter or may present 1–3 weeks later with urinary drainage per vagina.

      i) VVFs resulting from hysterectomy are usually located high in the vagina at the level of the vaginal cuff (Figure 12-1).

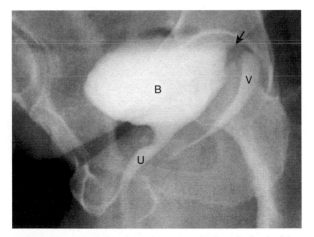

FIGURE 12-1. VCUG demonstrating a VVF high at the level of the vaginal cuff in a patient following hysterectomy. The arrow demonstrates the fistula tract (not well seen). B, urinary bladder; U, urethra; V, vagina.

d) VVF resulting from radiation therapy may not present for months to years following completion of radiation. These tend to represent some of the most challenging reconstructive cases in urology due to the size, complexity, and the associated voiding dysfunction due to the radiation effects on the urinary bladder. The endarteritis as a result of the radiation therapy may involve the surrounding tissues, limiting reconstructive options.

D. Evaluation (Figure 12-2)

1. History.
2. Physical examination.
    a) A pelvic exam with speculum should always be performed in an attempt to locate the fistula and assess the size and number of fistulas.
    b) Palpate for masses or other pelvic pathology, which may need to be addressed at the time of fistula repair.

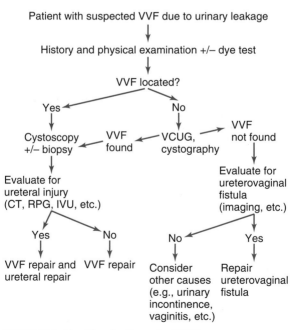

FIGURE 12-2. Algorithm for diagnosis of VVF.

    c) An assessment of inflammation surrounding the fistula is necessary as it may affect timing of the repair.

    d) The presence of a VVF may be confirmed by instilling a vital blue dye or sterile milk into the bladder per urethra and observing for discolored vaginal drainage.

        i) A double dye test may confirm the diagnosis of urinary fistula as well as suggest the possibility of an associated ureterovaginal or urethrovaginal fistula. A tampon is placed per vagina. Oral phenazopyridine is administered and vital blue dye is instilled into the bladder. If the tampon is discolored yellow-orange at the top, it is suggestive of a ureterovaginal fistula. Blue discoloration in the midportion of the tampon suggests VVF, whereas blue staining at the bottom suggests a urethrovaginal fistula.

3. Urine culture and urine analysis.

4. Cystoscopy and possible biopsy of the fistula tract are performed if malignancy is suspected.

    a) Note the location of fistula relative to ureters; repair of the fistula may require reimplantation of ureters if the fistula involves the ureteral orifice.

5. Voiding cystourethrography.

    a) Some small fistulas may not be seen radiographically unless the bladder is filled to capacity and a detrusor contraction is provoked during filling.

        i) Assesses for vesicoureteral reflux.

        ii) Examines for multiple fistulas including urethrovaginal fistula.

        iii) Assesses size and location of fistula.

6. Intravenous urography and/or retrograde pyeloureterography.

    a) Assesses for concomitant ureteral injury and/or ureterovaginal fistula, which has been reported to occur in up to 12% of patients.

7. Cross-sectional pelvic imaging (magnetic resonance imaging [MRI]/computed tomography [CT]) if malignancy is suspected.

E. Therapy

1. Nonsurgical management.

    a) Catheter drainage is the initial treatment in most cases when the VVF is recognized early in the clinical course. Antibiotics and topical estrogen creams are adjuvant measures to prevent infection and promote healing.

b) Fulguration of the fistula followed by catheter drainage has been shown to have some efficacy in small (<5 mm), uncomplicated fistulas.

c) Adjuvant measures such as fibrin glue and so forth have been used by some authors in conjunction with fulguration and catheter drainage as a "plug" in the fistula as well as a "scaffolding" to allow the ingrowth of healthy tissue.

2. Surgical management.

a) Success rates approach 90–98% regardless of surgical approach.

b) Adherence to basic surgical principles are essential to achieve success in the repair of all urinary fistula (Table 12-1).

c) Choice of the optimal surgical approach to VVF is controversial and there are numerous factors to consider (Table 12-2). No single approach is applicable to all VVFs.

i) Transabdominal approach: Generally performed as described by V.J. O'Conor. Through a midline infraumbilical incision, the bladder is exposed and opened in the sagittal plane down to the level of the fistula. The bladder is separated off the vagina beyond the level of the fistula. The fistu-

---

Table 12-1: Principles of Vesicovaginal Fistula Repair

1. Adequate exposure of the fistula tract with debridement of devitalized and ischemic tissue
2. Removal of involved foreign bodies or synthetic materials from region of fistula, if applicable
3. Careful dissection and/or anatomic separation of the involved organ cavities
4. Watertight closure
5. Use of well-vascularized, healthy tissue flaps for repair (atraumatic handling of tissue)
6. Multiple layer closure
7. Tension-free, nonoverlapping suture lines
8. Adequate urinary tract drainage and/or stenting after repair
9. Treatment and prevention of infection (appropriate use of antimicrobials)
10. Maintenance of hemostasis

Table 12-2: Abdominal Versus Transvaginal Repair of Vesicovaginal Fistula

	Abdominal	Transvaginal
Length of hospitalization	4–7 days	1–2 days
Timing of repair	Usually delayed 2–6 months from the time of initial injury	May be done immediately in the absence of infection
Location of ureters relative to fistula tract	Fistula located near ureteral orifice may necessitate reimplantation	Reimplantation may not be necessary even if fistula tract is located near ureteral orifice
Sexual function	No change in vaginal depth	Potential risk of vaginal shortening or stenosis
Location of fistula tract/ depth of vagina	Fistula located low on the trigone or near the bladder neck may be difficult to expose	Fistula located high at the vaginal cuff may be difficult to expose
Use of adjunctive flaps	Omentum, peritoneal flap, intestine	Labial fat pad (Martius fat pad), peritoneal flap, gracilis muscle, labial myocutaneous flap
Relative indications	Large fistulas, located high in a deep vagina, radiation fistulas, failed transvaginal approach, small capacity bladder requiring augmentation, need for ureteral reimplantation, inability to place patient in the lithotomy position	Uncomplicated fistulas, low fistulas Vaginal exposure may be difficult in some nulliparous patients

lous tract is debrided back to healthy tissue from both bladder and vaginal sides. The bladder and vagina are closed separately. Often, well-vascularized tissue such as omentum is interposed between the vagina and bladder as an additional layer to promote healing and prevent recurrence.

ii) Transvaginal approach: Many approaches have been described including Sims, Latzko, and Raz. Through a vaginal approach, the vaginal wall is mobilized circumferentially about the fistula tract. Either the fistula tract is excised with edges of the debrided tract forming the first layer of closure, or the tract is left in situ with fistula edges rolled over forming the primary layer of closure. The perivesical fascia on either side of the first layer of closure is then imbricated over the primary suture line forming the second layer. A labial fat pad (i.e., Martius flap), peritoneal flap, or gracilis muscle flap may be placed over the suture lines as a well-vascularized flap similar to the omental flap in the transabdominal approach. Finally, a flap of vaginal wall is advanced over the repair forming the final layer of closure.

d) Regardless of approach, maximal urinary drainage (urethral and suprapubic catheters) is maintained postoperatively. A cystogram is usually obtained 2–3 weeks following repair to confirm successful closure.

II. URETEROVAGINAL FISTULA

A. Etiology

Most ureterovaginal fistulas are secondary to unrecognized distal ureteral injuries sustained during gynecologic procedures including abdominal or vaginal hysterectomy, caesarean section, anti-incontinence surgery, and so forth. Occasionally, they may be secondary to endoscopic instrumentation, radiation therapy, pelvic malignancy, penetrating pelvic trauma, or other pelvic surgery (vascular, enteric, etc.).

1. Risk factors for ureteral injuries include a prior history of pelvic surgery, endometriosis, radiation therapy, and pelvic inflammatory disease (PID).
2. Up to 12% of vesicovaginal fistulas may have an associated ureterovaginal fistula.

B. Presentation

May present with clear drainage per vagina or unilateral hydroureteronephrosis and flank pain secondary to partial ureteral obstruction.

Flank pain, nausea, fever, and clear vaginal drainage following pelvic surgery are very suggestive of ureteral injury. Patients will have a normal voiding pattern if the contralateral kidney is unaffected.

C. Evaluation

1. Intravenous urography: A urogram may demonstrate partial obstruction, hydroureteronephrosis, and drainage into the vagina.
2. Cystoscopy and retrograde pyelography are performed to evaluate for bladder injury and to visualize the distal ureteral segment if not well seen on the urogram. An attempt at retrograde stenting is reasonable if the pyeloureterogram demonstrates ureteral continuity. Prolonged internal diversion with ureteral stenting may result in resolution of the fistula.
3. CT/MRI: Cross-sectional imaging may be useful to evaluate for pelvic malignancy when indicated or to evaluate for a urinoma in patients with persistent fevers.
4. Cystogram or cystometrogram: In cases in which a long segment of distal ureter is involved and a Boari flap is being considered for reconstruction, a cystogram or cystometrogram may be useful to evaluate the bladder capacity. In addition, a cystogram should evaluate for vesicoureteral reflux.
5. Percutaneous nephrostomy and antegrade nephrostogram: Percutaneous drainage of the involved kidney followed by antegrade instillation of contrast can provide decompression of a partially obstructed kidney as well as anatomic localization and demonstration of the fistula (Figure 12-3).

D. Therapy

1. Percutaneous drainage and possible antegrade stenting: If high-grade partial obstruction exists in the setting of sepsis, percutaneous drainage and a course of antibiotic therapy are indicated prior to definitive repair. If retrograde stenting is unsuccessful but the pyeloureterogram shows continuity of the ureteral lumen, then an attempt at antegrade stenting may be undertaken.

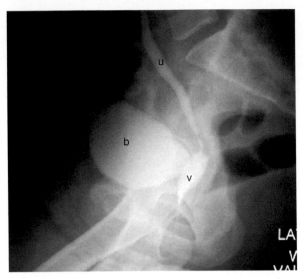

FIGURE 12-3. Antegrade nephrostogram demonstrating ureteral dilation and drainage into the vagina following abdominal hysterectomy. Contrast is seen entering the vagina (v) from the ureter (u) confirming the diagnosis of ureterovaginal fistula. A simultaneous cystogram demonstrates the bladder (b, bladder).

2. Ureteral stenting (see previous).
3. Surgery: When stenting is unsuccessful, ureteral reimplantation (with or without psoas hitch) is performed. It is not necessary to excise the distal ureteral segment or even close the fistula unless vesicoureteral reflux is present.
4. Fistulas resulting from advanced pelvic malignancy may best be treated by urinary diversion.

III. URETHROVAGINAL FISTULA

A. Etiology

Usually postsurgical (urethral diverticulectomy, antiincontinence surgery, etc.), although urethrovaginal fistulas may occur as a result of trauma, instrumentation (catheterization), radiation, and childbirth.

B. Presentation

Urethrovaginal fistulas are often asymptomatic if located in the distal third of the urethra (beyond the continence mechanism), otherwise the presentation is similar to VVF.

Occasionally, these patients may present with symptoms suggestive of stress or urgency incontinence and cystoure-thrography will be necessary to make the diagnosis. Dyspa-reunia or recurrent urinary tract infections (UTIs) are sometimes seen.

C. Evaluation

1. Voiding cystourethrogram (VCUG): Voiding images must be obtained in patients with a competent bladder neck and proximal sphincteric mechanism or the fistula will not be demonstrated.
2. Cystoscopy: Useful to evaluate for concurrent abnormalities of the bladder and urethra.

D. Therapy

1. Catheter drainage may be useful in a limited number of cases if the fistula is noted promptly following the causative event.
2. Transvaginal surgical excision with urethral reconstruc-tion, multiple layer closure using periurethral fascia, a labial fat pad (Martius flap), and vaginal wall flaps is usually highly successful.

IV. ENTEROVESICAL FISTULA

A. General Considerations

Enterovesical fistulas may form between any segment of bowel in the pelvis (colon, ileum, etc.) and the bladder.

B. Etiology

The most common cause of enterovesical fistula is diverti-cular disease of the colon (50–70%). Other common causes include neoplastic disease (colon cancer), inflammatory bowel disease (Crohn's disease), radiation therapy, and trauma.

C. Presentation

1. Enterovesical fistula may present with recurrent UTIs, fecaluria, pneumaturia, and hematuria.
2. Presentation with sepsis or GI symptoms is rare.
3. Gouverneur's syndrome (suprapubic pain, urinary frequency, dysuria, and tenesmus) is the hallmark of enterovesical fistula.

D. Evaluation

1. Charcoal test: The oral administration of activated charcoal may confirm the diagnosis of enterovesical fistula. Several hours after ingestion, flecks of charcoal may be noted in the urine.

2. Cystoscopy and possible biopsy: Endoscopic visualization has a very high yield for the identification of enterovesical fistula.
   a) 80–100% of cases demonstrate bullous edema, erythema, or exudation of feculent material from the fistula site.
   b) Generally, colonic fistulas occur on the left side and dome of the bladder, whereas small bowel fistulas occur on the dome and right side of the bladder.
   c) Biopsy of the fistula is indicated in cases in which malignancy is suspected.

3. Colonoscopy/barium enema: Although less common than diverticular disease, it is important to exclude primary intestinal malignancy as the cause for the fistula.

4. CT or MRI of the pelvis: Air in the bladder as seen on cross-sectional imaging in the absence of prior lower urinary instrumentation (cystoscopy, catheterization, etc.) is highly suggestive of an enterovesical fistula. CT scan with contrast is generally considered to have the best diagnostic yield.
   a) The triad of findings on CT that are suspicious for colovesical fistula consist of (1) bladder wall thickening adjacent to a loop of thickened colon, (2) air in the bladder (in the absence of previous lower urinary manipulation), and (3) the presence of colonic diverticula.

5. VCUG may demonstrate the fistulous connection. In some cases, however, the fistula may act as a "flap valve" and contrast will not be seen entering the bowel.

E. Therapy

1. Bowel rest and hyperalimentation (total parental nutrition [TPN]) may allow the spontaneous closure of some enterovesical fistulas.

2. Medical therapy: This is most applicable in enterovesical fistula secondary to Crohn's disease. Appropriate use of TPN, corticosteroids, sulfasalazine, and antibiotics may promote spontaneous resolution.

3. Surgery: The application of surgery may involve either a one-stage or multistage approach depending on the presence or absence of inflammation, malignancy, and adjacent organ involvement. In those cases managed with staged procedures, a temporary fecal diversion is performed at the time of fistula repair. Patients with an inflammatory cause of the fistula, but without gross contamination, can be treated with a one-stage procedure, whereas those with unprepared bowel, gross contamination, or abscess may require a two-stage procedure.

   a) The surgery involves laparotomy, separation of the bladder from the bowel, excision of the fistula tract, primary closure of the urinary tract, and either resection and reanastomosis of the involved bowel segment or a creation of a temporary ostomy.

   b) In some cases, partial cystectomy may be necessary.

   c) Interposition of well-vascularized tissue such as omentum between the bowel and bladder may promote healing and prevent recurrence.

V. RECTOURETHRAL FISTULA

A. Etiology

Rectourethral fistulas (RUFs) occur following radical prostatectomy, external beam radiotherapy for pelvic malignancy, pelvic brachytherapy or cryotherapy, inflammatory diseases of the pelvis (e.g., prostatic abscess, Crohn's disease), or following penetrating pelvic trauma.

1. During radical prostatectomy, the anterior rectal wall may be injured during dissection of the apical portion of the prostate. A postoperative RUF may form from the reconstructed vesicourethral anastomosis to the injured portion of the rectum. In the setting of radical prostatectomy, a prior history of pelvic radiation therapy, rectal surgery, or transurethral resection of the prostate (TURP) is associated with an increased risk of RUF.

B. Presentation

May present with recurrent UTIs, fecaluria, pneumaturia, or, rarely, urine per rectum. A defect may be palpable at the level of the vesicourethral anastomosis. If a Foley catheter is indwelling, it may be palpable on rectal exam.

C. Evaluation

1. Voiding cystourethrography will demonstrate a fistula between the rectum and urethra.
2. Intravenous urography may be utilized if there is concern for ureteral injury.
3. Barium enema may be helpful to rule out concurrent colonic malignancy.
4. Cystoscopy and/or colonoscopy.
5. CT or MRI of the pelvis may be utilized to evaluate for inflammatory collections or other pelvic masses (e.g., malignancy).

D. Therapy

Many approaches have been advocated for repair of this complex problem. Often, however, despite successful repair of the fistula and reconstitution of the GI and genitourinary (GU) tracts, the patient may have severe problems with urinary and fecal incontinence postoperatively and should be counseled regarding this possibility prior to attempted repair. Both staged repairs and one-stage repairs have been advocated, although most authors would agree that fecal diversion should be performed as an initial measure. In staged repairs, the GI tract is reconstituted only after the fistula has been repaired. Surgical options include:

1. Colostomy and urethral catheter drainage: An attempt at fecal diversion and urethral drainage is a reasonable option in most patients. With prolonged fecal diversion, the fistula may close over the urethral catheter.
2. Colostomy followed by a combined abdominal and/or perineal approach: The rectum is separated off the urethra and both are closed primarily. Well-vascularized tissue such as omentum is interposed between the layers.
3. Colostomy followed by a transrectal approach (York-Mason or trans-sphincteric approach): The fistula is exposed using either anal dilation and a speculum or transection of the anal sphincters. The fistula is then repaired in multiple layers by advancement and rotation of rectal wall flaps.

VI. OTHER URINARY FISTULA

A. Urovascular Fistula

Most commonly these fistulas occur between the ureter and surrounding blood vessels such as the iliacs. Vigorous hematuria in the setting of indwelling stents in a previously irradiated patient or a patient with a history of vascular surgery should alert the physician to the possibility of this type of fistula. If the patient is in extremis (exsanguinating, etc.), immediate surgical intervention is indicated. If the patient is stable, imaging studies including CT, MRI, or angiography may be indicated. In some cases, surgery may be avoided with the use of interventional radiologic techniques.

B. Vesicouterine Fistula

These rare fistulas most commonly occur following low-segment caesarean section. They may present with Youssef's syndrome: menouria, apparent amenorrhea, patent cervix, and urinary continence. Treatment is usually surgical and involves either hysterectomy and closure of the bladder (if the patient has completed childbearing) or excision of the fistula tract and separate closure of the bladder and uterus with interposition of omentum. Occasionally, successful treatment has been seen with hormonal induction of amenorrhea and catheter drainage.

SELF-ASSESSMENT QUESTIONS

1. What is the most common cause of vesicovaginal fistula in the United States?
2. What are the potential advantages and disadvantages of a transvaginal vesicovaginal fistula repair as compared to a transabdominal approach?
3. What diagnostic studies are indicated in the evaluation of urinary incontinence in a 45-year-old woman 6 months following radical hysterectomy and radiation therapy for cervical carcinoma?
4. What are the most common causes for colovesical fistula and what are the indications for a two-stage versus one-stage repair?
5. Describe the diagnostic evaluation and subsequent management of a suspected rectourethral fistula following radical prostatectomy.

SUGGESTED READINGS

1. Arrowsmith S, Hamlin EC, Wall LL: Obstructed labor injury complex: obstetric fistula formation and the multifaceted morbidity of maternal birth trauma in the developing world. *Obstet Gynecol Surv* 51:568–574, 1996.

2. Blaivas JG, Heritz DM, Romanzi LJ: Early versus late repair of vesicovaginal fistulas: vaginal and abdominal approaches. *J Urol* 153:1110–1112, 1995.

3. Cass AS, Odland M: Ureteroarterial fistula: case report and review of literature. *J Urol* 143:582–583, 1990.

4. Eilber KS, Kavaler E, Rodriguez LV, et al: Ten-year experience with transvaginal vesicovaginal fistula repair using tissue interposition. *J Urol* 169:1033–1036, 2003.

5. Gerber GS, Schoenberg HW: Female urinary tract fistulas,". *J Urol* 149:229–236, 1993.

6. Lee RA, Symmonds RE, Williams TJ: Current status of genitourinary fistula. *Obstet Gynecol* 72(3 Pt 1):313–319, 1988.

7. Margolis T, Mercer LJ: Vesicovaginal fistula. *Obstet Gynecol Surv* 49:840–847, 1994.

8. McConnell DB, Sasaki TM, Vetto RM: Experience with colovesical fistula. *Am J Surg* 140:80–84, 1980.

9. O'Conor VJ, Sokol JK, Bulkley GJ, Nanninga JB: Suprapubic closure of vesicovaginal fistula. *J Urol* 109:51–54, 1973.

10. Renschler TD, Middleton RG: 30 years of experience with York-Mason repair of recto-urinary fistulas. *J Urol* 170(4 Pt 1):1222–1225, 2003.

11. Tancer ML: Vesicouterine fistula—a review. *Obstet Gynecol Surv* 41:743–753, 1986.

Voiding Function and Dysfunction; Urinary Incontinence

Alan J. Wein, MD, PhD (hon) and
M. Louis Moy, MD

INTRODUCTION

The **lower urinary tract (LUT) functions as a group of inter-related structures with a joint function in the adult to bring about efficient and low-pressure bladder filling, low-pressure urine storage with perfect continence, and periodic complete voluntary urinary expulsion, again at low pressure.** Because in the adult the LUT is normally under voluntary neural control, it is clearly different from other visceral organs, which are regulated solely by involuntary mechanisms. **For description and teaching, the micturition cycle is best divided into two relatively discrete phases: bladder filling/urine storage and bladder emptying/voiding.** The micturition cycle normally displays these two modes of operation in a simple on-off fashion. The cycle involves switching from activation of storage reflexes and inhibition of the voiding reflex to inhibition of the storage reflexes and activation of the voiding reflex and back again. First some relevant facts regarding the anatomy, neuroanatomy, physiology, and pharmacology of the LUT are summarized. We then answer certain important functional questions related to the filling and storage phase and the emptying and voiding phase of micturition. Certain "rules" are formulated that must be satisfied for the LUT to function normally. By extrapolation, these rules are used as a basis for a very simple functional classification of voiding dysfunction and as a framework to understand urodynamic evaluation and the rationale for all types of treatment. The neurourologic evaluation, classification schemes for voiding dysfunction, and the more common types of neurogenic and non-neurogenic voiding dysfunction are considered, followed by a synopsis and summation of pertinent points relative to all types of treatment for filling/storage and for emptying/voiding disorders. Benign prostatic hypertrophy (BPH) and related issues are discussed in Chapter 14.

I. RELEVANT LOWER URINARY TRACT ANATOMY, PHYSIOLOGY, PHARMACOLOGY, AND TERMINOLOGY

A. Bladder, Urethra, Smooth and Striated Sphincter

1. The designation LUT includes the bladder, urethra, and periurethral striated muscle. Anatomically and embryologically, the bladder traditionally has been divided into detrusor and trigone regions. The terms bladder **body** and bladder **base** refer to a functional rather than anatomic division of bladder smooth muscle. This is based on distinct differences in neuromorphology and neuropharmacology between the smooth muscle lying circumferentially above (body) and below (base) the level of the ureterovesical junction. The **smooth sphincter** refers to the smooth muscle of the bladder neck and proximal urethra. This sphincter is not anatomic but physiologic and is not under voluntary control. Others refer to this area as the internal sphincter, the proximal sphincter, and, simply, the bladder neck sphincter. Although most would accept the facts that the proximal urethra is that portion of the LUT between the bladder neck and "urogenital diaphragm" in both genders and that it contains smooth muscle capable of affecting urethral resistance, there is virtually no physiologic or pharmacologic change that affects the smooth muscle of the most proximal urethra without also affecting the smooth muscle of the bladder neck. Normally, resistance increases in the area of the smooth sphincter during bladder filling and urine storage and decreases during an emptying bladder contraction. In the human proximal urethra, there is a thick, primarily longitudinal smooth muscle layer and a thinner outer circular layer. The longitudinal layer is believed by many, but not all, clinicians to be continuous with the musculature of the bladder base. Teleologically, this arrangement is consistent with a tonic role of the circular layer in maintaining closure during filling and storage and a phasic role for the longitudinal layer in contributing to the opening of the urethra during voiding. The bladder body does not contain discrete unidirectional layers of smooth muscle as suggested by some older texts. In the bladder base, there is a more or less layer-like arrangement of smooth muscle, loosely organized into inner and outer longitudinal and middle circular layers. The superficial and deep layers of the trigone musculature lie on the posterior bladder base smooth muscle.

2. The classic view of the **external urethral sphincter,** or **external sphincter,** is that of a striated muscle within the leaves of a urogenital diaphragm that extends horizontally across the pelvis. It is responsible for stopping the urinary stream when the command "stop voiding" is obeyed. The **striated sphincter** concept expands this definition to include intramural and extramural portions. The **extramural** portion is under voluntary control and corresponds roughly to the "classic" external urethral sphincter, although there is no unbroken sheet of muscle that extends across the pelvis in either male or female and, thus, there is no true urogenital diaphragm. The **intramural** portion denotes skeletal muscle that is intimately associated with part of the urethra in both sexes above the maximal condensation of extramural striated muscle and that is continuous from that level for a variable distance to the bladder neck in the female and at least to the apex of the prostate in the male, forming an integral part of the outer muscular layer of the urethra. Some call this intramural portion the intrinsic rhabdosphincter. Although differences of opinion exist regarding the ultrastructure and physiologic type of striated muscle fibers at various points within the striated sphincter mechanism, there is agreement on the general concept of a gradual increase in activity in the striated sphincter during bladder filling, maintenance with the potential of increases in this activity during bladder storage, and virtual disappearance of this activity just prior to normal emptying/voiding.

B. Innervation and Receptor Function

1. **Autonomic nervous system** (ANS). The physiology and pharmacology of the LUT cannot be separated from those of the ANS. There are many differences between the ANS and the **somatic nervous system** (SNS), but the one easiest for clinicians to understand and remember is that the ANS includes all efferent pathways having ganglionic synapses outside the central nervous system (CNS). There are no synapses between the CNS and the motor end plates of peripheral structures (striated muscle) in the SNS.

2. **Sympathetic** and **parasympathetic.** The terms sympathetic and parasympathetic refer simply to anatomic divisions of the ANS. The sympathetic division consists of those fibers that originate in the thoracic and lumbar regions of the spinal cord, whereas the parasympathetic

division refers to those fibers that originate in the cranial and sacral spinal nerves.

3. **Innervation and neuronal interaction.** The classic view of the peripheral ANS involves a two neuron system: preganglionic neurons emanating from the CNS and making synaptic contact with cells within ganglia, from which postganglionic neurons emerge to innervate peripheral organs (Figure 13-1). This relatively simply concept is still useful for the purposes of discussion but has undergone much expansion and modification. Most innervation of the LUT actually emanates from peripheral ganglia that are at a short distance from, adjacent to, or within the organs they innervate (the urogenital short neuron system). Additionally, the efferent autonomic pathways frequently do not conform to the classic two neuron model, as they are often interrupted by more than one synaptic relay. For many years, the only autonomic neurotransmitters recognized were acetylcholine and norepinephrine. It has become obvious that other transmitters are involved in various components of the ANS, and a once relatively simple concept of chemical neurotransmission has been expanded to include synaptic systems that involve modulator transmitter mechanisms, prejunctional inhibition or enhancement of transmitter release, postjunctional modulation of transmitter action, co-transmitter release, and secondary involvement of locally synthesized hormones and other substances. All of these are subject to neuronal and hormonal regulation, desensitization, and hypersensitization. Finally, these relationships may be altered by changes that occur secondary to disease or destruction in the neural axis, obstruction of the LUT, aging, and hormonal status.

4. **Bladder smooth muscle contraction and relaxation.** The classic model of smooth muscle contraction involves synaptic release of neurotransmitter in response to neural stimulation, with the transmitter agent subsequently combining with a recognition site, or receptor, on the postsynaptic smooth muscle cell membrane. The transmitter-receptor combination then initiates changes in the postsynaptic effector cell that ultimately results in what we consider the characteristic effect of that particular neurotransmitter on that particular smooth muscle.

   Excitation-contraction coupling in bladder smooth muscle has been classically described as mediated by mobilization of intracellular calcium via activation of

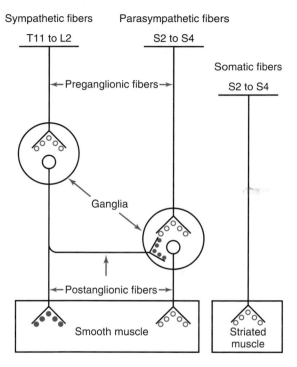

Sympathetic fibers   Parasympathetic fibers

T11 to L2   S2 to S4

Somatic fibers

←Preganglionic fibers→

S2 to S4

Ganglia

←Postanglionic fibers→

Smooth muscle

Striated muscle

Nature of primary chemical transmitter

Norepinephrine

Acetylcholine

FIGURE 13-1. Classical neuroanatomic and neuropharmacologic description of the innervation of the smooth muscle of the bladder and urethra and the striated muscle of the external urethral sphincter. Note the termination of some postganglionic sympathetic (adrenergic) fibers of parasympathetic ganglion cells, providing the morphologic substrate for sympathetic inhibition of parasympathetic ganglion cell transmission. Note also the lack of ganglia in the somatic innervation. (From Hanno P, Malkowicz SB, Wein A [eds]: *Voiding Function and Dysfunction, Clinical Manual of Urology.* McGraw Hill, New York, 2001, F14-1, p 341.)

phosphoinositide hydrolysis. The cytosolic calcium binds to calmodulin, initiating the cascade of events necessary to phosphorylate myosin and cause contraction. Relaxation is mediated by a decrease in intracellular calcium.

This is accomplished by extrusion extracellularly or reuptake into intracellular stores. Smooth muscle relaxation can also be produced by causing intracellular potassium efflux, resulting in membrane hyperpolarization. Both of these latter actions are potential pharmacologic targets for decreasing bladder contractility. Unfortunately, there are no bladder selective calcium channel blockers or potassium channel openers. Recently it has also been proposed that the main pathway for activation of bladder contraction is by calcium influx through L-type calcium channels and increased sensitivity to calcium of the contractile machinery by inhibition of myosin light chain phosphatase through activation of Rho kinase.

5. **Neurotransmitter terminology:** cholinergic and adrenergic subtypes. Clinicians are often confused because they assume that the terms sympathetic and parasympathetic imply particular neurotransmitters. These terms imply only anatomic origin within the ANS. Other adjectives are used to describe the nature of the neurotransmitter involved (see Figure 13-1).

The term **cholinergic** refers to those receptor sites where acetylcholine is a primary neurotransmitter. Peripheral cholinergic fibers include somatic motor fibers, all preganglionic autonomic fibers, and all postganglionic parasympathetic fibers. The cholinergic receptor sites on autonomic effector cells are termed **muscarinic.** Atropine and its congeners competitively inhibit muscarinic receptor sites. Cholinergic receptor sites on autonomic ganglia and on motor end plates of skeletal muscle are designated **nicotinic.** These are not atropine sensitive.

The term **adrenergic** is applied to those receptor sites where a catecholamine is the neurotransmitter. Most postganglionic sympathetic fibers are adrenergic receptor sites, including those to LUT smooth muscle, where the catecholamine responsible for neurotransmission is norepinephrine. Adrenergic receptor sites are further classified as **alpha (α) or beta (β)** on the basis of the differential effects elicited by a series of catecholamines and their antagonists. Classically, the term α-**adrenergic effect** designates vasoconstriction and/or contraction of smooth musculature in response to norepinephrine.

These effects are inhibited by phentolamine, phenoxybenzamine, prazosin, and related compounds. The term **β-adrenergic effect** implies smooth muscle relaxation in response to catecholamine stimulation and also includes cardiac stimulation, vasodilation, and bronchodilation.

These effects are stimulated most potently by isoproterenol (much more so than by norepinephrine) and antagonized by multiple β-blocker compounds, of which propranolol is a prototype.

Receptor subtyping is a relevant concept that explains why some neurotransmitters have differing effects in different organs or anatomic localizations. Subtyping can be based on functional assays, radioligand-binding affinity, or on cloning established genotypes. For instance, there are five different muscarinic receptor subtypes (M1–M5). Although it appears that the majority of these in human bladder smooth muscle are of the M_2 subtype, bladder smooth muscle contraction is mediated primarily by the M_3 subtype. There are multiple subtypes of α- and β-adrenergic receptors as well. Adding to the complexity is the fact that neurotransmitters may have differing (or no) effects at different sites (i.e., brain, pons, spinal cord, efferent ganglia, presynaptic and postsynaptic neural effector junction, sensory afferent fibers, and ganglia). In this chapter, we concentrate on peripheral smooth muscle actions.

6. **Other peripheral neurotransmitters.** Other nonadrenergic noncholinergic (NANC) peripheral neurotransmitters exist in the lower urinary tract and their role(s) in normal and abnormal states is the object of much current investigation. These are summarized in Table 13-1. Note, however, that the presence of a potential neurotransmitter and a laboratory tissue response to an agonist or/and antagonist does not necessarily imply physiologic function.

7. **Peripheral innervation.** The pelvic and hypogastric nerves supply the bladder and urethra with efferent parasympathetic and sympathetic innervation, and both convey afferent sensory impulses from these organs to the spinal cord (Figure 13-2). The **parasympathetic efferent supply** is classically described as originating in the grey matter of the interomediolateral cell column of sacral spinal cord segments S2-S4. This preganglionic supply is ultimately conveyed by the **pelvic nerve.** These fibers synapse with cholinergic postganglions in the pelvic plexus or in ganglia within the bladder wall. **Efferent sympathetic fibers** to the bladder and urethra are thought to originate in the interomediolateral cell column and nucleus intercalatus of spinal cord segments T11-L2 and are carried within the **hypogastric nerves.** Bilaterally, at a variable distance from the bladder and urethra, the hypogastric and pelvic nerves meet and branch to form the

Table 13-1: Possible Peripheral Transmitters and Modulators in the Lower Urinary Tract

Transmitter (Receptor)	Effect	Site of Action
Acetylcholine (M_3)	Contraction	Bladder smooth muscle
Acetylcholine (M_3, M_2)	Excitation (?)	Peripheral afferents
Acetylcholine (M_2)	Contraction (?)	Bladder smooth muscle
Acetylcholine (M_1, M_3)	Contraction (?)	Prejunctional
Acetylcholine (M_2, M_4)	Relaxation	Prejunctional
Norepinehphrine (β_3)	Relaxation	Bladder smooth muscle
Norepinehphrine (α_1)	Contraction	Bladder smooth muscle
Adenosine triphosphate ($P2X_1$)	Contraction	Bladder smooth muscle
Adenosine triphosphate ($P2X_3$)	Excitation	Peripheral afferents
Nitric oxide (NO)	Relaxation	Bladder base smooth muscle
Nitric oxide (NO)	Inhibition	Peripheral afferents
Serotonin ($5\text{-}HT_1$, $5\text{-}HT_2$)	Contraction	Bladder smooth muscle
Prostanoids	Contraction	Bladder smooth muscle
Prostanoids	Excitation	Peripheral afferents
Leukotrienes (LTB_4)	Contraction	Bladder smooth muscle
Angiotensin (AT1)	Contraction	Bladder smooth muscle
Bradykinin (B_2)	Contraction	Bladder smooth muscle
Endothelin (ETa)	Contraction	Bladder smooth muscle
Tachykinins (NK2)	Contraction	Bladder smooth muscle

Vasopressin (V1)	Contraction	Bladder smooth muscle
Vasoactive intestinal peptide (VPAC$_1$/VPC$_2$)	Relaxation	Bladder smooth muscle
Parathormone	Relaxation	Bladder smooth muscle

Adapted from Andersson K-E, Wein AJ: Pharmacology of the lower urinary tract: basis for current and future treatments of urinary incontinence. Pharmacol Rev 56:581–631, 2004.

pelvic plexus. Divergent branches of this pelvic plexus innervate the pelvic organs. Efferent innervation of the striated sphincter is classically thought to be somatic and to emanate from **Onuf's nucleus** in sacral spinal cord segments S2-S4, exiting the spinal cord as the pudendal nerve. Some clinicians believe that the striated sphincter is innervated by branches of the ANS as well.

The **afferents** traveling in the pelvic nerve are responsible for the initiation of the micturition reflex in the normal state. **Myelinated A-delta fibers** normally subserve this function and convey mechanoreceptor input. **Unmyelinated C fiber afferents** are more prevalent but remain relatively silent during normal filling and storage. These become "awakened" and functional under various conditions (i.e., responses to distention after spinal cord injury [SCI], to cold—the "ice water test," and to nociceptive stimuli). Myelinated somatic afferents from the striated sphincter travel in the pudendal nerve. Afferents also travel in the hypogastric nerve, but little is known about their specific function. The most important afferents for initiating and maintaining normal micturition are those in the pelvic nerve, relaying to the sacral spinal cord. These convey impulses from tension, volume, and nociceptors located in the serosal, muscle, and urothelial and suburothelial layers of the bladder and urethra. In a neurologically normal adult, the sensation of filling and distention is what develops during filling/storage and initiates the reflexes responsible for emptying/voiding.

8. **Cholinergic innervation and parasympathetic stimulation.** Cholinergic innervation is abundant to all areas of the bladder of animals and humans. Although most researchers agree on the existence of a cholinergic innervation at least of the proximal urethra in animals, there is disagreement regarding the extent (and in some cases existence) of a

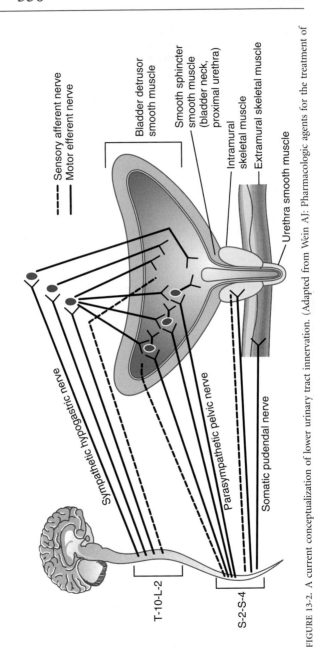

FIGURE 13-2. A current conceptualization of lower urinary tract innervation. (Adapted from Wein AJ: Pharmacologic agents for the treatment of incontinence due to overactive bladder. *Expert Opin Investig Drugs* 10:65–83, 2001.)

similar innervation in humans. It is generally agreed that abundant muscarinic cholinergic receptor sites exist throughout the bladder body and base musculature of various animal species and of humans and that they are more numerous in the bladder body. A sustained bladder contraction is produced by stimulation of the pelvic nerves, and it is generally agreed that reflex activation of this pelvic nerve excitatory tract is responsible for the emptying bladder contraction of normal micturition and for the involuntary bladder contractions seen with various neurologic and non-neurologic diseases/conditions. Whether acetylcholine is the sole neurotransmitter released during such stimulation is highly controversial. **Atropine resistance** refers to the incomplete antagonism produced by atropine of the bladder response to pelvic nerve stimulation or of isolated bladder strips to electrical field stimulation (producing intramural neural stimulation). This is in contrast to atropine's ability to completely block the response of bladder smooth muscle strips to exogenous acetylcholine. It is generally agreed that atropine resistance occurs in various experimental animal models, and the most logical explanation seems to be release of additional neurotransmitter(s) besides acetylcholine in response to nerve stimulation. Adenosine triphosphate (ATP) is most commonly mentioned as the prime candidate. Normally, atropine resistance does not occur in humans. However, one should not ignore the possibility that different types of atropine resistance may exist in various types of bladder overactivity, regardless of the normal state of affairs.

9. **Adrenergic innervation and sympathetic stimulation.** Adrenergic innervation of the bladder and urethral smooth musculature has been extensively demonstrated in animal studies. These studies have shown that the smooth musculature of the bladder base and proximal urethra possesses a rich adrenergic (norepinephrine containing) innervation, whereas the bladder body has a sparse but definite adrenergic innervation. The density of innervation seems, in all areas, to be less than that of the cholinergic systems. Considerable disagreement exists, however, as to even the presence of postganglionic sympathetic innervation in the human bladder and proximal urethra. There is general agreement that the smooth muscle of the human male bladder neck possesses a dense adrenergic innervation, but there is little consensus otherwise. Even those researchers who ascribe a significant influence on the micturition cycle to the sympathetic nervous system (SYNS) have difficulty demonstrating more than a sparse adrenergic innervation in other areas of the bladder and urethra. There is general agreement,

however, that the smooth muscle of the bladder and proximal urethra in a variety of animals and in humans contains both α- and ß-adrenergic receptors. α-Adrenergic contractile responses predominate in the bladder base and proximal urethra, whereas ß-adrenergic relaxation responses predominate in the bladder body.

Additionally, there is general agreement that, at least in certain animal (the cat, primarily) models, there is a significant inhibitory influence exerted on parasympathetic ganglionic transmission by postganglionic sympathetic fibers (see Figure 13-1). Those who advocate a major role of the SYNS in the micturition cycle summarize the influences as primarily to facilitate the filling and storage phase of micturition by three mechanisms.

a) Decreasing bladder contractility via an inhibitory effect on parasympathetic ganglionic transmission.

b) Increasing outlet resistance by stimulation of the predominantly α-adrenergic receptors in the bladder base and proximal urethra.

c) Increasing accommodation by stimulation of the predominantly β-adrenergic receptors in the bladder body. It should be noted, however, that some researchers are of the opinion that the SYNS plays a very minor role in the micturition cycle in the human.

II. CNS INFLUENCES ON MICTURITION

Micturition is basically a function of the peripheral ANS. However, the ultimate control of LUT function obviously resides at higher neurologic levels. There is general consensus that a micturition "center" in the spinal cord is localized to segments S2-S4, with the major portion at S3. Early workers believed that micturition was a simple sacral spinal reflex activity that was modulated by a number of central and peripheral reflexes. It is now acknowledged that the micturition cycle is coordinated in the **pontine mesencephalic reticular formation** (see Figure 13-2). Input to this area is derived from the cerebellum, basal ganglia, thalamus, hypothalamus, and cerebral cortex. Bladder contraction elicited by stimulation at or above this area seems to occur with a decrease in activity of the periurethral striated musculature, as in normal micturition. **In general, the tonic activity of the cerebral cortex and midbrain is inhibitory.** The regions of the cerebral hemispheres primarily concerned with bladder function are the superomedial portion of the frontal lobes and the genu of the corpus callosum. There is debate as to whether the cerebral areas controlling bladder and striated sphincter activity are geographically separate.

Table 13-2: Potential Central Nervous System Neurotransmitters Other than Opioids and Their Effects on the Micturition Reflex

Neurotransmitter	Site	Predominant Action
Glutamate	Brain, SC	+
Glycine	Brain, SC	−
GABA (gamma amino butyric acid)	Brain, SC	−
Serotonin	SC	−
Acetylcholine	Brain	±
Dopamine (D-2)	Brain	+
Dopamine (D-1)	Brain	−
Norepinephrine (α-1,α-2)	Brain, SC	±
Tachykinins (NK1, NK2)	Brain, SC	+

SC, spinal cord.

Evidence exists that endogenous opioid peptides influence micturition by a tonic inhibitory effect on detrusor reflex pathways. These inhibitory effects could be mediated at several levels, including the peripheral bladder ganglia, sacral spinal cord, and brain stem micturition center. Different types of opioid receptors may be responsible, at different sites, for different types of effects on bladder contractility. Numerous other potential neurotransmitters can be found in various areas of the CNS. A partial list is in Table 13-2.

III. NORMAL LOWER URINARY TRACT FUNCTION

A. What Determines Bladder Response During Filling?

The normal adult bladder response to filling at a physiologic rate is an almost imperceptible change in intravesical pressure. During at least the initial stages of bladder filling, this very high compliance (Δ volume/Δ pressure) is due primarily to passive properties of the bladder wall. The elastic and viscoelastic properties of the bladder wall allow it to stretch to a certain degree without any increase in tension exerted on its contents, and at physiologic filling rates, intravesical pressure remains virtually unchanged.

In the usual clinical setting, filling cystometry shows a slight increase in intravesical pressure, but this pressure rise is a function of the fact that cystometry filling is carried out at a greater than physiologic rate. **Compliance can be decreased clinically by (1) any process that alters the viscoelasticity or elasticity of the bladder wall components, (2) certain types of neurologic injury or disease, and (3) filling the bladder beyond its limit of distensibility.**

The viscoelastic properties of the stroma (bladder wall less smooth muscle and epithelium) and the relaxed detrusor muscle account for the passive mechanical properties seen during filling. The main components of stroma are collagen and elastin. When the collagen component increases, compliance decreases. This can occur with various types of injury, bladder outlet obstruction, and neurologic decentralization. Once decreased compliance occurs because of a replacement by collagen or other components of the stroma, it is generally unresponsive to pharmacologic manipulation, hydraulic distention, or nerve section. Most often under those circumstances, augmentation cystoplasty is required to achieve satisfactory reservoir function. There may also be an active but non-neurogenic component to the filling/storage properties of the bladder. Some have suggested that an as yet unidentified relaxing factor is released from the urothelium and others have suggested that urothelium released nitric oxide may exert an inhibitory effect on afferent mechanisms during filling.

At a certain level of bladder filling, spinal sympathetic reflexes are clearly evoked in all animals, and there is some indirect evidence to support such a role in humans. An inhibitory effect on bladder contractility is thought to be mediated primarily by sympathetic modulation of cholinergic ganglionic transmission (see section I.B.9). Through this sympathetic reflex, two other possibilities exist for promoting filling and storage. One is neurally mediated stimulation of the predominantly α-adrenergic receptors in the area of the smooth sphincter, the net result of which would be to cause an increase in resistance in that area. The other is neurally mediated stimulation of the predominantly ß-adrenergic receptors in the bladder body smooth musculature, causing a decrease in tension. Good evidence also seems to support a strong tonic inhibitory effect of endogenous opioids on bladder activity at the level of the spinal cord, the parasympathetic ganglia, and perhaps the brain stem as well. Finally, bladder filling and wall distention may release autocrine-like factors which themselves influence contractility, either by stimulation or inhibition.

B. What Determines Outlet Response During Filling?

There is a gradual increase in urethral pressure during bladder filling, contributed to by at least the striated sphincter element and perhaps, by the smooth sphincter element. The rise in urethral pressure seen during the filling and storage phase of micturition can be correlated with an increase in efferent pudendal nerve impulse frequency. This constitutes the efferent limb of a spinal somatic reflex that is initiated when a certain critical intravesical pressure is reached. This is the so-called **guarding reflex,** which results in an increase in striated sphincter activity (see Figure 13-8).

Although it seems logical, and certainly compatible with neuropharmacologic, neurophysiologic, and neuromorphologic data, to assume that the muscular component of the smooth sphincter also contributes to the change in urethral response during bladder filling, it is extremely difficult to prove this either experimentally or clinically. The passive properties of the urethral wall undoubtedly play a large role in the maintenance of continence. Urethral wall tension develops within the outer layers of the urethra; however, it is a product not only of the active characteristics of smooth and striated muscle but also of the passive characteristics of the elastic collagenous tissue that makes up the urethral wall. In addition, this tension must be exerted on a soft, plastic inner layer capable of being compressed to a closed configuration—the "filler material" representing the submucosal portion of the urethra. The softer and more plastic this area is, the less the pressure required by the tension-producing layers to produce continence.

Finally, whatever the compressive forces, the lumen of the urethra must be capable of being obliterated by a watertight seal. This mucosal seal mechanism explains why a very thin-walled rubber tube requires less pressure to close an open end when the inner layer is coated with a fine layer of grease than when it is not—the latter case being analogous to scarred or atrophic urethral mucosa.

C. Why Does Voiding Ensue with a Normal Bladder Contraction?

Normally, it is intravesical pressure producing the sensation of distention that is primarily responsible for the initiation of voluntary induced emptying of the LUT. **Although the origin** of the parasympathetic neural outflow to the bladder, the pelvic nerve, is in the sacral spinal cord, the actual organizational center for the micturition reflex in an intact neural axis is in the brain stem, and the complete neural circuit for normal micturition includes the ascending and descending spinal cord pathways to and from this area and the facilitory and inhibitory influences from other parts of the brain.

The final step in voluntarily induced micturition initially involves inhibition of the somatic neural efferent activity to the striated sphincter and an inhibition of all aspects of any spinal sympathetic reflex evoked during filling. Efferent parasympathetic pelvic nerve activity is ultimately what is responsible for a highly coordinated contraction of the bulk of the bladder smooth musculature. A decrease in outlet resistance occurs with adaptive shaping or funneling of the relaxed bladder outlet. In addition to the inhibition of any continence promoting reflexes that have occurred during bladder filling, the change in outlet resistance may also involve an active relaxation of the smooth sphincter through a mechanism mediated by nitric oxide. The adaptive changes that occur in the outlet are also in part due to the anatomic inter-relationships of the smooth muscle of the bladder base and proximal urethra (continuity). Other reflexes elicited by bladder contraction and by the passage of urine through the urethra may reinforce and facilitate complete bladder emptying. Superimposed on these autonomic and somatic reflexes is complex modifying supraspinal input from other central neuronal networks. These facilitory and inhibitory impulses, which originate from several areas of the nervous system, allow for the full conscious control of micturition in the adult.

D. Why Does Urinary Continence Persist During Abdominal Pressure Increases?

During voluntarily initiated micturition, the bladder pressure becomes higher than the outlet pressure and certain adaptive changes occur in the shape of the bladder outlet with consequent passage of urine into and through the proximal urethra. Why do such changes not occur with increases in pressure that are similar in magnitude but produced only by changes in intra-abdominal pressure, such as straining or coughing?

First, a coordinated bladder contraction does not occur in response to such stimuli, clearly emphasizing the fact that increases in total intravesical pressure are by no means equivalent to emptying ability. Normally, for urine to flow into the proximal urethra, not only must there be an increase in intravesical pressure but the increase must also be a product of a coordinated bladder contraction, occurring through a neurally mediated reflex mechanism and associated with characteristic conformational and tension changes in the bladder neck and proximal urethral area.

Assuming the bladder outlet is competent at rest, a major factor in the prevention of urinary leakage during increases in intra-abdominal pressure is the fact that there is normally at least equal pressure transmission to the proximal urethra during such activity. Failure of this mechanism, generally associated with hypermobility of the bladder neck and proximal urethra (another way of describing pathologic descent with abdominal straining), is an almost invariable correlate of "genuine" stress or effort-related urinary incontinence in the female. No such hypermobility occurs in the male. The increase in urethral closure pressure that is normally seen with increments in intra-abdominal pressure actually exceeds the extrinsic pressure increase, indicating that active muscular function due to a reflex increase in striated sphincter activity or other factors that increase urethral resistance, in addition to simple transmission of pressure, is also involved in preventing such leakage. A more complete description of the factors involved in sphincteric incontinence and its prevention can be found in the section on incontinence.

IV. OVERVIEW OF THE MICTURITION CYCLE: SIMPLIFICATION

Bladder accommodation during filling is a primarily passive phenomenon. It is dependent on the elastic and viscoelastic properties of the bladder wall and the lack of parasympathetic excitatory input. An increase in outlet resistance occurs via the striated sphincter somatic guarding reflex. In at least some species a sympathetic reflex also contributes to storage by (1) increasing outlet resistance by increasing tension on the smooth sphincter, (2) inhibiting bladder contractility through an inhibitory effect on parasympathetic ganglia, and (3) causing a decrease in tension of bladder body smooth muscle. Continence is maintained during increases in intra-abdominal pressure by the intrinsic competence of the bladder outlet and the pressure transmission ratio to this area with respect to the intravesical contents. A further increase in striated sphincter activity, on a reflex basis, is also contributory.

Emptying (voiding) can be voluntary or involuntary and involves an inhibition of the spinal somatic and sympathetic reflexes and activation of the vesical parasympathetic pathways, the organizational center for which is in the brain stem. Initially, there is a relaxation of the outlet musculature, mediated not only by the cessation of the somatic and sympathetic spinal reflexes but probably also by a relaxing factor, very possibly nitric oxide, released by parasympathetic stimulation or by some effect of bladder smooth muscle contraction itself.

A highly coordinated parasympathetically induced contraction of the bulk of the bladder smooth musculature occurs, with shaping or funneling of the relaxed outlet, due at least in part to a smooth muscle continuity between the bladder base and proximal urethra. With amplification and facilitation of the bladder contraction from other peripheral reflexes and from spinal cord supraspinal sources, and the absence of anatomic obstruction between the bladder and the urethral meatus, complete emptying will occur.

Whatever disagreements exist regarding the anatomic, morphologic, physiologic, pharmacologic, and mechanical details involved in both the storage and expulsion of urine by the LUT, we believe that agreement is found regarding certain points. First, the micturition cycle involves two relatively discrete processes: bladder filling/urine storage and bladder emptying/voiding. Second, whatever the details involved, these processes can be summarized succinctly from a conceptual point of view.

Bladder filling/urine storage require the following:

1. Accommodation of increasing volumes of urine at a low intravesical pressure (normal compliance) and with appropriate sensation.
2. A bladder outlet that is closed at rest and remains so during increases in intra-abdominal pressure.
3. Absence of involuntary bladder contractions (detrusor overactivity [DO]).

Bladder emptying/voiding require the following:

1. A coordinated contraction of the bladder smooth musculature of adequate magnitude and duration.
2. A concomitant lowering of resistance at the level of the smooth and striated sphincter.
3. Absence of anatomic (as opposed to functional) obstruction.

Any type of voiding dysfunction must result from an abnormality of one or more of the factors previously listed regardless of the exact pathophysiology involved. This division, with its implied subdivision under each category into causes related to the bladder and the outlet, provides a logical rationale for discussion and classification of all types of voiding dysfunction and disorders as related primarily to bladder filling/urine storage or to bladder emptying/voiding. There are some types of voiding dysfunction that represent combinations of filling and storage and emptying and voiding abnormalities. Within this scheme, however, these become readily understandable, and their detection and treatment can be logically described. Further, using this scheme, all aspects of urodynamic, radiologic, and video urodynamic evaluation can be conceptualized as to exactly what they evaluate in terms of either bladder or outlet activity during filling and storage or emptying and voiding. Treatments for voiding dysfunction can be classified under broad categories according to whether they facilitate filling and storage or emptying and voiding and whether they do so by acting primarily on the bladder or on one or more of the components of the bladder outlet. Finally, the individual disorders produced by various neuromuscular dysfunctions can be considered in terms of whether they produce primarily storage or emptying abnormalities or a combination.

V. ABNORMALITIES OF FILLING/STORAGE AND EMPTYING/VOIDING: OVERVIEW OF PATHOPHYSIOLOGY (TABLES 13-3 AND 13-4)

The pathophysiology of failure of the LUT to fill with or store urine adequately or to empty adequately must logically be secondary to reasons related to the bladder, the outlet, or both.

A. Filling/Storage Failure

Absolute or relative failure of the bladder to fill with and store urine adequately results from bladder overactivity (involuntary contraction or decreased compliance), decreased outlet resistance, heightened or altered sensation, or a combination.

1. Bladder Overactivity

Overactivity of the bladder during filling/storage can be expressed as phasic involuntary contractions, as low compliance,

Table 13-3: The Functional Classification of the Pathophysiology of Voiding Dysfunction
Failure to store
Because of the bladder
Because of the outlet
Failure to empty
Because of the bladder
Because of the outlet

Table 13-4: The Expanded Functional Classification of the Pathophysiology of Voiding Dysfunction

I. Failure to store
  A. Because of the bladder
    1. Overactivity
      a. Involuntary contractions
        Neurologic disease or injury
        Bladder outlet obstruction (myogenic)
        Inflammation
        Idiopathic
      b. Decreased compliance
        Neurologic disease or injury
        Fibrosis
        Idiopathic
      c. Combination
    2. Hypersensitivity
      a. Inflammatory/infectious
      b. Neurologic
      c. Psychologic
      d. Idiopathic
    3. Decreased pelvic floor activity (?)
  B. Because of the outlet
    1. Combination (GSI and ISD)
    2. Genuine stress urinary incontinence (GSI)
      a. Lack of suburethral support
      b. Pelvic floor laxity, hypermobility
    3. Intrinsic sphincter deficiency (ISD)
      a. Neurologic disease or injury
      b. Fibrosis
  C. Combination
II. Failure to empty
  A. Because of the bladder
    1. Neurogenic
    2. Myogenic
    3. Psychogenic
    4. Idiopathic
  B. Because of the outlet
    1. Anatomic
      a. Prostatic obstruction
      b. Bladder neck contracture
      c. Urethral stricture in the male
      d. Urethral compression, fibrosis in the female
    2. Functional
      a. Smooth sphincter dyssynergia
      b. Striated sphincter dyssynergia
  C. Combination

or as a combination. Involuntary contractions are most commonly seen in association with neurologic disease or injury; however, they may be associated with increased afferent input due to inflammation or irritation of the bladder or urethral wall, bladder outlet obstruction, stress urinary incontinence (UI) (perhaps due to sudden entry of urine into the proximal urethra), or aging (probably related to neural degeneration) or may be idiopathic. Others have hypothesized that decreased stimulation from the pelvic floor can contribute to phasic bladder overactivity. Decreased compliance during filling/storage may be secondary to neurologic injury or disease, usually at a sacral or infrasacral level, but may result from any process that destroys the viscoelastic or elastic properties of the bladder wall. Bladder-related storage failure may also occur in the absence of overactivity, due to increased afferent input from inflammation, irritation, other causes of hypersensitivity and pain. The causes may be chemical, psychologic, or idiopathic. One classic example is painful bladder syndrome, a term that is replacing "interstitial cystitis."

2. Outlet Underactivity

Decreased outlet resistance may result from any process that damages the innervation or structural elements of the smooth and/or striated sphincter or support of the bladder outlet in the female. This may occur with neurologic disease or injury, surgical or other mechanical trauma, or aging. Classically, sphincteric incontinence in the female was categorized into relatively discrete entities: (1) so-called genuine stress incontinence (GSI) and (2) intrinsic sphincter deficiency (ISD), originally described as "type III stress incontinence." Genuine stress incontinence in the female was described as associated with hypermobility of the bladder outlet because of poor pelvic support and with an outlet that was competent at rest but lost its competence only during increases in intra-abdominal pressure. ISD described a nonfunctional or very poorly functional bladder neck and proximal urethra at rest. The implication of classical ISD was that a surgical procedure designed to correct only urethral hypermobility would have a relatively high failure rate, as opposed to one designed to improve urethral coaptation and compression. The contemporary view is that the majority of cases of effort-related incontinence in the female involve varying proportions of support-related factors and ISD. It is possible to have outlet-related incontinence due only to ISD but not due solely to hypermobility or poor support—some ISD must exist.

Stress or effort-related UI is a symptom that arises primarily from damage to muscles and/or nerves and/or connective tissue within the pelvic floor. Urethral support is important in the female, the urethra normally being supported by the action of the levator ani muscles through their connection to the endopelvic fascia of the anterior vaginal wall. Damage to the connection between this fascia and this muscle, damage to the nerve supply, or direct muscle damage can therefore influence continence. Bladder neck function is likewise important, and loss of normal bladder neck closure can result in incontinence despite normal urethral support. In older writings, the urethra was sometimes ignored as a factor contributing to continence in the female, and the site of continence was thought to be exclusively the bladder neck. However, in approximately 50% of continent women, urine enters the urethra during increases in abdominal pressure. The continence point in these women (highest point of pressure transmission) is at the mid urethra.

Urethral hypermobility implies weakness of the pelvic floor supporting structures. During increases in intra-abdominal pressure, there is descent of the bladder neck and proximal urethra. If the outlet opens concomitantly, stress UI ensues. In the classic form of urethral hypermobility, there is rotational descent of the bladder neck and urethra. However, the urethra may also descend without rotation (it shortens and widens), or the posterior wall of the urethra may be pulled (sheared) open while the anterior wall remains fixed. However, urethral hypermobility is often present in women who are not incontinent, and thus the mere presence of urethral hypermobility is not sufficient to make a diagnosis of a sphincter abnormality unless UI is also demonstrated. The **"hammock hypothesis"** of John DeLancey (1994) proposes that for stress incontinence to occur with hypermobility, there must be a lack of stability of the suburethral supportive layer. This theory proposes that the effect of abdominal pressure increases on the normal bladder outlet, if the suburethral supportive layer is firm, is to compress the urethra rapidly and effectively. If the supportive suburethral layer is lax and/or movable, compression is not as effective. **Intrinsic sphincter dysfunction** denotes an intrinsic malfunction of the urethral sphincter mechanism itself. In its most overt form, it is characterized by a bladder neck that is open at rest and a low Valsalva leak point pressure (VLPP) and urethral closure pressure and is usually the result of prior surgery, trauma with scarring, or a neurologic lesion.

Urethral instability refers to the rare phenomenon of episodic decreases in outlet pressure unrelated to increases in bladder or abdominal pressure. The term urethral instability is probably a misnomer, because many believe that the drop in urethral pressure represents simply the urethral component of a normal voiding reflex in an individual whose bladder does not measurably contract, because of either myogenic or neurogenic reasons. Little has appeared in the literature about this entity since the last edition of this text.

In theory at least, categories of outlet related incontinence in the male are similar to those in the female. **Sphincteric incontinence in the male** is not, however, associated with hypermobility of the bladder neck and proximal urethra but is similar to what is termed intrinsic sphincter dysfunction in the female. There is essentially no information regarding the topic of urethral instability in the male.

The **treatment of filling/storage abnormalities** is directed toward inhibiting bladder contractility, decreasing sensory output, mechanically increasing bladder capacity, and/or toward increasing outlet resistance, the latter either continuously or just during increases in intra-abdominal pressure.

B. Emptying/Voiding Failure

Absolute or relative failure to empty the bladder results from decreased bladder contractility (a decrease in magnitude or duration), increased outlet resistance, or both.

1. Bladder Underactivity

Absolute or relative failure of bladder contractility may result from temporary or permanent alteration in one of the neuromuscular mechanisms necessary for initiating and maintaining a normal detrusor contraction. Inhibition of the voiding reflex in a neurologically normal individual may also occur; it may be by a reflex mechanism secondary to increased afferent input, especially from the pelvic and perineal areas, or may be psychogenic. Non-neurogenic causes also include impairment of bladder smooth muscle function, which may result from overdistention, various centrally or peripherally acting drugs, severe infection, or fibrosis.

2. Outlet Overactivity or Obstruction

Pathologically increased outlet resistance is much more common in men than in women. Although it is most often secondary to anatomic obstruction, it may be secondary to a failure of relaxation or active contraction of the striated or smooth sphincter during bladder contraction. Striated sphincter dyssynergia is a common cause of functional or nonanatomic (as opposed to fixed anatomic) obstruction in patients with neurologic disease or injury. A common cause of outlet obstruction in the female is compression or fibrosis following surgery for sphincteric incontinence.

The **treatment of emptying failure generally consists of maneuvers to increase intravesical/detrusor pressure, facilitate the micturition reflex, decrease outlet resistance, or a combination. If other means fail or are impractical, intermittent catheterization is an effective way to circumvent emptying failure.**

VI. THE NEUROUROLOGIC EVALUATION

A. History

Symptomatology can be valuable in suggesting whether voiding dysfunction represents an abnormality of storage, emptying, or both (Table 13-5). A complete history of the symptoms and their onset, duration, time course, and relationship to neurologic disease or other neurologic symptoms is essential. **Incontinence** is generally a primary symptom of filling and storage failure and may be bladder or outlet related; however, it can also result from ureteral ectopy and congenital or acquired fistulas. Leakage that is associated only with increases in intra-abdominal pressure implies **genuine stress urinary incontinence** (GSUI) at least in the female. Gravitational urethral incontinence that worsens on straining implies **intrinsic sphincter dysfunction.** **Precipitous incontinence** with a more sustained type of leakage similar to voiding is characteristic of involuntary

Table 13-5: Neurourologic Evaluation
History
Bladder diary
Quality of life assessment
Physical examination
Neurologic examination
Urine bacteriologic studies
Renal function studies
Radiologic evaluation
Upper tract
Lower tract
Urodynamic/video-urodynamic study
Endoscopic examination

bladder contractions. It can occur with sensation (urgency) or without urgency in the absence of sensation. Incontinence is not always, however, a primary symptom of filling and storage failure. **Overflow, or paradoxical incontinence,** can develop in a patient with insidious detrusor decompensation with emptying failure. The leakage in this case is generally most prominently associated with changes in position or sudden increases in intra-abdominal pressure and can mimic stress incontinence. **Urgency** is now defined in the International Continence Society (ICS) lexicon as a sudden compelling desire to void that is difficult to defer. Previously the definition included for fear of leaking. A perceived need to void solely because of pain is generally secondary to inflammatory disease.

An **increase in daytime urinary frequency** can be psychogenic, represent a response to pain on low-volume bladder distention (usually indicative of inflammatory disease), be due to DO, or simply be due to increased fluid intake. Increased frequency can also result from emptying failure with a substantial residual urine volume and therefore a decreased functional bladder capacity. It can also exist in association with outlet obstruction induced DO. **Nocturia** usually accompanies nonpsychogenic urinary frequency and can be associated, on the same basis as increased daytime frequency, with either storage or emptying failure. It can also be due, however, simply to an increased nocturnal urine output (nocturnal polyuria syndrome).

The symptom of **pressure** defies exact definition. It is not quite the urge to void but rather a feeling that the bladder is full or that the urge to void will occur shortly. There is often no discernible voiding dysfunction in patients who complain of this; however, such dysfunction can be due to an elevated intravesical pressure during filling, but one that is below the level necessary to elicit the sensation of distention or urgency. This symptom also may be representative of an accurate perception of inadequate emptying with a modest or large residual urine volume. A **bladder diary** is especially useful in accurately portraying symptoms due to a filling and storage abnormality. This should include at least the following: fluid intake, time and amount of voiding, association with urgency (or not), and leakage (or not), including type and amount. The diary will also allow estimation of the functional capacity, which should serve as a guide for filling volume during urodynamics.

Hesitancy, straining to void, and **poor stream** generally reflect a failure to empty adequately, but they can occur in an individual with frequency and urgency who, on toileting, simply has difficulty initiating a voluntary bladder contraction with a small intravesical urine content. A detailed history of prior medical and surgical treatment and the results should always be sought.

B. Physical and Neurologic Evaluation

Findings from a **general physical examination** are nonspecific. There may be cutaneous excoriation secondary to urinary leakage. A focused physical examination should include the lower abdomen, genitalia, and rectum in men and women. Prostate abnormalities must be detected. A careful pelvic examination in women is necessary to detect the presence and degree of pelvic organ prolapse: apical/uterine, anterior and posterior vaginal prolapse. The **neurologic examination** provides evidence of the presence or absence of a neurologic lesion and, if present, localizes it in an attempt to corroborate and explain a given voiding dysfunction. **Mental status** is determined by noting the level of consciousness, orientation, speech, comprehension, and memory. Mental status aberrations can be secondary to neurologic diseases that produce voiding dysfunction, such as senile and presenile dementia, brain tumors, and normal pressure hydrocephalus.

Cranial nerve dysfunction, except when indicative of a brain stem lesion, has little specific relevance to voiding dysfunction. Careful examination of **motor function and coordination** and a sensory examination (including touch, pain, temperature, vibration, and position) can have anatomic and etiologic significance. **Sensory** or motor deficits may suggest specific levels of spinal pathology, either unilateral or bilateral. The abnormalities associated with SCI, Parkinson's disease (PD), multiple sclerosis (MS), and cerebrovascular disease are usually obvious. The presence of lateralizing signs suggests that only one side of the neural axis is affected. Quadriplegia suggests an abnormality of the cervical or high thoracic spinal cord, whereas true paraplegia indicates a cord lesion below the upper thoracic segments. Specific dermatomal sensory alterations or deficits suggest localized pathology at the spinal cord or nerve root level.

Evaluation of the **deep tendon reflexes** provides an indication of segmental spinal cord function as well as suprasegmental function. **Hypoactivity** of the deep tendon reflexes generally is associated with a lower motor neuron (LMN) lesion (in this context, meaning from the anterior horn cells to the periphery), whereas **hyperactivity** generally indicates an upper motor neuron (UMN) lesion (between the brain and anterior horn cells of the spinal cord). These terms, **UMN and LMN**, refer, strictly speaking, only to the SNS (somatic nervous system). However, by convention, they are often applied by urologists and neurologists to the efferent portions of the ANS innervating the LUT. In this context, the terms are generally understood to mean the following: UMN, between the brain and anterior horn cells, and LMN, from anterior horn cells to the periphery, including all preganglionic and postganglionic fibers. Commonly tested deep tendon reflexes include the biceps (C5-C6), triceps (C6-C7), quadriceps or patellar (L2-L4), and Achilles (L5-S2). A pathologic toe sign (Babinski reflex) generally indicates a somatic UMN lesion but can be absent with a complete lesion and marked spasticity. A Babinski reflex may be present contralaterally with a unilateral lesion or may be present unilaterally with a bilateral lesion. The generic term **bulbocavernosus reflex** (BCR) describes contraction of the bulbocavernosus and ischiocavernosus muscles after penile glans or clitoral stimulation, or stimulation of the urethral or bladder mucosa by pulling an indwelling Foley catheter. These reflexes are mediated by pudendal and/or pelvic afferents and by pudendal nerve efferents and, as such, represent a local sacral spinal cord reflex. Most clinicians would agree that the BCR reflects activity in S2-S4, but some believe that this may involve segments as high as L5. Motor control of the external anal sphincter (EAS) is variously described as being served by sacral cord segments S2-S4 or S3-S5. A visible contraction the EAS after pinprick of the mucocutaneous junction constitutes the **anal reflex,** and its activity usually parallels that of the BCR. EAS tone, when strong, indicates that activity of the conus medullaris is present, whereas absent anal sphincter tone usually indicates absent conal activity. Volitional control of the EAS indicates intact control by supraspinal centers. The **cough reflex** (contraction of the EAS with cough) is a spinal reflex that depends on volitional innervation of the abdominal musculature T6-L1. The afferent limb is apparently from muscle receptors in the abdominal wall that enter the spinal cord and ascend. As long as one of these segments remains under volitional control, the cough reflex may be positive. If a lesion above the outflow to the abdominal musculature exists, the cough reflex is generally absent.

In regard to lesions that affect the spinal cord, it must be remembered that the **level of the vertebral lesion (such as in SCI or disk disease) usually differs from the spinal cord segmental level. Sacral spinal cord segments S2-S4 are generally at vertebral levels L1-L2.** Additionally, it must be remembered that after spinal cord trauma, descending degeneration of the cord may occur. In a complete spinal cord lesion above the conus medullaris (otherwise known as suprasegmental or UMN), there will generally be, after spinal shock has passed (see later), hyperactivity of the deep tendon reflexes, skeletal spasticity, and absent skin sensation below the level of the lesion; pathologic toe signs will exist. Following a complete spinal cord lesion at or below the conus (segmental or infrasegmental or LMN), after spinal shock has passed, there will generally be absent deep tendon reflexes, skeletal flaccidity, and absent skin sensation below the lesion level; pathologic toe signs will be absent.

C. Radiologic Evaluation

1. **Upper tracts** (see Chapter 3). Many urologists believe that the intravenous urogram is the optimal screening study of the upper tracts (kidneys and ureters) in patients with significant voiding dysfunction. Ultrasonography can give adequate information about hydronephrosis, the presence of calculi, and, occasionally, hydroureter. Isotope studies can be useful to evaluate renal blood flow and function and to establish the presence of renal or ureteral obstruction. Dilation of the ureters or renal collecting system, or a decrease in function, can represent significant complications of LUT dysfunction and as such are absolute indications for intervention. **Upper tract imaging, however, is generally recommended only in specific situations** in the adult: (1) decreased bladder compliance, (2) neurogenic incontinence, (3) severe urethral obstruction, (4) incontinence associated with significant post-void residual, (5) co-existing loin and flank pain, (6) severe untreated pelvic organ prolapse, and (7) suspected extraurethral UI.

2. **Lower tracts** (see Chapter 3). This portion of the chapter considers only basic cystourethrographic patterns that relate directly to voiding dysfunction caused by neuromuscular disease. There are only a few basic cystourethrographic radiologic configurations, but their significance can be fully ascertained only by concomitant urodynamic study. A **closed bladder neck** is normal in a resting individual whose bladder is undergoing either physiologic or urodynamic filling. However, it can also occur in an individual with an areflexic bladder who is straining to void and in an individual in whom a micturition reflex is occurring but whose smooth sphincter area is dysfunctional or dyssynergic. The closed appearance can sometimes be mimicked to a great degree by significant prostatic enlargement with bladder neck and urethral compression as

well. An **open bladder neck** is normal during voluntarily induced micturition and during most involuntary bladder contractions as well. However, this appearance may also be due to intrinsic sphincter dysfunction (ISD) or some types of neurologic illness or to endoscopic or open surgical alteration, and it may be seen transiently in some females with genuine stress incontinence.

A **closed striated sphincter** is normal during physiologic or urodynamic filling and with an attempt to stop normal urination or to abort an involuntary bladder contraction. The sphincter also normally remains closed during abdominal straining. During voluntary micturition or during micturition secondary to an involuntary bladder contraction caused by neurologic disease at or above the brain stem, the striated sphincter should open unless the patient is trying to abort the bladder contractions by voluntary sphincter contractions.

A cystogram in the erect position at rest and during straining may be useful in quantitating the degree of classical "genuine" stress incontinence (bladder neck closed at rest, open with straining, associated with hypermobility) versus classical ISD (bladder neck open at rest, more leakage with straining, no hypermobility). Voiding cystourethrography is useful to diagnose the site of obstruction in a patient with proven urodynamic evidence of obstruction.

D. Endoscopic Evaluation

Endoscopy is recommended only in specific situations in the adult: (1) when initial testing suggests other types of pathology (microscopic gross hematuria; pain, discomfort, and persistent or severe symptoms of bladder overactivity; and suspected extraurethral incontinence); (2) in patients who have previously undergone bladder, prostate, or other pelvic surgery; and (3) in men with incontinence. Bladder washings or a voided urine for cytology should be sent if symptoms suggest the possibility of neoplastic or preneoplastic changes in the bladder epithelium. The presence or absence of trabeculation (which is compatible with obstruction, involuntary bladder contractions, or neurologic decentralization) can also be determined. Endoscopic examination may likewise be confirmatory of or exclude anatomic obstruction at a particular site, but it should be recognized that not everything that appears obstructive endoscopically is obstructive urodynamically (all large prostates are not obstructive), and lack of a visually appreciated obstruction does not exclude functional obstruction (striated or smooth sphincter dyssynergia) during bladder emptying and voiding.

E. Urodynamic/Video Urodynamic Evaluation

1. General (Table 13-6). The studies that fall under the heading of LUT urodynamics consist simply of methods designed to generate quantitative data relevant to events taking place in the bladder and bladder outlet during the two relatively discrete phases of micturition described previously: filling/storage and emptying/voiding. This conceptualization fits nicely with the concept of two phases of micturition and the description of each phase requiring three components to occur normally.

Table 13-6:	Urodynamics Simplified	
	Bladder	**Outlet**
Filling/storage phase	Pves[1]Pdet[2] (FCMG[3])	UPP[5]
	DLPP[4]	VLPP[6]
		FLUORO[7]
Emptying phase	Pves[8]Pdet[9] (VCMG[10])	MUPP[11]
		FLUORO[12]
		EMG[13]
	(_____	_____)
	_____ FLOW[14] _____	
	_____ RU[15] _____	

This functional conceptualization of urodynamics categorizes each study as to whether it examines bladder or outlet activity during the filling/storage or emptying phase of micturition. In this scheme, uroflow and residual urine integrate the activity of the bladder and the outlet during the emptying phase.[1,2] Total bladder (Pves) and detrusor (Pdet) pressures during a filling cystometrogram (FCMG).
[3]Filling cystometrogram.
[4]Detrusor leak point pressure.
[5]Urethral pressure profilometry.
[6]Valsalva leak point pressure.
[7]Fluoroscopy of outlet during filling/storage.
[8,9]Total bladder and detrusor pressures during a voiding cystometrogram (VCMG).
[10]Voiding cystometrogram.
[11]Micturitional urethral pressure profilometry.
[12]Fluoroscopy of outlet during emptying.
[13]Electromyography of periurethral striated musculature.
[14]Flowmetry.
[15]Residual urine.

Ideally, the urodynamic/video urodynamic evaluation should be able to answer the implied questions regarding the normality or abnormality of each of the components of the two phases of micturition. Combined video urodynamic or separate cystourethrographic study (referred to as FLUORO in Table 13-6) also provides information regarding the presence or absence of vesicoureteral reflux (VUR). A **simple formulation of the commonly utilized urodynamic studies, based on the two phases of micturition concept, is presented in Table 13-6, the individual studies characterized as to whether they evaluate aspects of bladder or outlet activity during filling and storage or emptying.** Within this scheme, **flowmetry** and **residual urine** are simply **ways of integrating bladder and outlet activity during the emptying phase of micturition.**

The **purpose of urodynamic/video urodynamic evaluation is threefold**: (1) determine the precise etiology(ies) of the voiding dysfunction, (2) identify urodynamic risk factors for upper and lower urinary tract deterioration, and (3) identify factors that might affect the success of a particular therapy. The **study should ideally reproduce the patient's symptoms and/or accurately reflect bladder and outlet activity and sensation during filling/storage and emptying/voiding and provide a pathophysiologic basis for management.**

Certain very simple rules aid immeasurably in obtaining the maximum benefit from urodynamic and video urodynamic studies. Although these rules sound obvious, they are often ignored, sometimes even by experienced urodynamicists. **The prime directive is that the study must reproduce the clinical symptomatology or clinical abnormality being investigated.** If it does not, then, insofar as that particular patient is concerned, and despite the fact that the study may be perfectly done and the data beautifully reproduced, it may be worthless. Conversely, **the appropriate study done so as to reproduce the symptoms always yields pertinent information.** As a corollary, it is not necessary to perform the most complicated type of video urodynamic study with every patient. **The simplest, most readily reproducible, and least invasive study that gives the information desired is always the best.** The subject has become far more complicated than necessary. Up to 70–90% of voiding dysfunction problems can be diagnosed by a logical clinician using relatively simple urodynamic studies. As the complexity of the problem and the number of failed prior therapies increases, so does the need for more complicated or combined video urodynamic studies. Finally, it must be remembered that **urodynamics/video urodynamic evaluation must be an interactive process between the patient and examiner.** Information must be constantly exchanged and the study sequence tailored to a given patient and his or her LUT symptoms and signs.

2. **Flowmetry.** Flowmetry is a way to integrate the activity of the bladder and outlet during the emptying phase of micturition. The flow rates and pattern represent the recorded variables; if these are both normal, it is unlikely that there is any significant disorder of emptying. A normal flow, however, does not entirely exclude obstruction, which is strictly defined on the basis of a relationship between detrusor pressure and simultaneous flow. **Consistently low flow rates with adequate volumes voided generally indicate increased outlet resistance, decreased bladder contractility, or both. Flow rates considerably in excess of normal may indicate decreased outlet resistance.** There are only a few abnormal flow patterns. An abnormally broad plateau with a low mean and peak rate generally indicates outlet obstruction or decreased detrusor contractility or both. Intermittent flow is generally secondary to abdominal straining or sphincter dyssynergia, but in rare instances, it can be due to undulating low-amplitude detrusor contractions. An idealized normal flow curve is seen in Figure 13-3 and flow tracings from individuals with various characteristic abnormalities are seen in Figure 13-4.

The primary caveat in interpreting uroflow is to **make sure that the flow event closely approximates the usual voiding event for that patient. If not, it should be repeated with a comfortably full bladder.** In an adult, flow events of 100 mL or less should be interpreted with caution. An overfilled bladder may be accompanied by reduced flow rates as well, probably because of temporary dysfunction introduced by overstretching of detrusor fibers. Measurements of only one flow parameter, such as peak flow, may be misleading, as it is possible for patients with decreased outlet resistance to generate very high peak flows with straining. In comparisons of flow rates in a given individual from one time to another, either for the purposes of evaluating treatment or following a given condition, it is very important to standardize the rates to a given volume. Volume/rate nomograms can be useful in this regard. Most data from studies cite norms of 15 and 25 mL/sec for mean and maximum flow rates. However, flow rates should be standardized in terms of

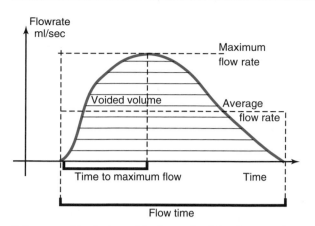

FIGURE 13-3. Terminology of the International Continence Society relating to the urodynamic description of urinary flow. (From Wein AJ, English WE, Whitmore KE: Office urodynamics. *Urol Clin North Am* 15:609, 1988.)

the minimum acceptable flow rates for given gender and age groups. Most "normal" data relate to flowmetry in patients younger than the age of 55 years.

3. **Residual urine volume.** Similarly, residual volume integrates the activity of the bladder and outlet during emptying. It can be measured directly or estimated by cystography or ultrasonography. A consistently increased residual urine volume that reflects the usual status of that patient generally indicates increased outlet resistance, decreased bladder contractility, or both. Negligible residual urine volume is compatible with normal function of the LUT but can also exist with significant disorders of filling and storage (i.e., incontinence) or emptying disorders in which the intravesical pressure is simply sufficient to overcome increases in outlet resistance up to a certain point. Generally, a significant residual urine volume is considered to be indicative of relative detrusor failure, with or without outlet obstruction. Residual urine volume may be expressed as an absolute number (mL) or as a percent of the functional bladder capacity.

4. **Filling cystometry.** Cystometry refers to the method by which changes in bladder pressure are measured. The test was designed originally to evaluate the filling and storage phase of bladder function and to measure changes in bladder pressure with slow progressive increases in volume. Strictly speaking, this is **filling**

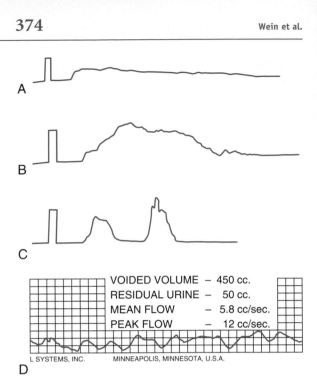

VOIDED VOLUME – 450 cc.
RESIDUAL URINE –   50 cc.
MEAN FLOW   – 5.8 cc./sec.
PEAK FLOW   –   12 cc./sec.

L SYSTEMS, INC.   MINNEAPOLIS, MINNESOTA, U.S.A.

FIGURE 13-4. A. Flowmetry in the patient with bladder outlet obstruction. Height of bar represents a flow of 10 mL/sec. Maximum flow if generally established soon after the onset of voiding. Peak and mean flow rates are decreased. Flow time is prolonged. Note that this diagnosis cannot be made from this flow event alone. However, this is most characteristic of bladder outlet obstruction in a patient with normal detrusor. **B.** Uroflow event from a patient with impaired detrusor contractility. Maximum flow is established near the middle of the flow event. Mean and peak flow rates are decreased. Flow time is somewhat prolonged. To establish this diagnosis beyond a doubt, especially because the therapeutic options differ, a pressure/flow study would be necessary to separate this entity from bladder outlet obstruction. **C.** Intermittent flow. This type of intermittent flow pattern is most commonly due to abdominal straining. In such a patient with decreased outlet resistance, the peak flow rate is often normal or may even be above normal. **D.** Another type of intermittent flow pattern. This can be due either to sphincter dyssynergia or low-amplitude fluctuating detrusor contractions. With sphincter dyssynergia, the changes in flow usually occur faster and are more staccato-like. This is actually from a patient with low-amplitude fluctuating detrusor contraction. (From Wein AJ, English WE, Whitmore KE: Office urodynamics. *Urol Clin North Am* 15:609, 1988.)

cystometry, as opposed to **voiding cystometry.** Unless the examiner clearly recognizes the distinction, erroneous conclusions regarding the activity of the bladder during the emptying phase of micturition may be made on the basis of what is commonly called a cystometrogram but which, in reality, represents only filling, and not voiding, cystometry. There is no single best method of performing cystometry or any urodynamic study, for that matter. All have their shortcomings. The "experts" often differ significantly in their choice of testing sequences and catheters, but their conclusions about an individual patient are usually remarkably similar. Liquid is preferred as a medium for filling cystometry. Few, if any, currently use gas (carbon dioxide). For full micturition studies (filling and voiding cystometry), a liquid medium is obviously required.

The first sensation of bladder filling and the first sensation of fullness, as well as the urge to void and the feeling of imminent micturition, are important data to record. When a phasic involuntary detrusor contraction occurs, it is important to note whether this coincides with a sensation of urgency and whether suppression is possible.

The pressure measured within the bladder is composed of that contributed by the detrusor plus intra-abdominal pressure. Thus, **any pressure increment recorded on a simple cystometrogram may at least partially, and sometimes totally, reflect intra-abdominal pressure. To eliminate such artifactual problems, it is desirable to measure intra-abdominal pressure simultaneously,** as reflected by a catheter-mounted intrarectal pressure balloon, a vaginal catheter, or a catheter inserted next to the bladder. It is true that an experienced operator can very often tell the difference between a true detrusor contraction and an increase in bladder pressure caused by an increase in intra-abdominal pressure by the configuration of the curve and by observation of the patient. However, if there is any question about this or if a significant decision is to be based on these data, electronic subtraction of the intra-abdominal pressure from the total bladder pressure (yielding detrusor pressure) is desirable. The normal adult cystometrogram can be divided into four phases (Figure 13-5).

a) Phase 1. The initial pressure rise represents the initial response to filling, and the level at which the bladder trace stabilizes is known as the initial filling pressure. The first phase of the curve is contributed to by the initial myogenic response to filling and by the elastic

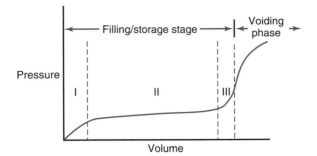

FIGURE 13-5. Idealized normal adult cystometrogram. (From Wein AJ, English WE, Whitmore KE: Office urodynamics. *Urol Clin North Am* 15:609, 1988.)

and viscoelastic response of the bladder wall to stretch, factors previously discussed. With liquid infusion, the initial filling pressure usually develops gradually and levels off between 0 and 8 cm of water in the supine position. With more rapid rates of filling, there may be an initially higher peak, which then levels off. This peak type of initial response is relatively common with gas cystometry. Although this is a detrusor response, its significance is not the same as that of an involuntary bladder contraction during phase 2.

b) Phase 2. Phase 2 is called the tonus limb, and compliance (Δ volume/Δ pressure) is normally high and uninterrupted by phasic rises. In practice, the compliance seen in the urodynamic laboratory is always lower than that existing during physiologic bladder filling. It must be remembered that in a normal individual, if the filling rate with liquid is 2.4 times or less than the hourly diuresis rate, phase 2 will be perfectly flat. Normally, in the urodynamic laboratory, the rise is less than 6 to 10 cm of water. It is difficult to find stated values for normal compliance.

c) Phase 3. Phase 3 is reached when the elastic and viscoelastic properties of the bladder wall have reached their limit. Any further increase in volume generates a substantial increase in pressure. This increase in pressure is not the same as a detrusor contraction. If a voluntary or involuntary contraction occurs, phase 3 can be obscured by the rise in pressure so generated.

d) Phase 4. Ideally, involuntary bladder contractions do not occur during either phase 2 or 3; phase 4 consists of the initiation of voluntary micturition. Many patients are unable to generate a voluntary detrusor contraction in the testing situation, especially in the supine position. This should not be called detrusor areflexia but, simply, absence of a detrusor contraction during cystometry, a finding that is not considered abnormal unless other clinical or urodynamic findings are present that substantiate the presence of neurologic or myogenic disease.

Involuntary bladder contractions (detrusor overactivity or DO) during filling are always significant. Detrusor hyperreflexia and detrusor instability are both terms no longer in use but previously defined by the International Continence Society to relate to the generic term involuntary bladder contraction. **Neurogenic DO (previously detrusor hyperreflexia)** refers to an involuntary contraction that is the result of associated neurologic disease; **idiopathic DO (previously detrusor instability)** refers to an involuntary contraction seen in the absence of neurologic disease. A number of representative adult filling cystometrograms (liquid) are diagrammed in Figure 13-6.

One of the most important urodynamic concepts to remember is that **adequate storage at low intravesical pressure will avoid deleterious upper urinary tract changes in patients with bladder outlet obstruction and/or neuromuscular LUT dysfunction.** Ed McGuire and co-workers have clearly shown that **upper tract deterioration is apt to occur when storage, even though adequate in terms of continence, occurs at sustained urodynamically generated intravesical pressures higher than 40 cm of water.** Application of this concept to patients with storage problems and specifically those with decreased compliance and incontinence has resulted in the concept of the **detrusor leak point pressure (DLPP)** as a very significant piece of urodynamic data. This is to be distinguished from the VLPP described subsequently.

The DLPP is also known as the bladder leak point pressure (BLPP). It is important to understand the context in which this test was originally described and the astute intuitive reasoning that went into describing the original concept. In the early 1980s, McGuire and associates studied a group of myelodysplastic children with decreased compliance and incontinence. Those children who did not leak on filling cystometry until their detrusor pressures exceeded 40 cm of water exhibited upper urinary tract deterioration on subsequent follow-up. Classically, the test was performed by passively filling the bladder through a

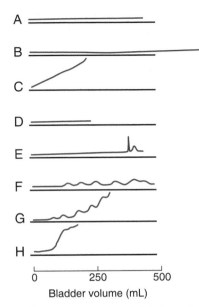

FIGURE 13-6. Various representative adult filling cystometrograms. **A.** Normal filling curve in a patient with a bladder capacity of 450 mL, normal compliance, and no involuntary bladder contractions. Nothing can be said about bladder activity during the emptying phase of micturition from this tracing. **B.** Large capacity bladder with increased compliance at medium fill rate. This type of curve is characteristic of an individual with decreased sensation and bladder decompensation. Although most individuals will in fact have no or poor detrusor contraction, that conclusion cannot be made on the basis of this curve. **C.** Decreased compliance. **D.** Small capacity bladder secondary to hypersensitivity without decreased compliance or involuntary bladder contraction. **E.** Bladder contraction provoked by cough. This particular tracing represents total bladder pressure. To make this diagnosis from this tracing alone, the clinician would need to be either a very astute examiner or review separate recordings of intravesical pressure and intra-abdominal pressure (intrarectal pressure). **F.** Low-amplitude detrusor contraction. This is a subtracted bladder pressure, and this type of recording may be seen most characteristically in a patient with suprasacral neurologic disease or idiopathic detrusor overactivity. **G.** Decreased compliance and involuntary bladder contractions. **H** High-amplitude early involuntary bladder contraction. (From Wein AJ, English WE, Whitmore KE: Office urodynamics. *Urol Clin North Am* 15:609, 1988.)

small-caliber urethral catheter with the patient at rest throughout the study, not attempting to volitionally void. The point at which leakage occurs around the catheter is measured as the DLPP. **If the DLPP in such an individual with decreased compliance and incontinence is greater than 40 cm of water, the patient is believed to be at risk for upper tract deterioration.** Thus, this test has become extremely useful in the management of such patients with neurogenic bladder dysfunction. An abnormal test dictates the necessity of reducing storage pressure to a point below which upper tract deterioration will subsequently be seen, even if this means combining measures to decrease bladder contractility and increase bladder capacity with intermittent catheterization. **The concept has been extended to cover patients who have decreased compliance and who do not have incontinence, but whose measured detrusor pressure at bladder volumes they often "carry" exceeds 40 cm of water.** Some apply the concept as well to patients with involuntary bladder contractions whose detrusor pressures exceed 40 cm of water. Whether this concept truly applies to this latter group of patients, except in instances where this occurs extremely frequently, or where the pressure is maintained once contraction has occurred, is unknown.

As a corollary, **in patients with decreased compliance and incontinence, one must remember that to accurately measure compliance urodynamically, the bladder outlet must be occluded.** This is especially important if there is a plan to correct outlet-related incontinence in an individual with neuromuscular dysfunction associated with decreased compliance (e.g., in the myelomeningocele patient). In other words, one may get a falsely reassuring sense of normal or only slightly decreased compliance in an individual with significant sphincteric insufficiency. Before correcting the sphincteric insufficiency, there needs to be an accurate idea of what bladder compliance will be when the outlet no longer leaks during filling and storage. This can be accomplished very simply by pulling a Foley balloon against the bladder outlet to occlude it during filling.

Cholinergic supersensitivity can be determined during cystometry (**bethanechol supersensitivity test**). This test is based on Cannon's law of denervation, which implies that when an organ is deprived of its nerve supply, it develops hypersensitivity to a variety of substances, including those that are normally excitatory neurotransmitters for that organ. Originally devised by Jack Lapides and associates, the test has remained virtually unaltered since 1962. It involves controlled liquid cystometry at an infusion rate of 1 mL/sec to a volume of 100 mL, when the bladder pressure is measured. After two or three such infusions, an average value is obtained, and this maneuver is repeated 10, 20, and 30 minutes after subcutaneous injection of 2.5 mg or 0.035 mg/kg of bethanechol chloride. A normal bladder shows a response of less than 15 cm of water pressure above the control value at the 100 mL volume. Under these circumstances, a positive result strongly suggests an interruption in the peripheral neural and/or distal spinal pathways to and from the bladder. The more distal and complete the lesion, the more frequently positive the test seems to be. A negative result in an individual with a normal bladder capacity and no detrusor decompensation (admittedly sometimes hard to judge) and in whom the bethanechol is administered on a weight basis, strongly suggests that there is no such lesion. Known factors that can give a falsely positive test include urinary tract infection, azotemia, detrusor hypertrophy, and emotional stress. A falsely negative study may result from the decompensated bladder that cannot respond to cholinergic stimulation under any circumstances. False-negative results may also be due to an insufficient dose of the cholinergic agonist in a very heavy person, and it is useful to administer bethanechol on a weight basis (0.035 mg/kg) to obviate this. The test is not very useful in individuals with involuntary bladder contractions. Under such circumstances, the cholinergic agonist often simply raises bladder pressure sufficiently to make the involuntary contraction occur at a lower volume than usual. It has never been clear whether this was originally intended to be interpreted as a positive test. If one administers the bethanechol on a weight basis and infection, detrusor hypertrophy, stress, and azotemia have been excluded, there should be a few false-positive results.

The **ice water test** was originally described by Bors and Blinn in 1957. Methodology differs amongst practitioners, but the gist is this. Sterile 0–4°C water or saline is rapidly instilled into the bladder (100 mL within 20 seconds or 200 mL/min to a volume of 30–50% of a previously determined cystometric capacity). A positive result is considered a detrusor contraction greater than 30 cm of water, with leakage around the catheter, expulsion of the catheter, or emptying immediately after removal of the catheter. The test has been described as a method of demonstrating a segmental reflex that is inhibited centrally in healthy subjects without neurologic lesions but which appears when suprasacral lesions are present and normally occurs in infants and young children. The afferent fibers for the ice water test are thought to be unmyelinated C-fiber afferents, which are normally silent during filling and storage but which become functional with various types of neurologic disease or injury (see I.B.7). Thus, a positive test can be considered indicative of a neurologic lesion, even though the neurologic lesion may not become manifest until a subsequent time. However, everyone with such a lesion may not have a positive ice water test.

5. **Voiding cystometry, combined pressure studies, video urodynamic studies.** Intravesical pressure, intra-abdominal pressure (generally reflected by intrarectal pressure), and flow are often measured simultaneously (Figure 13-7). The purposes of pressure/flow studies are

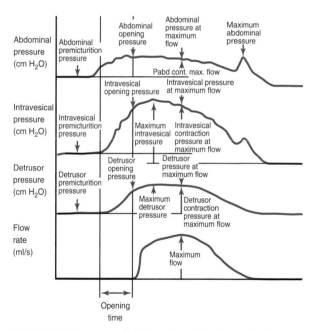

FIGURE 13-7. Recommended International Continence Society Registration of combined pressure(s) and flow recording. (From Wein AJ, English WE, Whitmore KE: Office urodynamics. *Urol Clin North Am* 15:609, 1988.)

to be able to better define whether obstruction is present and to assess detrusor contractility more precisely. By assessing patterns of detrusor pressure and flow, thereby inferring resistance and patterns of increased resistance, the examiner can often ascertain the exact pathology (e. g., anatomic obstruction versus dyssynergia). The normal adult male generally voids with a detrusor pressure of between 40 and 50 cm of water.

The normal adult female voids at a much lower pressure. Indeed, many women void with almost no detectable rise in detrusor pressure. This does not indicate that contraction is not occurring but simply that outlet resistance, lower in the female to begin with, drops to very low levels during bladder contraction. It should be remembered, however, as Derek Griffiths, a pioneer urodynamicist, has pointed out, that detrusor pressure alone is insufficient to assess the strength of a detrusor contraction. This is because a muscle can use energy to either generate force or shorten its length. With respect to the bladder, a relatively hollow viscus, the force developed contributes to detrusor pressure while the velocity of shortening contributes to flow. With significant obstruction, detrusor pressure can rise to high levels. If resistance is very low, detrusor pressure may be undetectable but the contractility may be equal in the two instances.

Urodynamically, obstruction is generally defined only by the relationship between detrusor pressure and flow-high pressure and low flow. Pressure flow studies can be analyzed according to a number of nomograms, a detailed description of which is beyond the scope of this chapter. We find that most often, a detailed visual analysis of the entire study is just as, or more, helpful. **Two easy and useful concepts to remember in this regard are the Abrams-Griffiths (AG) number and the bladder contractility index (BCI).** The AG number relates to whether outlet obstruction is present in the male. It is calculated as [Pdet @ Qmax − 2 Q max]. A value over 40 indicates obstruction, under 20 no obstruction, and 20–40 "equivocal." The BCI is calculated as [Pdet @ Qmax + 5Qmax]. Over 150 indicates a "strong" bladder, 100–150 a normal one, less than 100 a "weak" bladder.

Once obstruction is diagnosed, it is necessary to determine the site, and to do this, simultaneous fluoroscopy is often used. This **video urodynamic study** combines the cystourographic imaging described previously with simultaneous urodynamic studies, permitting a generally accurate determination of the site of obstruction at the time high pressure and low flow co-exist. The video urodynamic study is also extremely useful in assessing the etiology of complex cases of incontinence, as the precise pressure relationships existing in the bladder and urethra can be correlated with the cystourethrographic radiologic patterns, and a judgment, therefore, can be made of why involuntary leakage occurs at a particular time. In this case, the issue is generally whether the fluoroscopic demonstration of leakage occurs with or without DO or whether the incontinence is due in part to both detrusor and outlet related causes.

One of the most difficult problems in urodynamics is the clarification of whether contractile function is adequate; that is, whether it is sustained and coordinated. Phasic DO does not imply normal contractile function. There is a subset of patients with incontinence in whom DO and impaired contractile function co-exist (so-called DHIC, detrusor hyperactivity with impaired contractility). The bladder is overactive in these patients but empties ineffectively because of diminished detrusor contractile function and not necessarily because of outlet obstruction. In some patients, obstruction co-exists with impaired detrusor contractility, and this diagnosis often cannot be made. Several very sophisticated resistance formulas exist that attempt to calculate a number for outlet resistance utilizing data based on intravesical pressure, flow rate, and other mathematical factors. These formulas generally assume that the urethra is a rigid tube with a constant diameter and that the pressure always reflects that generated by a normal bladder not a decompensated one. If a bladder has normal contractility and the pressure that it generates during contraction is high and if the corresponding flow rate that results is low, one does not need a formula to diagnose obstruction. On the other hand, if the bladder is decompensated and incapable of producing a significant rise in pressure, obstruction cannot be quantitated by these formulas. More sophisticated and innovative methods of defining the relationship between intravesical pressure and uroflow have been devised, and these methods are beyond the scope of this discussion of urodynamics. The global question surrounding all noncomputer-assisted and computer-assisted characterizations and interpretations of pressure flow data is, what do these add? Is the evaluation of the average older man with LUT symptoms more likely to lead to a better treatment outcome if pressure flow urodynamic studies are performed, including the analysis of results in various mathematical ways with computer assistance? Do sophisticated or unsophisticated urodynamic studies predict the outcome of various treatments for LUTS, including watchful waiting? Are patients with LUTS in whom outlet ablation fails as treatment the same patients as those in whom detrusor contractility is judged ineffective by the criteria under consideration? Unfortunately, those of us who perform urodynamics have not done a terribly good job of looking into these aspects of outcome analysis. Figure 13-7 displays the International Continence Society's recommended registration of combined pressure and flow recording. Kinesiologic electromyography (see following discussion) is often added as an additional channel, and some investigators record urethral pressure at one or various sites along the urethra simultaneously as well. The typical video urodynamic configuration includes this and a fluoroscopic lower tract image.

6. **Electromyography.** For the majority of urologists, electromyography is a urodynamic study that permits evaluation of the striated sphincter during the emptying phase of micturition. Kinesiologic electromyography is the term that describes this application, that is, the study of the activity of one group of muscles (the striated musculature of the outlet) with respect to another (the bladder). **Normally, as the bladder fills with urine, there is a gradual and sustained increase in electromyographic (EMG) activity recruited from the pelvic floor muscles. This reaches a maximum just before voiding.** Compositely, this is known as the **guarding reflex.** The lack of a guarding reflex suggests neural pathology, as does the inability to produce a sphincter "flare" when given the command to "stop voiding." Voluntary voiding is normally followed by complete electrical silence-relaxation of the striated sphincter. There is a marked increase in EMG activity in response to a number of stimuli, including cough, Credé and Valsalva maneuvers, the BCR, and the request to stop voiding, a maneuver accomplished by most through forceful contraction of the pelvic floor musculature (Figure 13-8). Kinesiologic electromyography enables the urodynamic examiner to ascertain whether the striated sphincter appropriately increases its activity in a gradual fashion during bladder

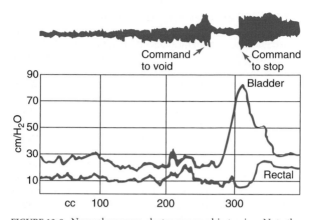

FIGURE 13-8. Normal pressure electromyographic tracing. Note the gradual increase in electromyographic activity during bladder filling with a decrease to control levels just before the onset of what is voluntary bladder contraction. Note that the command to stop voiding evokes a pelvic floor striated muscle contraction reflected by a flare in sphincter electromyography. (From Wein AJ, English WE, Whitmore KE: Office urodynamics. *Urol Clin North Am* 15:609, 1988.)

filling (whether the "guarding reflex" is normal) and whether quiescence occurs normally before and during bladder contraction. Kinesiologic electromyography can be performed with either needle electrodes or surface or patch electrodes. Needle electrodes certainly permit more accurate placement and more accurate recording, but in many cases, surface electrodes seem perfectly adequate to obtain the necessary information. When EMG activity gradually increases during filling cystometry and then ceases prior to or at the onset of attempted voiding, this is normal and can be taken as a reflection of what goes on during actual bladder filling and emptying. However, **a simultaneous increase of EMG activity with an increase in intravesical pressure during filling cystometry is not always indicative of detrusor-striated sphincter dyssynergia.** Abdominal straining or attempted inhibition of a bladder contraction will yield an identical pattern. For a patient with normal sensation, no matter how cooperative, it is extremely difficult to maintain true relaxation during an involuntary bladder contraction. In fact, the appropriate response is to try to suppress such a contraction by voluntary contraction of the anal sphincter, the pelvic floor musculature, or both. All of these circumstances represent types of **pseudodyssynergia** and are extremely difficult to differentiate from true dyssynergia on the basis of any type of urodynamic study done solely during bladder filling. The term **detrusor-striated sphincter dyssynergia** should refer to obstruction to the outflow of urine during bladder contraction caused by involuntary contraction of the striated sphincter. This is most often seen in patients with discrete neurologic disease, such as suprasacral spinal cord transection after spinal shock has passed. Individuals suspected of having detrusor-striated sphincter dyssynergia but who lack identifiable neurologic disease should always be further investigated with sophisticated video urodynamic evaluation during a full micturition study. True detrusor-striated sphincter dyssynergia is extremely uncommon (some examiners say that it does not exist) in patients without neurologic disease, and such a diagnosis deserves exhaustive study before it is in fact confirmed.

7. **Urethral profilometry.** The term urethral profilometry refers to many entities utilized in various settings. The most common usage refers to a **static infusion urethral pressure profile.** In this study, a small catheter with radially drilled side holes is placed in the bladder and through it a medium, usually liquid, is infused. The catheter is then withdrawn at a constant rate, and the pressure required to push the medium through the side holes is recorded from inside the bladder to a site where the pressure becomes essentially isobaric with bladder pressure. The infusion profile curve is thus a result of a number of factors, including urethral wall compliance, resistance to inflow of the medium, resistance to runoff of the medium into the bladder and out the urethral meatus, and artifact generated by the apparatus. Because the study is usually done at rest and not during bladder filling or emptying, it is difficult to associate the recorded events with bladder-urethral interaction during filling or emptying. Specifically with relevance to neuromuscular dysfunction, the static infusion profile has been cited as useful at various times in diagnosing stress incontinence, detrusor sphincter dyssynergia, and obstruction. In our opinion, it is not very useful for the specific diagnosis of any of these. There is much overlap in maximum urethral pressures and functional urethral lengths between individuals with stress incontinence and normal individuals, especially in the elderly population. The rationale of diagnosing either smooth or striated sphincter dyssynergia on the basis of a static infusion profile is difficult to understand. A high pressure at a given point in the

passage of the catheter from the bladder through the urethra can be secondary to a number of phenomena, and this result by no means indicates that there will always be contraction in this area during voluntary or involuntary micturition. The static infusion urethral profile is certainly useful for testing the function of an artificial genitourinary sphincter. With specific relevance to neuromuscular dysfunction, it is useful for suspecting intrinsic sphincter dysfunction. In an individual with such an abnormality (Figures 13-9 and 13-10), the proximal urethra is isobaric or almost isobaric with the bladder and the striated sphincter peak is generally lower than normal.

Stress urethral profilometry refers to a study done with a catheter with dual sensors, one in the bladder and one in the proximal urethra. With coughing or straining, the change in urethral pressure should always be equal to or greater than the change in bladder pressure. In patients with stress incontinence, along with much of the profile curve, the change in urethral pressure will be less than the change in bladder pressure. **Dynamic urethral profilometry** implies the use of a catheter with dual sensors—bladder and proximal urethra—with pressures recorded during bladder filling and emptying. An actual urethral pressure profile is not recorded. The interaction between bladder pressure and pressure in one area of the urethra, generally in the area

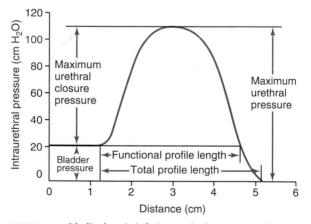

FIGURE 13-9. Idealized static infusion urethral pressure profile utilizing International Continence Society nomenclature (female). (From Wein AJ, English WE, Whitmore KE: Office urodynamics. *Urol Clin North Am* 15:609, 1988.)

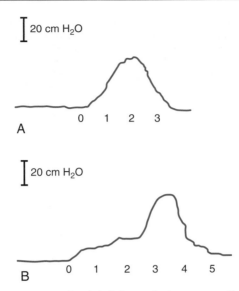

FIGURE 13-10. Actual static infusion urethral pressure profiles from normal female (**A**) and male (**B**) subjects. Numbers represent centimeters with 0 representing the level of the bladder neck. The maximum urethral pressure in both males and females is normally at the level of the urogenital diaphragm. The initial portion of the curve in the male, from the bladder neck to the pressure rise culminating at the maximum urethral pressure, is sometimes called prostatic plateau. The area under this portion of the curve corresponds roughly to prostatic size. (From Wein AJ, English WE, Whitmore KE: Office urodynamics. *Urol Clin North Am* 15:609, 1988.)

of maximal closure pressure, usually at the level of the striated sphincter is recorded. **Micturitional urethral profilometry** refers to a study in which a catheter with dual or triple sensors, one of which is in the bladder, is withdrawn during voiding in a patient with known obstruction. In such a patient, the area of the maximal pressure drop is the site of obstruction. Micturitional profilometry generally requires fluoroscopic monitoring to identify the anatomic location of this maximal pressure decrease.

8. **Abdominal leak point pressure.** The abdominal leak point pressure (ALPP) is a measure of the ability of the urethra to resist changes in abdominal pressure as an expulsive force. It has been popularized by Ed McGuire as a clinically useful test, perhaps the most useful one, to differentiate the extremes of ISD from hypermobility-related stress incontinence. It is easy to see why the concept of this test

appeals to straightforward logic: **If straining or increases in intra-abdominal pressure produce incontinence, and a filling study shows normal compliance, there must be a problem with the bladder outlet. The amount of abdominal pressure necessary to cause leakage under such circumstances is inversely proportional to the amount of outlet dysfunction.** A pressure catheter is placed in the bladder or rectum or both and the bladder is filled to a predetermined volume, usually 150 to 200 mL. The patient is then asked to perform a graded Valsalva maneuver until leakage is seen per urethra. If Valsalva does not produce leakage, the patient is asked to cough. The pressure at which leakage is first seen is the ALPP. The higher the ALPP, the better the intrinsic sphincter function, and, conversely, the lower the ALPP, the worse the intrinsic sphincter function.

There are still problems concerning standardization of technique, specification of variables, optimal location of pressure measurement, size of urethral catheter to be used, and the bladder volume at which the study is to be carried out. There is also disagreement about what "numbers" indicate a significant degree of intrinsic sphincter dysfunction. Originally, an ALPP of less than 60–65 cm of water was said to indicate ISD. One caveat to remember is that a large cystocele can invalidate the results, making the ALPP artificially higher.

9. **Ambulatory urodynamics.** An obvious limitation to routine or conventional urodynamic testing is the artificial environment and circumstances in which the test is conducted. Ambulatory urodynamics is an alternative technique in which the pressure transducing catheters are placed into the bladder and rectum but are attached to portable recording devices. The patient resumes his or her normal daily routine and cycles of natural bladder filling and storage. Emptying and voiding are recorded, while the patient writes down the time and qualitative nature of relevant subjective sensations. Provocative maneuvers such as coughing, climbing, jumping, and hand washing can be performed in an attempt to reproduce the patient's symptomatology. At the conclusion of the study, the data are downloaded to a computer, compared with the written record of symptomatology, and analyzed. Advocates of this type of study cite the ability to objectively confirm the complaints of many patients in whom nonambulatory urodynamics have been unrevealing. However, limitations of this study include the following: (1) the triggering effect of a catheter in the bladder can cause a higher incidence of

involuntary bladder contractions than in standard cystometry; (2) if one is recording urethral pressures as well,
small movements of the catheter are unavoidable in an
ambulatory patient, often resulting in artificial pressure
dips; (3) measurement of actual leakage is difficult or near
impossible; (4) the bladder filling rate depends on many
factors that are still not controllable (such as intake,
diuretic usage, congestive failure, etc.); (5) different
states of rectal filling and rectal catheter stimulation in
the ambulatory patient may exert reflex effects on the
bladder; (6) it is difficult to simultaneously measure flow
during ambulatory urodynamics, and so at present the
study is more useful in the evaluation of filling and storage abnormalities than emptying/voiding abnormalities;
(7) detrusor pressure values for certain parameters are
different during ambulatory urodynamics as opposed to
laboratory urodynamics (new agreed on standards for
normality and abnormality need to be developed); and
(8) a certain percent of records will be uninterpretable
because of artifacts. At present, ambulatory urodynamics
are utilized primarily as a research tool, although the
potential range of clinical applications, with some technologic improvements, are numerous.

VII. CLASSIFICATION OF VOIDING DYSFUNCTION

A. General

There are many classification systems for voiding dysfunction,
and these are based on neurologic, urodynamic, or functional
considerations, or on a combination of these. That there are
at least six to eight of these attests to the fact that none is
prefect. The purpose of any classification system should be
to facilitate understanding and management and to avoid
confusion among those who are concerned with the problem
for which the system was designed. A good classification
should serve as intellectual shorthand and should convey, in
a few key words or phrases, the essence of a clinical situation.
Most systems of classification for voiding dysfunction were
formulated primarily to describe dysfunction secondary to
neurologic disease or injury. The ideal system should be
applicable to all types of voiding dysfunction.

In this section, we describe the functional type of classification that we have found most useful, the International
Continence Society classification and the Lapides system.

B. The Functional System

Classification of voiding dysfunction can be formulated on a simple functional basis, describing the dysfunction in terms of whether the deficit produced is primarily one of the filling/storage or the emptying/voiding phase of micturition (see Tables 13-3 and 13-4). The genesis of such a system was proposed initially by F. Brantley Scott's group. This simple-minded scheme assumes only that, whatever their differences, all "experts" would agree on the two-phase concept of micturition (filling/storage and emptying/voiding) and on the simple overall mechanisms underlying the normality of each phase (see previous discussion).

Storage failure results because of either **bladder or outlet abnormalities or a combination.** The proven **bladder abnormalities** very simply include only involuntary bladder contractions, low compliance, and heightened or altered sensation. The **outlet abnormalities** can include only an intermittent or continuous decrease in outlet resistance.

Emptying failure, likewise, can occur because of **bladder or outlet abnormalities or a combination**. The bladder side includes only inadequate or unsustained bladder contractility, and the outlet side includes only anatomic obstruction and sphincter(s) dyssynergia.

There are indeed some types of voiding dysfunction that represent combinations of filling/storage and emptying/voiding abnormalities. Within this scheme, however, these become readily understandable and their detection and treatment can be logically described. Various aspects of physiology and pathophysiology are always related more to one phase of micturition than another. All aspects of urodynamic and videourodynamic evaluation can be conceptualized in this functional manner as to exactly what they evaluate in terms of either bladder or outlet activity during filling/storage and emptying/voiding (see Table 13-6). In addition, one can easily classify all known treatments for voiding dysfunction under the broad categories of whether they facilitate filling/storage and emptying/voiding and whether they do so by an action primarily on the bladder or on one or more of the components of the bladder outlet (Tables 13-7 and 13-8).

Failure in either category generally is not absolute, but more often is relative. Such a functional system can easily be "expanded" and made more complicated to include etiologic or specific urodynamic connotations (see Table 13-4). However, the simplified system is perfectly workable and avoids argument in those complex situations in which the

(Text continued on p. 394)

Table 13-7: Therapy to Facilitate Urine Storage/Bladder Filling

I. Bladder related (inhibiting bladder contractility, decreasing sensory input, and/or increasing bladder capacity)
   A. Behavioral therapy, including any or all of
      1. Education
      2. Bladder training
      3. Timed bladder emptying or prompted voiding
      4. Fluid restriction
      5. Pelvic floor physiotherapy ± biofeedback
   B. Pharmacologic therapy (oral, intravesical, intradetrusor)
      1. Anticholinergic agents
      2. Drugs with mixed actions
      3. Calcium antagonists
      4. Potassium channel openers
      5. Prostaglandin inhibitors
      6. β-Adrenergic agonists
      7. α-Adrenergic antagonists
      8. Tricyclic antidepressants; serotonin and norepinephrine reuptake inhibitors
      9. Dimethyl sulfoxide (DMSO)
      10. Polysynaptic inhibitors
      11. Capsaicin, resiniferatoxin, and like agents
      12. Botulinum toxin
   C. Bladder overdistention
   D. Electrical stimulation and neuromodulation
   E. Acupuncture and electroacupuncture
   F. Interruption of innervation
      1. Very central (subarachnoid block)
      2. Less central (sacral rhizotomy, selective sacral rhizotomy)
      3. Peripheral motor or/and sensory
   G. Augmentation cystoplasty (auto, bowel, tissue engineering)
II. Outlet related (increasing outlet resistance)
   A. Behavioral therapy
      1. Education
      2. Bladder training
      3. Timed bladder emptying or prompted voiding
      4. Fluid restriction
      5. Pelvic floor physiotherapy ± biofeedback
   B. Electrical stimulation
   C. Pharmacologic therapy
      1. α-Adrenergic agonists
      2. Tricyclic antidepressants; serotonin and norepinephrine reuptake inhibitors
      3. β-Adrenergic antagonists, agonists

D. Vaginal and perineal occlusive and/or supportive devices; urethral plugs

E. Nonsurgical periurethral bulking
   1. Collagen, synthetics, cell transfer

F. Vesicourethral suspension ± prolapse repair (female)

G. Sling procedures ± prolapse repair (female)

H. Closure of the bladder outlet
   1. Artificial urinary sphincter
   2. Bladder outlet reconstruction

I. Myoplasty (muscle transposition)

III. Circumventing the problem

A. Absorbent products

B. External collecting devices

C. Antidiuretic hormone-like agents

D. Short-acting diuretics

E. Intermittent catheterization

F. Continuous catheterization

G. Urinary diversion

Table 13-8: Therapy to Facilitate Bladder Emptying/Voiding

I. Bladder related (increasing intravesical pressure or facilitating bladder contractility)

A. External compression, Valsalva

B. Promotion or initiation of reflex contraction
   1. Trigger zones or maneuvers
   2. Bladder "training"; tidal drainage

C. Pharmacologic therapy (oral, intravesical)
   1. Parasympathomimetic agents
   2. Prostaglandins
   3. Blockers of inhibition
      a. α-Adrenergic antagonists
      b. Opioid antagonists

D. Electrical stimulation
   1. Directly to the bladder or spinal cord
   2. Directly to the nerve roots
   3. Intravesical (transurethral)
   4. Neuromodulation

E. Reduction cystoplasty

F. Bladder myoplasty (muscle wrap)

(Continued)

Table 13-8:—Cont'd

II. Outlet related (increasing outlet resistance)
  A. At a site of anatomic obstruction
    1. Pharmacologic therapy—decrease prostate size or tone
      a. α-Adrenergic antagonists
      b. 5 α-Reductase inhibitors
      c. Luteinizing hormone releasing hormone-agonists/
         antagonists
      d. Antiandrogens
    2. Prostatectomy, prostatotomy (diathermy, heat, laser)
    3. Bladder neck incision or resection
    4. Urethral stricture repair or dilation
    5. Intraurethral stent
    6. Balloon dilation of stricture/contracture
  B. At level of smooth sphincter
    1. Pharmacologic therapy
      a. α-Adrenergic antagonists
      b. β-Adrenergic agonists
    2. Transurethral resection or incision
    3. Y-V plasty
  C. At level of striated sphincter
    1. Behavioral therapy ± biofeedback
    2. Pharmacologic therapy
      a. Benzodiazepines
      b. Baclofen
      c. Dantrolene
      d. α-Adrenergic antagonists
      e. Botulinum toxin (injection)
    3. Urethral overdilation
    4. Surgical sphincterotomy
    5. Urethral stent
    6. Pudendal nerve interruption
III. Circumventing the problem
  A. Intermittent catheterization
  B. Continuous catheterization
  C. Urinary diversion (conduit)

exact etiology or urodynamic mechanism for a voiding dysfunction cannot be agreed on.

Proper use of the functional system for a given voiding dysfunction obviously requires a reasonably accurate notion of what the urodynamic data show. However, **an exact diagnosis is *not* required for treatment.** It should be recognized that **some patients do not have only a discrete storage or emptying failure, and the existence of combination deficits must be recognized to properly utilize**

this system of classification. For instance, the classic T10 paraplegic patient after spinal shock generally exhibits a relative failure to store because of involuntary bladder contraction and a relative failure to empty the bladder because of striated sphincter dyssynergia. With such a combination deficit, to utilize this classification system as a guide to treatment, one must assume that one of the deficits is primary and that significant improvement will result from its treatment alone or that the voiding dysfunction can be converted primarily to a disorder of either storage or emptying by means of nonsurgical or surgical therapy. The resultant deficit can then be treated or circumvented. Using this example, the combined deficit in a T10 paraplegic patient can be converted primarily to a storage failure by procedures directed at the dyssynergic striated sphincter; the resultant incontinence (secondary to involuntary contraction) can be circumvented (in a male) with an external collecting device. Alternatively, the deficit can be converted primarily to an emptying failure by pharmacologic or surgical measures designed to abolish or reduce the involuntary contraction, and the resultant emptying failure can then be circumvented with clean intermittent catheterization (CIC). Other examples of combination deficits include impaired bladder contractility or overactivity with sphincter dysfunction, bladder outlet obstruction with DO, bladder outlet obstruction with sphincter malfunction, and DO with impaired contractility.

One of the advantages of this functional classification is that it allows the clinician the liberty of "playing" with the system to suit his or her own preferences without an alteration in the basic concept of "keep it simple but accurate and informative." For instance, one could easily substitute the terms overactive or oversensitive bladder and underactive outlet for "because of the bladder" and "because of the outlet under" under "Failure to Store" in Table 13-3. One could choose to categorize the bladder reasons for overactivity (see Table 13-4) further in terms of neurogenic, myogenic, or anatomic causes and further subcategorize neurogenic in terms of decreased inhibitory control, increased afferent activity, increased sensitivity to efferent activity, and so on. The system is flexible.

C. International Continence Society Classification

The classification system proposed by the International Continence Society (ICS) (Table 13-9) is in **essence an extension of a urodynamic classification system.** The storage and voiding phases of micturition are described separately, and, within each, various designations are applied to describe bladder and urethral function. Some of the definitions were

Table 13-9: The International Continence Society Classification

Storage Phase	Voiding Phase
Bladder function	**Bladder function**
Detrusor activity	Detrusor activity
Normal or stable	Normal
Overactive	Underactive
Neurogenic	Acontractile
Idiopathic	Areflexic
Bladder sensation	
Normal	**Urethral function**
Increased or hypersensitive	Normal
Reduced or hyposensitive	Abnormal
Absent	Mechanical obstruction
Bladder capacity	Overactivity
Normal	Dysfunctional voiding
High	Detrusor sphincter
Low	dyssynergia
	Nonrelaxing urethral
	sphincter dysfunction
Urethral function	
Normal closure mechanism	
Incompetent closure mechanism	

changed by the standardization subcommittee of the ICS in 2002 and the relevant changes are indicated here. **Normal bladder function during filling/storage implies no significant rises in detrusor pressure (stability). Overactive detrusor function indicates the presence of "involuntary detrusor contractions during the filling phase which may be spontaneous or provoked."** If caused by neurologic disease, the term **neurogenic DO** (previously, detrusor hyperreflexia) is used; if not, the term **idiopathic DO** (previously, detrusor instability) is applied. **Bladder sensation** can be categorized only in qualitative terms as indicated. **Bladder capacity and compliance** (Δ volume/Δ pressure) are cystometric measurements. Bladder capacity can refer to cystometric capacity, maximum cystometric capacity, or maximum anesthetic cystometric capacity. **Normal urethral function during filling/storage indicates a positive urethral closure pressure (urethral pressure minus bladder pressure) even with increases in intra-abdominal pressure, although it may be overcome by DO. Incompetent**

urethral function during filling/storage implies urine leakage in the absence of a detrusor contraction. This may be secondary to genuine stress incontinence, intrinsic sphincter dysfunction, a combination, or an involuntary fall in urethral pressure in the absence of detrusor contraction.

During the voiding/emptying phase of micturition, normal detrusor activity implies voiding by a voluntarily initiated sustained contraction that leads to complete bladder emptying within a normal time span. An **underactive detrusor** defines a contraction of inadequate magnitude and/or duration to empty the bladder within a normal time span. An **acontractile detrusor** is one that cannot be demonstrated to contract during urodynamic testing. **Areflexia** is defined as acontractility due to an abnormality of neural control, implying the complete absence of centrally coordinated contraction. **Normal urethral function** during voiding indicates a urethra that opens and is continuously relaxed to allow bladder emptying at a normal pressure. **Abnormal urethra function during voiding may be due to either mechanical obstruction or urethral overactivity. Dysfunctional voiding** describes an intermittent or/ and fluctuating flow rate due to involuntary intermittent contractions of the periurethral striated muscle in neurologically normal individuals. **Detrusor sphincter dyssynergia** defines a detrusor contraction concurrent with an involuntary contraction of the urethral or periurethral striated muscle, or both. **Nonrelaxing urethral sphincter obstruction** usually occurs in individuals with a neurologic lesion and is characterized by a nonrelaxing obstructing urethra resulting in reduced urine flow.

LUT dysfunction in a classical T10 level paraplegic patient after spinal shock has passed would be classified in the ICS system as follows:

- Storage phase—overactive neurogenic detrusor function, absent sensation, low capacity, normal compliance, normal urethral closure function
- Voiding phase—overactive detrusor function, overactive obstructive urethral function

The micturition dysfunction of a stroke patient with urgency incontinence would most likely be classified during storage as overactive neurogenic detrusor function, normal sensation, low capacity, normal compliance, and normal urethral closure function. During voiding (this refers to voluntary micturition), the dysfunction would be classified as normal detrusor activity and normal urethral function, assuming that no anatomic obstruction existed.

D. Lapides Classification

Jack Lapides contributed significantly to the classification and care of the patient with neuropathic voiding dysfunction by slightly modifying and popularizing a system originally proposed by McLellan in 1939 (Table 13-10). Lapides' classification differs from that of McLellan in only one respect, and that is the division of the group of "atonic neurogenic bladder" into sensory neurogenic and motor neurogenic bladder. This remains one of the most familiar systems to urologists and nonurologists because it describes in recognizable shorthand the clinical and cystometric conditions of many types of neurogenic voiding dysfunction.

A **sensory neurogenic bladder** results from disease that selectively interrupts the sensory fibers between the bladder and the spinal cord or the afferent tracts to the brain. **Diabetes mellitus, tabes dorsalis, and pernicious anemia** are most commonly responsible. The first clinical changes are described as those of impaired sensation of bladder distention. Unless voiding is initiated on a timed basis, varying degrees of bladder overdistention can result with resultant hypotonicity. If bladder decompensation occurs, significant amounts of residual urine result, and at that time, the cystometric curve generally demonstrates a large capacity bladder with a flat, high-compliance, low-pressure filling curve.

A **motor paralytic bladder** results from disease processes that destroy the parasympathetic motor innervation of the bladder. **Extensive pelvic surgery or trauma** may produce this. **Herpes zoster** has been listed as a cause as well, but recent evidence suggests that the voiding dysfunction seen with herpes may be more related to a problem with afferent input. The early symptoms of a motor paralytic bladder may vary from painful urinary retention to only a relative inability to initiate and maintain normal micturition. Early cystometric filling is normal but without a voluntary bladder contraction at capacity. Chronic overdistention and decompensation may occur, resulting in a large capacity bladder with a flat, low-pressure filling curve; a large residual of urine may result.

Table 13-10: The Lapides Classification

Sensory neurogenic bladder
Motor paralytic bladder (motor neurogenic bladder)
Uninhibited neurogenic bladder
Reflex neurogenic bladder
Autonomous neurogenic bladder

An **uninhibited neurogenic bladder** was described originally as resulting from injury or disease to the "corticoregulatory tract." The sacral spinal cord was presumed to be the micturition reflex center, and this corticoregulatory tract was believed to normally exert an inhibitory influence on the sacral micturition reflex center. A destructive lesion in this tract would then result in overfacilitation of the micturition reflex. **Cerebrovascular accident (CVA), brain or spinal cord tumor, PD, and demyelinating disease** were listed as the most common causes in this category. The voiding dysfunction is most often characterized symptomatically by frequency, urgency, and urge incontinence and urodynamically by normal sensation with involuntary contraction at low filling volumes. Residual urine is characteristically low unless anatomic outlet obstruction or true smooth or striated sphincter dyssynergia occurs. The patient generally can initiate a bladder contraction voluntarily but is often unable to do so during cystometry because sufficient urine storage cannot occur before involuntary contraction is stimulated.

Reflex neurogenic bladder describes the post-spinal shock condition that exists after complete interruption of the sensory and motor pathways between the sacral spinal cord and the brain stem. Most commonly, this occurs in **traumatic SCI and transverse myelitis,** but it may occur with **extensive demyelinating disease or any process that produces significant spinal cord destruction.** Typically, there is no bladder sensation, and there is inability to initiate voluntary micturition. Incontinence without sensation generally results because of low volume involuntary contractions. Striated sphincter dyssynergia is the rule.

An **autonomous neurogenic bladder** results from complete motor and sensory separation of the bladder from the sacral spinal cord. This may be caused by any disease that destroys the sacral cord or causes extensive damage to the sacral roots or pelvic nerves. There is inability to voluntarily initiate micturition, no bladder reflex activity, and no specific bladder sensation. This is the type of dysfunction seen in patients with spinal shock. The characteristic cystometric pattern is initially similar to the late stages of the motor or sensory paralytic bladder, with a marked shift to the right of the cystometric filling curve and a large bladder capacity at low intravesical pressure. However, decreased compliance may develop, secondary either to chronic inflammatory change or to the effects of denervation/decentralization with secondary neuromorphologic and neuropharmacologic reorganizational changes. Emptying capacity may vary widely, depending on the ability of the patient to increase intravesical pressure and on the resistance offered during this increase by the smooth and striated sphincters.

These classic categories in their usual settings are generally easily understood and remembered, and this is why this system provides an excellent framework for teaching some fundamentals of neurogenic voiding dysfunction to students and nonurologists. Unfortunately, many patients do not exactly "fit" into one or another category. Gradations of sensory, motor, and mixed lesions occur, and the patterns produced after different types of peripheral denervation/decentralization may vary widely from those that are classically described. The **system is applicable only to neuropathic dysfunction.**

VIII. NEUROGENIC VOIDING DYSFUNCTION

A. General Patterns

Discrete neurologic lesions generally affect the filling/storage and emptying/voiding phases of LUT function in a relatively consistent fashion. This fashion is dependent on (1) the area(s) of the nervous system affected, (2) the physiologic function(s) and the contents and location of the area(s) affected, and (3) whether the lesion or process is destructive or irritative. The acute dysfunction produced may differ, for a variety of reasons, from the chronic one.

Table 13-11 summarizes many of these dysfunctions on the basis of the most common type of abnormal pattern that results from a given disease or injury, insofar as the parameters just listed are concerned. This abbreviated classification is not meant to be all inclusive but to simply indicate that, for the most part, an individual with a specific neurologic abnormality, and voiding dysfunction because of it, will, in general, have the type of dysfunction shown.

1. Lesions Above the Brain Stem

Neurologic lesions above the brain stem that affect micturition generally result in involuntary bladder contractions with coordinated sphincter function (smooth and striated sphincter synergy). Sensation and voluntary striated sphincter function are generally preserved but sensation may be deficient or delayed. Detrusor areflexia may, however, occur, either initially or as a permanent dysfunction. UI may occur due to the DO.

2. Complete Spinal Cord Lesions From Spinal Cord Level T6 to S2

Patients with complete lesions of the spinal cord between spinal cord level T6 and S2, after they recover from spinal shock, generally exhibit involuntary bladder contractions without

(Text continued on p. 405)

Table 13-11: Most Common Patterns of Typical Voiding Dysfunctions Seen with Various Types of Neurologic Disease or Injury

Disorder	Detrusor Activity	Compliance	Smooth Sphincter	Striated Sphincter	Other
Cerebrovascular accident	O	N	S	S ±VC	There may be decreased sensation of lower urinary tract events.
Brain tumor	O	N	S	S	There may be decreased sensation of lower urinary tract events.
Cerebral palsy	O	N	S	S D (25% of those with DO) ±VC	
Parkinson's disease	O I	N	S	S Bradykinesia	

(Continued)

Table 13-11:—Cont'd

Disorder	Detrusor Activity	Compliance	Smooth Sphincter	Striated Sphincter	Other
Multiple system atrophy	O I	N †	O	S	Striated sphincter may exhibit denervation.
Multiple sclerosis	O	N	S	S D (30–65%)	Dyssynergia figures refer to percentage of those with detrusor overactivity.
Spinal cord injury Suprasacral	O	N	S	D	Smooth sphincter may be dyssynergic if lesion is above T7.
Sacral	A	N † (may develop)	CNR O (may develop)	F	

			N	D	D	
Autonomic hyperreflexia	O					
Myelodysplasia	A		N O	O †(MA)	F	Findings vary widely in different series. Striated sphincter commonly shows some evidence of denervation.
Tabes, pernicious anemia	I A		N ‡	S	S	Primary problem is loss of sensation. Detrusor may become decompensated secondary to overdistention.
Disc disease	A		N	CNR	S	Striated sphincter may show evidence of denervation and fixed tone.

(Continued)

Table 13-11:—Cont'd

Disorder	Detrusor Activity	Compliance	Smooth Sphincter	Striated Sphincter	Other
Radical pelvic surgery	I A	† N	O	F	
Diabetes	I A O	N ‡	S	S	Sensory loss contributes, but there is a motor neuropathy as well.

Detrusor activity: I, impaired; O, overactive; A, areflexia.
Compliance: N, normal; †, decreased; ‡, increased.
Smooth sphincter: S, synergic; D, dyssynergic; O, open, incompetent at rest; CNR, competent, nonrelaxing.
§Striated sphincter: S, synergic; D, dyssynergic; ±VC, voluntary control may be impaired; F, fixed tone.

sensation or smooth sphincter synergy, but with striated sphincter dyssynergia. Those with lesions above T6 may experience, in addition, smooth sphincter dyssynergia and autonomic hyperreflexia (see later). Incontinence may occur due to DO but the outlet obstruction can also cause urinary retention.

3. Trauma Below Spinal Cord Level S2

Patients with significant spinal cord or nerve root trauma below spinal cord level S2 generally do not manifest involuntary bladder contractions per se. Detrusor areflexia is initially the rule after spinal shock, and, depending on the type and extent of neurologic injury, various forms of decreased compliance during filling may occur. An open smooth sphincter area may result, but whether this is caused by sympathetic or parasympathetic decentralization/defunctionalization (or both or neither) has never been determined. Various types of striated sphincter dysfunction may occur, but commonly the area retains a residual resting sphincter tone (not the same as dyssynergia) and is not under voluntary control.

4. Interruption of Peripheral Reflex Arc

The dysfunctions that occur with interruption of the peripheral reflex arc may be very similar to those of distal spinal cord or nerve root injury. Detrusor areflexia often develops, low compliance may result, the smooth sphincter area may be relatively incompetent, and the striated sphincter area may exhibit fixed residual tone not amenable to voluntary relaxation. True peripheral neuropathy can be motor or sensory, with the usual expected sequelae, at least initially.

B. Cerebrovascular Disease, CVA

Thrombus, occlusion, and hemorrhage are the most common causes of stroke, leading to ischemia and infarction of variably sized areas in the brain, usually around the internal capsule. **After the initial acute episode, urinary retention from detrusor areflexia may occur.** The neurophysiology of this "cerebral shock" is unclear. After a variable degree of recovery from the neurologic lesion, a fixed deficit may become apparent over a few weeks or months. **The most common long-term expression of LUT dysfunction after CVA is phasic DO. Sensation is variable but is classically described as generally intact, and thus the patient has urgency and frequency with DO. The appropriate response is to try to inhibit the involuntary bladder contraction by forceful voluntary contraction of the** striated sphincter. **If this can be accomplished, only urgency and frequency result; if not, urgency with incontinence results.**

The exact acute and chronic incidence of any voiding dysfunction after CVA, and specifically of incontinence, is not readily discernible. **The cited prevalence of UI on hospital admission for stroke ranges from 32–79%, on discharge from 25–28%, and some months later, from 12–19%. Previous descriptions of the voiding dysfunction after CVA have all cited the preponderance of DO with coordinated sphincter activity. It is difficult to reconcile this with the relatively high incontinence rate that occurs,** even considering the probability that a percentage of these patients had an incontinence problem before the CVA. **There are two possible mechanisms: (1) impaired sphincter control and (2) lack of appreciation of bladder filling and of impending bladder contraction.** It has been reported that the majority of patients with involvement of the cerebral cortex and/or internal capsule are unable to forcefully contract their striated sphincter when an impending involuntary bladder contraction is sensed. Reduced bladder sensation has been reported in patients with global underperfusion of the cerebral cortex, especially the frontal areas.

Detrusor underactivity or areflexia can also exist after CVA. **True detrusor-striated sphincter dyssynergia does not occur following a CVA. Pseudodyssynergia may occur** during urodynamic testing. **Smooth sphincter function is generally unaffected** by CVA. Poor flow rates and high residual urine volumes in a male with pre-CVA symptoms of prostatism generally indicate prostatic obstruction. A urodynamic evaluation is advisable before committing a patient to mechanical outlet reduction to exclude detrusor overactivity with impaired contractility (DHIC) as a cause of symptoms.

In the functional system of classification, the most common type of voiding dysfunction after stroke would then be characterized as a failure to store secondary to bladder overactivity, specifically involuntary bladder contractions.

In the ICS Classification System, the dysfunction would most likely be classified as overactive neurogenic detrusor function, normal sensation, low capacity, normal compliance, and normal urethral closure function during storage; during voiding the description would be normal detrusor activity and normal urethral function assuming that no anatomic obstruction existed. Treatment, in the absence of co-existing significant bladder obstruction or significantly impaired contractility, is directed at decreasing bladder contractility and increasing bladder capacity (see Table 13-7).

C. Dementia

Dementia is a poorly understood disease complex involving atrophy and the loss of grey and white matter of the brain, particularly the frontal lobes. **When voiding dysfunction occurs, the result is generally incontinence. It is difficult to ascertain whether this is due to DO with the type of disorder of voluntary striated sphincter control mentioned with CVA or whether it is a type of situation in which the individual has simply lost the awareness of the desirability of voluntary urinary control.**

D. Cerebral Palsy (CP)

CP is the rubric applied to a nonprogressive injury of the brain in the prenatal or perinatal period (some say up to 3 years) producing neuromuscular disability and/or specific symptom complexes of cerebral dysfunction. The etiology is generally infection or a period of hypoxia. **Most children and adults with only CP have urinary control and what seems to be normal filling and storage and normal emptying.**

The incidence of voiding dysfunction is vague because the few available series report mostly subcategorizations of those who present with symptoms. In those individuals with CP who exhibit significant dysfunction, the type of damage that one would suspect from the most common urodynamic abnormalities seems to be localized anatomically above the brain stem. This is commonly reflected by phasic DO and coordinated sphincters. However, spinal cord damage can occur, and perhaps this accounts for those individuals with CP who seem to have evidence of striated sphincter dyssynergia or of a more distal type of neural axis lesion.

E. Parkinson's Disease

This neurodegenerative disorder of unknown cause affects primarily the dopaminergic neurons of the substantia nigra, the origin of the dopaminergic nigrostriatal tract to the caudate nucleus and putamen. **Dopamine deficiency in the nigrostriatal pathway accounts for most of the classic clinical motor features of PD.** The classic major signs of PD consist of tremor, skeletal rigidity, and bradykinesia, a symptom complex often referred to as **parkinsonism.**

There are causes of parkinsonism other than PD. The combination of asymmetry of symptoms and signs, the presence of a resting tremor, and a good response to levodopa best differentiates PD from parkinsonism produced by other causes, although none of these is individually specific for PD. Multiple system atrophy (MSA; see next section) is the entity most commonly confused with PD. The following suggest MSA: (1) urinary symptoms precede or present with parkinsonism, (2) UI, (3) significant post-void residual, (4) initial erectile failure, and (5) abnormal striated sphincter EMG.

Voiding dysfunction occurs in 35–70% of patients with PD. Pre-existing detrusor or outlet abnormalities may be present, and the symptomatology may be affected by various types of treatment for the primary disease. **When voiding dysfunction occurs, symptoms generally (50–75%) consist of urgency, frequency, nocturia, and urge incontinence.** The remainder of patients have "obstructive" symptoms or a combination. **The most common urodynamic finding is DO. The smooth sphincter is synergic. There is some confusion regarding EMG interpretation.** Sporadic involuntary activity in the striated sphincter during involuntary bladder contraction has been reported in as many as 60% of patients; however, this does not cause obstruction and cannot be termed true dyssynergia, which generally does not occur. **Pseudodyssynergia may occur, as well as a delay in striated sphincter relaxation (bradykinesia) at the onset of voluntary micturition, both of which can be urodynamically misinterpreted as true dyssynergia. Impaired detrusor contractility may also occur, either in the form of low amplitude or poorly sustained contractions, or a combination. Detrusor areflexia is relatively uncommon in PD.**

Many cases of "PD" in the older literature may actually have been MSA, and citations regarding symptoms and urodynamic findings may not therefore be accurate. An example of this is the inference that transurethral prostatectomy (TURP) in the patient with PD is associated with a high incidence of UI (because of poor striated sphincter control). Retrospective interpretation has concluded that these were patients with MSA and not PD and that TURP should not be contraindicated in patients with PD, because external sphincter acontractility is extremely rare in such patients. However, one must be cautious with such patients, and a complete urodynamic or videourodynamic evaluation is advisable. Poorly sustained bladder contractions, sometimes with slow sphincter relaxation, should make one less optimistic regarding the results of outlet reduction in the male.

Voiding dysfunction secondary to PD defies "routine" classification within any system. It is most manifest by storage failure secondary to bladder overactivity, but detailed urodynamic evaluation is mandatory before any but the simplest and most reversible therapy. The therapeutic menus (see Tables 13-7 and 13-8) are perfectly applicable, but the disease itself may impose certain limitations on the use of certain treatments (e.g., limited mobility for rapid toilet access, hand control insufficient for CIC).

F. Multiple System Atrophy

MSA is a progressive neurodegenerative disease of unknown etiology. The symptoms encompass parkinsonism and cerebellar, autonomic (including urinary and erectile problems), and pyramidal cortical dysfunction in a multitude of combinations. The clinical features are separable from PD.

The neurologic lesions of MSA consist of cell loss and gliosis in widespread areas, much more so than with PD, and this more diffuse nature of cell loss probably explains why bladder symptoms may occur earlier than in PD and be more severe and why erection may be affected as well. Affected areas have been identified in the cerebellum, substantia nigra, globus pallidus, caudate, putamen, inferior olives, intermediolateral columns of the spinal cord, and Onuf's nucleus. Males and females are equally affected, with the onset in middle age. MSA is generally progressive and associated with a poor prognosis. Shy-Drager syndrome has been described in the past as characterized clinically by orthostatic hypotension, anhidrosis, and varying degrees of cerebellar and parkinsonian dysfunction. Voiding and erectile dysfunction are common. Some consider this as late stage MSA.

Clinical urogenital criteria favoring a diagnosis of MSA are (1) urinary symptoms precede or present with parkinsonism, (2) male erectile dysfunction precedes or presents with parkinsonism, (3) UI, (4) significant post-void residual, and (5) worsening LUT dysfunction after urologic surgery. The initial urinary symptoms of MSA are urgency, frequency, and urge incontinence, occurring up to 4 years before the diagnosis is made, as does erectile failure. DO is frequently found, as one would expect from the CNS areas affected, but decreased compliance may occur, reflecting distal spinal involvement of the locations of the cell bodies of autonomic neurons innervating the LUT. As the disease progresses, difficulty in initiating and maintaining voiding may occur, probably from pontine and sacral cord lesions, and this generally is associated with a poor prognosis. Cystourethrography or videourodynamic studies may reveal an open bladder neck (ISD) and many patients exhibit evidence of striated sphincter denervation on motor unit electromyography. The smooth and striated sphincter abnormalities predispose women to sphincteric incontinence and make prostatectomy hazardous in men.

The treatment of significant voiding dysfunction caused by MSA is difficult and seldom satisfactory. Treatment of DO during filling may worsen problems initiating voluntary micturition or worsen impaired contractility during emptying. Patients generally have sphincteric insufficiency and, rarely, therefore, is an outlet-reducing procedure indicated. Drug treatment for sphincteric incontinence may further worsen emptying problems. Generally, the goal in these patients is to facilitate storage, and CIC would often be desirable. Unfortunately, patients with advanced disease often are not candidates for CIC.

G. Multiple Sclerosis

MS is believed to be immune mediated and is characterized by neural demyelination, generally characterized by axonal sparing, in the brain and spinal cord. The demyelinating process most commonly involves the lateral corticospinal (pyramidal) and reticulospinal columns of the cervical spinal cord, but involvement of the lumbar and sacral cord occurs to a lesser extent. Lesions may also occur in the optic nerve and in the cerebral cortex and midbrain, the latter accounting for the intellectual deterioration and/or euphoria that may be seen as well.

The incidence of voiding dysfunction in MS is related to the disability status. Of patients with MS, **50–90% complain of voiding symptoms at some time; the prevalence of incontinence is cited as 37–72%.** LUT involvement may constitute the sole initial complaint or be part of the presenting symptom complex in up to 15% of patients, usually in the form of acute urinary retention of "unknown" etiology or as an acute onset of urgency and frequency, secondary to overactivity.

DO is the most common urodynamic abnormality detected, occurring in 34–99% of cases in reported series. Of the patients with overactivity, 30–65% have co-existent striated sphincter dyssynergia. Impaired detrusor contractility or areflexia may also exist, a phenomenon that can considerably complicate treatment efforts. Generally, the smooth sphincter is synergic. It is also possible to see relative degrees of sphincteric flaccidity caused by MS, which could predispose and contribute to sphincteric incontinence.

Because sensation is frequently intact in these patients, one must be careful to distinguish urodynamic pseudodyssynergia from true striated sphincter dyssynergia. Jerry Blaivas was the first to subcategorize true striated sphincter dyssynergia in patients with MS and identify some varieties that are more worrisome than others. For instance, in a female with MS, a brief period of striated sphincter dyssynergia during detrusor contraction but one that does not result in excessive intravesical pressure during voiding, substantial residual urine volume, or secondary detrusor hypertrophy may be relatively inconsequential, whereas those varieties that are more sustained—resulting in high bladder pressures of long duration—are most associated with urologic complications. A significant proportion of patients with MS with and without new symptoms will develop changes in their detrusor compliance and urodynamic pattern. Caution should therefore be exercised in recommending irreversible therapeutic options.

The most common functional classification applicable to patients with voiding dysfunction secondary to MS would thus be storage failure secondary to DO. This is commonly complicated by striated sphincter dyssynergia, with varying effects on the ability to empty completely at acceptable pressures. Other abnormalities, and other combined deficits, are obviously possible, however. Once the dysfunction is broadly characterized, the treatment options should be obvious from the therapeutic menus (see Tables 13-7 and 13-8).

H. Spinal Cord Injury

Altered LUT and sexual function frequently occur secondary to SCI and significantly affect quality of life; SCI patients are at risk urologically for urinary tract infection, sepsis, upper and lower urinary tract deterioration, upper and lower urinary tract calculi, autonomic hyperreflexia (dysreflexia), skin complications, and depression. Failure to properly address the LUT dysfunction can lead to significant morbidity and mortality.

1. **Spinal shock.** Following a significant SCI, a period of decreased excitability of spinal cord segments at and below the level of the lesion occurs, referred to as spinal shock. There is **absent somatic reflex activity and flaccid muscle paralysis below this level. Spinal shock includes a suppression of autonomic as well as somatic activity, and the bladder is acontractile and areflexic with a closed bladder neck. The smooth sphincter mechanism seems to be closed and competent but nonrelaxing, except in some cases of thoracolumbar injury. Some EMG activity can generally be recorded from the striated sphincter,** and the maximum urethral closure pressure is still maintained at the level of the external sphincter zone; **however, the normal guarding reflex is absent.** Because sphincter tone exists, UI generally does not result unless there is gross

overdistention with overflow. Urinary retention is the rule, and catheterization is necessary to circumvent this problem. Intermittent catheterization is an excellent method of management during this period.

If the distal spinal cord is intact but is simply isolated from higher centers, there is generally a return of detrusor contractility. At first, such reflex activity is poorly sustained and produces only low pressure changes, but the strength and duration of such involuntary contractions increase, producing involuntary voiding, usually with incomplete bladder emptying. Spinal shock generally lasts 6–12 weeks in complete suprasacral spinal cord lesions but can last for as long as a year or two. It can last for a shorter period of time in incomplete suprasacral lesions and only a few days in some patients. In evolving lesions, every attempt should be made to preserve as low a bladder storage pressure as possible.

2. **Suprasacral SCI.** The characteristic pattern that results when a patient has a complete lesion above the sacral spinal cord is **DO, smooth sphincter synergia (with lesions below the sympathetic outflow), and striated sphincter dyssynergia.** Neurologic examination shows spasticity of skeletal muscle distal to the lesion, hyperreflexic deep tendon reflexes, and abnormal plantar responses. There is impairment of superficial and deep sensation. The **guarding reflex is absent or weak in most patients** with a complete suprasacral SCI. In incomplete lesions the reflex is often preserved but very variable.

The striated sphincter dyssynergia causes a functional obstruction with poor emptying and high detrusor pressure. **Occasionally, incomplete bladder emptying may result from what seems to be a poorly sustained or absent detrusor contraction.** Once reflex voiding is established, it can be initiated or reinforced by the stimulation of certain dermatomes, as by tapping the suprapubic area. The urodynamic and upper tract consequences of the striated sphincter dyssynergia vary with severity (generally worse in complete lesions than in incomplete ones), duration (continuous contraction during detrusor activity is worse than intermittent contraction), and anatomy (male is worse than female).

From a functional standpoint the voiding dysfunction most commonly seen in suprasacral SCI represents both a filling/storage and an emptying failure. Although the urodynamics are "safe" enough in some individuals to allow only periodic stimulation of bladder reflex activity, many will require some treatment. If bladder pressures are suitably low or if they can be made suitably low with nonsurgical or surgical management, the problem can be treated primarily as an emptying failure, and CIC can be continued, when practical, as a safe and effective way of satisfying many of the goals of treatment. Alternatively, sphincterotomy, stenting, or intrasphincteric injection of botulinum toxin can be used in males to lower the detrusor leak point to an acceptable level, thus treating the dysfunction primarily as one of emptying. The resultant storage failure can be obviated either by timed stimulation or with an external collecting device. In the dexterous SCI patient, the former approach using CIC is becoming predominant. Electrical stimulation of the anterior sacral roots with some form of deafferentation is also now a distinct reality. As with all patients with neurologic impairment, a careful initial evaluation and periodic follow-up evaluation must be performed to identify and correct the following risk factors and potential complications: bladder overdistention, high-pressure storage, high DLPP, VUR, stone formation (lower and upper tracts), and complicating infection, especially in association with reflux.

3. **Sacral SCI.** Following recovery from spinal shock, there is usually a depression of deep tendon reflexes below the level of the lesion with varying degrees of flaccid paralysis. Sensation is generally absent below the lesion level. **Detrusor areflexia with high or normal compliance is the common initial result. Decreased compliance may develop, a change often seen with neurologic lesions at or distal to the sacral spinal cord and most likely representing a response to neurologic decentralization.**

The **classical outlet findings are described as a competent but nonrelaxing smooth sphincter and a striated sphincter that retains some fixed tone but is not under voluntary control.** Closure pressures are decreased in both areas. However, **the late appearance of the bladder neck may be open.** Attempted voiding by straining or Credé results in obstruction at the bladder neck (if closed) or at the distal sphincter area by fixed sphincter tone. Potential risk factors are those previously described, with particular emphasis on storage pressure, which can result in silent upper tract decompensation and deterioration in the absence of VUR. The treatment of such a patient is generally directed toward producing or maintaining low-pressure storage while circumventing emptying failure with CIC when possible. Pharmacologic and electric stimulation may be useful in promoting emptying in certain circumstances.

4. **Neurologic and urodynamic correlation in SCI.** Although generally correct, the correlation between somatic neurologic findings and urodynamic findings in suprasacral and sacral SCI patients is not exact. A number of factors should be considered in this regard. First, whether a lesion is complete or incomplete is sometimes a matter of definition. A complete lesion, somatically speaking, may not translate into a complete lesion autonomically, and vice versa. Multiple injuries may actually exist at different levels, even though what is seen somatically may reflect a single level of injury. Even considering these situations, however, all such discrepancies are not explained.

   Management of the urinary tract in such patients must be based on urodynamic principles and findings rather than inferences from the neurologic history and evaluation. Similarly, although the information regarding "classic" complete lesions is for the most part valid, neurologic conclusions should not be made solely on the basis of urodynamic findings.

5. **Autonomic hyperreflexia.** Autonomic hyperreflexia is a potentially fatal emergency unique to the SCI patient. **Autonomic hyperreflexia represents an acute massive disordered autonomic (primarily sympathetic) response to specific stimuli in patients with SCI above the level of T6 to T8 (the sympathetic outflow).** It is more common in cervical (60%) than thoracic (20%) injuries. Onset after injury is variable—usually soon after spinal shock but may be up to years after injury. Distal cord viability is a prerequisite.

   Symptomatically, autonomic hyperreflexia is a syndrome of exaggerated sympathetic activity in response to stimuli below the level of the lesion. The **symptoms** are **pounding headache, hypertension, and flushing of the face and body above the level of the lesion with sweating. Bradycardia is a usual accompaniment,** although tachycardia or arrhythmia may be present. **Hypertension may be of varying severity,** from causing a mild headache before the occurrence of voiding to life-threatening cerebral hemorrhage or seizure. The stimuli for this exaggerated response commonly arise from the bladder or rectum and generally involve distention, although other stimuli from these areas can be precipitating. Precipitation may be the result of simple LUT instrumentation, tube change, catheter obstruction, or clot retention; and, in such cases, the symptoms resolve quickly if the stimulus is withdrawn. Other causes or exacerbating factors may include other upper or lower urinary tract pathology (e.g., calculi), gastrointestinal pathology, long bone fracture, sexual activity, electrocoagulation, and decubiti.

Striated sphincter dyssynergia invariably occurs, and smooth sphincter dyssynergia is generally a part of the syndrome as well, at least in males. The pathophysiology is that of a nociceptive stimulation via afferent impulses that ascend through the cord and elicit reflex motor outflow, causing arteriolar, pilomotor, and pelvic visceral spasm and sweating. Normally, the reflexes would be inhibited by secondary output from the medulla, but because of the SCI this does not occur below the lesion level.

Ideally, any endoscopic procedure in susceptible patients should be done under spinal anesthesia or carefully monitored general anesthesia. Acutely, the hemodynamic effects of this syndrome may be managed with β- and/or α-adrenergic blocking agents. Ganglionic blockers had previously been the mainstay of treatment but their usage has essentially been abandoned.

Chronic prophylaxis with an α-1 adrenergic blocker has been recommended and found useful by some authorities. Such prophylaxis may be particularly important in view of the fact that significant elevations in blood pressure can occur without other symptoms of autonomic hyperreflexia. Prophylaxis, however, does not eliminate the need for careful monitoring during provocative procedures. There are patients with severe dysreflexia that is intractable to oral prophylaxis and correction by urologic procedures. For these unfortunate individuals, a number of neurologic ablative procedures have been used—sympathectomy, sacral neurectomy, sacral rhizotomy, cordectomy, and dorsal root ganglionectomy.

I. Neurospinal Dysraphism

Although primarily a pediatric problem, certain considerations regarding the adult with these abnormalities should be mentioned. Secondary to progress in the overall care of children with myelodysplasia, urologic dysfunction often becomes a problem of the adult with this disease. The **"typical" myelodysplastic patient** shows an **areflexic bladder with an open bladder neck. Decreased compliance may be present. The bladder generally fills until the resting residual fixed external sphincter pressure is** reached, and then leakage occurs. **Stress incontinence often occurs also. A small percentage of patients demonstrate detrusor-striated sphincter dyssynergia,** but these individuals show normal bladder neck function, which, if detrusor reflex activity is controlled, is associated with continence.

After puberty most male myelodysplastic patients note an improvement in continence. In adult patients, the problems encountered in myelodysplastic children still exist, but are often compounded by prior surgery, upper tract dysfunction, and one form of urinary diversion or another. In adult females, the goal is to increase urethral sphincter efficiency without causing an undue enough increase in urethral closing pressure, which will result in a change in bladder compliance. Periurethral injection therapy to achieve continence may give as good a result as a pubovaginal sling or artificial sphincter in this circumstance. Continence in adult male myelodysplastic individuals follows the same general rules as in females, and injectable materials may give good results in this group as well, unless the outlet is widely dilated. Dry individuals, of course, will be on intermittent self-catheterization. Nowhere is the failure of a neurologic examination to predict urodynamic behavior more obvious than in patients with myelomeningocele. The **prime directive of therapy remains the avoidance of high storage pressures.**

Tethered cord syndrome (TCS) is defined as a stretch-induced functional disorder of the spinal cord with its caudal part anchored by inelastic structures. Vertical movement is restricted. The anchoring structures can include scar from prior surgery, fibrous or fibroadipose filum terminale, a bony septum, or tumor. Adults with TCS can be divided into those with a prior history of spinal dysraphism with a previously stabilized neurologic status, who present with subtle progression in adulthood, and those without associated spinal dysraphism, who present with new subtle neurologic symptoms. Symptoms can include back pain, leg weakness, foot deformity, scoliosis, sensory loss, and bowel or LUT dysfunction. TCS is reported to occur in 3–15% of patients with myelomeningocele. There is no typical dysfunction in TCS, and treatment must be based on contemporary urodynamic evaluation.

J. Disk Disease; Cauda Equina Syndrome; Spinal Stenosis

Most **disk protrusions** compress the spinal roots in the L4–L5 or L5–S1 interspaces. Voiding dysfunction may occur as a result, and when present, generally occurs with the usual clinical manifestations of low back pain radiating in a girdle-like fashion along the involved spinal root areas. Examination may reveal reflex and sensory loss consistent with nerve root compression. The most characteristic findings on physical exam are sensory loss in the S2–4 dermatomes (perineum or perianal areas), S1–2 dermatomes (lateral foot), or both. The incidence of voiding dysfunction in disk prolapse ranges from 1–18%. The most consistent urodynamic finding is a normally compliant areflexic bladder associated with normal innervation or incomplete denervation of the perineal floor muscles. There is a lower incidence of decreased compliance in root damage secondary to disk prolapse, as opposed to myelomeningocele. Occasionally, patients may show DO, attributed to irritation of the nerve roots.

Patients with voiding dysfunction generally present with difficulty voiding, straining, or urinary retention. It should be noted that laminectomy may not improve bladder function, and prelaminectomy urodynamic evaluation is desirable because it may be difficult postoperatively to separate causation of voiding dysfunction due to the disk sequelae alone from changes secondary to the surgery.

Cauda equina syndrome is a term applied to the clinical picture of perineal sensory loss with loss of voluntary control of both anal and urethral sphincter and of sexual responsiveness. This can occur not only secondary to disk disease (severe central posterior disk protrusion) but to other spinal canal pathologies as well. Typically, patients have an acontractile detrusor with no bladder sensation.

Spinal stenosis is a term applied to any narrowing of the spinal canal, nerve root canals, or intervertebral foramina. It may be congenital, developmental, or acquired. Compression of the nerve roots or cord by such a problem may lead to neuronal damage, ischemia, or edema. **Spinal stenosis may occur without disk prolapse. Symptoms may range from those consequent to cervical spinal cord compression to a cauda equina syndrome, with corresponding urodynamic findings**. Back and lower extremity pain, cramping, and paresthesias related to exercise and relieved by rest are the classic symptoms of lumbar stenosis caused by lumbar spondylosis and are believed to result from a sacral nerve root ischemia. The urodynamic findings are dependent on the level and the amount of spinal cord or nerve root damage.

K. Radical Pelvic Surgery

Voiding dysfunction after pelvic plexus injury occurs most commonly after abdominoperineal resection and radical hysterectomy. The incidence has been estimated to range from

20–68% of patients after abdominoperineal resection, 16–80% after radical hysterectomy, 20–25% after anterior resection, and 10–20% after proctocolectomy. These are estimates drawn from past literature, and the current incidence is most likely significantly lower, owing to the use of nerve-sparing techniques during these types of pelvic surgery. It has been estimated, however, that in 15–20% of affected individuals, the voiding dysfunction is permanent. The injury may occur consequent to denervation or neurologic decentralization, tethering of the nerves or encasement in scar, direct bladder or urethral trauma, or bladder devascularization. Adjuvant treatment, such as chemotherapy or radiation, may play a role as well. The type of voiding dysfunction that occurs is dependent on the specific nerves involved, the degree of injury, and any pattern of reinnervation or altered innervation that results over time.

When permanent voiding dysfunction occurs after radical pelvic surgery, the **pattern is generally one of a failure of voluntary bladder contraction, or impaired bladder contractility, with obstruction by what seems urodynamically to be residual fixed striated sphincter tone,** which is not subject to voluntarily induced relaxation. **Often, the smooth sphincter area is open and nonfunctional.** Whether this appearance of the bladder neck-proximal urethra is caused by parasympathetic damage or terminal sympathetic damage or whether it results from the hydrodynamic effects of obstruction at the level of the striated sphincter is debated and unknown. **Decreased compliance is common** in these patients, and this, with the "obstruction" caused by fixed residual striated sphincter tone, results in both storage and emptying failure. **These patients often experience leaking across the distal sphincter area and, in addition, are unable to empty the bladder, because although intravesical pressure may be increased, there is nothing that approximates a true bladder contraction.** The patient often presents with UI that is characteristically most manifest with increases in intra-abdominal pressure. This is usually most obvious in females, because the prostatic bulk in males often masks an equivalent deficit in urethral closure function. Alternatively, patients may present with variable degrees of urinary retention.

Urodynamic studies may show decreased compliance, poor proximal urethral closure function, loss of voluntary control of the striated sphincter, and a positive bethanechol supersensitivity test. Upper tract risk factors are related to intravesical pressure and the DLPP, and the therapeutic goal is always low-pressure storage with periodic emptying. The temptation to perform a prostatectomy should be avoided unless a clear demonstration of outlet obstruction at this level is possible. Otherwise, prostatectomy simply decreases urethral sphincter function and thereby may result in the occurrence or worsening of sphincteric UI. Most of these dysfunctions will be transient, and the temptation to "do something" other than perform CIC initially after surgery in these patients, especially in those with little or no pre-existent history of voiding dysfunction, cannot be too strongly criticized.

L. Diabetes Mellitus

If specifically questioned, anywhere from 5–59% of patients with diabetes report symptoms of voiding dysfunction. However, the symptoms may or may not be caused by just the diabetes. In trying to come to conclusions regarding the incidence and types of voiding dysfunction specifically from diabetes, one has to carefully discriminate between articles that consider patients referred for voiding symptoms versus those that have evaluated unselected patients from a population known to have diabetes. Cai Frimodt-Moller coined the term **diabetic cystopathy** to describe the involvement of the LUT by this disease. **The classic description of voiding dysfunction secondary to diabetes is that of a peripheral autonomic neuropathy that first affects sensory afferent pathways, causing the insidious onset of impaired bladder sensation. As the classic description continues, a gradual increase in the time interval between voiding results, which may progress to the point at which the patient voids only once or twice a day without ever sensing any real urgency. If this continues, detrusor distention, overdistention, and decompensation ultimately occur. Detrusor contractility, therefore, is classically described as being decreased in the end-stage diabetic bladder.**

Current evidence points to both a sensory and a motor neuropathy as being involved in the pathogenesis, the motor aspect per se contributing to the impaired detrusor contractility. **The typically described classic urodynamic findings include impaired bladder sensation, increased cystometric capacity, decreased bladder contractility, impaired uroflow, and, later, increased residual urine volume.** The main differential diagnosis, at least in men, is generally bladder outlet obstruction, because both conditions commonly produce a low flow rate. Pressure/flow urodynamic studies easily differentiate the two. **Smooth or striated sphincter dyssynergia generally is not seen in classic diabetic cystopathy,** but these diagnoses can easily be erroneously made on a poor or incomplete urodynamic study—voiding may involve abdominal straining, which will produce an interference EMG pattern (pseudodyssynergia) and abdominal straining alone will not open the bladder neck area.

Other articles have appeared, however, suggesting that DO and not this "classic" diabetic cystopathy is the predominant form of LUT dysfunction. Although it is obvious that some (or even many) of the patients with diabetes who exhibited involuntary bladder contractions may have had factors other than diabetes to account for their bladder overactivity, the importance of urodynamic study in diabetic patients before institution of therapy cannot be overemphasized.

M. Tabes Dorsalis; Pernicious Anemia

Although syphilitic myelopathy is disappearing as a major neurologic problem, involvement of the spinal cord dorsal columns and posterior sacral roots can result in a loss of bladder sensation and large residual urine volumes and therefore be a cause of "sensory neurogenic bladder." Another spinal cord cause of the classic "sensory bladder" is the now uncommon pernicious anemia that produced this disorder by virtue of subacute combined degeneration of the dorsolateral columns of the spinal cord.

IX. COMMON NON-NEUROGENIC VOIDING DYSFUNCTIONS

A. Outlet Obstruction Secondary to BPH

This is probably the most common voiding dysfunction seen by the urologist (see Chapter 14). Classically, the patient complains of hesitancy and straining to void, with the **urodynamic correlates of low flow and high detrusor pressure during attempted voiding.** This situation represents a pure failure to empty. Approximately 50% of the time, the patient with significant prostatic obstruction develops DO, with resultant urgency, frequency, and, if the overactivity cannot be inhibited, urgency incontinence. Under such circumstances, the voiding dysfunction becomes a combined emptying and filling and storage problem. Treatment is relief of the obstruction either by reduction of prostatic bulk or tone. Relief of the outlet obstruction will result in the eventual disappearance of DO, where present, in approximately 70% of cases, although this may return years later.

B. Bladder Neck Dysfunction

Bladder neck dysfunction is characterized by an **incomplete opening of the bladder neck during voluntary or involuntary voiding.** It has also been referred to as smooth sphincter dyssynergia, proximal urethral obstruction, primary bladder neck obstruction, and dysfunctional bladder neck. The term **smooth sphincter dyssynergia or proximal sphincter dyssynergia is generally used when referring to this urodynamic finding in an individual with autonomic hyperreflexia. The term bladder neck dysfunction more often refers to a poorly understood non-neurogenic condition first described over a century ago** but first fully characterized by Richard Turner-Warwick and associates in 1973. The dysfunction is found almost exclusively in young and middle-aged men, and characteristically they complain of long-standing voiding/emptying (obstructive) and filling/storage (irritative) symptoms. These patients have often been seen by many urologists and have been diagnosed as having psychogenic voiding dysfunction because of a normal prostate on rectal examination, a negligible residual urine volume, and a normal endoscopic bladder appearance. The differential diagnosis also includes anatomic bladder neck contracture, BPH, dysfunctional voiding, prostatitis/prostatosis, neurogenic dysfunction, and low pressure/low flow (see later). Objective evidence of outlet obstruction in these patients is easily obtainable by urodynamic study. Once obstruction is diagnosed, it can be localized at the level of the bladder neck by video urodynamic study, cystourethrography during a bladder contraction, or micturitional urethral profilometry. The diagnosis may also be made indirectly by the urodynamic findings of outlet obstruction in the typical clinical situation in the absence of urethral stricture, prostatic enlargement, and striated sphincter dyssynergia. Involuntary bladder contractions or decreased compliance may occur. When prostatic enlargement develops in individuals with this problem, a double obstruction results, and Turner-Warwick has applied the term "trapped prostate" to this entity. The lobes of the prostate cannot expand the bladder neck and therefore expand into the urethra. A patient so affected generally has a lifelong history of voiding dysfunction that has gone relatively unnoticed because he has always accepted this as normal, and exacerbation of these symptoms occurs during a relatively short and early period of prostatic enlargement. **Although α-adrenergic–blocking agents provide improvement in some patients with bladder neck dysfunction, definitive relief in the male is best achieved by bladder neck incision.** In patients with this and a trapped prostate, marked relief is generally effected by a "small" prostatic resection or ablation that includes the bladder neck or a transurethral incision of the bladder neck and prostate.

Such patients often note afterward that they have "never" voided as well as after their treatment.

C. Bladder Outlet Obstruction in Women

The female counterpart of non-neurogenic bladder neck dysfunction in men does exist, although it is **rare**. Definitions and diagnostic criteria vary. Victor Nitti defines bladder outlet obstruction as radiographic evidence of obstruction between the bladder neck and the distal urethra in the presence of a sustained detrusor contraction of any magnitude, which is usually associated with a reduced or delayed urinary flow rate. Obstruction at the level of the bladder neck was diagnosed when the bladder neck was closed or narrowed during voiding. Strict pressure-flow criteria are not used to classify cases as obstructed or not obstructed. Jerry Blaivas' group defines obstruction as a persistent low, noninvasive maximum flow rate less than 12 mL/sec on repeated study combined with a detrusor pressure at maximum measured flow rate of more than 20 cm of water in a pressure-flow study. Most authors would agree that surgical treatment of this problem in women should be approached with caution, because sphincteric incontinence is a significant risk.

D. Low-Pressure/Low-Flow Voiding in Younger Men: The Bashful Bladder

Low-pressure/low-flow voiding can be the result of a number of causes, most notably a decompensating detrusor (generally from bladder outlet obstruction) or as a part of the syndrome known as DHIC (detrusor hyperactivity with impaired contractility). When this occurs in a young man, it is generally symptomatically characterized by frequency, hesitancy, and a poor stream. The entity is readily demonstrated on urodynamic assessment and with no co-existing endoscopic abnormality. The patient generally notes marked hesitancy when attempting to initiate micturition in the presence of others, and some have therefore described this condition as an "anxious bladder" or a "bashful bladder." Our experience has been similar to that of others who have stated that, in the younger nonobstructed male with this condition, neither empirical pharmacologic treatment nor transurethral surgery has had any consistent beneficial effect.

E. Dysfunctional Voiding

This syndrome, also known as non-neurogenic/neurogenic bladder, occult voiding dysfunction, or Hinman's syndrome, presents the unusual circumstance of what appears urodynamically to be involuntary obstruction at the striated sphincter level existing in the absence of demonstrable neurologic disease. It is very difficult to prove urodynamically that an individual has this entity. This requires simultaneous pressure/flow EMG evidence of bladder emptying occurring simultaneously with involuntary striated sphincter contraction in the absence of any element of abdominal straining component, either in an attempt to augment bladder contraction or as a response to discomfort during urination. The etiology is uncertain and may represent a persistent transitional phase in the development of micturitional control or persistence of a reaction phase to the stimulus of LUT discomfort during voiding, long after the initial problem that caused this has disappeared. The preferred treatment is biofeedback. Intermittent catheterization may be useful, both as therapy and as an aid to facilitating the ability to voluntarily relax the striated sphincter.

F. Decompensated Bladder

This situation may occur after a longstanding bladder outlet obstruction or as a chronic response to neurologic injury. Attempts to produce emptying pharmacologically with a cholinergic agonist and an α-adrenergic antagonist have been generally unsuccessful, and the best treatment is intermittent catheterization. The temptation to surgically decrease bladder outlet resistance in the hope of "tipping the balance" in favor of emptying should be resisted. This approach is seldom effective unless it produces a form of stress incontinence.

G. Postoperative Retention

Urinary retention can occur postoperatively for a number of reasons. Nociceptive impulses can inhibit the initiation of reflex bladder contraction, perhaps through an opioid-mediated mechanism or sympathetic mediated inhibition. Transient overdistention of the bladder can occur under anesthesia or under the influence of analgesic medication. Purely neurologic injury during abdominal and pelvic surgery can also occur. Generally, in the absence of neurologic injury and with proper decompression, a patient's voiding status will return pretty much to what it was prior to the surgery and anesthesia. Therefore the optimal treatment is intermittent catheterization. Return of bladder function may be facilitated by the use of an α-adrenergic antagonist. Treatment with cholinergic agonists alone has been generally unsuccessful. A patient with prostatism on the borderline of significant voiding dysfunction may have his previously ten-uous and abnormal ability to empty compromised. In these cases, prostatectomy may be justified.

H. Urinary Retention; The Fowler Syndrome in Young Women

The Fowler syndrome refers particularly to a syndrome of **urinary retention in young women in the absence of overt neurologic disease.** The **typical history** is that of a young woman younger than 30 years who has found her-self unable to void for a day or more with no urinary urgency but increasing lower abdominal discomfort. A bladder capacity of more than 1 L with no sensation of urgency is necessary for the diagnosis. There are no neuro-logic or laboratory features to support a diagnosis of any neurologic disease. MRI of the brain and the entire spinal cord is normal. The urodynamic problem is detrusor acon-tractility. **On concentric needle electrode examination** of the striated muscle of the urethral sphincter, however, Fowler and associates described a **unique EMG abnormality that impairs sphincter relaxation.** These patients often have poly-cystic ovaries. Efforts to treat this condition by hormonal manipulation, pharmacologic therapy, or injection of botuli-num toxin have been unsuccessful. This condition is said by some to be responsive to neuromodulation.

X. URINARY INCONTINENCE

UI is defined as the **involuntary loss of urine.** The term is used in various ways. It may denote a symptom, a sign, or a condition. The **symptom** is generally thought of as the patient's complaint of involuntary urine loss. The **sign** is the objective demonstration of urine loss. The **condition** is the underlying cause (pathophysiology). A simple classi-fication of the various subtypes of UI is seen in Table 13-12. The basic pathophysiology of incontinence and various related definitions are discussed in sections III, IV, and V.

There are situations in which urethral incontinence can-not be considered merely as an isolated abnormality of either bladder contractility or sphincter resistance. These situations, listed in Table 13-13, are more complicated to deal with, first, because they are more difficult to diagnose, and second, because one entity may adversely affect or compromise treatment of the other. The most common of these is **DO with outlet obstruction**. This occurs almost

Table 13-12: Classification of Incontinence

I. Extraurethral
  A. Fistula (vesicovaginal, ureterovaginal, urethrovaginal)
  B. Ectopic ureter
II. Urethral
  A. Functional
    1. Because of physical disability
    2. Due to lack of awareness or concern
  B. Bladder abnormalities
    1. Overactivity
      a. Involuntary contractions
      b. Decreased compliance
      c. Hypersensitivity with incontinence
  C. Outlet abnormalities
    1. Genuine stress incontinence
    2. Intrinsic sphincter deficiency
    3. Urethral instability
    4. Post-void dribbling
      a. Urethral diverticulum
      b. Vaginal pooling of urine
  D. Overflow incontinence

Table 13-13: Combined Problems Associated with Incontinence

Detrusor overactivity with outlet obstruction
Detrusor overactivity with impaired bladder contractility
Sphincteric incontinence with impaired bladder contractility
Sphincteric incontinence with detrusor overactivity

exclusively in the male. The incidence of DO in series of patients with outlet obstruction secondary to prostatic enlargement ranges from 50–80%. Treating only the DO in these patients may result in worsening symptoms. On the other hand, when the outlet obstruction is relieved in such patients, there is a high reversal rate of the bladder status, although this reversion generally takes between 1 and 6 months and may take as long as 12 months. Neil Resnick and Subbaro Yalla described the phenomenon of **DHIC** (detrusor hyperactivity and impaired contractility), especially in frail, elderly, incontinent patients. They found that one third of such patients and one half of those with an overactive detrusor had bladders that were poorly contractile despite extensive trabeculation. Because bladder contractility is impaired, a vigorous pharmacologic approach usually used for involuntary bladder contractions may not be appropriate for this entity.

Sphincter incontinence in an individual with impaired contractility should alert the clinician to the possibility of the requirement of permanent CIC following surgical repair. Depending on the patient's ability and willingness to carry out intermittent catheterization, this may drastically alter an individual's usual treatment program for sphincter incontinence if the simpler, noninvasive therapeutic measures have failed. **Sphincter incontinence can co-exist with DO** in a number of circumstances and with varying effects. Urgency often co-exists with stress incontinence. Such bladder overactivity has been cited as one of the most common causes of failure of a suspension operation for stress incontinence. Whether these urodynamic findings really do indicate that such an operation is likely to fail is an important question, as an affirmative answer would mandate a very careful urodynamic evaluation in all such patients and would doubtless decrease the enthusiasm for corrective surgery in such patients who have co-existent genuine stress incontinence. Patients with stress incontinence who also have decreased compliance do not seem to fare well after surgery to correct just the stress incontinence. The decreased compliance generally does not change, and if it was refractory to nonsurgical therapy before, it will remain that way, at least in our experience.

A **variant and more complicated form of such a combination may occur following radical pelvic surgery.** Such patients may have a combination of decreased compliance with impaired bladder contractility (from the standpoint of emptying potential) with an open and nonfunctional smooth sphincter area and obstruction by residual striated sphincter tone that is not subject to voluntary induced relaxation. These patients often leak across the distal sphincter area and, in addition, are unable to empty their bladders, because, although they have an increased intravesical pressure, they have nothing that approximates a true bladder contraction. They often present with UI, which is characteristically most manifest with increases in intra-abdominal pressure. This is usually most obvious in the female patient, as the prostatic bulk often masks a deficit in male urethral closure function.

One additional fact with respect to definition, however, bears mention. The traditional perspective on UI fails to account for instances in which symptoms of urinary frequency and urgency are present without the involuntary loss of urine. **Overactive bladder** is a term that describes the symptoms of urgency, with or without urgency incontinence, usually with frequency and nocturia. The management (evaluation and treatment) of overactive bladder should be the same as that of DO.

Prevalence rates for the most inclusive definitions of UI in women 15 years and older range from 5–69%, with daily rates ranging from 4–14%. In older women mixed and urgency incontinence predominate while in younger and middle-aged women stress (effort-related) incontinence predominates. Established and suggested risk factors for UI in women include age, pregnancy, parity, obstetric factors, hormonal status, LUT symptoms, neurologic disease, hysterectomy, obesity, functional impairment, cognitive impairment, and smoking. In men the prevalence of UI (inclusive definition) has been reported to range from 3–39%, with general agreement that the prevalence is less than half that in women. Urgency incontinence predominates (40–80%), followed by mixed UI (10–30%), and stress UI (less than 10%). Risk factors include age, LUT symptoms and infections, functional and cognitive impairment, neurologic disorder, and prostatectomy. In general the prevalence of some UI in nursing home residents of both sexes is estimated at 50% or higher.

A recent summary (3rd International Consultation on Incontinence 2004) reported the annual cost of UI in the United States as $16.3 billion in 1995 dollars and $19.5 billion in 2000 dollars. In addition to the financial costs, UI imposes a significant psychosocial impact on individuals, their families, and caregivers.

Quality of life, as measured by both generic and LUT-specific indices, is adversely affected to a significant degree. The primary spheres affected are (1) self-esteem, (2) ability to maintain an independent lifestyle, (3) social interactions with friends and family, (4) activities of daily life, and (5) sexual activity. A brief description of the more common types of UI follows.

A. Outlet-Related Incontinence in the Female

Classically, sphincteric incontinence in the female patient had been categorized into **(1) genuine stress incontinence (GSUI)** and (2) what was originally described by McGuire and Woodside as type III stress incontinence, now referred to as **ISD**. **GSUI** is associated with **hypermobility of the vesicourethral junction due to poor pelvic support and an outlet that is competent at rest but loses its competence** only during increases in intra-abdominal pressure. ISD describes a nonfunctional or very poorly functional bladder neck and proximal urethra at rest. **The division between these two situations, however, is not absolute, and virtually all "experts" agree that every case of sphincteric incontinence in the female involves varying proportions of GSUI and ISD.** The implication of classical ISD is that a surgical procedure designed to correct only urethral hypermobility will have a relatively high failure rate as opposed to one designed to improve urethral compression and/or coaptation.

Stress UI is a symptom that arises from damage to muscles and/or nerves and/or connective tissue within the pelvic floor. Urethral support is important—the urethra normally being supported by the action of the levator ani muscles through their connection to the endopelvic fascia of the anterior vaginal wall. Damage to the connection between this fascia and muscle, damage to the nerve supply, or direct muscle damage can therefore influence continence. Bladder neck function is similarly important, and loss of normal bladder neck closure can result in incontinence despite normal urethral support. **In older writings, the urethra was sometimes ignored as a factor contributing to continence in the female, and the site of continence was thought to be exclusively the bladder neck. However, in approximately 50% of continent women, urine enters the urethra during increases in abdominal pressure. The continence point in these women is at the mid urethra,** where urine is stopped before it can escape from the urethral meatus. With urethral hypermobility, there is weakness of the pelvic floor. During increases in intra-abdominal pressure, there is descent of the bladder neck and proximal urethra. If the outlet opens concomitantly, stress UI ensues. In the classic form of urethral hypermobility, there is rotational descent of the bladder neck and urethra. However, the urethra may also descend without rotation (it shortens and widens) or the posterior wall of the urethra may be pulled open while the anterior wall remains fixed. It should be noted, however, that **urethral hypermobility is often present in women who are not incontinent, and thus the mere presence of urethral hypermobility is not sufficient to make a diagnosis of a sphincter abnormality unless UI is also demonstrated.**

The **"hammock hypothesis"** of John DeLancey proposes that **for stress incontinence to occur with hypermobility, there must be a lack of stability of the suburethral supportive layer.** This theory proposes that the effect of abdominal pressure increases on the normal bladder outlet, if the suburethral supportive layer is firm, is to compress the urethra rapidly and effectively. If the supportive suburethral layer is lax and/or movable, compression is not as effective. **ISD** denotes an **intrinsic malfunction of the outlet sphincter mechanisms.** In its most overt form, it is characterized by a bladder neck that is open at rest and a low VLPP and urethral closure pressure and is usually the result of prior surgery, trauma with scarring, or a neurologic lesion. **Urethral instability** refers to the rare phenomenon of episodic decreases in outlet pressure unrelated to increases in bladder or abdominal pressure. The term urethral instability is probably a misnomer, because many believe that the drop in urethral pressure represents the urethral component of a normal voiding reflex in an individual whose bladder does not measurably contract, either because of myogenic or neurogenic reasons.

B. Outlet-Related Incontinence in the Male

In theory at least, categories of outlet-related incontinence in the male are similar to those in the female. In reality, there is little if any information regarding the topic of urethral instability in the male. **Sphincteric incontinence in the male is not associated with hypermobility of the bladder neck and proximal urethra but is rather more similar to what is termed ISD in the female.** It is generally due to prostatectomy, pelvic trauma, or neurologic diseases.

C. Bladder-Related Incontinence in the Female

Bladder-related abnormalities causing UI consist of either **DO or low bladder compliance. DO** is a generic term for involuntary bladder contractions. These can be either due to neurologic conditions (in which case neurogenic DO is the term applied) or non-neurologic in origin (in which case the term idiopathic DO is employed). Neurologically, involuntary bladder contractions can be due to any lesion occurring above the sacral spinal cord. The cause(s) of idiopathic DO in the female is (are) obscure. In addition to the etiologies noted previously (neurogenic voiding dysfunction), one subject that should be mentioned is the simultaneous occurrence of DO with stress UI. The fact that minor or moderate components of DO, and sometimes major ones, often disappear after successful surgery for stress incontinence suggests that these two phenomena are causally related in many patients in an as yet unknown fashion.

D. Bladder-Related Incontinence in the Male

The pathophysiology of bladder-related incontinence in the male is similar to that in the female except that there is **no**

known association between DO and stress incontinence in the male. There is, however, a unique association of DO with bladder outlet obstruction in the male. The incidence of DO in males with outlet obstruction secondary to prostatic enlargement is approximately 50%. When the outlet obstruction is relieved in such patients, there is a high reversion rate of the bladder status to stability (approximately 70%), although this reversion may take as long as 12 months.

E. Overflow Incontinence

This is a descriptive term that denotes **leakage of urine associated with urinary retention.** This is more common in the male than female. The **primary pathophysiology is actually a failure of emptying**, leading to urinary retention with "overflow" incontinence, resulting from either continuous or episodic elevation of intravesical pressure over urethral pressure. This generally results from outlet obstruction or detrusor inactivity, either neurologic or pharmacologic in origin, or may be secondary to inadvertent overdistention of the bladder.

F. Management of Incontinence

Management of incontinence includes the processes of evaluation and treatment. Various algorithms are available for each, ranging from the simplest to the most complicated.

What is appropriate for one patient/health care provider combination may not be appropriate for another. The level of complexity of the evaluation and management depends, as it does for all types of voiding dysfunction, on the following:

1. The clinical problem at hand.
2. The prior treatment experience(s).
3. The patient's desire for treatment.
4. The patient's goals of therapy.
5. The patient's desire to avoid invasive procedures and/or complications.
6. The patient's ability and desire to follow instructions or carry out specific tasks.
7. The expected level of improvement under optimal circumstances.
8. The health care provider's level of expertise.
9. Environmental considerations.
10. Economic considerations.

XI. TREATMENT OF VOIDING DYSFUNCTION

A. General

There are only a discrete number of therapies available, and these are easily categorized on a functional "menu" basis according to whether they are used primarily to facilitate urine storage or emptying and whether their primary effect is on the bladder or the outlet (see Tables 13-7 and 13-8). The algorithms for the management of UI in various populations endorsed by the third International Consultation on Incontinence (2004) (ICI) are reproduced in Tables 13-14, 13-15, 13-16, 13-17, 13-18, 13-19, and 13-20. The letter grades in the tables refer to the various committee assessments using the Oxford Guidelines (Table 13-21) adopted by the ICI. For any especially interested in this area, the most recent two-volume text is highly recommended (Abrams et al, 2005). Brief comments will be made about selected, more commonly used categories. Specific therapy for BPH is considered in Chapter 14.

Note that inclusion in the lists does not necessarily imply majority agreement on efficacy. Treatment should always begin with the simplest most reversible form(s) of therapy, proceeding gradually up the ladder of complexity, with the knowledge that it is only the patient (and/or family) who is (are) empowered to say when "enough is enough." A perfect result need not be achieved. Satisfaction and avoidance of adverse outcomes are the goals. At every step, the patient and/or family must understand the potential benefits, practicalities, and risks of further therapy.

B. Therapy to Facilitate Bladder Filling and Urine Storage

1. *Inhibiting Bladder Contractility/Decreasing Sensory Input/Increasing Bladder Capacity (see Table 13-7)*

a) Behavioral therapy, behavioral modification, and bladder training. These terms are sometimes used interchangeably in describing nonmedical, nonsurgical methods to treat various types of voiding dysfunction. The term **behavioral therapy** in our center includes (1) patient education about LUT function; (2) information about lifestyle changes or dietary modification (e.g., fluid restriction, avoidance of irritants); (3) so-called bladder training or retraining, which includes instituting intervals of timed voiding and gradually increasing these intervals;

(Text continued on p. 437)

Table 13-14: Management of Urinary Incontinence in Men (From Abrams et al, 2005, with permission)

A. Initial Management

1. Initial assessement should identify:

Men with "*complicated*" incontinence associated with *hematuria, pain, recurrent infection,* or who are known to have or who are thought to have *poor bladder emptying,* for example due to bladder outlet obstruction, are recommended for *specialized management.*

Poor bladder emptying may be suspected from symptoms, physical examination, or if imaging has been performed by x-ray or ultrasound after voiding.

Initial assessment aims to *identify 3 groups of men* suitable for *initial management.*

a. Those with *post-micturition dribble alone*

b. Those with symptoms of *urgency* with or without urge incontinence, together with frequency and nocturia (overactive bladder)

c. Those with *post-prostatectomy incontinence*

2. Treatment

a. Post-micturition dribble requires *no assessment* and can usually be effectively treated by pelvic floor muscle training and manual compression of the bulbous urethra directly after micturition (Grade A)

b. Urge incontinence and other overactive bladder symptoms should be treated by *noninvasive* means initially (Grade C)

- Lifestyle interventions (Grade C)
- Pelvic floor muscle training (Grade C)
- Bladder training (Grade C)
- Antimuscarinic drugs if detrusor overactivity is suspected as the cause for overactive bladder symptoms (Grade C)
- Alpha-adrenergic antagonists (α-blockers) can be considered if it is thought that there may also be bladder outlet obstruction (Grade C)

c. Post prostatectomy stress incontinence should also be treated initially by pelvic floor muscle training (Grade A) augmented by lifestyle interventions (Grade B) or bladder training (Grade C)

3. Outcome Assessment

Should *initial treatment* be *unsuccessful* after a reasonable period of time (8–12 weeks), referral for a *specialist's advice* is highly recommended.

Note: It may be necessary for patients to use (in)*continence products* while waiting for definitive treatment.

For *frail older men* with *neurogenic dysfunction* please see relevant algorithm and chapter.

Table 13-14:—Cont'd

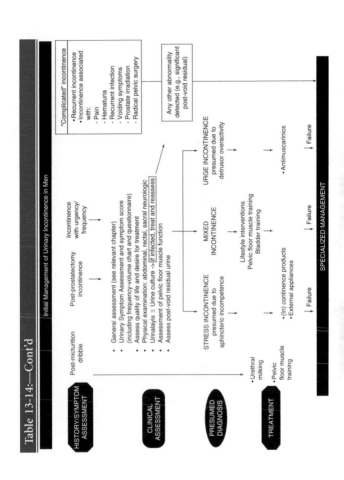

	Initial Management of Urinary Incontinence in Men			

HISTORY/SYMPTOM ASSESSMENT	Post-micturition dribble	Post-prostatectomy incontinence	Incontinence with urgency/ frequency	"Complicated" incontinence
				• Recurrent incontinence
				• Incontinence associated with:
				  - Pain
				  - Hematuria
				  - Recurrent infection
				  - Voiding symptoms
				  - Prostate irradiation
				  - Radical pelvic surgery

CLINICAL ASSESSMENT	• General assessment (see relevant chapter) • Urinary Symptom Assessment and symptom score (including frequency-volume chart and questionnaire) • Assess quality of life and desire for treatment • Physical examination: abdominal, rectal, sacral neurologic • Urinalysis ± Urine culture -> if infected, treat and reassess • Assessment of pelvic floor muscle function • Assess post-void residual urine			Any other abnormality detected (e.g., significant post-void residual)
PRESUMED DIAGNOSIS		STRESS INCONTINENCE presumed due to sphincteric incompetence	MIXED INCONTINENCE	URGE INCONTINENCE presumed due to detrusor overactivity
TREATMENT	• Urethral milking • Pelvic floor muscle training	• (In) continence products • External appliances ↓ Failure	Lifestyle interventions Pelvic floor muscle training Bladder training ↓ Failure	• Antimuscarinics ↓ Failure
			SPECIALIZED MANAGEMENT	

Table 13-15: Management of Urinary Incontinence in Men (From Abrams et al, 2005, with permission)

B. Specialized Management

The specialist may first *reinstitute initial management* if it is felt that previous therapy had been *inadequate.*

1. Assessment

Patients referred directly to specialized management are likely to require additional testing, cytology, cystourethroscopy, and urinary tract imaging.

If these tests prove normal then those individuals can be treated for incontinence by the initial or specialized management options as appropriate.

If symptoms suggestive of detrusor overactivity or of sphincter incompetence persist, then **urodynamic studies** are recommended in order to arrive at a precise diagnosis.

2. Treatment

When basic management has failed and if the patient's incontinence *markedly disrupts* his quality of life then *invasive therapies* should be considered.

For *sphincter incompetence* the recommended option is the *artificial urinary sphincter* (Grade B).

For the *idiopathic detrusor overactivity* (with intractible overactive bladder symptoms) the recommended therapies are bladder augmentation (Grade C), autoaugmentation (Grade D), neuromodulation and urinary diversion (Grade B).

When *incontinence* has been shown to be associated with *poor bladder emptying* and detrusor underactivity, it is recommended that effective means are used to ensure bladder emptying, for example, intermittent catheterization (Grade B/C).

If incontinence is associated with *bladder outlet obstruction,* then consideration should be given to surgical treatment to relieve obstruction (Grade B/C). α-Blockers or 5α reductase inhibitors would be an optional treatment (Grade C/D).

Note: At the time of writing, *botulinum toxin* was showing *promise* in the treatment of symptomatic detrusor *overactivity* unresponsive to other therapies.

Some evidence was emerging as to the safety of *antimuscarinics* for overactive bladder symptoms in *men,* chiefly in *combination with an α-blocker.*

Table 13-15:—Cont'd

Specialized Management of Urinary Incontinence in Men

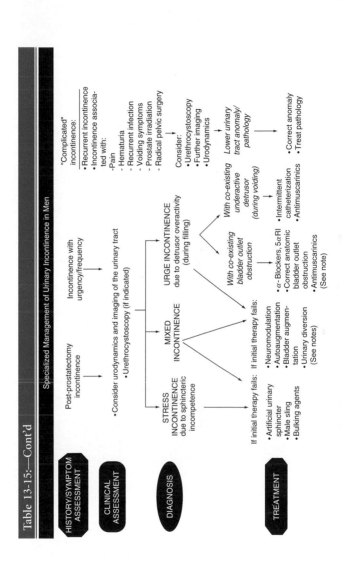

HISTORY/SYMPTOM ASSESSMENT	Post-prostatectomy incontinence	Incontinence with urgency/frequency	"Complicated" incontinence: • Recurrent incontinence • Incontinence associated with: -Pain - Hematuria - Recurrent infection - Voiding symptoms - Prostate irradiation - Radical pelvic surgery
CLINICAL ASSESSMENT	• Consider urodynamics and imaging of the urinary tract • Urethrocystoscopy (if indicated)		Consider: • Urethrocystoscopy • Further imaging • Urodynamics
DIAGNOSIS	STRESS INCONTINENCE due to sphincteric incompetence	MIXED INCONTINENCE	URGE INCONTINENCE due to detrusor overactivity (during filling)	Lower urinary tract anomaly/ pathology
			With co-existing bladder outlet obstruction	*With co-existing underactive detrusor (during voiding)*	
TREATMENT	If initial therapy fails: • Artificial urinary sphincter • Male sling • Bulking agents	If initial therapy fails: • Neuromodulation • Autoaugmentation • Bladder augmentation • Urinary diversion (See notes)	• α- Blockers, 5αRI • Correct anatomic bladder outlet obstruction • Antimuscarinics (See note)	• Intermittent catheterization • Antimuscarinics	• Correct anomaly • Treat pathology

Table 13-16:   Management of Urinary Incontinence in Women (From Abrams et al, 2005, with permission)

A. Initial Management

1. Initial assessment should identify:

- *"Complicated" incontinence group.*

In certain parts of the developing world, exceptionally severe incontinence results from childbirth injury and **urinary fistula.** These devastating injuries affect millions of women in sub-Saharan Africa. These women form a special group of women with **special needs** who must be identified at initial assessment and require **specialist management.**

Others include those who also have **pain** or **hematuria, recurrent infections,** suspected or proven **voiding problems, significant pelvic organ prolapse,** or who have persistent incontinence or recurrent incontinence after **previous surgery,** such as **pelvic irradiation, radical pelvic surgery,** or **previous surgery for incontinence.**

- **Three other main groups** of patients should be identified by initial assessment.

a. Women with **stress incontinence** on physical activity

b. Women with **urgency, frequency,** and **urge incontinence** (overactive bladder—OAB)

c. Those women with **mixed** urge and stress incontinence

In women, **abdominal, pelvic, and perineal examinations** should be a routine part of physical examination. Women should be asked to perform a "**stress test**" (cough and strain to detect leakage likely to be due to sphincter incompetence). Any **pelvic organ prolapse** or **urogenital atrophy** should be assessed. **Vaginal or rectal examination** allows the assessment of voluntary pelvic floor muscle contraction, an important step prior to the teaching of pelvic floor muscle training.

2. Treatment

Initial treatment should include lifestyle interventions, supervised pelvic floor muscle training, supervised bladder training, and for women with stress urinary incontinence, urge urinary incontinence or mixed urinary incontinence (Grade A).

Lifestyle interventions include weight reduction, smoking cessation, and dietary/fluid modification (including caffeine) (Grade A).

If **estrogen deficiency** and/or **UTI** is found, the patient should be treated at initial assessment and then **reassessed** after a suitable interval (Grade B).

Conservative treatment may be augmented with appropriate *drug therapy. Antimuscarinics* for OAB, *dual serotonin and noradrenaline reuptake inhibitors*[*] for stress urinary incontinence (Grade A).

Clinicians are likely to wish to *treat the predominant symptom first* in women with symptoms of *mixed incontinence* (Grade C).

Some women with co-existing *significant pelvic organ prolapse* can be treated by ring pessary.

Initial treatment should be *maintained for 8–12 weeks* before reassessment and possible specialist referral for further management.

Note: It may be necessary for patients to use *(in)continence products* while waiting for definitive treatment.

Some women with *significant pelvic organ prolapse* can be treated by *vaginal devices* that treat both incontinence and prolapse (incontinence rings and dishes).

---

[*]*Subject to local regulatory approval.*

(Continued)

(4) pelvic floor physiotherapy, with or without biofeedback, both to strengthen the pelvic floor musculature and to aid in the individual's ability to shut off an unwanted bladder contraction; and (5) for physically or mentally challenged individuals, scheduled toileting and/or prompted voiding. In patients with bladder overactivity, the pelvic floor physiotherapy is used primarily as an aid to patients in suppressing unwanted bladder contractions. They are taught to do "quick flicks" of the pelvic floor musculature in an effort to accomplish this. Putting all these things together involves establishing a regimen for the patient and combining all of these modalities, such that the patient voids according to a timed schedule that he or she can initially maintain. A bladder diary is useful in following the patient's progress. Periodically, the patient is asked to increase the intervals between micturition until an acceptable interval is reached without the symptoms of urgency or urge incontinence interfering. **Biofeedback** is a technique that provides visual and/or auditory signals to an individual with respect to his or her performance of a physiologic process, in this case pelvic floor muscle contraction. Electromyography or vaginal pressure measurements are generally used. Despite the logic of biofeedback, most comprehensive reviews have failed to demonstrate the superiority of pelvic floor muscle exercise instruction

(Text continued on p. 440)

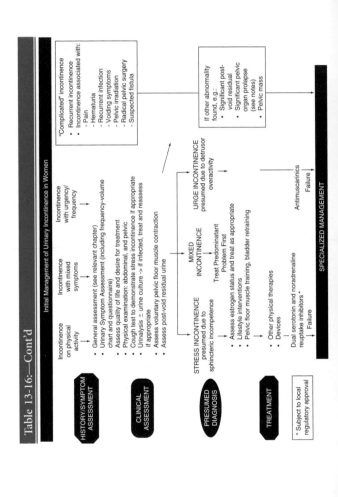

Table 13-16:—Cont'd

Table 13-17:   Management of Urinary Incontinence in Women (From Abrams et al, 2005, with permission)

B. Specialized Management

1. Assessment

Women who have *"complicated" incontinence* (see initial algorithm) may need to have *additional tests* such as cytology, cystourethroscopy, or urinary tract imaging. *If these tests are normal,* then they should be treated for incontinence by the initial or specialized management options as appropriate.

Those women who have failed initial management and whose *quality of life is impaired* are likely to request further treatment. If initial management has been given an adequate trial, then *interventional therapy may be desirable.* Prior to intervention *urodynamic testing is highly recommended,* because it is used to diagnose the type of incontinence and therefore inform the management plan. Within the urodynamic investigation *urethral function testing by urethral pressure profile or leak point pressure is optional.*

Systematic assessment for *pelvic organ prolapse* is highly recommended and it is suggested that the ICS method should be used in research studies. Women with *coexisting pelvic organ prolapse* should have their prolapse treated as appropriate

Women in developing countries with fistula due to *childbirth injuries* do not require urodynamic assessment and are best treated in specialist fistula units.

2. Treatment

If urodynamic stress incontinence is confirmed, then the treatment options that are recommended for patients with *some degree of bladder-neck and urethral mobility* include the full range of nonsurgical treatments, as well as retropubic suspension procedures and bladder neck/sub-urethral sling operations. The correction of symptomatic pelvic organ prolapse may be desirable at the same time.

For patients with *intrinsic sphincter* deficiency and limited bladder neck mobility, sling procedures, injectable bulking agents, and the artificial urinary sphincter can be considered.

Urge incontinence secondary to idiopathic detrusor overactivity (overactive bladder) may be treated by neuromodulation or bladder augmentation. Detrusor myectomy is an optional procedure (auto augmentation).

(Continued)

Table 13-17:—Cont'd

B. Specialized Management

Those patients with *voiding dysfunction* leading to *significant post-void residual urine* (for example, >30% of total bladder capacity) may have bladder *outlet obstruction or detrusor underactivity*. Prolapse is a common cause of voiding dysfunction.

Note: At the time of writing:
- Botulinum toxin was showing promise in the treatment of symptomatic detrusor overactivity unresponsive to other therapies.

(Continued)

with biofeedback over pelvic floor exercise instruction alone. It is clear, however, that, whether considering stress, urge, or mixed UI, and using the number of incontinence episodes or the amount of urine lost as primary outcome indicators, behavioral therapy is capable of causing a significant reduction. Quoted figures range from 40–80%. We think of behavioral therapy as an overall program that can be used for the treatment of UI or bladder overactivity without UI. With sphincteric related incontinence, obviously the patient should concentrate more on pelvic floor physiotherapy for the purpose of strengthening the pelvic floor musculature. With the overactive bladder, with or without urge incontinence, the patient should concentrate more on the behavioral modification, using pelvic floor physiotherapy more as a tool to abort involuntary bladder contractions. Biofeedback is optional in either case.

b) **Pharmacologic therapy.** In general, drug therapy for LUT dysfunction is hindered by a concept that can be expressed in one word: **uroselectivity,** a term originated by Karl-Erik Andersson. For instance, the clinical utility of available **antimuscarinic agents** is limited by their lack of selectivity, responsible for the classic peripheral antimuscarinic side effects of any dry mouth, constipation, blurred vision, tachycardia, and/or effects on cognitive function. **Calcium channel blockers** and **potassium channel openers** would be ideal for the treatment of bladder overactivity if a receptor or channel could be found that was bladder specific. At this point, the dosages needed to affect LUT function are so high that undesirable side effects, primarily cardiovascular, are produced elsewhere.

(Text continued on p. 444)

Table 13-17:—Cont'd

Specialized Management of Urinary Incontinence in Women

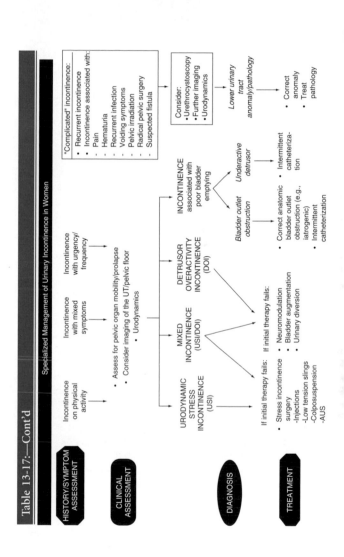

HISTORY/SYMPTOM ASSESSMENT

- Incontinence on physical activity
- Incontinence with mixed symptoms
- Incontinence with urgency/frequency

"Complicated" incontinence:
- Recurrent incontinence
- Incontinence associated with:
  - Pain
  - Hematuria
  - Recurrent infection
  - Voiding symptoms
  - Pelvic irradiation
  - Radical pelvic surgery
  - Suspected fistula

CLINICAL ASSESSMENT

- Assess for pelvic organ mobility/prolapse
- Consider imaging of the UT/pelvic floor
  - Urodynamics

Consider:
- Urethrocystoscopy
- Further imaging
- Urodynamics

Lower urinary tract anomaly/pathology

DIAGNOSIS

- URODYNAMIC STRESS INCONTINENCE (USI)
- MIXED INCONTINENCE (USI/DOI)
- DETRUSOR OVERACTIVITY INCONTINENCE (DOI)
- INCONTINENCE associated with poor bladder emptying
  - *Bladder outlet obstruction*
  - *Underactive detrusor*

TREATMENT

- Stress incontinence surgery
  - -Injections
  - -Low tension slings
  - -Colposuspension
  - -AUS

If initial therapy fails:

If initial therapy fails:
- Neuromodulation
- Bladder augmentation
- Urinary diversion

- Correct anatomic bladder outlet obstruction (e.g., iatrogenic)
- Intermittent catheterization

- Intermittent catheterization

- Correct anomaly
- Treat pathology

**Table 13-18:   Management of Urinary Incontinence in
Frail Older Men and Women (From Abrams et al, 2005,
with permission)**

Older persons in general should receive a *similar range of
treatment options* as younger persons. However, frail older
persons *present different problems* and challenges compared
with other fitter older patient populations. Implicit in the
term "frail" is that such individuals may *neither wish* nor *be
fit enough* to be considered for the full range of therapies
likely to be offered to healthier or younger persons. The
extent of investigation and *management* in frail older people
should take into account the *degree of bother* to the patient
and/or caregiver, their *motivation* and level of *cooperation/
compliance* as well as the *overall prognosis* and *life
expectancy*. At the same time, management effective to meet
their goals is possible for many frail persons [C].

I. History and Symptom Assessment

This algorithm applies to the evaluation of urinary
incontinence in frail persons. Many of the same principles
(especially assessment and treatment of potentially treatable
or modifiable conditions and medications that may cause or
worsen incontinence) also apply to fecal incontinence (FI) in
frail elderly.

Clinical assessment

Treatable or *potentially reversible* conditions should be
addressed first, followed by a *physical examination* targeted
to *comorbidity* and *functional assessment*. The "*DIAPPERS*"
mnemonic covers some of these conditions. Bowel symptom
history, rectal examination, and stool diary should be
considered. While most cases of fecal incontinence are
multifactoral, the primary goal of assessment is to distinguish
overflow fecal incontinence, associated with constipation,
from other causes.

While *post-void residual urine* (PVR) measurement is
recommended because it could influence the choice of
treatment, it is recognized that it is often impractical to
obtain a PVR, and in many cases may not change overall
management. Impaired bladder emptying may occur in older
men and women for various reasons including bladder *outlet
obstruction* and *detrusor underactivity*. Treatment of
co-existing conditions may reduce PVR (e.g., treatment of
constipation and stopping drugs with antimuscarinic action).
There is no specific "cut off" in this population, although
PVR over 100 mL (men) and 200 mL (women) is considered
elevated, and a low PVR does not exclude outlet obstruction.

Clinical diagnosis

Mixed UI (stress UI and urge UI symptoms) is common in older women. A cough stress test is appropriate if the diagnosis is likely to influence treatment choice (e.g., consideration of surgery). Combined urge UI and high PVR (without obstruction), known as detrusor hyperactivity with impaired contractility (DHIC) also is common in the frail elderly.

II. Initial Management

Initial treatment should be individualized and influenced by the most likely clinical diagnosis. *Conservative and behavioral* therapy for UI and FI include lifestyle changes [C], bladder training in the more fit or alert patient [B], assisted voiding for more disabled patients [C], and prompted voiding for frailer and more cognitively impaired patients [B]. For select, cognitively intact frail persons, pelvic muscle exercises may be considered, but they have not been well studied in this population [C]. A cautious trial of *antimuscarinic drugs* may be considered as an adjunct to conservative treatment of *urge UI* [C]. Similarly, *α-blockers* may be cautiously considered to assist bladder emptying in frail men with an *elevated PVR* [C], and topical estrogens considered for women with vaginal/urethral atrophy [C]. With all *drug treatment*, it is important to *start with a low dose* and titrate upwards with regular review of efficacy and tolerability until desired effect or unwanted side effects occur. For *constipation with overflow FI*, bowel clearout with combined suppositories/enemas and laxatives is recommended [C]. Loperamide can be used for FI in the absence of constipation [B].

III. Specialized Management

If after initial assessment a frail older person with UI is found to have *other significant factors* (e.g., pain, hematuria, rectal bleeding, persistent diarrhea), then referral for *specialist investigation* should be considered.

Referral to specialists also may be appropriate for individuals who have not responded adequately to initial management and if further investigation/treatment is desirable that could improve continence and quality of life.

Age per se is not a contraindication to incontinence surgery [C], but before surgery:

- All modifiable comorbidity should be addressed [C].
- An adequate trial of conservative therapy should be followed by reassessment of the need for surgery [C].
- Urodynamic testing should be done because clinical diagnosis may be inaccurate [A].

(Continued)

Table 13-18:—Cont'd

- Preoperative assessment plus careful perioperative care is essential to minimize geriatric complications such as delirium, infection, dehydration, and falls [A].

IV. Ongoing Management and Reassessment

If the patient cannot achieve *independent continence* (dry, not dependent on ongoing treatment) or *dependent continence* (dry with assistance, behavioral treatment, and/or medications) then *"Contained Incontinence"* (incontinence contained with use of appropriate aids and/or appliances) should be the treatment goal. Importantly, optimal care can usually be achieved by a combination of the previously discussed approaches [C].

(Continued)

At the Third International Consultation on Urinary Incontinence, the committee on pharmacology "graded" the various drugs used for the treatment of detrusor overactivity according to the Oxford system (Tables 13-21 and 13-22).

i) **Antimuscarinic agents.** The physiologic basis for the use of anticholinergic agents is that the major portion of the neurohumoral stimulus for physiologic and presumably involuntary bladder contraction is acetylcholine-induced stimulation of postganglionic parasympathetic cholinergic receptor sites on bladder smooth muscle.

In patients with overactive bladder, **the effects have been described as follows: (1) increase in the volume to the first involuntary bladder contraction, (2) decrease in the amplitude of involuntary bladder contractions, (3) increase in total bladder capacity, (4) decrease in urgency and urgency incontinence episodes.**

The common view is that in overactive bladder related detrusor overactivity (OAB-DO), the drugs act by blocking the muscarinic receptors on the detrusor muscle that are stimulated by acetylcholine, released from activated cholinergic (parasympathetic) nerves. Thereby, they decrease the ability of the bladder to contract. However, antimuscarinic drugs act mainly during the storage phase, decreasing urgency and increasing bladder capacity, and during this phase, there is normally no parasympathetic input to the LUT. Antimuscarinic drugs increase and anticholinesterase inhibitors decrease bladder capacity. Because antimuscarinic drugs do seem to affect the sensation of urgency during

(Text continued on p. 448)

Table 13-18:—Cont'd

MANAGEMENT OF URINARY INCONTINENCE IN FRAIL OLDER PERSONS (From Abrams et al, 2005, with permission)

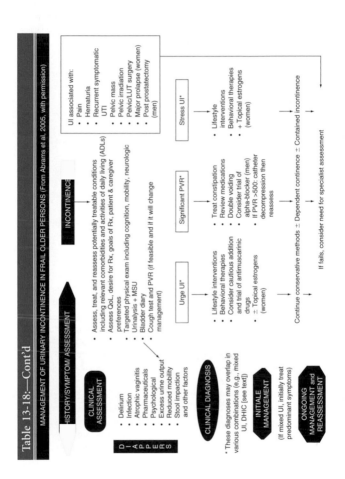

HISTORY/SYMPTOM/ ASSESSMENT

CLINICAL ASSESSMENT

D
I
A
P
P
E
R
S

- Delirium
- Infection
- Atrophic vaginitis
- Pharmaceuticals
- Psychological
- Excess urine output
- Reduced mobility
- Stool impaction and other factors

- Assess, treat, and reassess potentially treatable conditions including relevant comorbidities and activities of daily living (ADLs)
- Assess QoL, desire for Rx, goals of Rx, patient & caregiver preferences
- Targeted physical exam including cognition, mobility, neurologic
- Urinalysis + MSU
- Bladder diary
- Cough test and PVR (if feasible and if it will change management)

INCONTINENCE:

UI associated with:
- Pain
- Hematuria
- Recurrent symptomatic UTI
- Pelvic mass
- Pelvic irradiation
- Pelvic/LUT surgery
- Major prolapse (women)
- Post prostatectomy (men)

CLINICAL DIAGNOSIS

* These diagnoses may overlap in various combinations (e.g., mixed UI, DHIC [see text])

Urge UI*
- Lifestyle interventions
- Behavioral therapies
- Consider cautious addition and trial of antimuscarinic drugs
- ± Topical estrogens (women)

Significant PVR*
- Treat constipation
- Review medications
- Double voiding
- Consider trial of alpha-blocker (men)
- If PVR >500: catheter decompression then reassess

Stress UI*
- Lifestyle interventions
- Behavioral therapies
- + Topical estrogens (women)

INITIALE MANAGEMENT

(If mixed UI, initially treat predominant symptoms)

ONGOING MANAGEMENT and REASSESSMENT

Continue conservative methods ± Dependent continence ± Contained incontinence

If fails, consider need for specialist assessment

Table 13-19:   Management of Neurogenic Incontinence
(From Abrams et al, 2005, with permission)

A. Initial Management

1. Initial assessment

In assessing patients with incontinence due to neurogenic
vesicourethral dysfunction the management depends on an
**understanding of the likely mechanisms producing
incontinence,** which in turn depends on the **site of the
nervous system abnormality.** Therefore, neurogenic
incontinence patients can be divided as following:

Two groups of patients (a) with peripheral nerve lesions (b)
and the other with central lesions below the pons should be
managed by the specialist with a particular interest/training
in neurologic lower urinary tract dysfunction.

a. Peripheral lesions

Including **peripheral nerve lesions,** for example denervation
that occurs after major pelvic surgery such as for cancer of
the rectum or cervix. Also included are those lesions
involving the **lowest part of the spinal cord** (conus/cauda
equina lesions), e.g., lumbar disc prolapse.

b. Central lesions below the pons

Suprasacral infrapontine spinal cord lesions, e.g., traumatic
spinal cord lesions, should be treated according to the results
of urodynamic studies: the initial treatment should be
maintained for 8–12 weeks, before reassessment and possible
referral to the specialist.

c. Central lesions above the pons

Suprapontine central lesions include, for example, cerebrovascular accident, stroke, Parkinson's disease, and multiple
sclerosis

During initial assessment

• **Physical examination** is important in helping to
  distinguish these three groups and a **simple neurologic
  examination** should be routine.

• An estimate of **post-void residual (PVR) is highly
  recommended (preferably by ultrasound). If a significant
  PVR is found, then upper tract imaging is required.**

2. Treatment

Initial treatment is suitable for the large group of patients with
incontinence due to suprapontine conditions like strokes. At
initial assessment, these patients need to be assessed for their
degree of **mobility** and their **ability to cooperate,** as these two
factors will determine which therapies are possible.

The treatments recommended are behavioral (including timed
voiding) and **bladder-relaxant drugs** for presumed detrusor
overactivity. **Appliances** or catheters may be needed in
patients who are immobile or cannot cooperate.

Table 13-19.—Cont'd

Initial Management of Neurogenic Urinary Incontinence

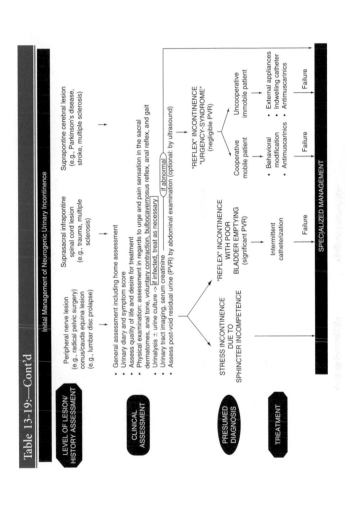

LEVEL OF LESION/HISTORY ASSESSMENT

Peripheral nerve lesion (e.g., radical pelvic surgery) conus/cauda equina lesion (e.g., lumbar disc prolapse)	Suprasacral infrapontine spinal cord lesion (e.g., trauma, multiple sclerosis)	Suprapontine cerebral lesion (e.g., Parkinson's disease, stroke, multiple sclerosis)

CLINICAL ASSESSMENT

- General assessment including home assessment
- Urinary diary and symptom score
- Assess quality of life and desire for treatment
- Physical examination: assessment in regards to urge and pain sensation in the sacral dermatomes, anal tone, voluntary contraction, bulbocavernosus reflex, anal reflex, and gait
- Urinalysis ± urine culture → if infected, treat as necessary
- Urinary tract imaging, serum creatinine
- Assess post-void residual urine (PVR) by abdominal examination (optional: by ultrasound) → if abnormal

PRESUMED DIAGNOSIS

STRESS INCONTINENCE DUE TO SPHINCTER INCOMPETENCE	"REFLEX" INCONTINENCE WITH POOR BLADDER EMPTYING (significant PVR)	"REFLEX" INCONTINENCE "URGENCY-SYNDROME" (negligible PVR)	
		Cooperative mobile patient	Uncooperative immobile patient

TREATMENT

	Intermittent catheterization	Behavioral modification • Antimuscarinics	External appliances • Indwelling catheter • Antimuscarinics
	Failure	Failure	Failure

SPECIALIZED MANAGEMENT

Table 13-20:   Management of Neurogenic Incontinence (From Abrams et al, 2005, with permission)

B. Specialized Management

1. Assessment

Most patients with ***peripheral lesion or central lesions below the pons*** require specialized assessment and management.

Urodynamic studies are highly recommended in these patients to establish both bladder and urethral function. ***Upper urinary tract imaging*** is needed in most patients and more detailed renal imaging or ***renal function studies*** will be desirable in some.

Urodynamics will define the filling function, with detrusor overactivity and neurogenic stress incontinence secondary to denervation being the most common abnormalities. During voiding, sphincter overactivity and detrusor underactivity are both likely to lead to persistent failure to empty.

2. Treatment

Management is straightforward in concept although the therapeutic options are extensive. The algorithm details the recommended options.

For ***sphincter incompetence*** the recommended options are the artificial urinary sphincter, sling procedures (in women), and injectables in selected patients.

Combinations of abnormalities are common (e.g., in meningomyelocele). Incontinence may be due to a combination of detrusor overactivity and neurogenic stress incontinence because of sphincter underactivity. Residual urine may be caused by detrusor underactivity as well as functional sphincter obstruction in the same patient. Each element of vesicourethral dysfunction needs to be dealt with. However, it must be remembered that ***preservation of upper tract function is of paramount importance.***

For detailed discussion on treatment, please read the relevant chapter from the consultation.

(Continued)

filling, this suggests an ongoing acetylcholine-mediated stimulation of detrusor tone (see later). If this is correct, agents inhibiting acetylcholine release or activity would be expected to contribute to bladder relaxation or the maintenance of low bladder tone during filling with a consequent decrease in filling and storage symptoms unrelated to the occurrence of an involuntary contraction. Outlet resistance, at least as reflected by

(Text continued on p. 451)

Table 13-20:—Cont'd

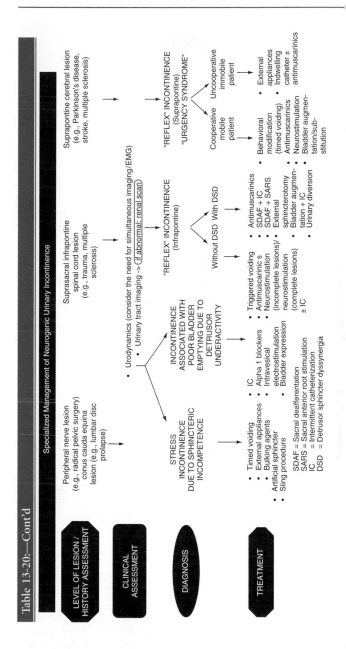

Specialized Management of Neurogenic Urinary Incontinence

LEVEL OF LESION / HISTORY ASSESSMENT

| Peripheral nerve lesion (e.g., radical pelvic surgery) conus cauda equina lesion (e.g., lumbar disc prolapse) | Suprasacral infrapontine spinal cord lesion (e.g., trauma, multiple sclerosis) | Suprapontine cerebral lesion (e.g., Parkinson's disease, stroke, multiple sclerosis) |

CLINICAL ASSESSMENT

• Urodynamics (consider the need for simultaneous imaging/EMG)
• Urinary tract imaging -> (if abnormal: renal scan)

DIAGNOSIS

STRESS INCONTINENCE DUE TO SPHINCTERIC INCOMPETENCE

INCONTINENCE ASSOCIATED WITH POOR BLADDER EMPTYING DUE TO DETRUSOR UNDERACTIVITY

"REFLEX" INCONTINENCE (Infrapontine)
- Without DSD
- With DSD

"REFLEX" INCONTINENCE (Suprapontine) "URGENCY SYNDROME"
- Cooperative mobile patient
- Uncooperative immobile patient

TREATMENT

STRESS INCONTINENCE DUE TO SPHINCTERIC INCOMPETENCE:
• Timed voiding
• External appliances
• Bulking agents
• Artificial sphincter
• Sling procedure

INCONTINENCE ASSOCIATED WITH POOR BLADDER EMPTYING:
• IC
• Alpha 1 blockers
• Intravesical electrostimulation
• Bladder expression

DETRUSOR UNDERACTIVITY:
• Triggered voiding
• Antimuscarinics
• Neurostimulation (incomplete lesions)/ neurostimulation (complete lesions) ± IC

Without DSD:
• Antimuscarinics
• SDAF + IC
• SDAF + SARS

With DSD:
• External sphincterotomy
• Bladder augmentation + IC
• Urinary diversion

Cooperative mobile patient:
• Behavioral modification (timed voiding)
• Antimuscarinics
• Neurostimulation
• Bladder augmentation/substitution

Uncooperative immobile patient:
• External appliances
• Indwelling catheter ± antimuscarinics

SDAF = Sacral deafferentation
SARS = Sacral anterior root stimulation
IC = Intermittent catheterization
DSD = Detrusor sphincter dyssynergia

Table 3-21: International Consultation on Incontinence Assessments, 2004: Oxford Guidelines (Modified)

Levels of Evidence
Level 1: Systematic reviews, meta-analyses, good quality randomized controlled clinical trials (RCTs)
Level 2: RCTs, good quality prospective cohort studies
Level 3: Case-control studies, case series
Level 4: Expert opinion
Grades of Recommendation
Grade A: Based on level 1 evidence (highly recommended)
Grade B: Consistent level 2 or 3 evidence (recommended)
Grade C: Level 4 studies or "majority evidence" (optional)
Grade D: Evidence inconsistent/inconclusive (no recommendation possible)

Table 3-22: Drugs Used in the Treatment of Detrusor Overactivity. Assessments According to the Oxford System (Modified from the 3rd International Consultation in Incontinence, 2004)

Antimuscarinic Drug	Level of Evidence	Grade of Recommendation
Tolterodine	1	A
Trospium	1	A
Solifenacin	1	A
Darifenacin	1	A
Propantheline	2	B
Atropine, hyoscyamine	3	C
Drugs with mixed actions		
Oxybutynin	1	A
Propiverine	1	A
Dicyclomine	3	C
Flavoxate	2	D
Antidepressants		
Imipramine	3	C
Alpha-AR antagonists		
Alfuzosin	3	C
Doxazosin	3	C
Prazosin	3	C
Terazosin	3	C
Tamsulosin	3	C

Beta-AR antagonists		
Terbutaline	3	C
Salbutamol	3	C
COX-inhibitors		
Indomethacin	2	C
Flurbiprofen	2	C
Other drugs		
Baclofen*	3	C
Capsaicin[†]	2	C
Resiniferatoxin[†]	2	C
Botulinum toxin[‡]	2	B
Estrogen	2	C
Desmopressin[§]	1	A

*, intrathecal; [†], intravesical; [‡], bladder wall; [§], nocturia.

urethral pressure measurements, does not seem to be clinically affected. **High doses of antimuscarinics can produce urinary retention in humans, but in the dose range needed for beneficial effects in OAB-DO, there is little evidence for a significant reduction of the voiding contraction.**

The only instance in which this is a consideration is in the patient with neurogenic DO who wets between intermittent catheterizations. In our experience it usually takes a higher than recommended dose of antimuscarinics to "quiet" the bladder and achieve continence between catheterizations. The pure antimuscarinics (and drugs with combined actions—see next section) and their "ratings" by the ICI are seen in Table 13-22.

There are many claims regarding superiority of one agent over another in terms of efficacy, tolerability, and safety. One must be careful to separate theoretical "edges" (marketing) from real ones.

ii) **Agents with combined action.** There are a number of agents that are grouped under the somewhat exotic term "musculotropic relaxant" or "antispasmodic" that are promoted as having more than an antimuscarinic action. These additional actions include smooth muscle inhibition at a site metabolically distal to the cholinergic receptor mechanism and what are referred to as local anesthetic properties. The former action may relate to some calcium channel blocking activity. It should be noted that these latter two activities can be demonstrated in vitro, but it is doubtful that when administered orally either of these activities contributes to the clinical efficacy of such agents, which is most likely due simply to the fact that the 1-A drugs in this category (see Table 13-22) are good antimuscarinic agents.

iii) **Tricyclic antidepressants.** The tricyclic antidepressants have been found by some to be useful agents for facilitating urine storage by both decreasing bladder contractility and increasing outlet resistance. There is disagreement about the latter function, but general agreement about their utility in decreasing bladder contractility. All of these agents possess varying degrees of three major pharmacologic actions: (1) they block the active transport system responsible for the reuptake of released amine neurotransmitters serotonin and norepinephrine; (2) they have central and peripheral anticholinergic effects at some, but not all, sites; and (3) they are sedatives, an action that occurs, presumably, on a central basis, but is perhaps related to antihistaminic properties. At histamine receptors, however, they also are antagonistic to some extent. Imipramine has prominent systemic anticholinergic effects, but only a weak antimuscarinic effect on bladder smooth muscle. This action could be mediated centrally, as an increase in serotonin concentration in the spinal cord could cause a decrease in bladder contractility, or it could be related to a direct inhibitory effect on bladder smooth muscle itself. In any case, the effects of imipramine on bladder smooth muscle do not appear to be mediated by an antimuscarinic effect. There is a rationale for combining the use of such agents with an antimuscarinic drug before abandoning pharmaceutical treatment in cases where antimuscarinics or agents with combined actions have not produced the desired effect. If imipramine is to be utilized one must pay careful attention to its adverse event profile, especially the potential for serious cardiac effects.

iv) **Intravesical therapy to decrease bladder contractility.** One way of achieving a more bladder-selective response is to administer a drug intravesically. This has been easily done in the laboratory with multiple agents and has been done clinically with oxybutynin.

Most series are small but report definite beneficial effects with seemingly fewer side effects. Although the drug is absorbed into the circulation and effective serum levels can be measured, the first-pass metabolism through the liver is less. It is thought that the primary liver metabolite of oxybutynin is responsible in large part for the side effects, and thus these would be less using this mode of administration. This is obviously cumbersome, requires catheterization to carry out, and there is no intravesical preparation. In addition, tablets must be dissolved in a vehicle to accomplish this. It may be, however, that with this mode of administration, those drugs with a theoretical combined action would be able to exert some direct effect on smooth muscle because of the high local concentration, whereas with oral administration they would not.

v) **Desmopressin.** This is a synthetic vasopressin analogue that lacks significant vasopressor action. It does exert a pronounced antidiuretic effect. It is widely used as a treatment for primary nocturnal enuresis and can be useful in adults with nocturia, particularly those who lack a normal nocturnal increase in plasma vasopressin (antidiuretic hormone). Attention should be paid to its adverse event profile, particularly the possibility of hyponatremia, especially in the elderly.

vi) **Botulinum toxin. Botulinum A toxin** (BTX-A) is an inhibitor of the release of acetylcholine and other neurotransmitters at the neuromuscular junction of autonomic nerves in smooth muscle and of somatic nerves in striated muscle. It does this by interacting with the protein complex necessary for docking vesicles. This results in decreased muscle contractility and muscle atrophy at the injection site. The chemical denervation is reversible, and regeneration takes place over 3–9 months. The intradetrusor injection of BTX-A has been reported by a number of investigators to be efficacious and safe in the treatment of both neurogenic and idiopathic DO. Dosage schedules and sites of injection vary, and a careful read of the source articles is recommended (see chapter by Andersson and Wein in *Campbell-Walsh Urology*, 9th edition). The botulinum toxin molecule cannot cross the blood-brain barrier. A potential side effect is spread to nearby muscles, particularly when high volumes are used. Distant effects can also occur but distant or generalized weakness due to intravascular spread is very rare. Caution is recommended in those with disturbed neuromuscular transmission or on treatment with aminoglycosides. Use of BTX-B has also been reported but data are few and dosing is different.

vii) **Drugs affecting sensory input.** One attractive modality of therapy for overactive bladder and bladder hypersensitivity, especially in an individual who retains the ability to voluntarily initiate a detrusor contraction, is to depress sensory neurotransmission. **Capsaicin** is the active ingredient of red peppers and, in sufficiently high concentrations, causes desensitization of C-fiber sensory afferents by initially releasing and emptying the stores of neuropeptides, which serve as sensory neurotransmitters and then by blocking further release. C-fiber afferents act as the primary sensory pathway in patients with voiding dysfunction secondary to SCI, some other neurologic diseases, and in response to other noxious stimuli. Due to the initial release of neuropeptides after intravesical administration of the drug, capsaicin causes intense local symptomatology and often requires anesthesia for administration. In addition, although beneficial effects have been reported, these effects are not universal, although positive effects, when they result, have been reported to last for 2–7 months. **Resiniferatoxin** is a compound with effects similar to those of capsaicin and is approximately 1000 times more potent than capsaicin in producing desensitization, but only 100–300 times more potent in producing inflammation. Available information suggests that this mode of intravesical therapy may be effective in both neurogenic and idiopathic DO. At present, apparent formulation and supply problems seem to have hindered further investigations.

viii) **Estrogens.** There are a number of reasons that estrogens may be useful in the treatment of postmenopausal women with both bladder and outlet related incontinence and in the treatment of the symptoms of OAB without incontinence, and they have been used for years in this manner. Even if it was concluded in a Cochrane review that "oestrogen treatment can improve or cure incontinence, and the evidence suggests that this is more likely with urge incontinence," there have been few controlled trials performed to confirm that it is of benefit. Estrogen has an important physiologic effect on the female LUT, and its deficiency may be an etiologic factor in the pathogenesis of a number of conditions. However, **the use of estrogens alone to treat UI has given disappointing results, in our opinion.**

It is surprising that, for a treatment with such a long history of usage, so little confirmatory evidence of efficacy exists (see chapters by Andersson and Wein in *Campbell-Walsh Urology,* 9th edition and the report of the Committee on Pharmacology of the ICI). In addition, the risks of oral hormone therapy have recently been highlighted, adding to the controversy. Whether local administration (vaginal) can produce beneficial LUT change is a question waiting to be answered in a double-blind controlled manner and, if a positive response results for stress or urge incontinence or for symptoms of OAB without incontinence, the proper dosing schedule and preparation need to be established along with proof that local therapy does not carry the apparent risk of systemic administration.

c) **Peripheral electrical stimulation.** Electrical stimulation is mentioned in three areas under the category of treatment, reflecting its potential use to facilitate storage by both the inhibition of bladder contractility and an increase in sphincter resistance and to facilitate emptying by stimulating a detrusor contraction. To inhibit bladder contractility, stimulation is generally applied to removable anal and vaginal devices, as well as peripherally through patch electrodes. The theory is that this induces an inhibitory pelvic to pudendal nerve reflex. Reported clinical results have been mixed, at best.

d) **Neuromodulation.** Neuromodulation implies modification of sensory and/or motor function through electrical stimulation. Currently there are two nerve stimulating modalities that are approved by the Food and Drug Administration (FDA): **sacral nerve stimulation (Interstim,** Medtronic, Minneapolis, MN) and **peripheral nerve stimulation (PNS).** Sacral nerve stimulation involves the stimulation of sacral nerves to modulate the neural reflexes that influence the bladder, sphincter, and pelvic floor. The exact mode of action of is still unclear. An electrode is placed through the S3 foramen with the aid of fluoroscopy and attached to a stimulator that the patient wears for a short trial period. Those reporting improvement ($>50\%$ improvement in symptoms) are suitable for permanent implantation of a pulse generator which can be adjusted using an external programming device. Sacral nerve stimulation has been approved for refractory urgency, frequency, and nonobstructive urinary retention.

Very promising results have been achieved to date in this difficult group of patients, all of whom have failed more conservative therapy, and for many of whom the next step would have been augmentation cystoplasty.

Depending on the definition and indication for the procedure, success rates have ranged anywhere from 50–80%. Only minor complications have been reported with the procedure. Overall, current neuromodulation gives patients a minimally invasive FDA approved option to control LUT symptoms, when previously only major bladder reconstructive surgery was an option. The success of existing neuromodulatory techniques has prompted other investigators to examine the effects of electrostimulation on other nerves, which may impact LUT function, such as the pudendal and dorsal genital nerves.

e) **Interruption of innervation.** Subarachnoid block is no longer used for urologic indications. Historically, this was used to convert a state of severe somatic spasticity to flaccidity and to abolish autonomic hyper-reflexia. As a by-product, bladder overactivity was acutely converted to areflexia. The obvious disadvantage of this type of procedure was a lack of neurologic selectivity. Additionally, the conceptually simple result of an areflexic bladder with normal compliance very often was not maintained, with decreased compliance occurring.

i) **Sacral rhizotomy, selective sacral rhizotomy.** Selective sacral rhizotomy was originally introduced as a treatment to increase bladder capacity by trying to abolish only the motor supply responsible for involuntary bladder contractions. Nonselective sacral rhizotomy often affected sphincter, sexual, and lower extremity function. There was still a problem in obtaining a truly selective result, and this procedure has fallen out of favor. Deafferentation using a **dorsal** or **posterior rhizotomy** is generally used as a part of an overall plan to simultaneously rehabilitate storage and emptying problems in patients with significant spinal cord injury or disease. Electrical stimulation is used to produce bladder emptying as well. **Dorsal root ganglionectomy** has also been mentioned in this regard. Surgical treatment of bladder hyperactivity by peripheral bladder denervation was popularized in the early 1980s. There were a variety of techniques proposed to partially or totally denervate (or more correctly neurologically decentralize) the bladder. These have been largely abandoned because, although some of these techniques had a high initial success rate in controlling bladder overactivity and related incontinence, the relapse rate was quite high. In addition, the long-term response to the neurologic procedure was sometimes associated with a type of neural plasticity, resulting in decreased bladder compliance.

f) **Augmentation cystoplasty**. Creation of a low-pressure high-capacity bladder reservoir by incorporation of a detubularized bowel segment is an important modality of treatment in LUT reconstruction and in the treatment of refractory filling and storage problems. Adequate reservoir function can generally be achieved by **augmentation enterocystoplasty.** Complications can arise including inadequate emptying or urinary retention, mucus accumulation and stones, electrolyte imbalance, recurrent infection, and the possibility of rare malignant change. Contraindications to augmentation enterocystoplasty include (1) urethral disease precluding intermittent catheterization, (2) unwillingness or inability to perform intermittent catheterization, (3) renal failure, (4) significant bowel disease, and (5) poor medical status precluding surgery. **Autoaugmentation** or **detrusor myomectomy** refers to a procedure whose purpose is to increase bladder capacity by, in essence, creating a large bladder diverticulum by removal of a section of the outer layer of the bladder wall down to the mucosa. This has the obvious advantage of not requiring bowel resection and anastomosis, but opinion is divided as to the efficacy of this procedure in increasing reservoir function in adults.

2. Increasing Outlet Resistance

a) **Behavioral therapy.** Although behavioral therapy without pelvic floor physiotherapy has been shown to significantly reduce the incidence and amount of stress incontinence in females, the **portion of a behavioral therapy program that has received most attention for sphincteric incontinence is the use of pelvic floor exercises.** The literature is remarkably consistent in describing a significant improvement rate in 50–65% of patients treated with this modality of therapy, sometimes known as Kegel's exercises (after Arnold Kegel, a gynecologist). For hypermobility-related stress incontinence in the female and for stress incontinence in the male, it is certainly worthwhile to try pelvic floor exercise along with the rest of the behavioral therapy program as an initial or adjunctive form of treatment. For female patients with a significant element of ISD, and for males with gross urinary leakage, it is conceptually doubtful whether significant improvement would occur in even a minority of such patients. However, it is also certain that such therapy would not hurt either, and such exercises may in fact allow the individual to be able to exert greater control over the detrusor reflex as well. As mentioned previously, it has never been objectively shown whether biofeedback, using either EMG or pressure displays, adds to careful and periodic personal instruction and supervision.

b) **Electrical stimulation. Intravaginal** and **anal electrical stimulation** have been used to treat storage failure by increasing outlet resistance as well as decreasing bladder contractility. In this case, the mechanism is said to involve stimulation of the striated pelvic floor musculature through branches of the pudendal nerve. Most reviews have come to the conclusion that there is not consistent objective evidence supporting the value of pelvic floor physiotherapy plus electrical stimulation over pelvic floor physiotherapy alone in the general population of patients with sphincteric incontinence. It may be that there are some subgroups that might benefit (i.e., those who cannot carry out pelvic floor exercises). **Sacral root stimulation,** by means of an implanted stimulator, has been described for the treatment of sphincteric weakness in patients with neurogenic difficulty. Long-term contemporary results are still forthcoming.

c) **Pharmacologic therapy.**

   i) **α-Adrenoreceptor agonists.** The theoretical basis for pharmacologic therapy of sphincteric incontinence is the preponderance of α-adrenergic receptor sites in the smooth muscle of the bladder neck and proximal urethra. When stimulated, these should produce smooth muscle contraction. Such stimulation can alter the urethral pressure profile by increasing maximum urethral profile and maximum urethral closure pressure. Current α-adrenergic agonists in use (ephedrine and phenylpropanolamine) lack selectivity for urethra alpha receptors and may increase blood pressure and cause sleep disturbances, headache, tremor, and palpitations. Although there are reports in the literature of efficacy with these agents, the Committee on Pharmacology of the Third International Consultation on Incontinence did not recommend any of these agents for the treatment of stress incontinence (Table 13-23).

   ii) **Estrogen.** The role of estrogen in the treatment of stress incontinence in the postmenopausal female has been controversial. Some studies have reported promising results, but this may be because they were observational and not randomized, blinded, or controlled.

Table 13-23: Drugs Used in the Treatment of Stress Incontinence. Assessments According to the Oxford System (Modified)

Drug	Level of Evidence	Grade of Recommendation
Duloxetine	1	A
Imipramine	3	D
Clenbuterol		
Methoxamine	2	D
Midodrine	2	C
Ephedrine	3	D
Norephedrine (phenylpro-panolamine)	3	D
Estrogen	2	D

There are several theoretical reasons why estrogen might be useful in the treatment of women with stress incontinence (and overactive bladder), but there is no consistent body of objective evidence to prove its efficacy per se in the treatment of stress incontinence.

iii) **Antidepressants.** Imipramine, among several other pharmacologic effects (see earlier), inhibits the reuptake of norepinephrine and 5-hydroxytryptamine (5-HT) in adrenergic nerve endings. In the urethra, this can be expected to enhance the contractile effects of norepinephrine on urethral smooth muscle. Theoretically, such an action may also influence the striated muscles in the urethra and pelvic floor by effects on the spinal cord level (Onuf's nucleus). Imipramine can cause a wide range of potentially dangerous side effects, especially regarding the cardiovascular system, and should be used with caution. No randomized controlled trials on the effects of imipramine in stress urinary incontinence (SUI) seem to be available.

Duloxetine hydrochloride, a combined norepinephrine and serotonin reuptake inhibitor, has been shown to significantly increase urethral sphincter muscle activity during the filling/storage phase of micturition in a cat model. Bladder capacity was also increased in this model, both effects mediated centrally through motor efferent and sensory afferent modulation. There are several randomized controlled trials documenting the efficacy of duloxetine in the treatment of stress incontinence. In one trial, the discontinuation rate for adverse events was 4% for placebo and 24% for duloxetine. The effectiveness of duloxetine for treatment of SUI is documented. Adverse effects occur but seem tolerable. Duloxetine is available in Europe but was withdrawn from the FDA approval process; at the time of this writing, it has not been resubmitted.

d) **Vaginal and perineal occlusive and supportive devices; urethral plugs.** Support of the bladder neck in the female resulting in improved continence is possible with intravaginal devices that have not been reported to cause significant LUT obstruction or morbidity. Tampons, traditional pessaries and contraceptive diaphragms, and intravaginal devices specifically designed for bladder neck support have been used. Ideally, **support devices** would reduce any degree of vaginal prolapse and, by supporting the anterior vaginal wall and therefore the urethrovesical junction and bladder neck, control incontinence. Although most individuals would agree that information about vaginal support devices should be included in the treatment options when counseling women with stress UI, most would also agree that studies performed on these devices in the acute laboratory setting demonstrate better performance than diary-based studies with respect to the amount and number of episodes of leakage. It is also generally agreed that such devices work best in individuals with minimal to moderate leakage. True pessary usage seems most effective and most common in the elderly woman with a major degree of anterior vaginal wall prolapse and hypermobility-related stress incontinence who is a poor surgical candidate. **Occlusive devices** can be broadly divided into external and internal devices, referring to whether the device itself occludes the urethra or bladder neck from the outside or has to be inserted per urethra. **There have been many patterns of external occlusive devices available for use in the male,** but all seem to take the form of a clamp that is applied across the penile urethra. The Baumrucker and Cunningham clamps are basically double-sided foam cushions that squeeze the penile urethra between the two arms. The Baumrucker clamp uses a Velcro-type system. Another type of compression device that is size adjustable encircles the penis and stops the flow of urine when it is inflated with air. Soft tissue damage by excess compression can occur with these clamps, and thus their use is extremely risky in patients with sensory impairment. Their prime use is in patients with sphincteric incontinence, although if applied tightly enough, the patient can occlude the urethra under any circumstances—although with a distinct danger of retrograde pressure damage. Occlusive devices for **female sphincteric incontinence** have been mentioned (and mostly discarded) since the late 1700s. Multiple **intravaginal occlusive devices** have been described, all of which historically consisted of rather bizarre looking configurations of silicone and plastic with a dual purpose: to stay in the vagina and to compress the urethra. None of these seem to have stood the test of time. Another interesting concept that proved to be poorly functional was an inflatable pad held firmly against the perineum by straps attached to a waistband, fitted to the individual patient. Inflation of the pad with a cuff resulted in an elevation and compression of the perineum. The simplest of the most recently introduced devices is a **continence control pad** or **external urethral occlusion device.** This hydrogen-coated foam pad is placed by the patient over the external urethral meatus. Another type of device is a **meatal suction** or **occlusion device.** The concept is to create, by suction, a measured amount of negative pressure, causing coaptation of the urethral wall.

Intraurethral devices are inserted into the urethra to block urinary leakage. Similarities among these devices include (1) a means to prevent intravesical migration (a meatal plate or tab at the meatus), (2) a mechanism to maintain the device in its proper place in the urethra (spheres, inflatable balloons, or flanges on the proximal end); and (3) a device or mechanism to permit removal for voiding (a string or pump). Most patients utilizing external meatal occlusive devices or intraurethral devices have reported dryness or improvement in the laboratory and on diaries. Long-term results, however, are limited, and the exact place of this therapy in the algorithm of conservative management of female sphincteric incontinence has not yet been determined. Certainly, the use of these devices is grossly out of proportion (lower) to the positive and optimistic reports in the literature.

The characteristics of an ideal occlusive or supportive device would include (1) efficacy, (2) comfort, (3) ease of application/insertion/removal, (4) lack of interference with adequate voiding, (5) lack of tissue damage, (6) lack of infection, (7) no compromise of subsequent therapy, (8) cosmetic acceptance (unobtrusive), and (9) lack of interference with sexual activity. Ideally, such a device could be used continuously during waking hours (for the majority who do not have sphincteric incontinence after bedtime), but many people would obviously be happy with a device that functioned well for "spot usage"—that is, usage only during those activities most provocative of incontinence. The perfect patient for an occlusive device would be one who has pure sphincteric incontinence that is mild to moderate; who has neither severe involuntary bladder contractions nor decreased compliance; who desires active involvement in her treatment program; who desires immediate results; and who has the body habitus, manual dexterity, and cognitive ability to apply or insert the device and remove it. Many of the devices recently introduced are already off the market, a fact that is certainly at odds with the conclusions from the reports in the literature. Reasons for failure, in our opinion, include (1) patient's reluctance to "put anything inside me or on me"; (2) inconvenience (frequent removal/self-insertion with a requirement for periodic replacement by health care provider); (3) discomfort, real or perceived; (4) fear of infection and/or bleeding; (5) association of such devices by the patient with "last resort" remedies and the implications which that association raises; (6) nonwillingness to pay out of pocket for these (poor coverage for these devices); (7) perceived lack of long-term success; and (8) nonincentive for the health care provider to promote the devices, except in a capitated environment.

e) **Nonsurgical periurethral compression.** Periurethral bulking by the percutaneous or transvesical injection of polytetrafluoroethylene particles, purified bovine cross-linked dermal collagen, or carbon-coated zirconium oxide beads to increase urethral resistance has been utilized in both women and men with sphincteric incontinence. In women, the results have ranged from quite good to not so good, with the best "success" and improvement rates ranging from 70–90%. Multiple therapy sessions may be necessary to achieve the desired result. The results obtained in men have not been as good, especially in patients with post radical prostatectomy incontinence. Originally, this therapy was recommended only for patients with intrinsic sphincter dysfunction and with a VLPP of less than 60 cm of water. The technique has been used with success, however, in other categories of incontinent patients, including those patients, especially elderly ones, with what seems to be a combination of hypermobility-related incontinence (see previous discussion) and ISD. The procedure can be carried out under local anesthesia or sedation, making it simple and relatively noninvasive. It does not seem to compromise further therapy.

f) **Retropubic suspension with or without prolapse repair (female).** The exact pathophysiology of stress incontinence is not known; however, loss of normal anatomic support of the urethra and bladder neck and ISD are both believed to be factors. The underlying principle of retropubic suspensions is to correct and prevent urethral hypermobility (posterior and inferior rotational descent with abdominal straining). Therefore, these procedures are typically only used when hypermobility is present and are generally less effective in those with predominantly ISD as seen in women with incontinence and a "lead pipe" urethra. This has been observed to correct genuine stress incontinence in the female in approximately 85% of those patients undergoing a first operation for this problem. There are more than 150 varieties of this operation and the names attached to many of these read like an honor roll of urologic and gynecologic superstars (Marshall, Marchetti, Krantz, Burch, Lapides, Tanagho, Raz, etc.). Each practitioner has his or her favorite suspension procedure, generally based on the site of residency or fellowship training, or on some recent development or product that promises to achieve the same end with less time and morbidity. The use of bone anchors for suture fixation, stapling devices, and laparoscopic techniques have added to the seemingly endless variations available for vesicourethral suspension.

The general technique for an open retropubic suspension consists of a low midline or Pfannenstiel incision, separating the rectus muscle and staying out of the peritoneum by sweeping it cephalad. The retropubic space is entered and developed until the urethra, bladder neck, and anterior vaginal wall are clearly identified. The choice of suture (absorbable or permanent) used for the suspension as well as the placement of the suture are variable. However, the basic principle is to support the urethra/bladder neck area in a more retropubic location.

If significant vaginal prolapse is present, this should be repaired at the same time, remembering that the pelvic floor in the female acts as a unit and that a surgical procedure should endeavor to correct all associated abnormalities. Failure to repair significant prolapse at the time of a retropubic suspension may result in post-operative voiding dysfunction. Suspension is rarely, if ever, used in patients with problems other than stress incontinence, and these procedures should be utilized only after more conservative therapy types have at least been attempted or suggested.

g) **Sling procedures.** Ed McGuire deserves, we believe, credit for popularizing the sling procedure and, more importantly, concepts that relate to its utilization. McGuire was among the first to conceptualize, in logical fashion, the fact that there was a category of patients who leaked with effort who were not well repaired by standard suspension procedures. These were patients who had poor sphincter function, irrespective of mobility, and whose urethral function at that time could be semiquantitated only with the urethral pressure profile. He later developed the concept of VLPP to better quantitate sphincteric resistance in patients with stress incontinence. The noncircumferential compression afforded by the sling is optimal treatment for patients with poor urethral closure function and poor urethral smooth muscle function. Although originally described through a retropubic approach, these are done most commonly through a vaginal approach today. Success rates as high as 90% with the pubovaginal sling procedure for sphincteric incontinence have been reported. Initially, the use of the sling procedure was restricted to patients who satisfied the definition of intrinsic sphincter dysfunction and who did not have stress incontinence associated with urethral hypermobility. However, **as individuals have come to believe that genuine stress incontinence (hypermobility related) and intrinsic sphincter dysfunction were but two ends of the spectrum and that the great majority of individuals had some combination of the two, the sling procedure became a logical choice for the correction of stress incontinence of all types.** The sling provides an adequate suburethral supporting layer (see prior description of the hammock hypothesis) and thus corrects hypermobility-related incontinence as well as ISD. The use of the sling for the surgical correction of all types of female sphincteric incontinence has been popularized mostly by Jerry Blaivas, with increasing support from others. The sling itself can be autologous fascia (rectus or fascia lata) and, recently, a variety of other materials (cadaveric fascia, dura, synthetic materials) have been used, some with success and some with problems. The various new devices utilized for suspension procedures (bone anchors, stapling devices, laparoscopic approaches) are all applicable to the sling procedure. As with suspension procedures, significant prolapse should be repaired simultaneously in the female.

h) **Synthetic midurethral slings.** The use of synthetic midurethral slings has taken off since the "integral theory" was introduced by Ulmsten and Petros. This theory suggest that laxity of the pubourethral ligaments allows the bladder neck to drop and open, which contributes to UI. To treat this they developed the **tension free vaginal tape** (TVT) procedure for the treatment of stress incontinence in previously surgery naïve patients. This involves placing a polypropylene tape under the mid urethra and tunneling the ends through the retropubic space without fixation. This is typically performed on an outpatient basis. With the increasing number of procedures performed, studies have shown objective cures rates ranging from 73–85%. The excellent results (equivalent to other retropubic suspensions) and minimally invasive nature of the procedure have fueled its growth. Because of the "blind" passage of the trocars through the retropubic space, major complications such as vascular and bowel injuries have been reported. Perforation of the bladder is not uncommon but can typically be managed by simple bladder drainage. Other potentially unique complications include vaginal and urethral erosions due to the use of a synthetic mesh. Many companies have since come out with similar mid urethral sling systems which at least in theory work via the same mechanism with similar results.

Even more recently the **transobturator synthetic midurethral sling** has been introduced. This is another minimally invasive technique, which utilizes a synthetic mesh placed under the mid urethra, but rather than tunneling the tape through the retropubic space, it is tunneled through the obturator foramen. The main potential advantage of this is that the abdominal cavity is never entered, therefore decreasing the chance of a bowel injury. Also the more lateral course that the trocars take minimizes the risk of bladder perforation. As with the retropubic mid urethral slings, a number of companies market similar versions of the transobturator sling. At this time, there are some initial studies that show that the transobturator sling may be equally effective to the retropubic mid urethral slings; however, larger studies with longer follow-up are needed to draw a definitive conclusion.

i) **Bladder outlet reconstruction.** This is primarily a historical treatment in adults. Reconstruction of the bladder outlet is one possible method of restoring sphincteric incontinence in patients with ISD. This technique was introduced by Young in 1907, and was subsequently modified by Dees, Leadbetter, and Tanagho. Procedures utilizing the Young-Dees principle involve construction of a neourethra from the posterior surface of the bladder wall and trigone. In the male, the prostatic urethra affords additional substance for closure and increase in outlet resistance. The Leadbetter modification involves proximal reimplantation of the ureters to allow more extensive tubularization of the trigone. Tanagho described a procedure based on a similar concept, but using the anterior bladder neck to create a functioning neourethral sphincter. "Success rates" of between 60% and 70% were reported, but it is difficult to know what success means and what the real long-term success rates are.

j) **Male perineal sling.** For the treatment of male stress UI, most often after radical prostatectomy, the male perineal sling has emerged as a viable patient option. The male perineal sling is a minimally invasive surgical technique that involves the placement of a compressive sling at the level of the bulbar urethra. This is anchored to the descending pubic rami, most often with bone screws. With this technique there is nothing for the patient to manipulate. Because of the minimal dissection that is needed, one theoretical benefit is less chance for any urethral complications. It also appears to be safe in those who have a previous artificial urinary sphincter or radiation therapy. Success rates have ranged from 39–80% depending on the end point. Few complications have been noted including perineal/scrotal numbness (usually self-limited), infection, and bone screw dislodgment. A review of the literature on male perineal slings suggests that this is another effective option in the treatment of male stress UI; however, it may be best reserved for those men with mild to moderate incontinence

k) **Artificial urinary sphincter.** Control of sphincteric UI with implantable prosthetics has evolved rapidly over the last 30 years. Clearly, the most significant contribution was the introduction, by Scott and co-workers, of a totally implantable artificial sphincter mechanism that could be used in adults and children of both genders. This was originally introduced in the early 1970s. The end result of the biomechanical evolution of this device currently is most frequently utilized for post prostatectomy incontinence, but use of the device has been championed by various clinicians for refractory sphincteric incontinence of virtually every etiology, assuming bladder storage is, or can be converted to, normal. The sphincter consists of an inflatable cuff that fits around the urethra (generally) or the bladder neck, a reservoir that generally is placed under the rectus muscle, and an inflate/deflate pump or bulb that transfers fluid from the cuff to the reservoir, allowing refilling of the cuff from the reservoir over a 3- to 4-minute period. The pump is placed in the scrotum or the labia. High success rates have been achieved by experienced surgeons. The incidence of mechanical malfunction and infection, although initially high, is quite low in contemporary series.

l) **Closure of the bladder outlet.** This is generally an end-stage procedure suitable for an individual whose outlet is totally incompetent and uncorrectable by medical or conventional surgical means. It is also sometimes used in individuals who can be put into retention but who cannot catheterize themselves per urethra. In this latter condition and in the circumstance of an incompetent urethra in an individual with adequate hand control who desires to be dry, a continent catheterizable abdominal stoma can be created. Augmentation cystoplasty can be carried out at the same time. For individuals lacking adequate hand control or the cognitive facilities necessary for intermittent catheterization or who simply do not want to carry out catheterization, a "chimney" type conduit of bowel is created emanating from the bladder with an abdominal stoma that drains into an appliance.

3. Circumventing the Problem

Antidiuretic hormone-like agents have been mentioned under the category of pharmacologic therapy. Another "trick" utilized in an individual with significant nocturia is to try to adjust diuretic dosage, utilizing a **short-acting diuretic** some time in the afternoon, the object being to reduce the amount of fluid mobilized after the individual goes to bed.

Popularization of **intermittent catheterization** as a treatment modality has made possible many of the other therapeutic options for the treatment of voiding dysfunction that are now commonplace. Originally introduced by Guttman in the treatment of SCI patients as a method of reducing urinary tract infection, credit needs to go to Jack Lapides for advocating and popularizing the use of CIC for all types of voiding dysfunction in which such circumvention of storage or emptying failure is necessary. The details (types of catheters, intervals, cleansing/sterilization regimens, prophylaxis or not) are practitioner and institutional specific.

Indwelling urethral catheters are generally used for short-term bladder drainage. The use of a small-bore catheter for a short time, does not, with proper care, seem to adversely affect the ultimate outcome. Occasionally, more often in female patients, an indwelling catheter is a last resort type of therapy for long-term bladder drainage. A contracted fibrotic bladder may be the ultimate result; bladder calculi may form on the catheter; urethral complications in the female may include urethral dilation because of the temptation to replace each catheter with a larger bore one to prevent leakage around the catheter consequent to bladder spasm. A suprapubic catheter does not obviate urethral leakage and does not provide better drainage in patients with sphincteric incontinence. There is still some controversy as to whether long-term indwelling catheterization, especially in the female, in the neurologically challenged population, is associated with a poorer outcome with respect to either significant upper and lower tract complications or quality of life. It must be kept in mind that development of carcinoma of the bladder in patients with long-term indwelling catheter drainage is possible.

External collecting devices are useful only in the male. A suitable external collecting device has not yet been devised for the female. Care must be taken in individuals with sensory impairment to avoid necrosis of the penis because of an inappropriately tightly fitting device. It is difficult to know whether to label **pads** and **absorbent products** as a treatment for refractory incontinence or as a convenient "bail-out." They are used for both. Approximately $2 billion is currently spent in the United States yearly for pads and absorbent products.

Urinary diversion is a last resort for these patients and is in a category known as "desperate measures." The diversion can utilize the patient's own bladder if the outlet is competent or closure can be accomplished, or a continent catheterizable reservoir can be constructed totally of bowel. Sometimes, the tried and true intestinal conduit (Bricker or bilateral ureteroileostomy) will represent, all things considered, the best choice for an individual patient. The usually listed standard indications for supravesical urinary diversion include (1) progressive hydronephrosis or intractable upper tract dilation (which may be due to obstruction at the ureterovesical junction or to VUR that does not respond to conservative measures), (2) recurrent episodes of sepsis, and (3) intractable filling and storage or emptying failure when CIC is impossible.

C. Therapy to Facilitate Bladder Emptying and Voiding

1. Bladder Related (Increasing Intravesical Pressure or Facilitating Bladder Contractility)

a) **External compression, Valsalva.** Such voiding is unphysiologic and is resisted by the same forces that normally resist stress incontinence. Adaptive changes (funneling) of the bladder outlet generally do not occur with external compression maneuvers of any kind. Increases in outlet resistance may actually occur. The greatest likelihood of success with this mode of therapy (although some would say it should never be used) is in the patient with an areflexic and hypotonic or atonic bladder and some outlet denervation (smooth or striated sphincter or both). Such a patient not uncommonly has stress incontinence as well. The continued use of external compression or Valsalva maneuver implies that the intravesical pressure between attempted voidings is consistently below that associated with upper tract deterioration. This may be an erroneous assumption, and close follow-up and periodic evaluation are necessary to avoid this complication.

b) **Promotion or initiation of reflex contractions.** In most types of SCI characterized by detrusor overactivity, manual stimulation of certain areas within sacral and lumbar dermatomes may provoke a reflex bladder contraction. The most effective classic method of doing so is rhythmic suprapubic manual pressure. If the pressure characteristics of such induced voiding are favorable, and induced emptying can be carried out frequently enough so as to keep bladder volume and pressure below the level dangerous for upper tract deterioration, the incontinence can be "controlled," and, conceptually, this amounts to a form of timed voiding in these neurologically impaired patients. Some clinicians still believe that the establishment of a rhythmic pattern of bladder filling and emptying by maintaining a copious fluid intake and by periodically clamping and unclamping an indwelling catheter or by intermittent catheterization can "condition" or "train" the micturition reflex. This concept, in our opinion, has yet to be proven, and it may be that the prime value of such programs is to focus attention on the urinary tract and ensure an adequate fluid intake.

c) **Pharmacologic therapy.**

   i) **Parasympathomimetic agents.** Many acetylcholine-like drugs exist. However, only bethanechol chloride exhibits a relatively selective action on the urinary bladder and gut with little or no action at therapeutic dosages on ganglia or the cardiovascular system. It is cholinesterase resistant and causes a contraction in vitro of smooth muscle from all areas of the bladder. Although anecdotal success in rare patients with voiding dysfunction seems to occur, attempts to facilitate bladder emptying in series of patients where bethanechol chloride was the only variable have been disappointing. In adequate doses, bethanechol chloride is capable of eliciting an increase in tension in bladder smooth muscle, as would be expected from in vitro studies, but its ability to stimulate or facilitate a physiologic bladder contraction in patients with voiding dysfunction has been unimpressive. **It is difficult to find reproducible urodynamic data that support a general recommendation for the use of bethanechol chloride in any specific category of patients.**

ii) **Other pharmacologic treatments.** One could construct a "wish list" of other potential pharmacologic avenues for facilitating bladder contractility or the micturition reflex. In the cat at least (see previous discussion) there is a sympathetic reflex elicited during filling that promotes urine storage partially by exerting an α-adrenergic inhibitory effect on pelvic parasympathetic ganglionic transmission. **α-Adrenergic blockade,** theoretically, then could facilitate transmission through these ganglia and thereby enhance bladder contractility. α-Adrenergic blockers are sometimes given for the "treatment" of urinary retention, using this rationale, but whether relief of retention occurs because of the use of these agents or simply simultaneously is unknown. Because endogenous opioids have been hypothesized to exert a tonic inhibitory effect on the micturition reflex at various levels, **narcotic antagonists** offer possibilities for stimulating reflex bladder activity. This concept has never been translated into successful clinical use. **Prostaglandins** contribute to the maintenance of bladder tone and bladder contractile activity. Some cause an in vitro and in vivo bladder contractile response and some cause a decrease in urethral smooth muscle tone. Intravesical prostaglandin use has been reported to facilitate voiding in postsurgical patients. A number of conflicting positive and negative reports exist, and double-blind placebo studies are obviously necessary to settle this controversy.

d) **Electrical stimulation.** Stimulation directly to the bladder or spinal cord originated in the 1940s but met with failure. Fibrosis related to the electrodes, bladder erosion, electrode malfunction, or other equipment malfunction was common. The spread of current to other pelvic structures with stimulus thresholds lower than that of the bladder resulted in undesirable stimulation of a number of bodily processes.

Stimulation to the nerve roots has been pursued for the last 30 years by Brindley, Tanagho, and Schmidt for the treatment of voiding dysfunction. **Anterior sacral root stimulation, in combination with dorsal rhizotomy or dorsal root ganglionectomy,** has become a practicality and a reality, especially in patients with SCI. Prerequisites for such usage are (1) intact neural pathways between the sacral cord nuclei of the pelvic nerve and the bladder and (2) a bladder that is capable of contracting. The champions of these techniques deserve much credit for pursuing and developing their ideas over the years, in the face of much negative opinion as to the possibility of their ultimate success. Although these techniques are still in a phase of evolution, they are currently practical and hold much promise for the future.

Intravesical electrostimulation is an old technique that has been resurrected with some very interesting and promising results. The mechanism of action is totally unknown, and it is similar to neuromodulation in two respects: the vague way in which it is defined and the definition of its mechanism of action. Patients with incomplete central or peripheral nerve lesions and with at least some neural pathways between the bladder and cerebral centers are candidates for this technique. One conceptualization of the mechanism of efficacy invokes the involvement of an artificial activation of the micturition reflex, with repeated activation producing an "upgrade" of the micturition reflex.

e) **Reduction cystoplasty.** The problem of myogenic decompensation has suggested surgical reduction to some investigators, as the chronic overstretching affects mainly the upper free part of the bladder, and as the nerve and vessel supply enter primarily from below. Thus, resection of the dome (or doubling this over) does not influence the function of the spared bladder base and lower bladder body. This technique would seem to be most effective when the detrusor was underactive rather than acontractile, and measures to decrease outlet resistance might be required in addition to achieve adequate emptying. Anecdotal success stories aside, the risk-benefit ratio of this procedure has not been established.

2. Outlet Related (Decreasing Outlet Resistance)

a) **At a site of anatomic obstruction.** These measures are all discussed in the chapters on benign prostatic (Chapter 14) hyperplasia and urethral stricture disease (Chapter 11).

b) **At the level of the smooth sphincter.**

   i) **Pharmacologic therapy.** Bob Krane and Carl Olsson promoted the concept of a physiologic internal sphincter partially controlled by tonic sympathetic stimulation of contractile α-adrenergic receptors in the smooth musculature of the bladder neck and proximal urethra. Further, they hypothesized that some obstructions at this level are a result of inadequate opening of the bladder neck and/or inadequate decrease in resistance in the area of the proximal urethra. They also theorized and presented evidence that **α-adrenergic blockade** could be useful in promoting bladder emptying in such a patient with an adequate detrusor contraction but without anatomic obstruction or detrusor-striated sphincter dyssynergia. Although most would agree that α-adrenergic blocking agents exert at least some of their favorable effects on voiding dysfunction by affecting the smooth muscle of the bladder neck and proximal urethra, other information in the literature suggests that they may affect striated sphincter tone as well. These agents are also used to treat obstruction due to BPH by lowering prostatic "tone" and may have some secondary effects on bladder contractility in these patients as well, mediated through as of yet poorly characterized neurohumoral or neurologic pathways.

      Phenoxybenzamine was the α-AR (adrenergic receptor) antagonist originally used for the treatment of voiding dysfunction. Side effects affect approximately 30% of patients and include orthostatic hypotension, reflex tachycardia, nasal congestion, diarrhea, miosis, sedation, nausea, and vomiting (secondary to local irritation).

      Prazosin was the first potent selective α_1-AR antagonist used to lower outlet resistance. The potential side effects of prazosin are consequent to its α_1-AR blockade. Occasionally, there occurs a "first-dose phenomenon," a symptom complex of faintness, dizziness, palpitation, and, infrequently, syncope, thought to be caused by acute postural hypotension.

Terazosin and **doxazosin** are two highly selective postsynaptic α_1-AR antagonists. They are readily absorbed with high bioavailability and a long plasma half-life, enabling their activity to be maintained over 24 hours after a single oral dose. Both of these agents have been evaluated with respect to their efficacy in patients with LUT symptoms and decreased flow rates presumed secondary to BPH. Their efficacy in decreasing symptoms and raising flow rates has been shown to be superior to placebo. Their safety profiles have been well documented as a result of their widespread use over several years for the treatment of hypertension. Side effects are related to peripheral vasodilatation (postural hypotension), and both drugs have to be started at a low dose and titrated to obtain an optimal balance between efficacy and tolerability. Dizziness and weakness are sometimes observed, and these are presumed secondary to CNS actions.

Most recently, **alfuzosin** and **tamsulosin,** both highly selective α_1-AR blockers, have appeared and are marketed solely for the treatment of BPH because of some reports suggesting preferential action on prostatic rather than vascular smooth muscle. Marketing claims aside, whether there is any difference in the efficacy/side effect profiles of these individual agents remains a topic of controversy. Tamsulosin and alfuzosin have the advantage of being able to be administered once daily and without titration. Available data suggest that retrograde ejaculation and rhinitis are more common with tamsulosin, whereas dizziness and asthenia are more common with terazosin and doxazosin.

ii) **Transurethral resection or incision of the bladder neck/smooth sphincter.** The prime indication for transurethral resection or incision of the bladder neck is the demonstration of true obstruction at the bladder neck or proximal urethra by combining urodynamic studies, with either fluoroscopic demonstration of failure of opening of the smooth sphincter area or a micturitional profile showing that the pressure falls off sharply at some point between the bladder neck and the area of the striated sphincter. Bladder neck or smooth sphincter dyssynergia has been previously discussed, and it is this entity (occurring almost exclusively in males) that is the most common indication for the current performance of transurethral incision or resection of the bladder neck. The preferred technique at this time is incision of the bladder neck at the 5 o'clock and/or 7 o'clock position, with a single full-thickness incision extending from the bladder base down to the level of the verumontanum. Most clinicians would place the incidence of retrograde or diminished ejaculation somewhere between the reported incidences of 10% and 50%.

iii) **Y-V plasty of the bladder neck.** This is recommended or suggested only when a bladder neck resection or incision is desired and an open surgical procedure is simultaneously required to correct a concomitant disorder. This is rarely carried out.

c) **At the level of the striated sphincter.**

i) **Behavioral therapy with or without biofeedback.** Behavioral therapy in this case is used to facilitate emptying in an individual with occult voiding dysfunction (characteristics of striated sphincter dyssynergia, but neurologically normal). A urodynamic display of striated sphincter activity can facilitate clinical improvement in a strongly motivated patient capable of understanding the instructions of biofeedback assisted therapy.

ii) **Pharmacologic therapy.** There is no class of pharmacologic agents that selectively relaxes the striated musculature of the pelvic floor. Three different types of drugs have been used to treat voiding dysfunction secondary to outlet obstruction at the level of the striated sphincter: (1) the **benzodiazepines,** (2) **baclofen,** and (3) **dantrolene,** all of which have been characterized under the general heading of antispasticity drugs. Baclofen and the benzodiazepines exert their actions predominantly within the CNS, whereas dantrolene acts directly on skeletal muscle. Unfortunately, there is no completely satisfactory oral form of therapy for alleviation of skeletal muscle spasticity. Although these drugs are capable of providing variable relief of spasticity in some circumstances, their efficacy is far from complete, and this, along with troublesome muscle weakness, adverse effects on gait, and a variety of other side effects, minimizes their overall usefulness. α-Adrenergic blocking agents have also been hypothesized to exert an inhibitory effect on the striated sphincter, and this may be especially pronounced in those cases in which neuroplasticity with altered innervation of this area has occurred. Finally, **botulinum toxin** has been injected directly into the striated sphincter to reduce its tone and the results have been impressive (see prior section on BTX).

iii) **Urethral overdilation.** Overdilation to 40–50 French in female patients can achieve the same objective as external sphincterotomy but is rarely used because of the lack of a suitable external collecting device. It is sometimes used in young boys, when sphincterotomy is contemplated, and a similar stretching of the posterior urethra can be accomplished through a perineal urethrostomy. Observations indicate that, in myelomeningocele patients treated by this method, compliance can be improved by decreasing the outlet resistance.

iv) **Surgical sphincterotomy.** The primary indication for this procedure is detrusor-striated sphincter dyssynergia in a male patient when other types of management have been unsuccessful or are not possible. A substantial improvement in bladder emptying occurs in 70–90% of cases. Upper tract deterioration is rare following successful sphincterotomy; VUR, if present preoperatively, often disappears because of decreased bladder pressures and a reduced incidence of infection in a catheter-free patient with a low residual urine volume. An external collecting device is generally worn postoperatively, although total dripping incontinence or severe stress incontinence is unusual unless the proximal sphincter mechanism (the bladder neck and proximal urethra) has been compromised—by prior surgical therapy, the neurologic lesion itself, or as a secondary effect of the striated sphincter dyssynergia (presumably a hydraulic effect on the bladder neck itself). The 12 o'clock sphincterotomy remains the procedure of choice for a number of reasons. The anatomy of the striated sphincter is such that its main bulk is anteromedial. The blood supply is primarily lateral, and thus there is less chance of significant hemorrhage with a 12 o'clock incision. There is some disagreement about the rate of postoperative erectile dysfunction in those individuals who preoperatively have erections. Estimates utilizing the 3 o'clock and 9 o'clock technique vary from 5–30%, but whatever the true figure is, it is clear that most would agree that this complication is far less common (approximately 5%) with incision in the anteromedial position. Other complications may include significant hemorrhage and urinary extravasation. Failure to attain satisfactory bladder emptying following external sphincterotomy may be due to inadequate or poorly sustained bladder contractility, a poorly done sphincterotomy, or persistent obstruction at the level of the bladder neck from unrecognized coexistent smooth sphincter dyssynergia. In these latter patients, bladder neck incisions, as described previously, may facilitate bladder emptying.

v) **Urethral stent.** Permanent urethral stents to bypass the sphincter area have been utilized and results have become available over the last 10 years. There is little question that a significant decrease in detrusor leak pressure and residual urine volume occurs. Certainly, compared to sphincterotomy, this would seem to be conceptually less morbid. The questions are long-term efficacy, ease of removal/replacement when required, and the true incidence of the development of bladder outlet obstruction.

vi) **Pudendal nerve interruption.** This procedure, first described in the late 1890s, is seldom if ever used today because of the potential of undesirable effects consequent to even a unilateral nerve section (impotence, and fecal and stress incontinence).

SELF-ASSESSMENT QUESTIONS

1. Regardless of differences regarding physiologic and pharmacologic details, what would most experts agree are the requirements for normal bladder filling/storage and emptying/voiding? Discuss the main points relating to the anatomy, neurophysiology, and neuropharmacology of each of these factors.

2. Characterize the most common types of voiding dysfunction seen with the following neurologic injury(ies) and disease(s) in terms of sensation, bladder activity, smooth sphincter activity, and striated sphincter activity: (1) cerebrovascular accident, (2) Parkinson's disease, (3) multiple sclerosis, (4) suprasacral spinal cord injury, (5) sacral spinal cord injury, (6) radical pelvic surgery, and (7) diabetes.

3. Describe and discuss the use of pressure flow urodynamic studies and video urodynamic studies.

4. Discuss the possibilities and practicalities of pharmacologic therapy and neuromodulation for (1) bladder overactivity, (2) decreased outlet resistance, (3) increased outlet resistance, and (4) decreased bladder contractility.

5. Discuss the pathophysiology and surgical options for treating sphincteric incontinence in adults.

SUGGESTED READINGS

1. Abrams P, Cardozo L, Khoury S, Wein A (eds): *Incontinence*, vol 1 and 2. Health Publication Ltd, Editions 21 (distributor), Paris, 2005.
   Chapters:
   2. Continence Promotion: Prevention, Education and Organisation. Newman D,k, Denis L, Gruenwald I, Ee CH, Millard R, Roberts R, Sampselle C, Williams K, Muller, Norton N. pp 35–72
   5. Epidemiology of Urinary and Faecal Incontinence and Pelvic Organ Prolapse. Hunskaar S, Burgio K, Clark A, Lapitan MC, Nelson R, Sillen U, Thom D. pp 255–312
   14. Pharmacological Treatment of Urinary Incontinence. Andersson KE, Appell R, Cardozo L, Chapple C, Drutz H, Fourcroy J, Nishizawa O, Vela Naverette R, Wein A. pp 809–854
   19. Surgical Treatment of Urinary Incontinence in Men. Herschorn S, Thuroff J, Bruschini W, Grise P, Hanus T, Kakizaki H, Kirshner Hermanns R, Schick E, Nitti V. pp 1241–1296
   20. Surgery for Urinary Incontinence in Women. Smith A, Daneshgari F, Dmochowski R, Milani R, Miller K, Paraiso MF, Rovner E. pp 1297–1370

2. Abrams P, Cardozo L, Fall M, et al: The standardization of terminology in lower urinary tract function: report from the standardization subcommittee of the International Continence Society. *Neurourol Urodyn* 21:167–178, 2002; *Urology* 61:37–49, 2003.

3. Andersson K-E, Arner A: Urinary bladder contraction and relaxation: physiology and pathophysiology. *Physiol Rev* 84:935–988, 2004.

4. Andersson K-E, Wein AJ: Pharmacology of the lower urinary tract: basis for current and future treatments of urinary incontinence. *Pharmacol Rev* 56:581–631, 2004.

5. Wein AJ, Barrett DM: *Voiding Function and Dysfunction: A Logical and Practical Approach*. Year Book Medical, Chicago, 1988.

6. Wein AJ, Kavoussi LR, Novick AC, et al (eds): *Campbell-Walsh Urology*, 9th ed. Elsevier Science, Philadelphia, 2007.
   Chapters:
   57. Pathophysiology, Categorization, and Management of Voiding Dysfunction, Wein AJ, pp 1973–1985
   58. Urodynamic and Videourodynamic Evaluation of Voiding Dysfunction, Webster GD, pp 1986–2010
   59. Lower Urinary Tract Dysfunction in Neurologic Injury and Disease, Wein AJ, pp 2011–2045

C H A P T E R 14

Benign Prostatic Hyperplasia and Related Entities

Alan J. Wein, MD, PhD (hon) and
David I. Lee, MD

I. GENERAL CONSIDERATIONS

The evaluation and management of symptoms related to bladder outlet and urethral obstruction are responsible for a large portion of any given urology practice. An etiologic categorization is seen in Table 14-1. Although some of these entities may be associated with abnormalities of the urinary sediment or a characteristic finding on physical examination, most present only with lower urinary tract symptoms (LUTS). The symptoms are remarkably nonspecific and are associated more so with some entities rather than others strictly because of their prevalence.

This chapter considers the most common of these, benign prostatic hyperplasia (BPH), and its related entities: benign prostatic enlargement (BPE) and benign prostatic obstruction (BPO). Bladder neck/smooth sphincter dyssynergia or dysfunction and striated sphincter dyssynergia have been previously considered in Chapter 13, and urethral stricture disease in Chapter 11.

II. DEFINITIONS AND EPIDEMIOLOGY

BPH refers to a regional nodular growth of varying combinations of glandular and stromal proliferation that occurs in almost all men who have testes and who live long enough. Because of the anatomic localization of the prostatic growth that characterizes BPH—surrounding and adjacent to the proximal urethra—clinical problems can result. BPH can be defined in a number of ways, depending on the orientation of the user of the term. **Microscopic BPH** refers to the histologic evidence of cellular proliferation. **Macroscopic BPH** refers to organ enlargement due to the cellular changes. BPH histopathologically is characterized by an increased number of epithelial and stromal cells in the periurethral area of the prostate, the molecular etiology of which is

479

Table 14-1:   Bladder Outlet and Urethral Obstruction: Etiology

Prostate
  Benign prostatic enlargement
  Cancer
  Other infiltrative processes
Bladder neck and proximal urethra
  Contracture, fibrosis, stricture, stenosis
  Dyssynergia/dysfunction
    Smooth sphincter
    Striated sphincter
  Secondary hypertrophy of bladder neck
  Compression
  Distended vagina and uterus
  Extrinsic tumor
  Calculus, mucus, foreign body
  Ectopic ureterocele
  Polyp
  Posterior urethral valve
Distal urethra
  Contracture, fibrosis, stricture, stenosis, calculus, foreign body
  Anterior urethral valve

uncertain. The incidence of histologic or microscopic BPH is far greater than that of clinical or macroscopic BPH. BPH has also been referred to as hyperplasia, benign prostatic hypertrophy, adenomatous hypertrophy, glandular hyperplasia, and stromal hyperplasia.

Historically, the term prostatism was applied to almost all symptoms that reflected a micturition disorder in the older man. The term unfortunately implied that the cause of the problem was the prostate, which, in later years, was found clearly not to be the case in many instances. The World Health Organization (WHO) sponsored consultations on BPH and has recommended changes to the terminology related to urinary symptoms and the prostate in elderly men. The term LUTS (lower urinary tract symptoms) was introduced by Paul Abrams and has been adopted as the proper terminology to apply to any patient, regardless of age or sex, with urinary symptoms but without implying the underlying problem. **LUTS were initially divided into "irritative" and "obstructive" symptoms, but it became obvious that there was a poor correlation between so-called obstructive symptoms and a urodynamic diagnosis of bladder outlet obstruction (BOO) and**

also between so-called irritative symptoms and a urody-namic diagnosis that related to definable abnormalities seen during filling/storage. Additionally, the term "irritative" implied to some people as infectious or inflammatory process. Thus, **the division of LUTS into "filling/storage symptoms and emptying/voiding symptoms" evolved.** (See Chapter 13.)

The terminology with respect to prostate characteristics has also changed. Paul Abrams was the first to suggest a reconsideration of the use of the term BPH and a redefinition of the terminology. He pointed out that BPH was a histologic diagnosis that had been shown to occur in 88% of men older than 80 years. He added that, in some patients, the prostate gland enlarged, and this condition should be distinguished from BPH and referred to as BPE. In approximately half of these patients with BPE, he stated that true BOO resulted, a condition that should be termed BPO. BPH was previously an all-encompassing term that included prostate size, benign prostate histology, and all filling/storage or voiding/emptying symptoms thought related to the prostate pathophysiologi-cally in the adult male. The current terminology recognizes the imprecise and misleading implications of the initial usage of this phrase. The terminology related to the prostate is currently expressed as follows:

1. **BPH**—Benign prostatic hyperplasia. This term is used and reserved for the typical histopathologic pattern that defines the condition.
2. **BPE**—Benign prostatic enlargement. This refers to the size of the prostate, specifically the prostatic enlargement due to a benign cause, generally histologic BPH. If there is no prostatic histologic examination available, the term prostatic enlargement should be used.
3. **BPO**—Benign prostatic obstruction. This is a form of BOO. This term may be applied when the cause of the outlet obstruction is known to be BPE due to a benign cause, generally histologic BPH. BOO is a functional term for any cause of subvesical obstruction. The WHO-sponsored consultation on BPH recommended the generic phrase "LUTS suggestive of BPO" to describe elderly men with filling/storage or voiding/emptying pro-blems likely to be caused by an obstructing prostate. It should be noted that there are other causes of BOO than prostatic enlargement (see Table 14-1).

Autopsy data indicate that anatomic (microscopic) evidence of BPH is seen in about 25% of men of 40 to 50 years, 50% of men of ages 50 to 60, 65% of men of ages 60 to 70, 80% of men of ages 70 to 80, and 90% of men of ages 80 to 90.

Estimates of the prevalence of clinical BPH vary widely, probably because of the varying thresholds used to define the presence of BPH on the basis of symptoms and/or urodynamics (no uniform definition) or on the basis of the rate of prostatic surgery. It has been classically stated that 25–50% of individuals with microscopic and macroscopic evidence of BPH will progress to clinical BPH. Depending on which definition is used, the prevalence of clinical BPH in an individual community in men ages 55–74 years may vary from less than 5% to more than 30%. Only 40% of this group, however, complain of LUTS, and only about 20% seek medical advice because of them. The number of individuals who receive treatment for clinical BPH varies according to the threshold for providing such treatment, a threshold that can vary widely in different parts of the world and in different parts of the United States. As treatments become less invasive, this number can be expected to rise.

Only age and the presence of testes are positively correlated with the development of BPH. Obesity may be positively correlated with prostate volume. Most agree that cirrhosis is inversely correlated, probably because of decreased plasma testosterone (T) levels. **A positive association between LUTS secondary to BPO and erectile dysfunction seems to be real, but whether this is simply age related or not is less certain.** There are no consistent correlations for dietary factors, vasectomy, prior sexual history, smoking, or other disease states. **BPH does appear to have an inheritable genetic component,** although the specifics are yet to be elucidated.

III. PROSTATIC SIZE AND MORPHOLOGY PERTINENT TO BPH

Although some prostatic growth occurs throughout life, the prostate changes relatively little in size until puberty, when it undergoes rapid growth. Autopsy studies indicate that the normal adult prostate plateaus at a volume of approximately 25 mL at age 30. This remains relatively stable until approximately age 50, after which increasing volume is observed, such that the average prostate volume is approximately 35–45 mL at age 80.

Throughout developmental life the prostate maintains its ability to respond to endocrine signals, undergoes rapid growth at puberty, and maintains its size and tissue androgen receptor levels. In some individuals, abnormal growth subsequently occurs, which may be either benign or malignant.

The mechanisms of normal and abnormal growth have yet to be resolved but are thought to involve multiple growth promoting and inhibiting factors ultimately controlling cell replication, cell cycle control, cell aging, cell senescence, and cell death, both necrosis and apoptosis. A full discussion of the factors relating to prostate physiology and growth can be found in *Campbell-Walsh Urology*, 9th edition, Chapter 85, "Molecular Biology, Endocrinology and Physiology of the Prostate and Seminal Vesicles."

The size of the prostate is not linearly correlated to either urodynamic evidence of BOO or the severity of symptoms.

The adult prostate is a truncated cone with its base at the urethrovesical junction and its apex at the urogenital diaphragm. The prostate is pierced by the urethra, which angles forward at the verumontanum, and by the paired ejaculatory ducts, which join the urethra at its point of angulation. A lobular configuration of the prostate was originally described by Lowsley, based on studies of the human fetal prostate. A posterior, two lateral, an anterior, and a middle lobe were described. Although this description was used by urologists for years because it seemed to bear some relationship to endoscopic and gross surgical anatomy, **distinct lobes do not exist in the prepubertal and normal adult prostate.** The concept of a lobular structure has been replaced by one based on concentric zones that have morphologic, functional, and pathologic significance. McNeal and associates from Stanford have done the most to expand our understanding of adult prostate morphology, describing the zonal anatomy based on examination of the gland in different planes of section (Figure 14-1). The urethra represents the primary reference point, dividing the prostate into an anterior fibromuscular and a posterior glandular portion. The anterior fibromuscular stroma comprises up to one third of the total bulk of the prostate. It contains no glandular element. This fibromuscular stroma has not been linked to a specific pathologic process. The two principal regions of the glandular prostate are defined as the peripheral zone (approximately 75% of total glandular volume) and the central zone (approximately 25%), each morphometrically distinct. The central zone makes up about 25% of the functioning glandular prostate. It contains the urethra only at the upper end of the veru, where its ducts open. The development of carcinoma is relatively uncommon in this area. **The peripheral zone is the site of origin of most prostate cancer. The glandular tissue that participates in the BPH nodule formation is derived exclusively from the branches of a few small ducts, representing approximately 5–10%**

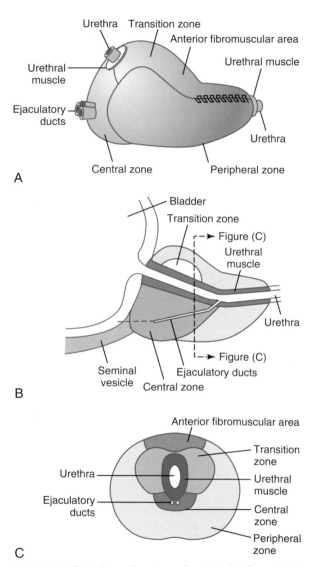

FIGURE 14-1. Prostatic zonal anatomy after McNeal. Schematic (**A**), sagittal cross-section (**B**), transverse cross-section (**C**). (From Hanno P, Malkowicz SB, Wein A [eds]: *Benign Prostatic Hyperplasia, Clinical Manual of Urology.* McGraw Hill, 2001, F15-1, p. 441.)

of the glandular prostate, that join the urethra at or proximal to its point of angulation. Urethral angulation at the most proximal extent of the verumontanum displaces the proximal urethral segment from the secretory gland mass anteriorly and into the anterior fibromuscular stroma. The resulting space between the urethra and glandular prostate accommodates a cylindrical smooth muscle sphincter that surrounds the proximal segment of the urethra from the base of the verumontanum to the bladder neck. All nodules of BPH develop within or immediately adjacent to this smooth muscle layer, and this tissue is subdivided by this muscle into two discrete regions. The transitional zone comprises less than 5–10% of the total glandular volume and consists of two separate lobules of tissue immediately outside of the smooth muscle layer, located laterally and extending somewhat ventrally. A tiny periurethral region (less than 1% of the total glandular prostate) contains glands that are entirely contained within the smooth muscle layer from just proximal to the point of urethral angulation to the bladder neck. This periurethral zone is so small that it is not pictured in many other renditions of McNeal's zonal anatomy. The origin of BPH is confined exclusively to these areas and some cancers may also originate here. Between the transitional and peripheral zones are the central zones, which have not been implicated in the origin of a specific pathologic process.

IV. ETIOLOGIC THEORIES OF BPH: PATHOPHYSIOLOGY

Clinically detectable BPH nodules arise from a variety of adenomas in the transitional and periurethral zones. As these grow they may outwardly compress the anterior fibromuscular stroma and areas in the peripheral and central zones. A so-called **surgical capsule** develops between the hyperplastic nodules and the compressed glandular tissue and serves as a plane of cleavage. This serves as a useful landmark in open or transurethral surgical treatment. The etiologic factors responsible for BPH nodule induction and further development are unclear. However, there are a number of factors that are obviously involved, although the magnitude of their importance and their interactions remains to be fully elucidated. What follows is the briefest of descriptions of the major factors mentioned, gleaned, mostly from the work of Walsh, Coffey, and their group at Johns Hopkins; Grayhack, Lee, and the group at Northwestern; and Cunha and others. A complete discussion of prostate physiology and the pathophysiology of

BPH can be found in Chapters 85 and 86 of *Campbell's-Walsh Urology,* 9th edition ("Molecular Biology, Endocrinology, and Physiology of the Prostate and Seminal Vesicles" and "Etiology, Pathophysiology, Epidemiology, and Natural History of Benign Prostatic Hyperplasia").

A. Hormones

There is no question that a functioning testis is a prerequisite for the normal development of the prostate in animals and humans. Males castrated before puberty do not develop BPH. BPH is rare in males castrated before the age of 40. Androgen deprivation in older men reduces prostate size. Patients with diseases that result in impaired androgenic production or metabolism have reduced or minimal prostatic growth. Although other endocrine factors are no doubt involved, the androgenic influence on prostatic growth and function is obviously central, although endocrine evaluation of the aging male has disclosed no recognizable surge in androgen secretion. The prostate develops from the urogenital sinus during the third fetal month under the influence of dihydrotestosterone (DHT) produced from fetal T via 5α-reductase. During development there is a close but as yet incompletely understood interaction between the stromal and epithelial components. DHT is produced from T in the stroma cell and has an autocrine effect there and a paracrine effect in the epithelial cell. These effects are thought to include induction of multiple growth factors and alteration in the extracellular matrix. Prostate growth and maintenance of size and secretory function are stimulated by serum T, converted within the prostate to DHT, a compound whose relative androgenicity is higher. Free plasma T enters prostatic cells by diffusion and is rapidly metabolized to other steroids. More than 90% is irreversibly converted to the main prostatic androgen, DHT, by the enzyme 5α-reductase. DHT or T is bound to specific androgen receptors in the nucleus, when activation of the steroid receptor occurs.

Originally, an abnormal accumulation of DHT in the prostate was hypothesized as a primary cause of BPH development. However, Coffey and Walsh showed that human BPH occurs in the presence of normal prostatic levels of DHT. Estrogen-androgen synergism has been postulated as necessary for prostatic growth, as well as other steroid hormones and growth factors. Although much remains to be elucidated regarding the hormonal interactions and necessities for the induction and maintenance of BPH, it is clear that clinically a reduction in prostate size of approximately

20–30% can be induced by either interfering with androgen receptor binding or metabolism.

B. Stromal-Epithelial Interaction Theory

This theory, first introduced by Cunha and associates, postulates that there is a delicate stromal-epithelial balance in the prostate and that stroma may mediate the effects of androgen and on the epithelial component, perhaps by the production of various growth factors and/or autocrine and paracrine messengers.

C. Stem-Cell Theory

This is attributed to Issacs and associates and hypothesizes that BPH may result from abnormal maturation and regulation of the cell renewal process. In simple terms, this postulates that abnormal size in an aged prostate is maintained not by the increase in the rate of cell replication but rather by a decrease in the rate of cell death. Hormonal factors, growth factors, and oncogenes all influence this balance of replication and cell death. The exact interaction of these and possibly other factors and what determines the setting points for the level of cells in the prostate and their rates of growth, replication, and death are of major importance in understanding both BPH and prostate cancer.

D. Static and Dynamic Components of Prostatic Obstruction

It is extremely important to understand the concepts of the two prostatic components contributing to BOO caused by BPO. The **static component** is due to bulk and includes elements of the stromal and epithelial cells as well as extracellular matrix. Androgen ablation, at least in short-term studies, affects primarily the epithelial cell population volume. Long-term effects on stromal and matrix volume and effects on aspects of stroma and matrix other than volume have not been excluded, however. Therapeutic modalities that reduce the size of the prostate or "make a hole" or enlarge one are directed primarily toward this bulk component.

The **dynamic component** of obstruction refers to the contribution of prostatic smooth muscle. The tension of prostatic smooth muscle is mediated by α_1-adrenergic receptors, most of which are in the prostatic stroma. α_1-Receptors also exist in the smooth muscle of the bladder neck and the prostatic capsule. Activation of these contractile receptors can occur either through circulating catecholamine levels or through adrenergic innervation. Prostatic intraurethral pressure can be reduced experimentally by as much as 40% after systemic administration of an α-receptor antagonist. This dynamic component may be responsible for the well-recognized variation in symptoms over time experienced by many patients and may account for exacerbation of symptoms experienced by some individuals in response to certain foods, beverages, change in temperature, and levels of stress.

This two-component idea was first popularized by Marco Caine and later developed by Herb Lepor and Ellen Shapiro, resulting in the successful application of selective α-adrenergic blocking agents for the treatment of BPH symptoms. **The ratio of stroma to epithelium in the normal prostate is approximately 2:1, and in BPH approximately 5:1.** These data for BPH are derived primarily from small resected prostates; the ratio for larger glands with epithelial nodules may be lower. Although the smooth muscle content of stroma has not been precisely determined, a significant proportion of the stroma is in fact smooth muscle.

V. LOWER URINARY TRACT SYMPTOMS (LUTS)

LUTS is a rubric, introduced by Abrams, to replace the term "prostatism," which implied that the prostate was responsible for most (or all) symptomatic voiding complaints in men. LUTS with its subdivisions, filling/storage symptoms and voiding/emptying symptoms, have replaced the terminology of "irritative" and "obstructive" symptoms, both rather imprecise terms that imply an etiology that may be incorrect. **Voiding/emptying symptoms include impairment in the size/force of the urinary stream, hesitancy and/or straining to void, intermittent or interrupted flow, a sensation of incomplete emptying, and terminal dribbling, although the last by itself seems to have little clinical significance. Filling/storage symptoms include nocturia, daytime frequency, urgency, and urgency incontinence. Emptying/voiding symptoms are the most prevalent but filling/storage symptoms are the most bothersome to the patient** and interfere to the greatest extent with daily life activities.

LUTS associated with BPE/BPO are, however, not simply solely due to BOO. Such symptoms are due, in varying proportions in different individuals, to obstruction, obstruction-related changes in detrusor structure and function, age-related changes in detrusor structure and function, and changes in neural circuitry that may occur secondary to these factors.

VI. SIGNS OF BPH

A. Detectable anatomic **enlargement of the prostate** on physical examination or imaging is generally, but not always, the correlate of symptom-producing BPH. However, **there is no clear relationship between the degree of anatomic enlargement and the severity of urodynamic changes.**

B. **Bladder changes** secondary to obstruction can occur. These consist of **bladder wall thickening, trabeculations** (which are also associated with involuntary bladder contractions), and **bladder diverticula** (which could also be congenital). Bladder **calculi** can develop. Bladder **decompensation** can occur and gross bladder **distention** can result. Chronically increased residual urine volumes may result and may contribute to frequency and urgency and persistent urinary infection. Acute urinary retention may supervene. Azotemia may result from upper tract changes. There is an increased incidence of lower urinary tract infections (UTIs) in obstructed patients.

C. **Upper tract changes** of ureterectasis, hydroureter, and/or hydronephrosis can result. These can result either from secondary vesicoureteral reflux, sustained high-pressure bladder storage without reflux, and sustained high-pressure attempts at emptying. Ureteral obstruction could also occur secondary to muscular hypertrophy or angulation at the ureterovesical junction. Hematuria may arise from dilated veins coursing over the surface of the enlarged adenomatous prostate.

VII. URODYNAMICS OF BOO

The urodynamics of BOO are described in Chapter 13. Patients with BPO characteristically exhibit decreased mean and peak flow rates, an abnormal flow pattern characterized by a long, low plateau, and elevated detrusor pressures at the initiation of and during flow. They may or may not have residual urine. Approximately 50% of such patients are found to have detrusor overactivity during filling. Pressure-flow UDS can demonstrate detrusor underactivity. In this circumstance, it usually cannot be determined whether obstruction exists or existed prior, accounting for the detrusor dysfunction—a major issue. Specialized variations of UDS, either with or without video, are often helpful to separate BPO from other forms of outlet obstruction (see Chapter 13).

A. Residual Urine Volume

If the residual urine volume is significant, its reduction is important in the evaluation of results of treatment of BPO. For many with a significant residual volume, it is impossible to differentiate deficient bladder contractility from outlet obstruction as the primary cause, without a pressure-flow study. Most agree that a large residual urine volume reflects a degree of bladder dysfunction, but it is difficult to correlate residual urine with either specific symptomatology or other urodynamic abnormalities. The most popular noninvasive method of measurement is ultrasonography. The error for ultrasound has been estimated at 10–25% for bladder volumes greater than 100 mL and somewhat worse for smaller volumes. Residual urine volumes in an individual patient at different times can vary widely. Reflux and large diverticula may complicate the accuracy of measurement. Paul Abrams and colleagues, after a thorough review of the subject, concluded that elevated residual urine has a relation to prostatic obstruction, although not a strong one, as supported by the following observations.

1. Elevated residual urine is common in the elderly of both genders.
2. The absence of residual urine does not rule out severe obstruction.
3. Elevated residual urine does not have a significant prognostic factor for a good operative outcome. Volume of more than 300 mL may correlate with unfavorable outcome.

What constitutes an abnormal residual urine? The International Consultation on BPH concluded that a range of 50 to 100 mL represents the lower threshold to define abnormal. There is discussion ongoing as to the concept that it may be more clinically meaningful to describe residual urine volume as a percent of bladder capacity rather than as an absolute number.

B. Uroflowmetry

Significant disagreement exists regarding what constitutes an adequate urodynamic evaluation of LUTS in the male and whether a urodynamically quantifiable definition of obstruction is necessary or desirable before beginning treatment. Of all these urodynamic studies, uroflowmetry seems to excite the least controversy. **Although diminished flow may be caused by either outlet obstruction or impairment of detrusor contractility and outlet obstruction** may certainly exist in the presence of a normal flow, it is acknowledged that most men with BOO do have a diminished flow rate and altered flow pattern.

What is a normal flow rate? Paul Abrams and Derek Griffiths originally proposed that, empirically, peak flow rates of less than 10 mL/sec were associated with obstruction, that peak flow rates greater than 15 mL/sec were not associated with obstructed voiding, and that peak flow rates between 10 and 15 mL/sec were equivocal. Although this proposal has been widely used, it is generally acknowledged that flow rates at any level may be associated with either obstruction or lack of obstruction. Studies are cited showing that 7–25% of patients referred with LUTS had high flow BOO.

Potential problems related to uroflow include the following:

1. Many patients do not or will not void in a volume sufficient for accurate measurement.
2. Others void with an interrupted stream or with post-void dribbling, which makes interpretation of the endpoint of micturition difficult, casting some element of subjectivity into the calculation of average flow rate.
3. Some patients are unable to relax sufficiently to void in the same manner in which they would in the privacy of their own bathroom.
4. A considerable discrepancy may exist between the first and subsequent measures of mean and peak flow.
5. The flow parameter measured noninvasively and in the course of pressure flow studies in the same individual may vary considerably.

Flow data changes can be expressed in terms of absolute change, percent change, or as cumulative frequency distribution. Clearly important is the initial flow number, the value of which may make the absolute or percent change look better or worse. In other words, raw data must be expressed as well as the other frills that may be added to embellish flow data. It should be noted as well that **it is unknown what change in flow is necessary to give the impression of mild, moderate, or marked improvement.**

Because voiding events may be different from point to point in an individual's life, a variety of flow nomograms have been constructed to facilitate comparison of them. It should be noted that there are many nomograms and tables of "acceptable flow rates" available for various age groups. Many believe that the Siroky nomogram, commonly used in the United States, overestimates peak and average flow rates for older men and therefore underestimates the number of older men with BOO. Other nomograms include the Drach peak flow nomogram and the Liverpool and Bristol nomograms. It is doubtful that consistency will be achieved among flow nomogram makers. However, one of the systems supported by at least a portion of urodynamicists should be utilized for comparison following treatment of BPO.

C. Cystometry and Pressure-Flow Studies

Filling cystometry provides information on sensation, compliance, and the presence of and threshold for involuntary bladder contractions and urodynamic bladder capacity. Compliance is generally not affected in patients with BPO, but as mentioned previously, approximately 50% of such patients will have involuntary bladder contractions.

On a logical basis, BOO would seem to be defined by the relationship between flow rate and detrusor contractility. **Outlet obstruction is best characterized by a poor flow rate in the presence of a detrusor contraction of adequate force, duration, and speed. With obstruction, detrusor pressure during attempted voiding generally rises, flow rates generally fall, and the shape of the flow curve becomes more plateau than parabola-like.** There is, however, marked disagreement about the utility of pressure-flow urodynamic measurements in the prediction of success of a given treatment, and in the assessment of treatment results. Authorities who make an excellent case for the use of various types of pressure-flow studies in evaluating patients with LUTS and favorably affecting outcomes include Abrams and associates; Blaivas, Coolsaet, and Blok; Jensen, Neal, and colleagues; Schafer and co-workers; and Rollema and Van Mastrigt. Some add other mathematical means to augment the relationships observed on a simple plot of detrusor pressure versus flow. Equally forceful arguments against the utility of such measurements are made by Andersen, Bruskewitz, and colleagues; Graverson and co-workers; and McConnell. Jensen did an exhaustive review of the subject of urodynamic efficacy in the evaluation of elderly men with prostatism. One conclusion was that, in this group, interpretation of pressure-flow data using the nomogram of Abrams and Griffiths (see Chapter 13) revealed a significantly better subjective outcome for surgery in patients classified as "obstructed" than in those classified as "unobstructed" (93.1% versus 77.8%, $p < .02$). Others have also demonstrated better outcomes for surgery in urodynamically obstructed men than in those with no obstruction.

Successful treatment of BPO by prostatectomy is generally correlated with a reduction in the detrusor pressure (P_{DET}), and the corresponding detrusor pressure at maximum flow (P_{DET} at Q_{MAX}) and the peak flow rate (Q_{MAX}) are the most common and most important pressure-flow variables reported. Consideration of the entire pressure-flow plot or other complex mathematical manipulations and graphic representation may, in fact, prove to be more accurate and informative ways of looking at this relationship and may narrow further the diagnostic grey zone between BOO and decreased detrusor function. The problem is that there is not just one such program, but a number of them, with intense competition among their creators in the literature. We totaled more than 12 at last count.

D. Symptomatic Versus Urodynamic Improvement

The data from pressure-flow studies can be reported either as raw changes in individual parameters (e.g., Q_{MAX}, P_{DET}, P_{DET} at Q_{MAX}), as a change in category or number designating the grade or severity of obstruction, or by a visual demonstration of change on the nomogram itself. Aside from the utility (or nonutility) of these measurements in assessing the outcome of BPH treatment, a **global question referable to these studies seems to be whether the evaluation of the average older man with LUTS is more likely to lead to a better treatment outcome if urodynamic studies are performed.** In other words, can urodynamic studies predict the outcome of various treatments for LUTS, including watchful waiting? The critical question, when considering a given analysis of pressure-flow data, is: Are patients with LUTS in whom treatment in the form of outlet ablation fails the same as those whose detrusor contractility is judged ineffective by the criteria under consideration? If the answer to this question is no, then the relevance of the analysis is in question, unless it can predict which patients will worsen or which patients will have undesirable sequelae, or it can predict which modalities are apt to be more successful in treatment than others. In our opinion, we who perform urodynamics have done a remarkably poor job of looking into this aspect of outcome analysis.

One final consideration should be mentioned—a seeming dissociation that may occur between symptomatic and urodynamic improvement. This has been most noticeable in data concerning pharmacologic agents. The fact that symptomatic improvement occurs that is seemingly out of proportion to the amount of urodynamic improvement may, in fact, indicate that a given treatment is not equal to the current gold standard of prostatectomy or that the results will be of shorter duration. However, **one important possibility to consider is that the actual symptoms which we will attribute to BPO have much less to do with urodynamically defined obstruction than is thought, and their relief with these other types of treatment has to do more with the correction of some ill-defined mechanism within the prostate and/or prostatic urethra that is not directly related to the amount of mechanical obstruction. Alternatively, it may not be necessary to reduce outlet obstruction by the amount achievable by prostatectomy to significantly improve symptomatology and prevent bladder or upper tract deterioration**.

VIII. THE NATURAL HISTORY OF BPH AND ITS ALTERATION

Although LUTS due to BPO may be progressive over time, spontaneous improvement can occur in an untreated patient, and thus the course may be highly variable. Combining data from a number of reports of the natural history of untreated LUTS/BPO, one can conclude that over a 1- to 5-year period, approximately 15–30% of patients with clinical BPH will experience subjective improvement, 15–55% will have no change, and 15–50% will experience some worsening in their symptomatology. Data suggest that over 3 to 5 years 15–25% of patients will show an increase in flow rates, 15% will have no change, and 60–70% will have some worsening. Placebo responses of 20–40% have consistently been reported over the years for drug therapy.

Although BPH is rarely life threatening, it is generally considered to be a slowly progressive disease. Although many patients may do perfectly well with watchful waiting over long periods of time, the natural history of the disease can include undesirable outcomes. More recently, attention has been focused not only on evaluating the acute positive effects of treatment but on stabilizing symptoms, reversing the natural progression of BPH, and avoiding acute or undesirable events. The outcome measures recorded generally include (1) progression of symptoms, or signs, or both; (2) the occurrence of acute urinary retention; and (3) the need for surgical intervention. Progression can be measured in terms of any of the parameters used to assess outcome acutely or subacutely. A matched control group is obviously valuable in this regard, as the use of historical control subjects is less than ideal. Acute urinary retention is probably the event most feared by men with BPH as range from 0.004 to 0.13 episodes per person-year, with a 10-year cumulative incidence rate ranging from 4–73%! Others report the incidence of retention in 3 years to be 2.9% and cite incidences in the literature as low as 2% in 5 years and as high as 35% in 3 years! Progression to the point of requiring surgical intervention is an obvious undesirable outcome, but there are little data available regarding the incidence of this outcome, especially because the definitions of "surgery" and the indications and triggers for different types of "make a hole" therapy other than prostatectomy are continually changing.

IX. EVALUATION OF LUTS SUSPECTED TO BE DUE TO BPH

The essentials of our initial evaluation include history, digital rectal and focused physical examinations, urinalysis, urine cytology in those with significant irritative symptoms, serum creatinine, renal ultrasound if creatinine is abnormal, and a standardized symptom assessment, such as the American Urological Association symptom score (AUASS) or International Prostate Symptom Score (IPSS) (Figure 14-2). **Currently there is no absolute consensus as to routine prostate-specific antigen (PSA) measurement in men with LUTS. PSA can be useful for two reasons: prostate cancer screening and as a parameter for prognostic value for BPH progression and response to treatment.** Prostate cancer screening is addressed in Chapter 15. **PSA is a surrogate for prostate volume in the absence of cancer and a predictor of the risk of acute urinary retention and the ultimate need for surgery in men with LUTS secondary to BPO.** In any case the benefits and risks of PSA measurement should be discussed with the patient including the issues of false negative and positive results. Our belief is that PSA should be measured in men older than 50 years with a life expectancy of 10 years or more and in whom prostate cancer would be treated. For African Americans or those with a family history (first-degree relative), we drop this threshold age to 40.

Men who do not have absolute or near-absolute indications for treatment (see the following discussion), and have an AUASS of less than or equal to 7 (mild symptoms) do not need further evaluation or active treatment but should

(Text continued on p. 498)

AUA Symptom Index (range from 0 to 35 points).

	NOT AT ALL	LESS THAN 1 TIME IN 5	LESS THAN HALF THE TIME	ABOUT HALF THE TIME	MORE THAN HALF THE TIME	ALMOST ALWAYS
1. Over the last month how often have you had a sensation of not emptying your bladder completely after you finished urinating?	0	1	2	3	4	5
2. Over the last month, how often have you had to urinate again less than 2 hours after you finished urinating?	0	1	2	3	4	5
3. Over the last month, how often have you found you stopped and started again several times while urinating?	0	1	2	3	4	5
4. Over the last month, how often have you found it difficult to postpone urinating?	0	1	2	3	4	5
5. Over the last month, how often have you had a weak stream while urinating?	0	1	2	3	4	5
6. Over the last month, how often have you had to push or strain to begin urinating?	0	1	2	3	4	5

FIGURE 14-2. (Continued)

7. Over the last month, how many times did you most typically get up to urinate from the time you went to bed until the time you got up in the morning?

| 0, none | 1 time | 2 times | 3 times | 4 times | 5 or more times |

TOTAL ☐

AUA symptom index score: 0–7 mild; 8–18 moderate; 19–35 severe symptoms.

QUALITY OF LIFE DUE TO URINARY SYSTOMS

	DELIGHTED	PLEASED	MOSTLY SATISFIED	MIXED ABOUT EQUALLY SATISFIED AND DISSATISFIED	MOSTLY DISSATISFIED	UNHAPPY	TERRIBLE
1. If you were to spend the rest of your life with your urinary condition just the way it is now, how would you feel about that?	0	1	2	3	4	5	6

QUALITY OF LIFE ASSESSMENT INDEX (QOL) =

B. Quality of life assessment recommended by the World Health Organization.

FIGURE 14-2. AUA Symptom Index for benign prostatic hyperplasia. (From Hanno P, Malkowicz SB, Wein A [eds]: *Benign Prostatic Hyperplasia. Clinical Manual of Urology.* McGraw Hill, 2001, T15-2, pp. 389–90.)

be followed on a watchful waiting program. In patients with more severe symptoms or who are being considered for active treatment, urodynamics may be desirable. The simplest of these, flowmetry and residual urine volume, are now considered optional in primary management by the American Urological Association (AUA) (Practice Guideline Committee) and the 6th International Consultation on BPH. We consider endoscopic examination of the lower urinary tract to be reasonable if other lower urinary tract pathology is suspected or prior to invasive treatment when the choice of treatment or changes of success or failure depends on the anatomic configuration and/or intraurethral size of the prostate. Algorithms from the AUA Guidelines Committee and the 6th International Consultation on New Developments in Prostate Cancer and Prostate Diseases are seen in Figures 14-3 and 14-4.

A. Symptoms and Symptom Scores

Symptoms have classically formed the initial database on which to formulate (1) evaluation of potential outlet obstruction, (2) indications for active treatment, and (3) evaluation of the results of treatment. Symptom quantitation is difficult, and meaningful comparison of symptoms before and after treatment is even harder. The concept of a symptom score or severity table for BPH was first developed by an ad hoc group formed by the Food and Drug Administration (FDA) in 1975; the initial recommendations were published in 1977. Investigators can and have evaluated every factor imaginable with such scoring tables, eliminating some symptoms and adding others, changing the weights and definitions of the severity of various symptoms, considering some symptoms separately, or dividing the symptoms into storage and voiding groups. **There is generally no provision in a symptom score for considering what actually changed most recently to bring the patient to the physician, what is in fact most annoying to him, and what he wants corrected most, or what effect the overall symptom complex, or any one symptom, has on his quality of life, general activities of daily living, or any activity in particular such as sexual activity.**

Through its original Measurement Committee, the AUA formulated indices that address many of the issues relevant to symptom scores and produced a symptom index that has become widely utilized (see Figure 14-2). **This index correlates highly with the global rating by a subject of**

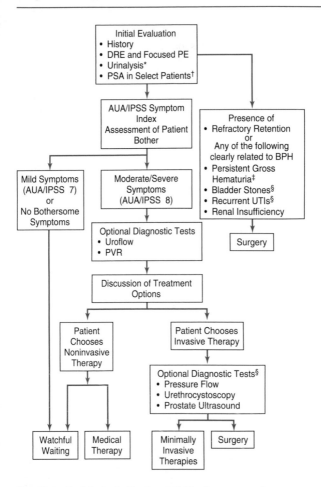

*In patients with clinically significant prostatic bleeding, a course of a 5α-reductase inhibitor may be used. If bleeding persists, tissue ablative surgery is indicated.

†Patients with at least a 10-year life expectancy for whom knowledge of the presence of prostate cancer would change management or patients for whom the PSA measurement may change the management of voiding symptoms.

‡After exhausting other therapeutic options as discussed in detail in the text.

§Some diagnostic tests are used in predicting response to therapy. Pressure-flow studies are most useful in men prior to surgery.

AUA, American Urological Association; DRE, digital rectal exam; IPSS, International Prostate Symptom Score; PE, physical exam; PSA, prostate-specific antigen; PVR, post-void residual urine; UTI, urinary tract infection.

FIGURE 14-3. AUA Practice Guidelines Committee algorithm for benign prostatic hyperplasia diagnosis and treatment. (From Claus G. Roehrborn, MD; John D. McConnell, MD; Michael J. Barry MD; Elie A. Benaim, MD; Michael L. Blute, MD; Reginald Bruskewitz, MD; H. Logan Holtgrewe, MD, FACS; Steven A. Kaplan, MD; John L. Lange, MD; Franklin C. Lowe, MD, MPH; Richard G. Roberts, MD, JD; and Barry Stein, MD. AUA Guidelines on the Management of Benign Prostatic Hyperplasia. American Urological Association Education and Research, Inc. © 2003.)

---

the magnitude of urinary problems attributed to BPH and has been reported to satisfy the requirements of validity, reliability, and responsiveness. The WHO Consultation on BPH has adopted this index, and in this context, it is referred to as the IPSS. **This measure of voiding symptoms is useful to ascertain symptom severity and treatment of response, or change over time without treatment.**

The AUASS/IPSS was originally introduced in 1992 as a symptom index specifically designed for what was called BPH at that time. In the years that followed, the questionnaires were administered to samples of men and women, however, and it became obvious that there is **indeed a lack of specificity for LUTS attributed to BPO/BPE. The AUASS/IPSS is neither gender specific nor disease specific, as symptomatology found in men and women are similar.** This argues for an age- or detrusor-related rather than an obstruction-related etiology of LUTS in at least a substantial portion of patients.

The AUASS/IPSS is sensitive to change. If rating patients' estimate of treatment as markedly, moderately, or slightly improved, unchanged, or worse, slight improvement in general equates to a mean reduction of 3, moderate improvement to 5.1, and marked improvement to 8.8. However, those who begin with a higher symptom score require a greater numerical decrease to achieve the same subjective improvement rating.

The AUASS/IPSS does not make the diagnosis of BPH and it cannot be used to screen for BPH. A variety of primary and secondary bladder abnormalities and nonprostatic causes of obstruction can produce similar symptoms and high symptom scores. In our practice, some of the highest scores are generated by women with filling/storage LUTS. **AUASS/IPSS does not correlate with or predict urodynamically documented BOO. Bothersomeness and effect on**

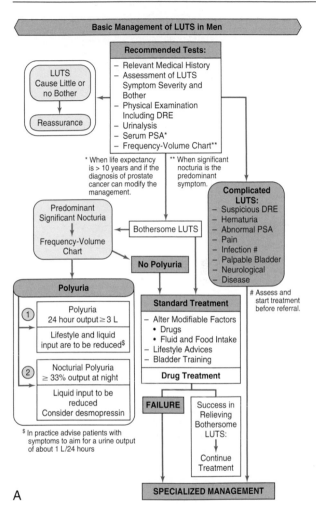

A

FIGURE 14-4. Algorithms for basic (**A**) and specialization (**B**) management of LUTS in men. (From the 6th International Consultation on New Developments in Prostate Cancer and Prostate Disease.)

the quality of life are not addressed by the AUA question-naire. Jerry Blaivas has questioned the accepted statements that the purpose of the AUASS is to quantify severity of disease, document response to therapy, assess patient

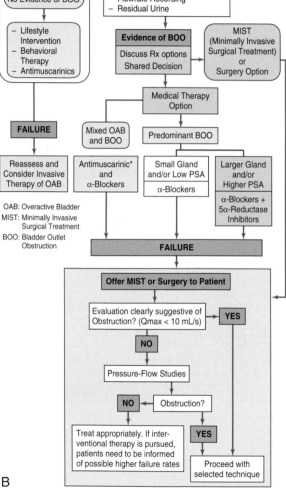

B

FIGURE 14-4. (Continued)

symptoms, follow the patient with time to determine disease progression, and follow comparison of the effectiveness of various interventions. He lists four reasons why, in his opinion, the AUASS is not a good tool for accomplishing these purposes:

1. There is an undue emphasis on emptying/voiding compared with filling/storage symptoms. In most series on LUTS in older men, urinary frequency and nocturia are the most common symptoms, and coupled with urge and urge incontinence, they seem to be the most troublesome. Only three of the seven questions relate to these symptoms. Urgency incontinence, which most would consider the most bothersome symptom, is not mentioned.

2. There is no means of quantitating how badly the symptoms bother the patient. An example cited is that a man who voids every half hour during the day, has urgency and urge incontinence half of the time, and gets up three times a night to void scores only 11 of 35 points, yet has severe symptoms. A man who voids three times daily, hesitates, stops and starts, and has a weak stream and sensation of incomplete emptying but no nocturia, urgency, or incontinence scores 20 of 35 points, even if he empties completely, yet has mild to moderate symptoms.

3. The symptom score does not consider the possibility that urinary frequency and nocturia may not reflect any dysfunction or may not be related to the lower urinary tract, because many persons void frequently by habit or by choice and do not consider daytime frequency or nocturia to be a symptom.

4. Changes in the symptom score are not necessarily a good measure of therapeutic efficacy because treatment of the most bothersome symptoms may be diluted by the response of symptoms that cause relatively no bother. An example cited is that in many of the original studies on drug treatment of BPH there was no effect whatever of drug versus placebo on the two most troublesome symptoms (nocturia and frequency) and yet there was a statistically significant effect on overall symptom score.

Change in symptom score is currently the most featured data in any clinical trial but what constitutes a significant change may be viewed differently by patient, investigator, gatekeeper or specialty physician, statistician, manufacturer, and the FDA. In the original publication about the AUASS, the index was noted to decrease from a preoperative mean of 17.6 to 7.1 in 4 weeks after prostatectomy and to 5 at 3 months. (Results of symptom scores can be reported in terms of absolute change or percent change from the pretreatment value.) The higher the pretreatment symptom score, the lower the percent change of a given absolute change. To compare symptom score changes, either absolute numbers or percentages, between groups, the pretreatment symptom scores clearly must be about the same.

B. Quality of Life Indices

Perhaps the softest, but maybe the most important, outcome measure to gauge the overall effect of clinical BPH on an individual and the efficacy of treatment for BPH is quality of life. **Most men seek treatment for BPH because of the bothersome nature of their symptoms, which affect the quality of their lives.** Symptom severity does not necessarily correlate with bothersomeness or quality of life indices. No consensus has been reached as to the optimal tool to record and compare disease-specific quality of life measures in patients with LUTS.

One question on the quality of life issue has been included by the International Consensus Committee to assess the impact of symptoms on quality of life in clinical practice (see Figure 14-2). This has been a consistent recommendation since the first WHO consultation on BPH in 1991. Although the Committee recognized that this single question could not capture the global impact of LUTS on quality of life, it was believed that this might serve as a valuable starting point for a physician-patient conversation concerning this issue.

X. INDICATION FOR TREATMENT

Indications for **surgery** have varied widely over time, and the current climate is much more conservative than existed 10–20 years ago. **Certain absolute or near absolute indications exist;** they are refractory or repeated urinary retention, related azotemia, significant recurrent gross hematuria, related recurrent or residual infection, bladder calculi, and large related bladder diverticula. All of these assume that the bladder is indeed contractile. In our opinion, a large residual urine volume that is increasing can also be considered an indication.

Without an absolute or near absolute indication, or combinations of these, the bothersome nature of the symptomatology is generally what prompts the patient to request, or the physician to suggest, treatment. Pathologic urodynamic findings may certainly be influential as well. Once the option of treatment is chosen, the risks and benefits of all applicable modalities must be discussed with the patient, and the patient must ultimately decide among these. General medical status and comorbid conditions may significantly influence this decision. **In general, the more definitive the expectation of a positive outcome is, the more invasive the procedure and the greater the risk.** The term "watchful waiting" has replaced "no treatment." Ideally each patient would be presented with a chart or other informational medium that describes each possible accepted treatment in terms of the expected likelihood of improvement, the magnitude of improvement, the likelihood of side effects (incontinence, impotence, retrograde ejaculation, and others), and the incidence of reoperation (if a procedure).

XI. TREATMENT OF BPH AND RELATED ENTITIES

The treatment options are summarized in Table 14-2. The natural determines the results that can be expected from watchful waiting. There are few studies that actually describe the natural history of this condition, and only a few more that look at the results of placebo treatment. It is clear that symptoms do tend to wax and wane and that a substantial number of men will have at least short-term stability or improvement of symptoms. The literature would suggest that, at least over a 5-year period, more than 50% of patients have either improved or have exhibited no change on the basis of subjective criteria. Development of urodynamic parameters to predict those patients who will worsen is clearly of paramount importance. The most commonly used, but not all, therapies are discussed.

A. Assessing the Results of Treatment

The outcome measures utilized to assess the results of treatment are seen in Table 14-3. Symptom scores and urodynamic parameters are most commonly used. Quality of life improvement and alteration of natural history are currently rarely utilized, an unfortunate state of affairs.

Table 14-2: Treatment Options for Clinical BPH

Watchful waiting (observation)
Pharmacologic
  Reducing prostate smooth muscle tone (the dynamic
  component)
    α-1 adrenergic antagonists
  Reducing prostate bulk (the static component primarily)
    Estrogen
    LHRH agonists/antagonists
    5-α reductase inhibitors
    Antiandrogens
    Aromatase inhibitors
    Growth factor inhibitors (theoretical)
  Unknown mechanisms
    Phytotherapy
    Other
Mechanical and Surgical
  Prostatic urethral stents
  Transurethral microwave thermotherapy (TUMT)
  Transurethral water induced thermotherapy (WIT)
  Interstitial therapy
    Radiofrequency energy (TUNA)
    Laser energy
    High intensity focused ultrasound
    Ethanol injection
  Transurethral resection and incision by
    Laser (laser TURP, TUIBN-P)
    Electrosurgery (TURP, TUIBN-P)
    Electrovaporization (TUVP)
    Ultrasound aspiration
  Open prostatectomy

LHRH, leutinizing hormone releasing hormone; TUMT, transurethral
microwave thermotherapy; TUNA, transurethral needle ablution;
TURP, transurethral prostatectomy; TUIBN-P, transurethral incision
bladder neck-prostate; TUVP, transurethral vaporization of prostate.

It must be recognized, however, that different segments of the
population will have different priorities and orientations and
may draw different conclusions regarding relative value or
efficacy from the same set of outcomes (Table 14-4).

Table 14-3: Outcome Measures to Assess the Results of Treatment for Benign Prostatic Hyperplasia and Related Entities

Symptoms and symptom scores
Quality of life indices
Correction of undesirable sequelae (e.g., azotemia)
Urodynamic indices
Size (for bulk reducing therapy)
Alteration of natural history
Adverse effects
Cost and cost-effectiveness

Table 14-4: Populations with Different Viewpoints on Evaluation of Outcomes Following Any Type of Treatment

Patient
Family
Treater
Referrer
Friend
Manufacturer
Competitor
Person in the street
Agency for Health Care Policy and Research
Food and Drug Administration

B. Alpha-Adrenergic Antagonists

Pharmacologic studies and receptor cloning have identified at least three α-1 adrenergic receptor subtypes in the lower urinary tract: α-1_a, α-1_b, α-1_d. In the prostate, α-1_a receptors are found predominantly in the stroma, α-1_b in the glandular epithelium, and the α-1_d in stroma and blood vessels. The α-1_a subtype is the predominant (about 70%) one in stromal tissue. The α-1 receptors are found also in the smooth muscle of the bladder base and proximal urethra, and α receptors are found in the spinal cord and ganglia as well. The extra-prostatic sites of α receptors and the lack of absolute receptor or organ selectivity account for their side effects when used for the treatment of LUTS. **The beneficial effects of α-blockers in the treatment of BPH are assumed primarily to result from a direct antagonism of α-adrenergic induced tone in the stromal smooth muscle, resulting in a decrease in outlet resistance.** Recently longer term effects on apoptosis and prostate cellular differentiation have been proposed as well.

Some of the history of the development of the use of α-blockers for the male LUTS patient can be found in Chapter 13. Commonly used preparations now include alfuzosin, doxazosin, doxazosin GITS (gastrointestinal therapeutic system), terazosin (once daily), and tamsulosin (once daily). **with these agents ranges from 30–45%, with a placebo effect of 10–30%. The improvement in maximum flow varies from 15–30%, with placebo showing 5–15%. It should be noted that numerically these translate into relatively small increments. Potential side effects include dizziness, asthenia, orthostatic hypotension, nasal congestion, and abnormal ejaculation.** The 6th International Consultation on BPH reports α-1 blockers as first-line medical treatment for BPH, stating further that they are efficacious, produce quality of life improvements, and have acceptable safety. Claims abound as to superiority of individual products. The AUA guidelines committee concluded that the α-blockers mentioned previously are appropriate treatment options for patients with LUTS secondary to BPH and that all four agents had equal clinical effectiveness with slight differences in the adverse event profiles. Acceptable head to head trials are scarce.

C. 5-α Reductase Inhibitors

The rationale for the use of 5-α reductase inhibitors (5 ARI) is that the embryonic development of the prostate is dependent on DHT, to which T is converted by the enzyme 5 AR. **Two isoenzymes exist. Type 2 is found mainly in the prostate, and type 1 in extraprostatic tissues. Finasteride is a competitive type 2 inhibitor; dutasteride inhibits both types 1 and 2 5 AR.** Finasteride reduces serum DHT by about 70%, prostate DHT by 80–90%, and dutasteride reduces serum DHT by more than 90%. **Both reduce serum PSA levels by approximately 50%.** Although the number of clinical trials with finasteride is much greater, most agree that clinical efficacy seems comparable at this point: volume reduction of 18–26% (placebo −2 to +14), IPSS reduction of 3.3 to 4.5 (placebo 1.3 to 2.3), and peak flow increase of 1.9 to 2.2 (placebo 0.2 to 0.6). **Both are reported to decrease the long-term risk of acute urinary retention and the need for surgery by up to 50–60% in patients with enlarged prostates (baseline numbers were, however, small). These benefits are seen primarily in men with enlarged prostates (over 30 to 40 cc). Side effects include decreased libido, ejaculatory disorders, and erectile dysfunction, all with a reported incidence of 5–6% and reversible on discontinuation** of therapy (data primarily from finasteride studies). The two agents have not been directly compared specifically with respect to efficacy and tolerability.

D. Combined Therapy

Is combination therapy (alpha blocker plus finasteride) more effective than either alone? A Veterans Administration Cooperative Study by Herb Lepor compared placebo, finasteride, terazosin, and finasteride plus terazosin. The mean group differences for all patients between finasteride and placebo were not statistically significant for AUA symptom index, symptom problem index, BPH impact index, and peak flow rate. The changes for terazosin were significant versus placebo and versus finasteride. The group mean differences between combination therapy and terazosin for all measures other than prostate volume were significantly in favor of terazosin. The volume decrease was 20% in their finasteride and combination groups. The AUA symptom index components were 2.6 units for placebo, 3.2 for finasteride, 6.6 for terazosin, and 6.2 for the combination. Finasteride supporters argue that the apparent lack of efficacy in this study was due to a relatively small mean prostate volume in the population studied. For the men with volumes larger than 50 mL, there was a mean increase in Q_{MAX} of 2.5 mL/sec and a mean decrease in AUA SS of 2.9, both significantly different from those of comparable men in the placebo group.

The **MTOPS (Medical Therapy of Prostate Symptoms)** study looked at the question of whether long-term therapy of BPH with placebo, doxazosin, finasteride, or doxazosin plus finasteride would prevent or delay disease progression. **The AUA Guidelines Committee cites this study as the primary reason for the conclusion that combination therapy is an appropriate and effective therapy for patients with LUTS and prostatic enlargement.** Combination therapy appeared more effective than α-blocker monotherapy in relieving and preventing the progression of symptoms. **The overall risk of progression was reduced** by 39% for doxazosin (D), 34% for finasteride (F), and by 67% for a combination. The risk of retention was reduced by 31% for D, 67% for F, and 79% for D + F. **The risk of surgery was reduced by 64% for F and 67% for F + D. Doxazosin alone did not reduce the risk of surgery over placebo. Patients more likely to benefit are those with larger pros-tates and higher non-cancer related PSA values,** although absolute thresholds are yet uncertain.

E. Balloon Dilation

Variable balloon lengths and diameters are available, and dilation occurs over 5 to 20 minutes with a pressure of 2–5 atmospheres. Treatment can be performed under local or short general anesthesia, and the balloon positioned endo-scopically, radiologically, or ultrasonographically, or by rectal palpation. Improvement rates of 14.3–84% were reported. A recent study by Lepor using a sham arm concluded that improvement after balloon dilation was no greater than that after simple cystoscopy. **This treatment has fallen out of favor**.

F. Prostatic Urethral Stents

A bewildering array of prostatic urethral stents has become available. These include temporary metallic, temporary poly-mer, biodegradable, and permanent metallic stents. **The per-manent metallic stents are the only commercially available types that are FDA approved for use in the Uni-ted States.** The AMS UroLume (Minnetonka, MN) is **approved for use in BPH, urethral stricture disease, and detrusor-sphincter dyssynergia.** These are implanted by endoscopic control with one end at the bladder and the other at the mid verumontanum, and the ideal result is a stent completely covered by urothelium, making encrustation impossible. Alleviation of voiding symptoms occurs in as many as 85% of patients in the short term, with correspond-ing improvement in objective parameters as well. Durability is now demonstrated with 7-year data. **Removal of the stent may be extremely difficult** creating concern regarding subsequent procedures and thus patient selection is crucial. Relatively elderly and unhealthy patients who may be unable to undergo other more aggressive therapy are usually consid-ered. The consensus of the International Consultation on BPH is that the absence of randomized controlled clinical trials and cost-effectiveness studies makes it difficult to offer recommendations for this mode of treatment.

G. Resection and Modalities Producing Vaporization and/or Coagulation Necrosis

Traditional electrocautery, laser, microwave, and radiofrequency energy can be utilized to resect, vaporize, or cause coagulation necrosis of prostatic tissue. At temperatures lower than 45°C, coagulation necrosis of normal tissue does not occur. **Irreversible cellular damage begins to occur above 45°C.** Coagulation can take up to an hour to occur at temperatures minimally above this level. At 60°–100°C, coagulation is rapid and at 100°C is virtually instantaneous. **At temperatures higher than 100°C, tissue vaporization is produced**.

H. Transurethral Microwave Thermotherapy (TUMT)

This is the most commonly utilized method of energy ablation in the **office setting.** There now exists a large body of literature that supports both the efficacy and the very low rate of significant side effects of these therapies. These are systems are based on urethral catheters that house a microwave transducer just proximal to the anchoring balloon and thus dwell within the prostate during treatment. After placement of this catheter and a rectal temperature sensor, **the microwave is activated to heat the prostate adenoma to a target temperature of at least 45°C for an extended period of time (30–45 minutes).** This causes coagulation necrosis and subsequent reduction in the size of the adenoma allowing for improved peak flow and reduction of symptom score that is durable even up to 48 months. **Results are encouraging but still do not match those of transurethral resection of the prostate (TURP).** Representative results include an increase in Q_{MAX} from 8 to 12 mL/sec, and a decrease in AUASS from 22 to 12 and 17.5 to 9. These procedures are performed in the office setting with only local anesthesia via lidocaine jelly. However, many patients do initially require an indwelling urethral catheter for a few days post procedure due to problems with urinary retention caused initially by edema. Additionally, urinary symptoms require 6–12 weeks to improve post treatment. Some systems feature water flow through the catheter during heating to cool the urethral wall thus preventing sloughing and possibly reducing side effects such as urgency. Side effects and complication profiles are generally very low with this form of therapy. Minimal erectile dysfunction, stricture, and incontinence have been reported in 0–44% of treated patients.

I. Transurethral Needle Ablation of the Prostate (TUNA)

TUNA is also an **office-based procedure in which radio-frequency energy is used to ablate prostatic adenoma.** The system is based on a cystoscope-like device that allows the surgeon to visualize the prostatic urethra and then deploy electrodes into the parenchyma of the prostate that deliver radiofrequency to heat the prostate to 80°–100°C. Each cycle, lasting about 5 minutes, creates an area of necrosis that is rather small and thus requires multiple lesions to be created in a systematic fashion to effectively debulk the prostate. Total treatment times range from 30–60 minutes. **A number of randomized trials have shown effectiveness both subjectively and objectively.** Representative results include Q_{MAX} changes from 7.8 to 14.4 and 8.8 to 15.5 mL/sec and AUASS changes from 24 to 11, 22 to 9, and 20 to 5.4. By 12 months post treatment, a decrease of AUASS of 77% and peak flow increases of 6 mL/sec can be expected. **Side effects are also mild and include retention and hematuria.** Sexual dysfunction and stricture are rare.

J. Transurethral Water-Induced Thermotherapy (WIT)

This is a variation of an old theme, balloon dilation, with the addition of thermal energy to augment effect. A specialized balloon catheter is placed under local anesthesia. **A treatment balloon is then inflated within the prostate to 50 F thereby compressing the prostatic urethra. This also tamponades intraprostatic blood flow to allow better thermal effect. Water heated to 60°C is then circulated inside the balloon.** Coagulative necrosis then occurs; however, urethral sloughing is common and troublesome for patients. Initial trials report a 71% increase in Q_{MAX} and a 24 to 11 reduction in AUASS. Longer term studies are lacking.

K. Laser Usage

The tissue effects of laser energy are produced by the virtually instantaneous attainment of temperatures higher than 60°C to create coagulation necrosis and above 100°C to create vaporization. The types of laser utilized for clinical BPH treatment include:

1. Neodynium yttrium-aluminum-garnet (Nd:YAG). This is generally applied transurethrally through contact or noncontact fibers. At low power density, this laser penetrates deeply and produces coagulation necrosis. At higher energy levels, vaporization and coagulation occur. Interstitial fibers can also be placed to produce coagulation necrosis with interstitial application; post procedure, the lesions result in secondary atrophy and regression of the prostatic "lobes." Internal scarring with retraction of the periurethral tissue also probably occurs.
2. Semiconductor diode. This can be used with either a free beam low energy technique or an interstitial technique.
3. Potassium titanyl phosphate laser (KTP). This uses a free beam treatment with high energy density to create vaporization without concurrent deep coagulation.
4. Pulsed holmium:YAG. This causes thermomechanical vaporization and can be used as a cutting tool.

L. Nd:YAG Ablation Via Side Firing Fiber

The Nd:YAG laser produces wavelengths of 1064 nm that can penetrate tissue to a depth of 15–20 mm. Energy levels of 40–60 W can cause coagulative necrosis. Initial means to deliver Nd:YAG energy was performed cystoscopically with direct application via a side firing laser fiber. **Although initial reports seemed promising, patient tolerance was low due to delayed sloughing, significant local symptoms, and prolonged time until maximal improvement**.

M. Interstitial Laser Coagulation (ILC)

This procedure utilizes a standard cystoscope that allows passage of a laser fiber that is then inserted directly into the prostate in a fashion similar to TUNA. **This is typically a diode type laser with wavelength of 830 nm. Once proper depth is established, the laser energy is activated to create an elliptical lesion of necrosis. There is no limit to the number of lesions that can be created; however, increasing numbers create more edema and longer retention times.** Procedures typically take 30 minutes. These are outpatient procedures and catheters are left indwelling for 48 hours. Results at 12 months from multicenter experience demonstrate AUASS improvement from 21.4 to 9.25 and peak flow rates from 9.55 to 16.5 mL/sec.

Few complications have been reported and do include hemorrhage, incontinence, and impotence; however, retrograde ejaculation is seen in only 10% of patients.

N. Photoselective Vaporization of the Prostate (PVP)

The KTP laser (wavelength 532 nm) is utilized during this procedure. **This wavelength is highly absorbed by oxyhemoglobin thus allowing efficient tissue vaporization with excellent hemostasis.** A specialized side firing laser fiber is utilized cystoscopically to focus the energy into the prostate causing vaporization of all vascularized tissue. Representative results at one year versus TURP show a 171% versus 102% improvement in Q_{MAX}, 54% versus 47% decrease in IPSS, and catheterization time of 13.5 versus 40.1 hours. Advantages include excellent hemostasis allowing use on anticoagulated patients, no risk of TUR syndrome, and quick learning curve. Side effects are minimal. Drawbacks include difficulty of resection of very large glands (>80 gm).

O. Holmium Laser Enucleation of the Prostate (HOLEP)

The addition of high-powered holmium lasers (80–100 W) has enabled urologists to perform prostate resection. Holmium energy (wavelength 2100 nm) allows actual resection and debulking of adenoma in a similar fashion to standard TURP. Holmium energy has a minimal depth of penetration (0.5 mm) but divides tissue in a nearly bloodless fashion. **The HOLEP procedure utilizes a continuous flow resectoscope with an end-firing 550 micron fiber that enables enucleation of the prostate in a fashion similar to open suprapubic prostatectomy. The laser fiber is used to incise the prostate adenoma down to capsule and then entire lobes of the prostate are enucleated and pushed into the bladder. Once the entire adenoma is resected, a tissue morcellator is used cystoscopically to remove the prostate piecemeal. Significant advantages include excellent hemostasis, results equivalent to standard TURP, no risk of TUR syndrome (saline irrigation), and shortened hospital stay.** Patients who are fully anticoagulated can be treated using this approach. **Drawbacks are a significant learning curve, need for a high-power laser, and the need for morcellation.**

P. Holmium Laser Ablation of the Prostate (HOLAP)

The HOLAP procedure is a modification of the HOLEP that also requires a continuous flow resectoscope, high-powered holmium laser, but, instead of an end firing laser fiber, a side firing laser fiber. During this procedure, the laser fiber is employed to vaporize the surface tissue of the adenoma via continuous delivery of laser energy. With the minimal depth of penetration of the holmium energy, this approach can be time consuming; however, it does provide bloodless, immediate debulking of adenoma. Benefits include excellent short-term results and shorter hospital and catheter time. Drawbacks include difficulty in treatment of prostates greater than 80 gm in size.

Q. Transurethral Resection of the Prostate (TURP)

This remains the gold standard of treatment for symptoms of BPH. This technique uses a resection loop and electrosurgical generator capable of delivering cutting and coagulating current. The lower voltage continuous cutting wave form instantaneously vaporizes a path through the tissue and does not result in significant coagulation. The coagulation current consists of short segments of higher voltage lower current energy, resulting in deeper penetrative heating and hemostasis. **Resection via electrocautery loop by a transurethral route has, on literature review, a 75–96% chance of improvement of symptoms, with the degree of improvement 4 on a scale of 4. Modern series reporting risks of TURP have shown significant improvement.** The recent AUA guidelines on BPH have quoted total urinary incontinence as occurring in less than 1%, stress incontinence at 1–2%, urge incontinence at 5–25%, and impotence is cited at 3%. Retrograde ejaculation occurs 50–95% of the time, and the incidence of bladder neck contracture and urethral stricture is cited at 3–5% and 2–5%, respectively. Other significant intraoperative and perioperative risks include TUR syndrome, hemorrhage, and even death. **TUR syndrome is a potential devastating complication that is caused by intravascular absorption of irrigating fluids. Dilutional hyponatremia and fluid overload can occur leading to bradycardia, neuromuscular dysfunction, seizures, coma, and death. If suspected, immediate treatment with intravenous saline, IV mannitol, and loop diuretics should be instituted.** Additionally, patients can expect to stay in the hospital for 1–3 days post surgery with an indwelling catheter during that time. Thus, newer procedures are being refined to help decrease these risks and morbidity. The risk/benefit ratio of TURP was held up to significant scrutiny by articles appearing in 1987 to 1989 that cited a mortality rate of 2.5% within 90 days after surgery and a requirement for re-resection of approximately 2% per year or 16% at 8 years when compared with open prostatectomy. The relative risk of death was 1.45 at up to 5 years after TURP. The risk of reoperation was approximately double. Since that time, a number of individuals have cited significant problems with these data because of comorbidity issues and because other populations have failed to confirm these problems as sequelae of electrosurgical TURP.

R. Transurethral Electrovaporization of the Prostate (TUVP)

This technique that is very similar to TURP involves substitution of the resection loop of the resectoscope with a broad-based, rolling electrode that can be swept over the surface of the prostate while the electrical current is activated. The high power density that is transmitted literally vaporizes the underlying tissue. This technique requires more time than resection but greatly decreases risks of hemorrhage and TUR syndrome as vessels are sealed during vaporization. The desiccated base, however, is less susceptible to further vaporization. Other advantages include shorter hospitalization and shortened learning curve and catheter time. No tissue is recovered during the procedure. Representative results include increases of Q_{MAX} from 9 to 24.3 mL/sec and 7.4 to 17 mL/sec and decreases in AUASS from 24 to 8 and 23 to 5. Sexual side effects and incontinence rates are similar to those following TURP.

S. Transurethral Electrosurgical Incision of the Bladder Neck and Prostate (TUIBN-P)

For patients with smaller prostates (less than 30 gm) this procedure involves simply incising through the bladder neck from a point distal to the ureteral orifices to the lateral edge of the verumontanum. The incisions can be performed with either electrocautery or holmium laser energy. **Ideal candidates are those with little lateral lobe hypertrophy, no median lobe hypertrophy, and a high posterior lip of**

the bladder neck. In suitable candidates, improvement in peak flow rates is approximately the same, global improvement rates slightly less (80–95% versus 85–100%), retrograde ejaculation much less (0–37%), and bladder neck contracture much less (1%). Impotence has been rarely reported, and incontinence is seen in 0–1% of patients. This is certainly an underutilized procedure; based on historical statistics, nearly 80% of patients undergoing TURP in the United States have less than 30 gm of tissue resected.

T. High Intensity Focused Ultrasound (HIFU)

This procedure is based on the principle of focusing ultrasound beams via a transducer or lens to create high temperatures ($>70°C$) in target tissues. The experience in the United States is very limited; however, there is growing European data. **Transrectal devices are placed under general or regional anesthesia. Short bursts of HIFU energy are guided by computer placement via ultrasound imaging.** Limited and selective experience has reported Q_{MAX} increases from 6.4 to 12.8 and 9.2 to 13.7 mL/sec along with AUASS decreases from 18 to 6.3, 20.3 to 9.6, and 26 to 14. Cross-over treatment by TURP was fairly significant at 44% by 4 years. Complications have included urinary retention, infection, epididymitis, and in one early series, a rectourethral fistula developed postoperatively. FDA clinical trials are now under way.

U. Ethanol Interstitial Injection

This involves the transurethral injection of ethanol into the prostate to create an ovoid space of necrosis. Clinical trials are planned.

V. Open Prostatectomy

This increasingly infrequently utilized option for BPH is clearly the most invasive but may still be the treatment of choice for prostates larger than 100 gm. This operation, first described by Fuller in 1894, is performed through a lower midline incision and allows complete, intact removal either through the bladder or through the anterior capsule of the prostate. However, the morbidity of the procedure stemming from complications including retrograde ejaculation, impotence, UTI, transfusion, stricture, incontinence, bladder neck contracture, ureteral obstruction, and persistent urine leak makes this operation generally less attractive and thus less often performed. Recent publications report the viability of laparoscopic transvesical prostatectomy with minimally morbidity and excellent symptom improvement. However, this experience is still limited.

It is clear that the age of significant morbidity for treatment for BPH is coming to a close. More data over longer periods of follow-up are necessary to fully describe the natural history and advantages and disadvantages of other methods of therapy including watchful waiting. In the future, patients will likely be presented with a checklist of the advantages and disadvantages of each type of management. The number of surgical and mechanical therapies dictates, however, that no one practitioner will have expertise with all of these, but rather each will have his or her "favorites," hopefully based on sound reasoning and results. Patients with minimal to moderate symptoms and bother, who do not have an absolute indication for surgery, will doubtless choose less invasive therapy, at least initially. Minimally invasive therapies offer many patients significant durable relief of BPH related symptoms as an outpatient with minimal morbidity. Even TURP, the traditional gold standard, with its significant improvement in morbidity over open prostatectomy, is rapidly becoming replaced by less invasive treatments. Even those patients with extremely large prostates may be able to select a laparoscopic approach to prostatectomy in the near future. Finally, it remains to be seen how much, if anything, is "lost" by utilizing those surgical mechanical methods that do not yield tissue for pathologic analysis because prior to the PSA era, approximately 10–12% of prostatectomy specimens were found to contain unsuspected cancer. Although this is probably less with the advent of widespread PSA testing, it remains to be seen whether any noticeable delays in the diagnosis of cancer occur and, if so, whether outcome is adversely influenced.

SELF-ASSESSMENT QUESTIONS

1. Discuss the varying definition of BPH (microscopic, macroscopic, and clinical) and the epidemiology of each.
2. Discuss the origin and meaning of the term LUTS, the subdivisions of LUTS, and their potential etiologies.
3. Discuss the typical urodynamic changes seen in moderate to severe bladder outlet obstruction secondary to BPH.

4. Discuss the outcome measures for evaluating the efficacy of therapy for clinical BPH and their relative importance.
5. Discuss the pharmacologic and ablative therapies of clinical BPH, including expected changes in symptom scores and flowmetry.

SUGGESTED READINGS

1. Abrams P: In support of pressure-flow studies for evaluating men with lower urinary tract symptoms. *Urology* 44:153–155, 1994.
2. Abrams, P, D'Ancona, C, Griffiths, D, et al: Lower urinary tract symptoms: etiology, assessment and predictive outcome from therapy. From 6th International Consultation on New Developments in Prostate Cancer and Prostate Disease. Plymouth, United Kingdom, Plymbridge Distributors, Ltd., in press.
3. Ball AJ, Fenely RCL, Abrams PH: The natural history of untreated "prostatism." *Br J Urol* 53:613–616, 1981.
4. Barry MJ: Epidemiology of benign prostatic hyperplasia. *AUA Update Series* 16:274–279, 1997.
5. Barry MJ, Fowler FJ, Bin L, et al: The natural history of patients with benign prostatic hyperplasia as diagnosed by North American urologists. *J Urol* 157:10–15, 1997.
6. Barry MJ, Fowler FJ, O'Leary MP, and the Measurement Committee of the AUA: The America Urological Association symptom index for benign prostatic hyperplasia. *J Urol* 148:1549–1557, 1992.
7. Barry MJ, Williford WO, Chang Y, et al: Benign prostatic hyperplasia specific health status measures in clinical research: how much change in the AUA symptom index and the BPH impact index is perceptible to patients? *J Urol* 154:1770–1774, 1995.
8. Blaivas J: The bladder is an unreliable witness. *Neurourol Urodyn* 15:443–445, 1996.
9. Chatelain C, Denis L, Foo KT, et al. (eds): 5th International Consultation on Benign Prostatic Hyperplasia (BPH). Plymouth, United Kingdom, Plymbridge Distributors, Ltd., 2001.
   Chapter 1: Epidemiology and Natural History. Boyle P, Liu F, Jacobsen S, et al.
   Chapter 3: Regulation of Prostate Growth. Lee C, Cockett A, Cussenot K, et al.
   Chapter 5: Initial Evaluation of LUTS. Resnick M, Ackermann R, Bosch J, et al.

Chapter 7: The Urodynamic Assessment of Lower Urinary Tract Symptoms. Abrams P, Griffiths D, Hofner K, et al.

Chapter 10: Interventional Therapy for Benign Prostatic Hyperplasia. Debruyne FMJ, Djavan B, De la Rosette J, et al.

Chapter 11: Endocrine Treatment of Benign Prostatic Hyperplasia. Bartsch G, McConnell JD, Mahler C, et al.

Chapter 12: Alpha1-Adrenoceptor Antagonist in the Treatment of BPH. Jardin A, Andersson KE, Chapple C, et al.

10. Lepor H, Williford WO, Barry MJ, et al: The efficacy of terazosin, finasteride, or both in BPH. Veterans Affairs Cooperative Studies Benign Prostatic Hyperplasia Study Group. *N Engl J Med* 335:533–539, 1996.

11. McConnell J: Why pressure flow studies should be optional and not mandatory for evaluating men with benign prostatic hyperplasia. *Urology* 44:156–158, 1994.

12. McConnell JD, Barry MJ, Bruskewitz R, et al: Benign prostatic hyperplasia: diagnosis and treatment. *Clinical Practice Guideline, no 8. AHCPR publication No. 94–0583.* Rockville, MD, Agency for Health Care Policy Research, Public Health Service, US Dept. of Health and Human Services, 1994.

13. McConnell JD, and the MTOPS Steering Committee: The long term effects of medical therapy on the progression of BPH: results for the MTOPS trial. *J Urol* 167:1042, 2002.

14. Roehrborn CG, McConnell JD, Barry MJ, et al: *AUA Guidelines for the Management of Benign Prostatic Hyperplasia.* Baltimore, MD, American Urological Association, 2003.

15. Wasson JH, Reda DJ, Bruskewitz RC, et al: A comparison of transurethral surgery with watchful waiting for moderate symptoms of BPH. *N Engl J Med* 332:75–79, 1995.

16. Wein AJ, Kavoussi LR, Novick AC, et al (eds): *Campbell-Walsh Urology,* Philadelphia, Elsevier Science, 2007.

Chapter 85: Molecular Biology, Endocrinology, and Physiology of the Prostate and Seminal Vesicles. Rodriguez R, Veltri R.

Chapter 86: Etiology, Pathophysiology, Epidemiology, and Natural History of Benign Prostatic Hyperplasia. Roehrborn CG, McConnell JD.

Chapter 87: Evaluation and Nonsurgical Management of Benign Prostatic Hyperplasia. Kirby R, Lepor H.

Chapter 88: Minimally Invasive and Endoscopic Management of Benign Prostatic Hyperplasia. Fitzpatrick JJ.

Chapter 89: Retropubic and Suprapubic Open Radical Prostatectomy. Han M, Partin A.

17. Wein JA: Criteria for assessing outcome following intervention for benign prostatic hyperplasia. In Lepor H (ed): *Prostatic Diseases*. Saunders, Philadelphia, 1999, pp 210–231.

C H A P T E R 15

Adult Genitourinary Cancer—Prostate and Bladder

S. Bruce Malkowicz, MD,
David J. Vaughn, MD, and
Alan J. Wein, MD, PhD (hon)

I. PROSTATE CANCER

A. General Considerations

Prostate cancer is the most common cancer in men and the second greatest cause of cancer mortality in men. Disease awareness has grown considerably in the past two decades leading to a greater emphasis on early disease detection. Currently one in six men will be diagnosed with prostate cancer. The major factor in this has been the introduction of prostate-specific antigen (PSA) testing as part of the detection and management of prostate disease. The refinement in diagnosis by ultrasound-guided needle biopsy has also aided in the rapid identification of the disease. Early detection has been further complemented by refinements in several approaches to the treatment of clinically localized disease. Those patients with intermediate or high risk for disease recurrence after local therapy may benefit from combined modality at the outset. The nature of biochemical recurrence after local treatment is being better defined, allowing for the stratification of these patients. Treatment of initial advanced disease has classically been provided through some form of androgen ablation, and cytoreductive chemotherapy has recently been demonstrated to have a statistical improvement on survival in patients with androgen resistant disease. Such therapy will hopefully be further augmented by the addition of newer molecular agents with the ability to target specific particular cellular pathways involved in angiogenesis and signal transduction.

B. Incidence

In the United States there will be an estimated 232,000 new cases of prostate cancer in the coming year with approximately 29,000 cancer-related deaths. In general there is a prevalence of approximately 1.8 million individuals with prostate cancer. Worldwide there are approximately 700,000 new cases per year with 220,000 deaths, making it responsible for almost 12% of all new cancers and nearly 6% of cancer deaths. After the rapid increase in detected cases after the introduction of PSA testing, the number of incident cases has decreased to its present level. The death rate from prostate cancer has also been decreasing by approximately 25% in the past decade, yet it cannot be said with certainty at this time that this is the result of earlier detection and therapy.

C. Epidemiology

Prostate cancer is distributed in a very uneven manner with regard to race. African-Americans have the highest mortality rate from this disease, which is also highly prevalent in the Caribbean and Africa. There is a significant contrast to native Asian men who have the lowest disease incidence and death rate from this condition. Although lower than in other ethnic groups, prostate cancer incidence and disease mortality demonstrate an upward trend in these Asian countries. Caucasian men in the United States and Europe have an intermediate rate of disease expression, with the highest incidence rate and disease mortality found in northern Europeans.

1. Age. The autopsy incidence of prostate cancer can be significant by the fourth decade of life and is at least 30% in men older than the age of 50 years, which climbs to more than 70% by the eighth decade of life. Clinical detection occurs at earlier ages due to increased awareness and more intense disease screening. More significant disease may be found in African-Americans at an earlier age.
2. Family history. A twofold greater risk for developing prostate cancer exists in those individuals with a first-degree relative with prostate cancer. This climbs to almost ninefold if three first-degree relatives are affected. Risk also exists if second-degree relatives have a diagnosis of prostate cancer. Alterations in specific genes or genetic loci may contribute to the development of disease. Hereditary prostate cancer is usually defined as multiple affected family members and a distribution along several generations. Approximately 20% of patients may have a familial association with another individual with prostate cancer.

3. Geography. Data suggest an inverse relationship between latitude and the incidence of prostate cancer. Northern populations have a greater level of disease, and it is hypothesized that it is related to the lower vitamin D levels secondary to less exposure to ultraviolet radiation. This may be due to dietary changes or other factors. Native black populations in Zaire have lower levels of prostate cancer compared to ethnic Zairians living in Belgium.

D. Etiology

1. The genetic factors responsible for prostate cancer are being actively investigated. At this time a few candidate prostate cancer genes have been identified, yet the majority of data suggests that subtle changes in several different genes involved in such vital areas as steroid metabolism or detoxification may have an aggregate affect on prostate cancer disposition.
    a) HPC1/RNASEL (1q24–25) and PG1/MSR1 (8p22–23) are potential prostate-cancer specific susceptibility genes, which functionally deal with inflammatory and infectious processes. Their exact roles in cancer etiology are under intense scrutiny.
    b) Recently chromosomal rearrangements similar to that seen in certain sarcomas have been identified in prostate tumors. Gene fusions resulting in androgen driven oncogenic gene products suggest a new method of tumor pathogenesis. This is exemplified in the fusion/rearrangement of TMPRSS2 with ETS transcription factor genes.
    c) Androgen receptor CAG repeat length, alterations in SRD5A2 (5-α reductase-2), and cytochrome p450 genes associated with steroid metabolism (Cyp 3A4, Cyp 19A1, Cyp 17A1) have some relative impact on prostate cancer susceptibility alone or in concert.
    d) Data suggest that the GSTM1-null phenotype may increase prostate cancer risk in smokers.
2. Androgens. Studies on androgen levels have been conflicting but have suggested higher testosterone levels or dihydrotestosterone/testosterone ratios in African-American men. Mutations or alterations in the androgen receptor (CAG repeats) may also be unequally distributed among individuals in populations, affecting response to testosterone.
3. Diet. High intake of animal fat is associated with increased prostate cancer risk. Conversely the intake of soy products (isoflavenoids, phytoestrogens, Bowman-Birk inhibitor)

may affect the development and progression of prostate cancer. Migration studies of Asians moving west demonstrate an increase in prostate cancer incidence compared to that of white populations in the same area. Studies in other tumor systems on vitamin E and selenium showed a one-third to two-third decrease in prostate cancer incidence, respectively. Intake of carotenoids such as lycopene (responsible for the red color of tomatoes) may be associated with the decreased prostate cancer risk.

4. IGF (insulin-like growth factor) system. These are peptides similar in structure to proinsulin which modulate proliferation, apoptosis, and tissue repair. IGF-I and IGF-II combine with one of six binding proteins (usually IGFBP3). Several studies have demonstrated that elevated serum levels of IGF-I are associated with a higher risk of prostate cancer. The relative impact of the IGF axis on prostate cancer development or detection is currently unclear.

5. Inflammation. A growing body of investigation suggests that chronic inflammatory processes may play a role in the pathogenesis of prostate cancer. A pathway from normal tissue to proliferative inflammatory atrophy (PIA), to prostatic intraepithelial neoplasia (PIN), with resultant invasive prostate cancer has been proposed.

E. Pathology

The proposed pathway from inflammatory atrophy to invasive disease is a working hypothesis under investigation. Evidence for high-grade PIN as a precursor of invasive disease has grown stronger with further genetic and biochemical research. PIN is the proliferation of the acinar epithelium and high-grade PIN is associated with the detection of prostate cancer in 20–40% of repeat needle biopsies. Although the natural history of this condition is incompletely defined, patients with high-grade PIN have a 30–50% chance of developing overt prostate cancer over 5 to 10 years.

1. Adenocarcinoma. The majority of prostate tumors are adenocarcinoma, which develops from the acinar glands. The majority of these arise from the peripheral zone of the prostate gland, yet up to 25% may originate in the central gland from the central and transitional zones.

2. Mucinous variant. If more than 25% of the representative tissue has mucin-containing glands, this designation may be given. It is purported to have an equal or worse outcome than classic adenocarcinoma.

3. Signet cell carcinoma. Another adenovariant with rapid progression and poor prognosis.
4. Endometrioid or ductal carcinoma. A variant that usually presents at advanced stage with papillary-like growth. Generally poor prognosis.
5. Small cell carcinoma. Neuroendocrine variant of prostate carcinoma. They often present with normal PSA values. Although general prognosis is poor, they may respond to platinum based therapy.
6. Transitional cell carcinoma (TCC) may arise from the distal prostatic ducts. It is usually manifest as an extension of primary bladder cancer. Stromal invasion carries a poorer prognosis than ductal infiltration.
7. Prostate sarcoma. Very rare tumors. Generally designated as leiomyosarcomas. Recent data demonstrate c-kit positive staining in several cases suggesting potential therapy with Gleevac.
8. Hematologic malignancies. Leukemia and lymphoma variants are rare.
9. Metastases. Malignant melanoma, colorectal carcinoma, and pulmonary metastases have been documented.

F. Grading and Staging System

1. The Gleason grading system has emerged as the standard grading nomenclature for prostate cancer over the past several years. It is a system based on the glandular structure of the tumor graded from 1 to 5. When tumors were diagnosed as incidental findings after transurethral resection of prostate (TURP), lower grade designations were commonly assigned. Contemporarily, needle biopsy specimens and surgical specimens are usually assigned a grade from 3 to 5. The two most common patterns are added together to provide a Gleason score with the grade of the most predominant tumor listed first. This provides stratification of score 7 lesions as 3+4 or 4+3, which can have some prognostic implications.
2. Staging is generally designated by the TMN system (Tables 15-1 and 15-2). This provides a general description of tumor extent, yet may not fully represent the degree of tumor volume or the significance or insignificance of microscopic tumor extension beyond the prostatic capsule. Oftentimes the designation of organ confinement, extracapsular extension, and the degree of margin positivity, with some sense of the overall tumor volume, better describes lesions that are similar yet might be categorized more divergently.

TNM 2002	Histologic Description
Tis	Carcinoma in situ
Ta	Epithelial confined, usually papillary
T1	Invading lamina propria
T2a,b	Invasion of the muscularis propria:
	2A: superficial invasion
	2B: deep invasion
T3a,b	Perivesical fat invasion:
	3A: microscopically
	3B: macroscopically
T4a,b	Invasion of contiguous organs:
	4A: prostate, vagina, uterus
	4B: pelvic sidewall, abdominal wall
N0	No lymph node involvement
N1	Single ≤2 cm
N2	Single >2 cm, ≤5 cm
	Multiple ≤5 cm
N3	Single or multiple >5 cm
M0	No distant metastases
M1	Distant metastases

Table 15-1: TNM Classification

G. Signs and Symptoms

This disease has few dramatic primary signs or symptoms. It may be associated with urinary obstructive symptoms or hematuria, although these findings are usually due to other causes. Bone pain can unfortunately be an initial symptom, but it represents very late disease. A nodule on the prostate or induration of the gland is a hallmark sign on physical examination. It is not always specific for a carcinoma and can underestimate the extent of disease when it does represent a carcinoma

H. Natural History

1. Until recently the natural history of prostate cancer, especially for earlier stage disease, has been difficult to discern. Several longitudinal studies and clinical trials have provided greater information in that regard. Information regarding high-grade PIN continues to accrue and suggests that there is a progression rate from this entity to clinical cancer in a reasonable number of patients.

Table 15-2:	TNM Definitions
TNM 2002	**Definitions**
T1	Tumor an incidental histologic finding
T1a	<3 chips
	<5% of tissue resected
	Tumor an incidental histologic finding
T1b	>3 chips
	>5% of tissue resected
T1c	Tumor identified by needle biopsy (e.g., for elevated serum PSA)
T2	Tumor confined within the prostate
T2a	Tumor involves half of a lobe or less
T2b	Tumor involves more than half of a lobe but not both lobes
T2c	Tumor involves both lobes
T3	Tumor extends through and beyond the prostate capsule
T3a	Unilateral extracapsular extension
T3b	Bilateral extracapsular extension
T3c	Tumor invades seminal vesicle(s)
T4	Tumor is fixed or invades adjacent structures other than seminal vesicles

PSA, prostate-specific antigen.

2. The data from the Connecticut tumor registry provide reasonable information for natural history and depict significantly worse outcomes in those individuals with higher Gleason scores.
3. Follow-up from Scandinavian patient cohorts suggest that 40% of patients with localized disease demonstrate progression over this time and a cancer-related mortality of 16% is noted in all patients with a 22% mortality in those diagnosed younger than the age of 70 years.
4. In a study of active observation vs. surgery, 14.4% of men in the observation group died of prostate cancer during a median period of 8.2 years. Nearly 25% of the men in the observation group developed metastasis during that time.
5. In patients with classic metastatic bone disease, the median survival is 27–33 months. Mortality is 75% at 5 years and 90% at 10 years. Recent data suggest that androgen independent prostate cancer in the presence of metastatic disease has a median survival of 16 months.

I. Diagnosis and Staging/PSA Screening

1. Digital rectal examination (DRE). This is a classic component of the physical examination that, by itself, is not as sensitive or specific for prostate cancer as one might think. Any palpable irregularity has an approximately 50% chance of being a carcinoma. Conversely, a normal DRE does not exclude the possibility of prostate cancer.

2. Transrectal ultrasound (TRUS). Multiple studies have demonstrated that TRUS is sensitive yet not specific for the detection of prostate cancer. The classic finding is a hypoechoic lesion that in general has a 30% chance of being positive for carcinoma. Prostate cancer can also present as a isoechoic or hyperechoic lesion. The most important use of TRUS is in aiding transrectal guided needle biopsies of the prostate gland.

3. Serum markers. The classic marker for prostate cancer was acid phosphatase. The enzymatic test was elevated in 70% of patients with extracapsular and metastatic prostate cancer. The more sensitive radioimmunoassay of this enzyme is not as useful for detecting extracapsular disease and has no value as a screening test for prostate cancer. PSA is the most useful marker in the detection and monitoring of prostate cancer and is discussed in detail separately.

4. Prostate needle biopsy. Spring-loaded gun is used to obtain prostate needle biopsy cores. Contemporarily 10–12 cores of tissue are obtained. The procedure is well tolerated with the major side effect being prolonged hematospermia; hematochezia and sepsis are rare. The percentage of positive cores, line length, or line percentage of cancer per core can provide further predictive information with regard to staging and outcomes. In difficult diagnostic cases, saturation biopsies in which 20–30 cores of tissue may be sampled at one time under anesthesia may be performed.

5. Bone scan. Before a lesion can be seen on a conventional radiograph, it must have replaced bone mass by 30–50% and be 10–15 mm in diameter. Plain film correlates of suspicious areas are often obtained. In some cases dedicated magnetic resonance imaging (MRI) or computed tomography (CT) imaging can resolve equivocal cases. Patients with a PSA value less than 10 ng/mL rarely demonstrate metastases.

6. CT/MRI. CT scans of the pelvis have poor performance characteristics for assessing metastatic disease and are not part of standard staging. Body coil MRI is performed

similarly. Endorectal MRI may provide additional staging information in those patients with intermediate PSAs, and greater than 50% are positive needle core biopsies. Additionally, data obtained by MRI spectroscopy may provide further information regarding the location and nature of malignant lesions.

7. PSA

    a) Biochemical characteristics. PSA is a 240 amino acid single chain glycoprotein that has a molecular weight of 34 kD. It is coded on chromosome 19 (6 Kb: 4 introns, 5 exons) and is homologous to members of the kallikrein gene superfamily and is designated human kallikrein3 (hK3). It is as a serine protease.

    b) Physiology. PSA liquefies the seminal coagulum that is formed after ejaculation. A substrate produced in the seminal vesicles has been identified. PSA has chymotrypsin- and trypsin-like activity. The half-life of PSA is 2.2–3.2 days.

    c) Marker properties. The generally used monoclonal assay (two murine MAbs for two specific epitopes) suggests a normal value of 4.0 ng/mL in serum. Serum values are not generally altered by DRE but can be affected by recumbency, urologic instrumentation, ejaculation, and prostate biopsy. Nonmalignant conditions that affect PSA levels include prostatitis, prostate infarction, and benign prostatic hypertrophy (BPH).

    d) General clinical use. The principle use of PSA is in disease detection. The most specific use for PSA is the monitoring of patients after radical prostatectomy. Postoperative baseline values should be in the undetectable range. Residual disease is suggested by any detectable postoperative levels, and values greater than 0.4 ng/mL suggest biochemical failure of therapy. It is also used to monitor the response to radiation therapy.

8. Screening and disease detection.

    a) The major goal of any screening strategy is to decrease the number of deaths caused by that particular cancer. Technically, screening is the evaluation of asymptomatic subjects. PSA determinations are used as part of the overall evaluation of urology patients and represents an effort at disease detection in populations that may be at greater risk for disease. Because of the long time to progression and death from prostate cancer, it is not known whether present screening strategies are absolutely effective. The continuing decrease in the prostate cancer death rate and stage shift in disease is indirect positive proof for the value of early disease detection.

b) DRE (base screening) demonstrated that more than two thirds of patients had extraprostatic tumor at the time of surgery; therefore, any tumor marker had a fairly low threshold to exceed to prove some value in disease detection.

c) Using a threshold of 4.0 ng/mL, 5–8% of a screening population will demonstrate an abnormal PSA. A serum PSA between 4 to 10 ng/mL suggests a 16–30% chance of a positive needle biopsy. A serum PSA greater than 10 ng/mL is associated with a 67% chance of a positive biopsy. In general 1–5% of participants of a screening trial are found to have cancer (significantly lower than the incidental pathologic incidence). Lowering the threshold for biopsy to 2.5 ng/mL can aid in the further detection of significant disease especially in younger patients, those with family histories of prostate cancer, and African-American patients. Research indicates there is no absolute lower "normal" value for PSA with regard to disease detection, yet the number of negative evaluations will increase significantly in these ranges.

d) PSA velocity. Several studies suggest that if serum PSA increases greater than 0.75 ng/mL/year the potential for prostate cancer is greater. Unfortunately PSA variability can be as high as 25% per reading; therefore, three separate readings several months apart are necessary to establish a true trend. Even so, relatively abrupt rises in PSA within the usual "normal" ranges warrant an evaluation. Furthermore, PSA kinetics (PSA rise of greater than 2.0 ng/mL) prior to surgery can predict disease-related mortality.

e) The American Cancer Society, AUA, and ARS now recommend that a serum PSA and DRE be performed yearly in men older than the age of 50 in the context of a physician-patient dialogue. Confirmation of this recommendation as an effective screening tool is pending. African-Americans and individuals with a family history of prostate cancer may benefit from detection strategies starting at age 40. Other government agencies and professional societies do not recommend screening at this time.

f) Other PSA species. Free PSA is an isoform that does not bind to other serum proteins and provides information with regard to the potential for a cancer diagnosis when the PSA is elevated. When the free PSA fraction of the total PSA is greater than 25%, the potential for an abnormal value between 4 to 10 ng/mL to indicate cancer is as low as 5–7%. Conversely, free PSA values below 10% suggest a significant potential that the abnormal total PSA value represents cancer. Similar information can be obtained by measuring the complex PSA, which is the PSA isoform that binds to proteins. Other cleaved forms of free PSA such as BPSA and proPSA are being evaluated for their ability to refine cancer detection.

g) Other markers. Markers such as early prostate cancer antigen (EPCA 1 and 2) are being evaluated for potential superior operational characteristics to PSA. Ongoing research using DNA microarrays have demonstrated the consistent up-regulation of several genes such as Hepsin and AMACR (α-methylacyl-CoA). The gene EZH2 has also been identified as a potential marker to distinguish metastatic from local cancer. Additionally, work in proteomics and antibody arrays suggests the potential to demonstrate novel marker approaches to disease detection and monitoring.

J. Cancer Prevention

1. General considerations. Because prostate cancer is relatively common, chemoprevention strategies for this disease are reasonable. However, because such therapies are delivered to large groups of cancer-free subjects, toxicity must be extremely low or nonexistent. Estimates for the number of patients requiring treatment to prevent one case of cancer demonstrate the broad range of such therapies. Given the incidence of prostate cancer in the United States, 500 men would have to be treated with an agent that could reduce cancer of the prostate by 50% to avoid one cancer. Chemoprevention strategies may therefore require additional considerations such as a focus toward higher risk populations.

2. 5α-reductase inhibition. A major phase III chemoprevention trial, the Prostate Cancer Prevention Trial (PCPT), demonstrated a 24.8% reduction in period prevalence of prostate cancer in patients using 5 mg of finasteride (type II) daily compared to placebo. However, the prevalence of higher grade prostate cancer was 25% higher (6.4 versus 5.1%), dampening this overall positive result. The reasons for this increase in higher grade disease remain to be fully explained but may in part be due to the unmasking effect

of finasteride to shrink the prostate and make small volume, higher grade disease accessible to biopsy. The REDUCE trial using dutasteride, a type I and type II 5α-reductase, is in progress.

3. Toremifene. This agent is a synthetic estrogen receptor modulator (SERM) that in phase IIb/III trials demonstrated the ability to reduce the progression of those patients with high-grade PIN to prostate cancer by 22%. It is currently being studied in a larger phase III trial.

4. Selenium and vitamin E. In large phase III chemoprevention trials targeting other primary tumors, a secondary endpoint analysis demonstrated that selenium reduced the incidence of prostate cancer by 63% in a study targeting skin cancer, and vitamin E reduced prostate cancer by 32% in a lung cancer study. This provided the basis of the SELECT trial, which is ongoing and evaluating the chemopreventative effect of these agents alone or in combination on prostate cancer.

5. Lycopene. This agent is a water-soluble antioxidant. There are several lines of evidence, but there is no conclusive proof that it may have an impact on prostate cancer chemoprevention.

6. Anti-inflammatory agents. General nonsteroidal anti-inflammatory drugs (NSAIDs) and cyclo-oxygenase (COX)-2 inhibitors demonstrate antiprostate cancer activity in the laboratory but are not under current consideration for study as chemopreventative agents due to their additional side effects.

7. Soy and other isoflavones. The components of soy may have anticancer properties, and epidemiologic studies support the potential for risk reduction by the inclusion of these substances in the diet.

K. Outcome Prognosis and Stratification

Several statistical approaches to the stratification of patients with regard to outcomes based on clinical data have been developed. Approaches using multiple regression analysis, nomograms (Figure 15-1), and neural networks have been employed for several different scenarios for prostate cancer. Hybrids of these methods have also been tested. In general the correlation of these models to individual outcomes is in the 0.7 to 0.75 range. Nomogram strategies may provide more individualized information. All of these methods may be useful in better directing patient choices and the use of additional therapies in the future.

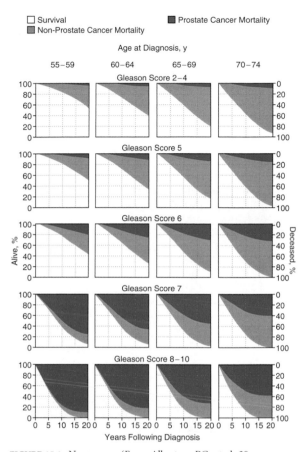

FIGURE 15-1. Nonogram. (From Albertsen PC, et al: 20-year outcomes following conservative management of clinically localized prostate cancer. *JAMA* 293[17]:2095–2101, 2005.)

L. Treatment of Localized Disease

1. General considerations. In discussing treatment for prostate cancer it is important to consider patient factors such as age and general performance status as well as tumor factors such as Gleason score, initial serum PSA, and estimated clinical volumes/stage of the tumor. If a patient has less than a 50% chance for surviving 10 years due to other comorbidities, it is difficult to measure the positive effect of treatment. Patient tolerance for the side

effects of different therapies also has to be considered. It is best when patients come to a treatment decision based on consultation and input from both surgical and radiation oncology services. The stage shift in tumors due to PSA detection strategies has resulted in 5-year disease-free survival in active therapies of nearly 100%.

2. Active observation/watchful waiting. This approach has generally been reserved for men with significant comorbidities that limit their overall survival and those unwilling to consider other forms of treatment. Recent 8-year follow-up on a trial of surgery versus watchful waiting demonstrated advantages to metastasis rate (10% risk reduction), disease-specific survival (5.3% reduction), and overall survival at 10 years (5% reduction). These findings were more pronounced in patients younger than the age of 65 years.

   With the significant stage shift in prostate cancer, however, smaller potential volumes of disease are being detected, and in those individuals with low-volume moderate-grade disease based on percent positive needle biopsy cores, trials of watchful waiting are demonstrating good 5-year disease-free survival.

3. Radical prostatectomy. This is an appropriate treatment choice for younger patients as well as older patients who are very fit and desire this form of treatment. Generally, a chronologic age of 70 is used as a relative cutoff point, but decisions need to be individualized. Surgical mortality is less than 0.2% but 1–2% of patients may experience a pulmonary embolus or deep vein thrombosis. Surgical approaches include a retropubic or perineal approach. Laparoscopic and robotic approaches have been developed and are described elsewhere in this manual. Urinary incontinence may occur in 2–10% of patients. The potential for erectile dysfunction can be decreased with surgical approaches that spare the cavernosal nerves. A bladder neck contracture can occur in 2–3% of patients. Disease-specific survival is in the 95% range over 10 years.

4. Radiation therapy
   a) External beam radiation therapy. This is an option for localized prostate cancer and is the treatment of choice for T3 disease. This modality is discussed in greater depth in Chapter X. Significant technical advances such as conformal radiation and intensity modulated radiation therapy (IMRT) have allowed for the increase in dose intensity yet a decrease in overall side effects. In general, it is administered in

divided doses ranging from 70 to 80 Gy and is well tolerated. Approximately 3–5% of patients will experience persistent rectal or bladder symptomatology; greater than 60% of patients develop erectile dysfunction within 2 years. Hematuria or hemorrhagic cystitis is a late development in a small percentage of patients.

b) Interstitial brachytherapy. Ultrasound guided transperineal brachytherapy has become an accepted modality for the treatment of localized prostate cancer. Optimal candidates have a serum PSA of less than 10 ng/mL and a Gleason score of 6 or lower. It is difficult to treat large prostate glands (greater than 50 cm^3) with this technique. Intermediate term results (10 years) suggest similar outcomes to surgery or external beam radiation therapy in selected patients. ^{125}I or ^{103}Pd are the usual radiation sources. The principle urologic side effect is voiding dysfunction, which is usually short term but may be persistent. Those individuals with high ISSP scores should not be considered for this technique.

5. Cryosurgical ablation of the prostate. This technique has undergone multiple modifications and is currently performed with small-caliber needles using freeze-thaw cycles employing argon and helium gas. More recent series show less morbidity and a decrease in chronic pelvic pain noted in early reports.

6. High intensity focused ultrasound (HIFU). HIFU is currently under investigation for treatment of localized disease. Early data demonstrate feasibility yet data on intermediate- and long-term outcomes and side effects are pending.

7. Post treatment follow-up. Serum PSA is the single most important follow-up parameter in evaluating post treatment patients with either surgery or radiation.

a) In surgery patients, the serum PSA should nadir to an undetectable level. Occasionally very low persistent PSA findings that do not progress are noted. In most cases, if the serum PSA becomes detectable and rises above 0.4 ng/mL, the patient continues to show disease progression. Biochemical failure can predate clinical failure by 4–6 years. Newer data suggest that biochemical failure is a surrogate marker for ultimate clinical failure and survival. Outcomes are heterogenic. Patients with high-grade disease who fail early and display a short doubling time may have a survival as short as 7 years, whereas patients who are late failures with lower moderate grade disease who are progressing slowly may live as long as 19 years. Further follow-up is necessary to clearly define the true impact of biochemical failure.

b) In general, response to radiation therapy is predicated on the pretreatment PSA and can be predicted by the post treatment PSA. The closer to an undetectable value post treatment the better the overall outcome. Nadir values of 4.0 ng/mL or less generally demonstrate treatment failure.

c) There is a role for radiation therapy after post surgical biochemical failures. Success is best when therapy is instituted before the PSA is greater than 1.0 ng/mL. Percentage for cure ranges between 30 and 50% in different series. Salvage surgery can be employed in radiation therapy failures. The major side effect is significant incontinence in more than 50% of patients.

M. Treatment of Biochemical and Clinical Failure

1. In general, 25% of patients will experience a PSA recurrence in 10 years after local therapy. The exact definition of recurrence and the clinical significance of these outcomes have become somewhat clearer in the past several years. The yearly incidence of such patients in the United States is 50,000.

2. PSA failure in surgery. This definition ranges from any detectable PSA to 0.4 ng/mL. Low, stable detection of PSA may occur in postoperative patients and is often attributed to persistent benign tissue. Once the PSA value rises above 0.4 ng/mL, it rarely recedes. This value is therefore considered an absolute threshold for biochemical failure.

3. PSA failure in radiation patients. A strong definition for these patients has been more difficult to define due to the persistence of PSA detection after therapy and the kinetics involved in defining true progression from variations about a mean value. Nadir value plus two consecutive rises is the current operational definition, yet other definitions may be employed in the future.

4. Significance of biochemical failure. A rough guide to PSA failure in surgery patients suggests that there is approximately 8 years from biochemical failure to clinical failure, and 5 years from that point to cancer-related death. This could be stratified by time to failure from surgery, initial PSA and Gleason score of the tumor, and PSA doubling time. The range of values was from 7 to 19 years. Recent

analysis places significant import on PSA doubling times, with a doubling time of 3 months as a surrogate marker for cancer-related death. This was noted in approximately 12% of surgery patients and 20% of radiation patients. A more recent analysis based on the stratification of time to failure (greater or less than 3 years), less or greater than Gleason score 8 cancer, and a PSA doubling time ranging from 3 to 15 months could separate out patients with a 2–99% chance of experiencing a prostate cancer related death.

5. Treatment for biochemical failure.
   a) Watchful waiting for late recurrence, slow velocity, long doubling time tumors.
   b) Salvage radiation therapy for surgery patients; 90% response and 70% sustained response for patients treated for an absolute PSA at or below 1.5 ng/mL.
   c) Androgen blockade for radiation patients with persistently rising PSA.

N. Treatment of Advanced Disease

Patients with metastatic prostate cancer are initially treated with androgen ablation therapy. This can be accomplished with gonadotropin releasing hormone (GnRH) agonists, bilateral orchiectomy, and more recently GnRH antagonists. Diethylstilbestrol (DES) is no longer used due to increased cardiovascular risk associated with this agent. Present controversies being addressed in ongoing clinical trials include (1) early versus delayed androgen ablation and (2) intermittent versus continuous androgen ablation. Toxicities of androgen ablation therapy include hot flashes, loss of libido, impotency, muscular atrophy, and osteopenia/osteoporosis.

Antiandrogens block the intracytoplasmic androgen receptor. Multiple trials have compared castration alone to castration plus an antiandrogen (termed total or maximal androgen blockade). Meta-analysis demonstrated that total androgen blockade is associated with a very small survival advantage at 5 years. However, the antiandrogens may cause toxicity (gastrointestinal [GI], liver) and are very expensive. Patients with a rising PSA on total androgen blockade may respond to withdrawal of the antiandrogen. Ketoconazole suppresses production of adrenal steroids and may be helpful in some patients who progress despite castration.

Patients with metastatic disease who progress despite castration have hormone-refractory disease (also called androgen-independent or castrate metastatic). Options for these HRPC patients include systemic chemotherapy, palliative external beam radiation therapy to treat painful bone metastases, and radionuclide therapy for control of more diffuse skeletal pain.

For years, systemic chemotherapy was believed to be ineffective for prostate cancer. A randomized trial comparing mitoxantrone/prednisone to prednisone alone demonstrated improved pain scores in men with HRPC and painful bone metastases resulting in mitoxantrone/prednisone being approved by the Food and Drug Administration (FDA). A more recent randomized trial compared docetaxel/prednisone to mitoxantrone/prednisone in men with HRPC. This trial demonstrated a survival advantage to docetaxel/prednisone, leading to FDA approval as the standard chemotherapy regimen for first-line HRPC.

The utilization of systemic chemotherapy in the early disease setting continues to be investigated but a role has not yet been established.

Experimental approaches being developed for HRPC include novel cytotoxics, vaccine based therapies, angiogenesis inhibitors, and targeted therapy.

Role of bisphosphonates. HRPC patients with bone metastases are at increased risk of skeletal complications including pathologic fracture and bone pain. A randomized trial demonstrated that administration of the biphosphate zoledronic acid decreases the risk of skeletal complications in men with progressive HRPC and bone metastases compared to placebo.

An important complication of androgen ablation therapy is osteopenia/osteoporosis. Some advocate that baseline DEXA scan be obtained prior to initiating androgen ablation therapy in hormone-naïve patients. Studies have demonstrated that bisphosphonate therapy can prevent the loss of bone mineral density in these patients. However, studies have not yet demonstrated that this treatment decreases the skeletal complication rate in these patients.

Important morbidity associated with bisphosphonate therapy includes renal toxicity and osteonecrosis of the jaw.

II. CARCINOMA OF THE BLADDER

A. General Considerations

Bladder cancer is the second most common urologic malignancy. The majority of cases are TCC histology, and 65–75% of new cases are Ta (mucosal only), T1 (lamina propria invasion), or carcinoma in situ (CIS) (flat, noninvasive). These lesions were previously grouped as "superficial" tumors, but their distinct biology warrants the stratification of these lesions. The remainder are muscle-invasive tumors. Transurethral resection of these lesions is the principle form of diagnosis and therapy for bladder cancer. Non-muscle invasive lesions may be treated with intravesical chemotherapy, which is most effective when administered immediately after tumor resection. Recurrent Ta, initial T1, and CIS lesions may be treated with bacille Calmette-Guérin (BCG) intravesical immunotherapy, which can decrease tumor recurrence and reduce tumor progression. Muscle-invasive disease and treatment-resistant T1 and CIS lesions are best treated with radical cystectomy and some form of urinary diversion. Combined chemotherapy and radiation approaches are useful in select patients and those who cannot tolerate surgery. Advanced disease responds to platinum and paclitaxel-based chemotherapy regimens, but sustained complete responses are rare.

B. Epidemiology

In the United States there are more than 60,000 new cases of bladder cancer yearly with approximately 13,000 cancer deaths. Bladder cancer accounts for approximately 5–8% of male cancers and is the fourth most common cancer in men. It accounts for 2% of female cancers (eighth most common) and that percentage is rising. Bladder cancer is the ninth most frequent cancer worldwide with a yearly incidence of 356,000 new cases and a worldwide prevalence (5 year) of 1.1 million (U.S. estimate 500,000). Over the past 15 years, a 40% increase in the incidence of bladder cancer has been observed in the United States.

It is three to four times more common in women, and disease risk is half as common in African-Americans. Survival among women and African-Americans appears to be worse than in white men.

C. Etiology

1. Tobacco exposure. Tobacco use confers a two- to three-fold increased risk of developing bladder cancer. The polycyclic aromatic hydrocarbon, 4-aminobiphenyl, has been suggested as the most significant carcinogen in tobacco. Latency is approximately 20 years and risk reduction does occur with smoking cessation.
2. Industrial exposure. The first link of industrial exposure and cancer was made between bladder cancer and aniline dyes. Textile printing and rubber manufacturing have

also been established with this tumor. 2-Naphtylamine, 4-aminobiphenyl, and 4-nitrobiphenyl are major carcinogens found in such environments.

3. Chemotherapy. Cyclophosphamide and ifosfamide have been associated with the development of bladder cancer. The presence or absence of hemorrhagic cystitis is not associated with the likelihood of developing cancer. The use of reducing agents (mesna), hydration, and catheter drainage during therapy have probably decreased the development of cancer with these agents.

4. *Schistosoma haematobium.* Infection is common in many areas of North Africa and the deposition of ova in the bladder lead to inflammation and the development of carcinoma. Inflammation in the presence of nitrites from bacterial activity is also implicated. Additionally heavy tobacco use is endemic in these areas as well as exposure to nitrate-containing fertilizers. The majority of these tumors are squamous carcinoma.

5. Chronic irritation and infection. Chronic infection carries a slightly increased risk of developing bladder cancer, and those patients with a chronic indwelling Foley catheter have a 10- to 20-fold increase in developing bladder cancer (primarily squamous). Premalignant changes can be noted after a few years, and yearly cystoscopic evaluations are recommended.

6. Genetic predisposition. Differences in metabolism of toxins rather than germline mutations play a role. N acetyl transferase 2 (slow acetylators), glutathione S transferase M1 homozygous deletions, and *CYP 2A1* expression all add to risk.

7. Pelvic irradiation. This is associated with an approximate 10% increased risk of developing bladder cancer. Newer methods of conformal radiation may lessen the risk to non-target organs.

8. Additional risks. Arsenic in the water supply, the ingestion of the Chinese herb *Aristolochia fangchi,* and ingestion of ochratoxin A (in Bracken fern) may also contribute to the development of bladder tumors. Ingestion of phenacetin is associated with the development of upper urinary tract TCC.

D. Pathology

1. Normal urothelium demonstrates basal, intermediate, and superficial cells. There are usually seven cell layers.

2. Hyperplasia is generally described as thickened mucosa without cellular atypia.

3. Urothelial dysplasia. Preneoplastic changes in the basal and intermediate layers with the presence of cell cohesion, yet some architectural disruption. Progresses to frank neoplasia in 15–20% of cases.

4. CIS. Cytologically malignant flat lesion with prominent disorganization of cells. Loss of cell cohesion. Loss of cellular polarity and coarse chromatin. Pagetoid, small cell, and large cell variants have been described.

5. Urothelial papilloma. A benign exophytic neoplasia with normal appearing urothelium on a fibrovascular core. Usually appear as solitary lesions. Inverted papilloma growth variant also exists.

6. Papillary urothelial neoplasm of low malignant potential (PUNLMP). Similar to papilloma yet with increased cellularity. Associated with greater propensity for recurrence progression and rare mortality.

7. Papillary urothelial neoplasm low grade. Papillary morphology with variable architecture and mitoses at all levels. Altered CK20 expression FGFR3 mutations in 80% of cases.

8. Papillary urothelial neoplasm high grade. Marked architectural disorder with papillary fusion and variable cell number thickness. Demonstrate significantly more molecular alterations.

9. Stromal invasion (T1). Tumor invades the lamina propria but not the muscularis propria. Attempts at subdivision have been made with regard to depth of lesion, vascular invasion, and muscularis mucosa involvement.

10. Invasive urothelial carcinoma. Tumor invasion into true muscularis propria. Almost exclusively high grade. Tumor front may be "pushing" or tentacular.

11. Squamous carcinoma. Uncommon cancer (3–7%). Distinct from squamous metaplasia. Associated with chronic irritation or schistosomiasis. Greater tendency for local recurrence when treated.

12. Adenocarcinoma. Rare tumor (1–2%). Associated with urachal carcinoma at the bladder dome. Necessary to rule out GI tract or breast metastases before designating it as a primary tumor.

13. Small cell carcinoma. Neuroendocrine origin. Highly aggressive with presentation at high pathologic stage. Responds poorly to any therapy.

14. Micropapillary carcinoma. Aggressive variant of bladder cancer that resembles papillary serous carcinoma of the ovary. Noninvasive and invasive presentations have been reported.

E. Grading and Staging System

1. Tumor grading was codified by the 1973 World Health Organization (WHO) system of urothelial papilloma and grade 1 to 3 designations for progressive cell abnormality. The WHO/ISUP classification originally proposed in 1998 segregates PUNLMP from papilloma and low-grade lesions. Hybrid classifications have also been used.
2. Staging is currently best achieved with the TNM classification, which subdivides the different levels of muscle invasion and extravesical extension.

F. Natural History

The natural history of bladder tumors with regard to recurrence and progression is closely related to the stage and grade of the lesion. The distinct classifications of noninvasive tumors as opposed to lumping them as superficial lesions demonstrate these differences.

1. Low-Grade Ta Lesions

a) Noninvasive low-grade lesions account for 25–50% of bladder tumors. Those lesions defined as PUNLMP demonstrate a recurrence rate of 30–50%, but with 5- to 10-year follow-up no episodes of progression are noted. In low-grade lesions, tumor multiplicity, recurrence at 3-month cystoscopy, and tumor size greater than 3 cm are factors favoring recurrence.
b) In G1Ta lesions there is a 16–25% rate of grade progression with a stage progression to muscle invasion of 2–3%.

2. High-Grade Ta Lesions

a) These lesions account for 3–18% of most series with an average incidence of 6%. This is a difficult tumor to distinguish pathologically and on comparative review many of these lesions (up to three fourths) are restaged as T1 lesions.
b) These lesions demonstrate a 20–25% risk of tumor stage progression.

3. CIS

a) These lesions account for 5–10% of all superficial bladder cancer and by definition are high-grade tumors.
b) A suggestion of clinical subtypes has been made: primary disease, secondary CIS (detected after prior papillary

disease), and concurrent CIS (CIS in the presence of papillary tumors). Primary disease accounts for 30% of cases, secondary 42%, and concurrent 28% of cases. The distinction of primary asymptomatic unifocal CIS and symptomatic multifocal primary CIS has also been advanced.

c) Overall, 54% of patients with CIS progress to muscle-invasive disease. Concurrent CIS has the highest (60%) progression rate to T1 disease and primary CIS the lowest (8–28%).

d) Asymptomatic patients account for 25% of patients, whereas 40–75% of patients will have irritative bladder symptoms.

4. T1 Bladder Tumors

a) T1 lesions comprise 25–30% of superficial bladder tumors. They will recur in up to 80% of cases and demonstrate tumor progression in 20–50% of cases. Those with deep invasion to the layer of the muscularis mucosa have a more aggressive history with a progression rate of 40% and 5-year survival of 50%.

b) Rebiopsy of T1 lesions can result in upstaging of the initial lesion in 30–60% of cases. This is especially the case when no muscle is noted on the initial biopsy. Persistent tumor on repeat biopsy can also be a poor prognostic indicator for response to therapy.

5. Muscle-Invasive Disease

Patients with muscle-invasive disease demonstrate stage progression and tumor metastases to lymph nodes, lung, liver, and bone. The majority of untreated patients (80–90%) will demonstrate a cancer-related death in 2–3 years.

G. Signs and Symptoms

1. The most common symptom of bladder cancer is microscopic or gross hematuria followed by irritative bladder symptoms. Bladder masses can also be found as incidental findings on imaging examinations or as incidental findings during a cystoscopic examination.

2. Hematuria in some form is noted in 85% of cases of bladder cancer. Bladder masses on imaging can represent stones or polypoid cystis. Additionally, the absence of a mass on imaging does not rule out the presence of a

bladder tumor, which may not be detected due to tumor size or incomplete filling of the bladder.

H. Diagnosis of Bladder Cancer

1. The evaluation of a suspected bladder mass should consist of an imaging exam, visual inspection of the urothelium, and cytologic evaluation of the urine. A role for protein-based or genomic-based tumor markers is also developing for diagnosis of this condition.
2. The classic imaging modality for the urinary tract has been the intravenous urogram (pyelogram). With improvements in technology, the CT urogram and MR urogram have become very popular. Ultrasound resolution is too low to discern small upper tract lesions or many bladder lesions and does not evaluate the ureters. In the case of renal insufficiency, an ultrasound can evaluate the renal parenchyma and the urinary tract can be evaluated with retrograde pyelograms and cystoscopy.
3. Urinary cytology. This cellular evaluation has poor overall sensitivity yet is very specific for high-grade disease and CIS. Although the performance characteristics are rather poor for low-grade, low-stage lesions, high-grade tumors and CIS, which may not be easily seen on cystoscopy, can be detected with a sensitivity in the 80% range and a specificity of 90–95%.
4. Cystoscopy. Endoscopic evaluation of the urothelium can be carried out by rigid or flexible optical scopes that allow one to examine the urethra, prostatic fossa, and bladder lining. It is the "gold standard" for the evaluation of the urinary tract lining; however, it is not 100% accurate. Small tumors and areas of CIS may be missed on exam. Enhanced imaging with fluorescent imaging may improve detection and is currently being evaluated.

I. Disease Screening and Tumor Markers

1. Hematuria screening. There are no prospective studies that demonstrate a decrease in bladder cancer related deaths as a function of screening. Comparisons of screened and unscreened populations suggest a shift in the detection from T2 to high-grade noninvasive disease with serial dipstick hematuria screening. This suggests that high-risk populations such as male smokers older than 50 years may benefit from this activity.
2. Tumor markers. Several protein-based and genomic-based markers have been evaluated for their role in the

detection and surveillance of bladder cancer. A few have FDA approval for the monitoring of bladder cancer. In general, the protein markers have high sensitivity yet lack specificity as tumor markers. They are more sensitive than urine cytology for the detection of lower grade tumors and oftentimes less sensitive than cytology for high-grade disease or CIS. The performance of the protein-based markers can be degraded by inflammation and hematuria. False-positive tests create test anxiety but in some cases may detect disease before it is clinically evident. False-negative tests result in missed diagnosis and tumor progression. In general, these markers have the potential to make detection and monitoring of bladder cancer more precise, yet no marker has been definitively established in this role.

a) Protein-based markers.

 i) NMP22. This is a nuclear mitotic protein that is released in urine. It has been available as a laboratory test and now a point of contact test. A general cutoff value has been 10 U/mL, but different values have been used. The specificity ranges between 60 and 80% and the sensitivity ranges between 18 and 100%. It is approved as an aid in the diagnosis of patients at risk for bladder cancer and for disease monitoring.

 ii) BTA. This test detects a complement factor H-related protein and complement factor H. It exists as a point of contact test and a standard enzyme linked immunosorbent assay (ELISA). Sensitivity ranges from 10–90% and sensitivity is near 90% in healthy patients. This, however, is degraded by inflammation and hematuria to the 50% range. It is not useful for the detection of disease and is approved as an aid in managing bladder cancer.

 iii) Hyaluronic acid-hyaluronidase (HA-HAase). This test measures HA and HAase ELISA assays. It has an 83% sensitivity and 90% specificity in detecting bladder cancer. It appears to be less affected by inflammation or hematuria, and false-positive studies have a 10-fold risk of tumor recurrence within 5 months. It is yet to undergo multicenter trials.

 iv) ImmunoCyt. An immunocytologic evaluation of exfoliated cells with three antibodies. This test in conjunction with cytology has a combined sensitivity of 90% and specificity of 79%. This falls off, however, in patients with hematuria, cystitis, or BPH.

b) Genomic-based markers.
    i) UroVysion test, fluorescence in situ hybridization (FISH). A multitarget FISH assay that evaluates alterations in ploidy with three chromosome enumeration probes 3, 7, and 17 and one locus specific identifier 9p21 (p16 locus). Sensitivity is between 60 and 100% for low- to high-grade tumors and specificity is approximately 95%. It is approved for the detection and monitoring of bladder cancer.
    ii) Microsatellite analysis. This assay evaluates loss of heterozygosity at several loci in the genome. Sensitivity ranges between 72 and 97%. Specificity is high in healthy populations but may be altered in cystitis and BPH. No standardized set of markers is in use and prospective studies are in progress.

J. Clinical Staging and Imaging

1. Transurethral resection (TUR). TUR by the method of electrocautery is the classic method for initial treatment and staging of bladder tumors. A blended current of cutting and cautery is employed and an effort to resect the entire tumor with deep muscle biopsy is made. The potential for bladder perforation exists and generally may be treated by prolonged catheterization when extraperitoneal. Intraperitoneal perforation may require an open repair. Patients can demonstrate hematuria and irritative symptoms for several weeks after the procedure.
2. Random biopsies. The routine use of random biopsies has not been established, yet they can be useful in determining the extent of disease such as CIS and the presence of disease in sites such as the prostatic urethra. The have a greater role in higher grade and stage noninvasive lesions. It is less common to detect disease from normal-appearing areas of the bladder when low-grade Ta lesions are present.
3. CT scanning and MRI scanning do not provide precise information regarding clinical stage [invasive]. Sensitivity is in the 70–90% range with specificity in the similar range. Accuracy is in the 55–85% range. Operational characteristics for defining lymph node status is somewhat higher. These modalities are also useful for demonstrating the absence or presence of hydronephrosis.
4. Bimanual examination under anesthesia. This maneuver is still valuable in assessing the status of patients with muscle-invasive tumors and provides information with regard to tumor extent as well as pelvic or abdominal wall involvement.

K. Therapy in General

1. TUR

Surgical excision alone may be adequate in the treatment of low-grade Ta disease. Fulguration about the perimeter of resection and care in avoiding gross perforation enhance the effectiveness of this technique.

2. Laser Ablation of Bladder Tumors

An effective method of treating bladder lesions. Major drawback is the lack of pathologic specimen. Advantages for patients on anticoagulation therapy. Less pain and lack of obturator reflex. Neodymium:yttrium-aluminum-garnet (Nd:YAG) laser is popular for this purpose.

3. Intravesical Chemotherapy Instillation

a) General considerations. Cytotoxic chemotherapy agents have been administered within the bladder with the objective of eradicating existing tumors, preventing the recurrence of treated tumors, and possibly preventing or delaying tumor progression. The ideal agent would be nontoxic, be effective in a single dose, achieve the objectives listed previously, and be inexpensive. No such ideal agents exists, yet several agents demonstrate activity against noninvasive TCC lesions.

b) The summary analysis of multiple studies looking at the efficacy of chemotherapy demonstrates that in the short term these agents reduce recurrence by 14–17%. Over 3–5 years, this effect is reduced to approximately 7%. Several large series of intravesical chemotherapy with a median survival follow-up of nearly 8 years demonstrate that there is no advantage to inhibiting tumor progression with this form of therapy. Most of these data are compiled from six course administrations. Data evaluating combined or sequential chemotherapy generally demonstrate no therapeutic advantage but an increase in side effects. Some work on sequential mitomycin and gemcitabine suggests some potential synergy. Combined chemotherapy and immunotherapy have likewise shown additive value.

c) Immediate instillation of single dose therapy. The meta-analysis of seven clinical trials demonstrates that immediate instillation of a single dose of intravesical chemotherapy can decrease Ta and T1 tumor recurrence by approximately 39%. This was most effective in those patients with a single tumor, but it had some effect on patients with multiple lesions. The principle impact on recurrence occurred over the first 2 years. The mechanism is probably through an inhibition of tumor reimplantation after TUR. This form of therapy is contraindicated if a bladder perforation is noted during tumor resection. BCG cannot be used in this approach due to the possibility of intravascular inoculation and possible sepsis.

4. Optimization of Therapy

Attempts to optimize therapy include dehydration prior to instillation, alkalinization of urine, administration of small volumes of intravesical fluid, and maximum dwell times. Studies with mitomycin C suggest that this can improve time to recurrence and recurrence-free survival. Additionally, research is progressing with drug delivery enhanced by electromotive administration and thermotherapy.

5. Common Intravesical Chemotherapy Agents

a) Mitomycin C. An alkylating agent that inhibits DNA synthesis by cross-linking, it is cell cycle nonspecific. The molecular weight is 334 kD; therefore, there is negligible systemic absorption. The most frequent side effects are chemical cystitis in up to 40% of patients and palmar rash or other cutaneous symptoms in up to 10% of patients. It is usually administered as 40 mg in 40 mL of solution.

b) Doxorubicin. An anthracycline antibiotic that binds DNA base pairs and inhibits topoisomerase II as well as protein synthesis. It has a high molecular weight of 580 kD, and 25–50% of patients can develop chemical cystitis. The usual dose is 50 mg in 30 mL of solution with ranges reported from 30–100 mg.

c) Thiotepa. One of the first intravesical agents. It is an alkylating agent and is not cell cycle specific. At a molecular weight of 189 kD, it can be absorbed systemically causing thrombocytopenia in 3–13% of patients and leucopenia in –55% of patients. The usual dose is 30 mg in 15 mL of sterile water.

d) Valrubicin. A lipophilic, semisynthetic analogue of doxorubicin that demonstrates a 21% response in BCG refractory patients. It has been intermittently available.

e) Newer agents: gemcitabine and taxanes. Gemcitabine is a novel deoxycytidine analogue (2′,2′-difluoro-2′ deoxycytidine) that has shown single agent activity in advanced bladder cancer. The molecular weight is 299.7 kD. Dose range has been 1000–2000 mg. It is active in phase I and II trials and currently in phase III testing. Grade 1 hematologic complications have been noted in 5–15% of patients. In phase II testing, response rates have been greater than 50% in pretreated tumor populations. Early phase I data have been reported on the taxane paclitaxel, which has activity in advanced disease.

6. BCG Therapy

BCG is an attenuated strain of *Mycobacterium bovis* developed in 1921 and used as a tuberculosis vaccine. In 1976, BCG's efficacy against non-muscle invasive bladder cancer was demonstrated by Morales. Collective series demonstrate a 60–80% response rate against CIS, a 45–60% chance of eradicating residual papillary disease, and a 40% improvement over TUR alone for disease prophylaxis.

The exact mechanism of BCG action is incompletely understood. Direct cell contact is necessary and it appears that a TH1 immune pathway is predominant. Some activation of TH2 pathways are also seen as is nitric oxide synthetase (NOS) activity. Recruitment of polymorphonucleocytes to the area of inflammation may provide further cytotoxic agents for tumor cell killing.

Currently, there are no data to demonstrate the optimal schedule for BCG therapy. The most commonly accepted program has been designated the "6+3" program consisting of a 6-week induction therapy followed by three booster treatments at 6-month intervals anywhere from 2 to 3 years. Irritative side effects can be significant and limit the long-term application of this strategy.

BCG appears to be the only intravesical agent that can decrease tumor progression. This has been demonstrated in meta-analysis and is powered by those clinical series in which maintenance BCG in some form was administered. The persistence of this effect over the long term (10–15 years) is questionable. The effect of BCG on overall patient survival so far demonstrates no advantage.

BCG produces irritative bladder symptoms in 90% of patients. Other symptoms include hematuria, low-grade fever, malaise, and nausea. Treatment with isoniazid and fluoroquinolones may be required. Patients with high fever ($>$103°F/ 39.4°C) require hospitalization and treatment with isoniazid 300 mg and rifampin 600 mg. A fluoroquinolone may also be used. BCG sepsis is rare, occurring in early series in 0.4% of patients. Patients with sepsis are treated with isoniazid, rifampin, and ethambutol 1200 mg daily plus a fluoroquinolone. Steroid therapy may be added. Additionally, one should consider and cover for gram-negative sepsis. Severe side effects may be reduced by avoiding situations when direct intravascular absorption can be avoided such as traumatic catheterization, administration of BCG in the presence of an active urinary tract infection (UTI), or administration early after TUR.

Anatomically protected sites include the prostatic urethra and the distal ureters. Limited series suggest that a TUR of the prostatic fossa can provide better access for BCG allowing a response in 50–80% of patients with superficial or ductal involvement.

L. Treatment of Low-Grade Ta Disease

1. The contemporary data suggest that such patients should be treated with a single intravesical instillation of a chemotherapeutic agent as described previously, unless there is evidence of a bladder perforation.

2. Resection and repeat cystoscopy only has also been performed, yet the potential for recurrence is higher.

3. There is little evidence for the use of BCG in these patients. Patients with recurrent disease, especially multiple recurrences and/or associated CIS, may benefit from BCG therapy.

4. Small low-grade recurrences may be treated by office fulguration.

5. Cystoscopy disease status at 3 months and tumor size greater than 3 cm predict recurrence and possible progression.

M. Treatment of High-Grade Ta Disease and CIS

1. Evidence-based data are sparse for treatment of high-grade Ta lesions due to small percentage of overall tumors.

2. Immediate intravesical instillation warranted with second look cysto and TURBT with possible bladder mapping and BCG therapy with maintenance for persistent or recurrent high-grade Ta disease.

3. Consider cystectomy for original high-grade Ta, if there is progression to T1 disease or CIS after BCG.

4. Maintain long-term close (6 month) follow-up.

5. BCG demonstrates a 72–90% complete response in CIS only patients. Initial response does not predict durability because up to 50% of patients may recur or progress.

6. Intravesical chemotherapy demonstrates a 35–53% response rate with wide variance about that interval given the studies evaluated.

7. TUR alone demonstrates a 0% durable response at 3 years.
8. In trials comparing BCG to chemotherapy, 68% of BCG and 49% of chemotherapy patients demonstrate a complete response. The BCG response is durable in 68% of patients compared to 47% of chemotherapy patients. Overall disease-free rates at nearly 4 years are 51% for BCG and 27% for chemotherapy.
9. Maintenance therapy with BCG results in an improvement in complete response from 55 to 84%. Maintenance consists of a 3-week course of therapy for 2–3 years. Patients may experience complications of bladder dysfunction. Decreased dose therapy ($\frac{1}{3}$, $\frac{1}{10}$, $\frac{1}{30}$, $\frac{1}{100}$ of normal dose) may allow completion of therapy.
10. Disease progression in CIS is reduced by at least 35% with BCG. This effect is more prominent early. Long-term effects are less clear.
11. Treatment of BCG failures includes further therapy with valrubicin, additional therapy with intravesical interferon and BCG, or cystectomy. Valrubicin responses are in the 20% range. Forty to 50% of BCG failures may respond to combined BCG and interferon. Photodynamic therapy is a historical option.

N. Treatment of T1 Disease

1. Repeat TURBT for staging is mandatory. Intravesical immediate instillation of chemotherapy should be performed even with suspected T1 lesions.
2. Immediate cystectomy versus BCG.
   a) Argument for cystectomy is 30% upstaging in multiple series. Chemotherapy is associated with 33% progression and is not a good option unless patient cannot tolerate it.
   b) BCG treated T1 disease associated with an average of only 12% recurrence (0–35%). Overall treatment failure including any recurrence is 40–50%.
   c) Immediate cystectomy carries the morbidity and mortality of cystectomy. Surgery does not provide 100% 5-year survival (85–90%).
   d) Some stratification of T1G3 may be useful. Those with accessible, unifocal tumors, no CIS, and less than T1 disease on reTURBT may benefit from initial therapy. Those with multifocal disease, concomitant CIS, residual T1 on reTURBT, and tumors in difficult locations may benefit from cystectomy.

3. BCG therapy.
    a) BCG failure may require stratification.
        i) Refractory disease: worsening or non improved disease at 3 months or persistent disease at 6 months.
        ii) Resistant disease: recurrent or persistent at 3 months but of lesser intensity. Cleared at 6 months.
        iii) Relapsing: recurrent after disease-free status achieved at 6 months.
        iv) Intolerant: persistent or recurrent disease after less than adequate treatment due to patient tolerance.
    b) Overall a second course of BCG may be useful in T1G3 patients, but therapy should not persist beyond two courses.

O. Cystoscopic Schedule and Upper Urinary Tract Follow-Up

1. Cystoscopic schedules have been developed on the basis of authority opinion. Usually patients undergo cystoscopy every 3 months for the first 1–2 years, every 6 months for the next year, and either yearly thereafter exams or an exam every 6 months for 5 years in high-risk patients. A return to every-3-month evaluations occurs after a recurrence.
2. Data on low-grade Ta disease suggest that evaluations can be of lesser intensity. Although irritating, patients are willing to forego regular cystoscopy on the basis of the results of a tumor marker only if that marker would be 95% accurate. Cystoscopy findings at 3 months also influence pattern of recurrences.
3. Upper tract disease is uncommon in low-grade Ta disease yet can occur in more than 20% of patients with high-grade disease or CIS. Actuarial recurrence of upper tract disease has been reported as high as 40% over 15 years in high-risk patients. Yearly or every other year upper tract imaging is indicated for the intermediate time frame for such patients.

P. Treatment of T2 and Greater Disease

1. Radical Cystectomy

This is the standard of care in treating muscle-invasive bladder cancer. A radical cystectomy entails en bloc removal of the bladder, prostate, seminal vesicles, and proximal urethra. If the prostatic urethra is involved with tumor, a total urethrectomy is also carried out. This can also be performed

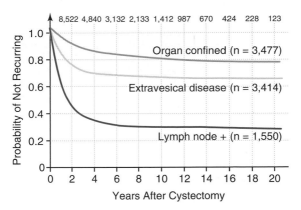

FIGURE 15-2. KM curve. (From Bochner BH, et al: Postoperative nomogram predicting risk of recurrence after radical cystectomy for bladder cancer. *J Clin Oncol* 24[24]:3967–3972, 2006. Epub July 24, 2006.)

as a subsequent separate procedure. An intact urethra is monitored by routine urethral cytology and/or urethroscopy in the postoperative period.

In females, an anterior exenteration is performed that includes removal of the bladder, entire urethra, anterior vaginal wall, and a total abdominal hysterectomy/bilateral salpingo-oophorectomy. An en bloc pelvic lymph node dissection starting at the aortic bifurcation or common iliac vessels is performed in both sexes. Survival for patients with radical cystectomy alone is shown in Figure 15-2.

Urinary diversion is an integral component of the procedure and accounts for most of the long-term postoperative morbidity. The major forms of diversion include a standard ileal conduit, colon conduit, or continent urinary diversion, which may be cutaneous or orthotopic. Operative mortality for radical cystectomy and urinary diversion is roughly 1–3%. Early and late postoperative complications range from 10–30%.

2. Partial Cystectomy

This technique may be employed on a very selective basis for circumscribed lesions usually in the dome of the bladder where a 2-cm free margin may be obtained without requiring a further procedure such as ureteral reimplantation. This procedure can be overextended in the hope of preserving a normal lower urinary tract. This should not be the case in the present era of continent urinary diversion.

3. Radiation Therapy

Definitive radiation therapy has been employed in invasive bladder cancer. Overall, durable complete responses are 40% and are much poorer stage for stage than those obtained with surgery. Interstitial radiation therapy (iridium needles) has been employed primarily in Europe. Careful patient selection is necessary to obtain success.

4. TUR

In the case of patients who are severely medically compromised, TUR may be an appropriate form of therapy for invasive lesions. In addition, laser irradiation may be employed in this situation. A complete response may be obtained in as many as 20–30% of patients. Reports of greater success also incorporate salvage cystectomy as part of the therapy.

5. Combined Modality Therapy

TUR, platinum based combination chemotherapy, and external beam radiation therapy have been employed on a protocol basis. Select patients have experienced good short-term complete responses while preserving their bladders. Long-term follow-up is necessary to gauge duration of response and side effects on lower tract urinary function.

Q. Urinary Diversion

1. General Considerations

Urinary diversion is an integral part of urinary reconstruction and urologic oncology. Such surgery can be technically advanced and is associated with potential long-term as well as short-term complications. Additionally, careful consideration must be given to the physiologic costs of diverting the urinary tract and the appropriate selection of patients for a particular procedure. Urinary diversion can consist of simple diversion of the ureters to the skin, diversion of urine into the alimentary tract, or diversion of urine into an isolated segment of bowel serving as a conduit or reservoir for urine. There is no one pre-ferred method of performing urinary diversion; therefore, fundamental principles of reconstruction must be understood to appropriately apply these techniques in a given situation.

2. History

During the mid and late 19th century many efforts were made to divert urine into the alimentary tract in an attempt to treat congenital malformations such as bladder exstrophy or conditions such as bladder cancer. Although innovative, multiple complications occurred due to technical limitations in the preantibiotic era. The ureterosigmoidostomy of Coffey provided one of the first reasonable methods of diverting the urinary system. Metabolic complications and the development of adenocarcinoma at the ureter-bowel junction discouraged further widespread use of this technique. The ileal loop urinary conduit described by Bricker in 1950 became the standard form of urinary diversion over the next several decades. Different techniques of continent urinary diversion have since been developed and modified by multiple individuals. The application of continent diversion has been further aided by the acceptance of clean intermittent catheterization as an appropriate form of urinary drainage.

3. General Physiologic Considerations

a. Renal Function

Approximately 30% of patients will experience long-term (5 to 15 years) renal deterioration after urinary diversion. It must be remembered, however, that not all renal units associated with a diversion are normal preoperatively. This deterioration can be hastened by high static pressures within the reconstructed urinary tract, reflux, or chronic infection. Many of the metabolic abnormalities described below first became manifest or are exacerbated by patients displaying a serum creatinine greater than 2 ng/dL. Care must therefore be taken when considering such patients for urinary diversion.

b. Infection

The majority of patients with a urinary diversion will display urine colonized with bacteria. In general there is no concomitant symptomatic infection, and this situation is best left untreated. Repeated therapy for asymptomatic colonization can lead to infection with stone formation or severely resistant strains of bacteria. This may necessitate the use of parenteral antibiotics. Classically 4–6% of patients with urinary diversions may eventually die of urosepsis.

c. Urolithiasis

This may occur in 2–10% of patients with urinary diversions. The presence of foreign bodies, especially staples, provides a nidus for stone formation. Stones also have a greater tendency to form in patients with *Proteus* UTIs and in patients with hyperchloremic metabolic acidosis.

4. Metabolic Considerations

a. Electrolyte Abnormalities

These occur secondary to the interaction of urine with a particular bowel epithelium. The altered transport of different ions gives rise to particular metabolic abnormalities.

i) Colon. The classic abnormality seen in ureterosigmoidostomy is hyperchloremic metabolic acidosis. It was first recognized by Ferris and Odel in 1950. The condition can be seen in as many as 80% of patients and is exacerbated by the large surface area of the colon exposed to urine. Essentially, a significant amount of bicarbonate equivalents is lost into the colonic urine with the absorption of chloride from the urine. This condition can lead to a severe acidosis that is exacerbated by compromised baseline renal function. Another less recognized complication can be total body potassium depletion and hypokalemia. Furthermore, elevated ammonia levels may develop in patients secondary to bacterial overgrowth. This is best treated by adequate urinary drainage and/or treatment with neomycin or lactulose.

ii) Ileum. Hyperchloremic metabolic acidosis is also seen in patients with ileal conduits. Although the findings are less severe, they can be present in as many as 70% of patients with ileal conduits. Again, patients with impaired baseline renal function will display a greater propensity toward metabolic derangement.

    a) Monitoring. McDougal and Koch emphasize the potential implications of long-term subtle metabolic abnormalities such as growth retardation and osteomalacia. The exact timing for intervention in subtle acidosis is not clear, especially in elderly adults treated for cancer, yet these issues are of great concern in the pediatric and young adult population.

    b) Treatment. Hyperchloremic acidosis is treated by alkalizing agents such as oral sodium bicarbonate, Polycitra, or Shohl's solution. If a sodium cannot be tolerated, cyclic adenosine monophosphate (cAMP) inhibitors such as nicotinic acid and chlorpromazine, may be employed. Although sodium overload is avoided with such therapies, potential side effects such as peptic ulcer disease and tardive dyskinesia can occur.

iii) Jejunum. Use of this bowel segment is associated with a hyponatremic, hypochloremic, hyperkalemic, metabolic acidosis. This is due to a loss of salt and an increase in potassium and hydrogen ions. A feed-forward mechanism is established by the initial loss of salt and water, followed by a renin-aldosterone response to the hypovolemia. The permeable jejunal epithelium is presented with a low-sodium, high-potassium urine, which facilitates further body loss of sodium into the conduit and reabsorption of potassium. Initial management requires fluid resuscitation followed by long-term sodium chloride supplementation.

iv) Stomach. This bowel segment has been employed in urinary diversion or bladder augmentation in several different configurations. It has been employed predominantly in the pediatric population. The advantages of using stomach include compensation for pre-existing metabolic acidosis, conversation of GI absorptive area, and decreased mucus production. The most common metabolic side effect is a hypokalemic, hypochloremic, metabolic alkalosis such as that seen with prolonged nasogastric suction. It is best managed with good oral fluid intake.

5. Other Considerations

a. Neoplasia

Reports of adenocarcinoma in patients with ureterosigmoidostomies were first made in 1929. This event will occur in approximately 10% of such patients with a latency period of 10–20 years. Because serial screening was not performed, original reports displayed generally advanced disease with up to a 36% mortality rate. Although the lesion is usually at the ureter-colon junction, it is difficult to discern the issue of origin. The etiology of these carcinomas is poorly understood. Cases of carcinoma have been reported in ileal conduits and cystoplasties. The long-term implications for continent diversion are unknown.

b. Drug Absorption

A large bowel segment provides a significant reabsorptive area for many chemicals. This is important because many patients undergoing chemotherapy for bladder cancer may be at risk for intoxication. Methotrexate, which is employed in the methotrexate, vinblastine, Adriamycin, cisplatin (MVAC) regimen, has reported to cause toxicity. Anticonvulsant agents may also be reabsorbed by the bowel of a urinary diversion.

c. Vitamin B_{12} Metabolism

Vitamin B_{12} is absorbed primarily in the terminal ileum, which is often isolated from the alimentary tract when constructing a continent reservoir. Because usual body reserves are adequate for approximately 5 years, this is not an immediate postoperative concern, but it must be addressed with regard to replacement therapy in patients over the long term. The 15–20 cm segment employed in a standard ileal conduit usually does not deplete the absorptive distal ileum still in continuity with the alimentary tract.

d. Hematuria-Dysuria Syndrome

This is a complex of symptoms in patients with a diversion or bladder augment from a gastric segment, which includes bladder spasm, urethral pain, gross hematuria, and skin irritation. The etiology is incompletely understood yet is probably related to the secretion of gastric acid. The activation of pepsinogen to pepsin at a low pH has been proposed as the urothelial irritant. It is best treated by oral hydration and histamine blockade. This syndrome is partially related to hypergastrinemia, which can be demonstrated in gastric segment diversions. Ulceration is another possible problem with these segments.

6. Mechanical Considerations

a. Neuromuscular Activity

Bowel segments have an intrinsic coordinated contractile activity that must be taken into consideration when constructing conduits. It is a physiologic property that is disadvantageous for the active storage of urine. For continent reconstruction, the splitting of bowel on its antimesenteric border and its reconfiguration are meant to cause a zero net resultant pressure vector, thus preventing directional flow of urine. Additionally, a general dyscoordination of contraction activity occurs and thus lowers intraluminal pressure. This discoordination is the primary mechanical effect of reconfiguration, but its long-term efficacy is questionable because several studies suggest the return of coordinated activity fronts over time.

b. Geometric Aspects

Much of the effectiveness in creating high-volume, low-pressure reservoirs by bowel reconfiguration may be accomplished by the fact that detubularization essentially approximates a sphere. This is the maximized volume for a given surface area, and the sphere has a larger radius than the tube of the bowel. The law of Laplace states that for a given wall tension, a larger radius will result in lower intra-luminal pressure, which is the goal of a continent pouch with regard to continence and the prevention of upper tract deterioration.

7. Forms of Urinary Diversion (Non-Continent)

a. Ileal Conduit

Since its introduction in 1950, the ileal conduit has become reference standard for urinary diversion. Approximately 15–20 cm of terminal ileum are isolated bowel continuity, allowing this bowel segment to serve as a conduit or passageway to the skin. General complications are listed in the following.

i) Cutaneous considerations. The loop may be matured at the skin as a Brooke ostomy or as a Turnbull loop. The latter is useful in patients with a thick abdominal wall. One of the several ostomy appliances are attached to this site. Appropriate preoperative marking on the abdominal wall and care in constructing the stoma bud are important to avoid difficulties with patient comfort and skin care. Stomal stenosis is the most common long-term complication of cutaneous urinary diversion.

ii) Ureteral considerations. The ureteral/enteral anastomosis is a potential site for complications. A direct anastomosis between the bowel and ureter with mucosa-to-mucosa apposition is the preferred method of construction. Early ureteral leakage was a significant and morbid complication of this procedure that has been reduced by greater attention to technique and the use of ureteral diversion stents in the perioperative period. Ureteral stenosis is not uncommon and may require balloon dilation or reanastomosis.

b. Colon Conduit

A portion of colon may be employed as a urinary conduit. The potential for hyperchloremic acidosis exists but is reduced if short segments of colon are used. When employed in conjunction with a full pelvic exenteration, a bowel anastomosis may be avoided. A transverse colon conduit is a very useful alternative in patients with heavily irradiated bowel. This segment is usually away from most radiation fields and provides a healthy alternative to possibly damaged ileum. Nonrefluxing ureteral anastomoses may be constructed with the use of tinea coli, but the potential for ureteral obstruction exists.

c. Jejunal Conduit

The jejunum has been employed as an alternative segment in cases of irradicated bowel. Due to its permeability characteristics, it is prone to severe metabolic complications previously described and is not generally employed in urinary diversion.

d. Cutaneous Ureteral Diversion

This is a direct form of urinary diversion generally complicated by stenosis at the level of the skin and by potential difficulties with collection appliances.

8. *Continent Urinary Diversion*

a. General Goals

  i) Adequate capacity reservoir.
 ii) Low-pressure reservoir.
iii) Urinary continence during normal activities.
 iv) Volitional emptying.

b. General Construction

  i) Cutaneous urinary diversion.
 ii) Orthotopic urinary diversion.

c. Continence Mechanisms

  i) Intussuscepted nipple valve.
 ii) Fixed resistance.
iii) Flap valve—Mitrofanoff principle.
 iv) Pelvic floor external sphincter (orthotopic).

d. Ureterosigmoidostomy

This is one of the original forms of urinary diversion and can be considered continent urinary diversion in the broad sense. It is rarely applied in developed countries due to the metabolic and neoplastic complications previously described. Recent modifications of this procedure have included J-pouch alteration of the sigmoid colon or the use of detubularized ileal patches to increase local capacity and decrease tenesmus.

e. Cutaneous Continent Diversion

In this form of diversion a reservoir or ileum, colon, or a combination of both is constructed from detubularized bowel and brought to the skin as a discrete flush, catheterizable stoma. The site may be paraumbilical of just above the pubic hairline. In the case of a thick or distorted abdominal wall, the umbilicus is the preferred site. The site must be catheterized every 4–6 hours to avoid overdistention. In addition to the standard complications of urinary diversion, patients may develop eccentricity of the catheterization pathway or incontinence requiring revision of the site. Initial series reported revision rates of 25–30% but these have decreased to a 5–15% range.

i) Indiana pouch. A detubularized segment of cecum and colon acts as a storage reservoir whose continence is maintained by fixed resistance established at the ileocecal valve and distal ileum. The tapered distal ileum serves as the catheterizable limb. Ease of construction and a low complication profile make this a popular form of diversion. Capacity is lower than that seen with ileal pouches, and a potential for chronic diarrhea exists (5%) due the removal of the ileocecal valve and colonic tissue.

ii) Penn pouch. In this form of diversion the appendix is used in a tunneled method and acts as a flap valve (Mitrofanoff principle) to provide urinary continence. This recapitulates the natural course and mechanism of the ureter as it enters the bladder. Issues of pouch capacity and diarrhea are similar to those seen in the Indiana pouch. The appendix may not be a suitable catheterizable limb in all adults.

iii) Monti procedure. The use of a transversely tubularized bowel segment (TTBS) increases the range and flexibility for the construction of a catheterizable limb in a cutaneous continent urinary reconstruction. A 2.5-cm segment of small bowel can be detubularized and transversely retubularized to create long, relatively narrow bowel segments, which can be implanted in a urinary reservoir and brought to the skin. When necessary, two segments can be attached in series to gain additional length. This is an extension of the Mitrofanoff principle, which uses a small-diameter tube implanted in a flap valve fashion to provide continence.

iv) Pouch hygiene. As previously stated, forms of urinary diversion are subject to bacterial colonization. In continent reservoirs this may proceed to frank "pouchitis" and pyelonephritis if emptying is inefficient or incomplete. Furthermore, most bowel segments continue to produce mucus for at least 1 year, which can be a source of obstruction leading to dysfunction and infection. The potential for such difficulties can be reduced by simple maneuvers such as daily pouch irrigation with saline solution by the patient after a routine catheterization.

f. Orthotopic Continent Diversion

This is a form of continent reconstruction based on the striated external sphincter as the primary continence mechanism. A high-capacity, low-pressure system is essential for an optimal result. Potential complications include enuresis in 5–10% of patients (due to relaxation of the pelvic floor during deep stages of sleep) and tumor recurrence at the urethral margin necessitating major surgical revision. Pouches may be constructed of pure ileum (hemi-Kock pouch, ileal neobladder) or mixed segments of large and small bowel (Mainz pouch).

- Urodynamics. Functional studies reveal excellent capacity and storage as well as efficient emptying with a combination of pelvic floor relaxation and abdominal straining. The potentially large capacity of these pouches can make a patient inattentive to the need for voiding. If the reservoir is chronically overdistended, the ability to empty is compromised and may necessitate the need for intermittent catheterization. Upper tract deterioration is primarily avoided by having low static pressures in the pouch and avoiding pouch-ureter reflux. Reflux may be further prevented by an intussuscepted nipple.
- Female orthotopic diversion. The technique of orthotopic diversion has recently been extended to female patients. Careful pathologic studies have suggested that the absence of CIS or lack of tumor involvement in the trigone or bladder neck is associated with a lack of tumor in the female urethra. Although a concern for urinary incontinence was an initial issue, it has been noticed that many of these patients will develop partial or complete urinary retention. Patients tend to be equally divided: one third void normally with or without occasional catheterization, one third experience complete urinary retention, and one third have stress urinary incontinence. No significant problems with urethral recurrence have been reported.

R. Treatment of Advanced Disease

1. Chemotherapy for Metastatic Disease

Urothelial cancer is a moderately chemotherapy sensitive malignancy. Prognostic risk factors (sometimes called the Bajorin risk factors) for patients with metastatic disease include (1) visceral metastases (bone, lung, liver) and (2) Karnofsky performance status <80% (>ECOG 2). Patients are classified as having zero, one, or two risk factors. Patients with zero risk factors treated with cisplatin-based chemotherapy have a median survival of 33 months and some derive long-term benefit from chemotherapy. Patients with two risk factors have a median survival of 9 months and are unlikely to derive long-term benefit from chemotherapy. An important point is that results of chemotherapy trials including response rate and survival are clearly influenced by patient selection; randomized trials should stratify for these risk factors.

MVAC is the historic standard of care. MVAC is associated with significant toxicity. Recently, the combination of gemcitabine/cisplatin has been demonstrated to result in similar survival to but less toxicity than MVAC. A regimen of dose-intense MVAC has not demonstrated improved survival over standard dose MVAC.

Because cisplatin is nephrotoxic, this agent should not be used in patients with significant renal impairment. Approximately one quarter of patients with advanced urothelial cancer are not candidates for cisplatin because of renal insufficiency. The combination of paclitaxel plus carboplatin can be used in these patients.

There is no standard effective second-line chemotherapy option for patients with advanced urothelial cancer. Patients should be encouraged to participate in clinical trials investigating novel agents.

2. Neoadjuvant/Adjuvant Chemotherapy

Patients with muscle-invasive bladder cancer are at risk of developing metastatic disease, even after cystectomy. Postcystectomy pathology demonstrating extravesical disease or lymph node metastases is associated with an increased risk of recurrence and distant metastases. Systemic chemotherapy has been studied to determine if it can eradicate micrometastatic disease in the earlier disease setting.

Neoadjuvant chemotherapy refers to chemotherapy given before cystectomy. A meta-analysis of multiple randomized trials demonstrated that neoadjuvant chemotherapy is associated with an absolute survival advantage of about 5%

at 5 years. Neoadjuvant therapy can also be given to down-stage locally advanced tumors.

Adjuvant chemotherapy refers to systemic chemotherapy administered after cystectomy. Small trials suggest benefit, but to date a sufficiently powered randomized trial of surgery alone versus surgery plus adjuvant chemotherapy has not been performed. The EORTC is performing such a trial, but the results are not available.

Finally, a small trial from MD Anderson compared neoadjuvant MVAC with adjuvant MVAC and determined that survival was similar with both approaches.

3. Chemoradiation Therapy for Muscle-Invasive Bladder Cancer

An alternative to radical cystectomy for patients with muscle-invasive bladder cancer is a multimodality approach incorporating surgery, chemotherapy, and radiation therapy. Patients first undergo maximal transurethral resection of the bladder tumor followed by a combination of radiation therapy and radiosensitization with chemotherapy (drugs used have included cisplatin, 5-fluorouracil [FU], paclitaxel). Studies have demonstrated that approximately 40% of patients treated with this approach will be alive with an intact bladder at 5 years. Five-year overall survival is approximately 50%. Factors that decrease the chance of successful outcome include extravesical disease and/or hydronephrosis.

SELF-ASSESSMENT QUESTIONS

1. Has the case for prostate cancer screening/disease detection been proven?
2. What are the principle issues that should be considered by the physician and patient in the choice of therapy for clinically localized bladder cancer?
3. What are the side effects of androgen blockade therapy?
4. What are the alternatives for the treatment of high-grade T1 bladder cancer?
5. Describe the general complications of urinary diversion.

SUGGESTED READINGS

Prostate Cancer

1. Albertsen PC, Hanley J, Fine J: Twenty year outcomes following conservative management of clinically localized prostate cancer. *JAMA* 293:2095–2101, 2005.

2. Bill-Axelson A, Holmberg L, Ruutu M, Haggman M, et al: Scandinavian prostate cancer group study No. 4. Radical prostatectomy versus watchful waiting in early prostate cancer. *N Engl J Med* 352:1977–1984, 2005.

3. Bostwick DG, Burke HB, Djakiew D, et al: Human prostate cancer risk factors. *Cancer* 101:2371–2490, 2004.

4. Catalona WJ, Smith DS, Wolfert RL, et al: Evaluation of percentage of free serum prostate-specific antigen to improve specificity of prostate cancer screening. *JAMA* 274:1214–1220, 1995.

5. Freeland SJ, Humphreys EB, Mangold LA, et al: Risk of prostate cancer-specific mortality following biochemical recurrence after radical prostatectomy. *JAMA* 294:433–439, 2005.

6. Eisenberger MA, Blumenstein BA, Crawford ED, et al: Bilateral orchiectomy with or without flutamide for metastatic prostate cancer. *N Engl J Med* 339:1036–1042, 1998.

7. Han M, Partin AW, Pound CR, et al: Long-term biochemical disease-free and cancer-specific survival following anatomic radical retropubic prostatectomy. The 15-year Johns Hopkins experience. *Urol Clin North Am* 28:555–565, 2001.

8. Kattan MW, Eastham JA, Stapleton AM, et al: A preoperative nomogram for disease recurrence following radical prostatectomy for prostate cancer. *J Natl Cancer Inst* 90:766–771, 1998.

9. Pound CR, Partin AW, Eisenberger MA, et al: Natural history of progression after PSA elevation following radical prostatectomy. *JAMA* 281:1591–1597, 1999.

10. Stephenson RA: Prostate cancer trends in the era of prostate specific antigen: an update of incidence, mortality, and clinical factors from the SEER database. *Urol Clin North Am* 29:173–178, 2002.

11. Thompson IM, Goodman PJ, Tangen CM, et al: The influence of finasteride on the development of prostate cancer. *N Engl J Med* 349:215–224, 2003.

12. Zelefsky MJ, Fuks Z, Hunt M, et al: High-dose intensity modulated radiation therapy for prostate cancer: early toxicity and biochemical outcome in 772 patients. *Int J Radiat Oncol Biol Phys* 53:1111–1116, 2002.

Bladder Cancer

1. Au L-SJ, Badalament RA, Wientjes MG, et al: Methods to improve efficacy of intravesical mitomycin C: results of a randomized phase III trial. *J Natl Inst* 93:597–604, 2001.

2. Bohle A, Jocham D, Bock PR: Intravesical bacillus Calmette-Guérin versus mitomycin C in superficial bladder cancer: formal meta-analysis of comparative studies on recurrence and toxicity. *J Urol* 169:90–95, 2003.

3. Lamm DL: Complications of bacillus Calmette-Guérin immunotherapy. *Urol Clin North Am* 19:265–572, 1992.

4. Lamm DL, Blumenstein BA, Crissman JD, et al: Maintenance bacillus Calmette-Guérin immunotherapy for recurrent TA, T1 and carcinoma in situ transitional cell carcinoma of the bladder: a randomized Southwest Oncology Group Study. *J Urol* 163:1124–1129, 2000.

5. Leissner J, Ghoneim MA, Abol-Enein H, et al: Extended radical lymphadenectomy in patients with urothelial bladder cancer: results of a postoperative multicenter study. *J Urol* 171:139–144, 2004.

6. Logothetis CJ, Finn LD, Smith T, et al: Escalated MVAC with or without recombinant human granulocyte-macrophage colony-stimulating factor for the initial treatment of advanced malignant urothelial tumors: results of a randomized trial. *J Clin Oncol* 13:2272–2277, 1995.

7. Pansadoro V, Emiliozzi P, Defidio L, et al: Bacillus Calmette-Guérin in the treatment of stage T1 grade 3 transitional cell carcinoma of the bladder; long-term results. *J Urol* 154:2054–2058, 1995.

8. Pawinski A, Sylvester R, Kurth KH, et al: A combined analysis of European Organization for Research and Treatment of Cancer and Medical Research Council randomized clinical trials for the prophylactic treatment of stage TaT1 bladder cancer. *J Urol* 156:1934–1941, 1996.

9. Rodel C, Grabenbauer CG, Kuhn R, et al: Combined-modality treatment and selective organ preservation in invasive bladder cancer: long-term results. *J Clin Oncol* 20:3061–3071, 2002.

10. Stein JP, Lieskovsky G, Cote R, et al: Radical cystectomy in the treatment of invasive bladder cancer: long-term results in 1054 patients. *J Clin Oncol* 19:666–675, 2001.

11. Stein JP, Quek MD, Skinner DG: Contemporary surgical techniques for continence urinary diversion: continence and potency preservation. *Atlas Urol Clin North Am* 9:147–173, 2001.

12. Sylvester RJ, Oosterlinck W, van der Meljden APM: A single immediate postoperative instillation of chemotherapy decreases the risk of recurrence in patients with stage Ta T1 bladder cancer: a meta-analysis of published results of randomized clinical trials. *J Urol* 171:2186–2190, 2004.

13. Vaughn DJ, Malkowicz SB, Zoltick B, et al: Phase I trial of paclitaxel/carboplatin in advanced carcinoma of the urothelium. *Semin Oncol* 24(1 Suppl 2):S2–47, S2–50, 1997.
14. von der Maase H, Hansen SW, Roberts JT, et al: Gemcitabine and cisplatin versus methotrexate, vinblastine, doxorubicin, and cisplatin in advanced or metastatic bladder cancer: results of a large, randomized multinational, multicenter, phase III study. *J Clin Oncol* 18:3068–3077, 2000.

C H A P T E R 16

Renal, Testicular, and Penile Cancer

Ricardo F. Sánchez-Ortiz, MD and
David J. Vaughn, MD

I. NEOPLASMS OF THE KIDNEY

A. General Considerations

Although renal cell carcinoma (RCC) is primarily a surgical disease, its diagnosis may involve several medical specialists because these tumors have multiple presenting signs and symptoms. In the era of contemporary imaging, however, its initial diagnosis is most commonly made incidentally during an abdominal ultrasound, computed tomography (CT) scan, or magnetic resonance imaging (MRI) performed for other reasons. Tumors are radioresistant and unresponsive to traditional forms of chemotherapy. Complete responses to immunotherapeutic agents are rare in advanced disease. Since late 2005 and early 2006, new agents such as sunitinib and sorafenib have become available and have shown response in selected patients.

B. Incidence

1. U.S. incidence is 38,000 new cases annually (12,840 cancer-related deaths).
2. Incidence has risen in the past 20 years. Represent 2–4% of human neoplasms.
3. The majority of tumors (85–90%) are renal parenchymal lesions, most commonly clear cell adenocarcinoma.
4. Traditionally 30% of patients have presented with metastatic disease. This number has decreased in an era of contemporary imaging as the number of incidentally discovered renal masses has increased.

C. Epidemiology

1. Male-to-female ratio is approximately 2:1.
2. Most patients present in the fifth to seventh decades of life.
3. Racial distribution is equal.

4. The highest incidence is in Scandinavia; the lowest is in Asia.
5. It is more common in urban settings.
6. Although most cases are sporadic, conventional RCC is associated with von Hippel-Lindau (VHL) disease and less commonly with the tuberous sclerosis complex (TSC). VHL disease is a rare multiorgan syndrome of autosomal dominant inheritance associated with RCC (40%), renal cysts (75%), cysts of the epididymis and pancreas, as well as cerebellar hemangioblastomas, retinal angiomas, and pheochromocytoma (14%). Occurs in 1/36,000 live births. The protein produced by the VHL gene ($3p^{25-26}$) has been isolated and found to bind to the cellular transcription protein elongin, inhibiting transcriptional activity in vitro via RNA polymerase II dysfunction. Hereditary papillary RCC not associated with mutations in the VHL gene has also been described. Multiple renal oncocytomas have also been described in the Birt-Hogg-Dubé syndrome.

D. Etiology

1. The strongest risk factor is tobacco use (twofold increased relative risk).
2. Arterial hypertension and obesity have been associated with RCC in large epidemiologic studies.
3. Industrial exposure (except coke oven workers) is not a significant risk.
4. Acquired renal cystic disease in dialysis patients with 4–9% incidence.

E. Pathology: Renal Tumors

1. Renal Cell Carcinoma

a) Represents up to 90% of solid renal tumors.
b) Classic histologic patterns include conventional (clear cell) RCC (60–75%), papillary RCC (15%), chromophobe RCC (5%), collecting duct carcinoma (<1%), and unclassified carcinoma (up to 5%). Arises from proximal tubular renal cells. Occurs in familial and sporadic forms. The Heidelberg system has gained acceptance. As genetic mutations are identified, a genotypic classification of tumors will likely be adopted in the future.
c) Conventional (clear cell) RCC. Most common histology. Associated with a point mutation or allelic loss of the VHL gene, which maps to $3p^{25-26}$. Grossly, tumors appear

yellow or gray-tan in color with variable areas of hemorrhage, necrosis, or cystic change. Microscopically, they are
composed predominantly of cells with clear eosinophilic
or granular cytoplasm. These tumors are usually unilateral
but may occur bilaterally in 1–2% of cases. The prognosis is
worse in patients with metachronous as opposed to synchronous presentation.

d) Papillary RCC: comprises 5–15% of renal carcinomas.
May occur in both inherited and noninherited forms,
but the VHL gene mutation is not involved. Hereditary
papillary RCC is related to a defect in c-met on the
long arm of chromosome 7. Other genetic alterations
identified include Y-chromosome loss and trisomies
of chromosomes 7, 16, and 17. Age and sex predilec-
tions are similar to conventional RCC. It is multifocal
in up to 40% of cases and bilateral in up to 6% of
patients. Some studies have shown a slight increase
in papillary histology in African-American patients
and in patients with renal insufficiency.

e) Chromophobe tumors are associated with multiple chromosome losses excluding 3p. Age and sex distributions
are similar to conventional RCC. Grossly, these tumors
appear well circumscribed, and tan or beige in color.
Microscopically, an admixture of clear and eosinophilic
cells is common. Its histology may be confused with
oncocytoma, a benign renal lesion. They are multifocal
in less than 10% of cases. Bilaterality is exceedingly rare.

2. Oncocytoma

Accounting for approximately 5% of all renal parenchymal
tumors, oncocytomas are well-circumscribed parenchymal
masses composed of densely acidophilic cells that show mitochondrial hyperplasia on electron microscopy. Bilaterality has
been reported in up to 5% of cases. They may also be seen
in the adrenal, thyroid, parathyroid, and salivary glands. In
contrast to RCC, the principal genetic alteration appears to
involve changes in mitochondrial DNA and translocation of
chromosome 14. Grossly, they are usually mahogany brown
in color, encapsulated, and contain a dense central scar extending in a stellate pattern (seen in one third of cases) which may
be seen in cross-sectional imaging studies. Angiographically,
there is often a "spoke wheel" appearance to the vessels that
surround the tumor. Several case reports in the 1980s suggested
the potential for metastasis before the realization that oncocytoma is difficult to distinguish from chromophobe RCC histologically. Therefore, oncocytomas are benign and merit

conservative treatment. Unfortunately, their preoperative diagnosis based on imaging is unreliable, and a definitive diagnosis cannot be made on frozen section. Radical or partial nephrectomy is the safest method of treatment unless other factors argue for a conservative approach. Although percutaneous renal biopsies are unreliable in making a tissue diagnosis, perhaps future genetic markers may assist in differentiating RCC from oncocytoma. The Birt-Hogg-Dubé syndrome has been recently described, consisting of bilateral renal oncocytomas or chromophobe RCCs and cutaneous lesions (fibrofolliculomas, trichodiscomas, acrochordons) in the scalp, forehead, or neck. It has also been associated with spontaneous pneumothorax.

3. Angiomyolipoma (AML) (Renal Hamartoma)

These benign lesions composed of fat, muscle, and blood vessels can usually be definitively diagnosed by the presence of fat on computerized tomography (CT) (negative Hounsfield CT attenuation units). Lesions may also appear hyperechoic on renal sonography due to their high fat content and may have arterial microaneurysms detected on angiography. Isolated AMLs usually present at a mean age of 50 years with a 4:1 female predominance. Although they are generally noted as incidental radiographic findings, they may present dramatically with acute flank pain or shock due to spontaneous renal or retroperitoneal hemorrhage. Multiple and often bilateral AMLs are seen in the tuberous sclerosis complex (TSC), a condition of autosomal dominant inheritance associated with seizures, mental retardation, and adenoma sebaceum. Eighty percent of patients with the TSC will develop AMLs. Patients with pulmonary lymphangiomyomatosis, a progressive global pulmonary condition, also exhibit renal AMLs in 40% of cases. Treatment is based on tumor size and patient symptoms. Asymptomatic tumors smaller than 4 cm may be followed closely with serial imaging. However, symptomatic tumors or those greater than 4 cm should undergo selective embolization, percutaneous ablation, or nephron-sparing surgery. Some large central tumors not amenable to nephron-sparing strategies may require radical nephrectomy.

4. Sarcoma

Sarcomas constitute 2–3% of malignant renal parenchymal tumors. They are more common in women. Differentiation from RCC is difficult. The predominant subcategory is leiomyosarcoma. The treatment of choice is radical nephrectomy, because chemotherapy does not improve survival in adults.

5. Hemangiopericytoma

This is a rare, usually small, renin-secreting lesion that is profusely vascular and may have regional or distant metastases in 15% of cases. It may produce severe hypertension.

6. Lymphoma

B cell non-Hodgkin's lymphoma will occasionally present as an infiltrative renal mass. It is uncommon for leukemia to present as a primary renal lesion.

7. Metastasis

The most common tumors that metastasize to the kidneys are carcinomas of the lung, breast, and uterus. Metastatic melanoma is often noted on autopsy. Metastatic lesions appear poorly vascularized and display irregular borders on imaging studies. Recent studies suggest that when patients with other secondary malignancies present with a renal mass, the histology of the mass may be predicted based on the status of the secondary malignancy. If the patient is disease-free from his or her secondary malignancy (e.g., breast cancer), the mass is rarely, if ever, a metastasis to the kidney. A percutaneous biopsy of the renal mass may be warranted in patients with signs of progression from their secondary malignancy or in masses that do not demonstrate contrast enhancement on imaging studies.

8. Xanthogranulomatous pyelonephritis (XGP)

XGP is a rare renal infection that may mimic a renal tumor. It is more commonly seen in women (3:1) in the fifth to seventh decade of life. Diabetes mellitus is found in up to 15% of patients. Usually infection (*Escherichia coli* or *Proteus mirabilis*) and obstructing renal calculi are present. The lesions demonstrate lipid-laden macrophages that resemble clear cell RCC. Patients are generally best treated with nephrectomy rather than incision or drainage.

F. Grading and Staging

1. Fuhrman grading system generally used in the United States (I–IV).
2. General classification systems include the Robson system and TNM system (Tables 16-1 and 16-2).

Table 16-1:—Robson Staging System for Renal Cancer

Stage I   Tumor confined within capsule of kidney
Stage II Tumor invading perinephric fat but still contained within the Gerota fascia
Stage III Tumor invading the renal vein or inferior vena cava (A), or regional lymph-node involvement (B), or both (C)
Stage IV Tumor invading adjacent viscera (excluding ipsilateral adrenal) or distant metastases

Table 16-2:—AJCC TNM Staging System for Renal Cell Carcinoma

Primary tumor (T)
TX - Primary tumor cannot be assessed
T0 - No evidence of primary tumor
T1 - Tumor 7 cm or smaller in greatest dimension, limited to the kidney
T2 - Tumor larger than 7 cm in greatest dimension, limited to the kidney
T3 - Tumor extends into major veins or invades adrenal gland or perinephric tissues but not beyond the Gerota fascia
T3a - Tumor invades adrenal gland or perinephric tissues but not beyond the Gerota fascia
T3b - Tumor grossly extends into the renal vein(s) or vena cava below the diaphragm
T3c - Tumor grossly extends into the renal vein(s) or vena cava above the diaphragm
T4 - Tumor invading beyond the Gerota fascia

Regional lymph nodes (N)
NX - Regional lymph nodes cannot be assessed
N0 - No regional lymph node metastasis
N1 - Metastasis in a single regional lymph node
N2 - Metastasis in more than 1 regional lymph node

Distant metastasis (M)
MX - Distant metastasis cannot be assessed
M0 - No distant metastasis
M1 - Distant metastasis

AJCC stages
AJCC stage I - T1, N0, M0
AJCC stage II - T2, N0, M0
AJCC stage III - T1–2, N1, M0 or T3a-c, N0–1, M0
AJCC stage IV - T4; or any T, N2, M0; or any T, any N, M1

G. Clinical Presentation

1. An increasing number of renal cell tumors are found as asymptomatic incidental masses on imaging studies obtained for another purpose.
2. Classic triad. Only 11% of RCC patients present with the classic triad of hematuria, flank pain, and a palpable mass. These patients generally have advanced disease. Most patients will present with one or two components of the triad. Gross or microscopic hematuria is present in 40–60%, flank pain in 40–50%, and a flank mass in 20–35%.
3. General symptoms. Weight loss (33%), fever (15%), anemia (33%), and night sweats (7%) are common systemic manifestations. The lesion may present by a manifestation of metastasis. Growth along the left renal vein or vena cava can block the testicular vein, producing a varicocele. The sudden appearance of a right-sided varicocele or a varicocele in a man older than 40 years (especially if it does not disappear on recumbency) warrants renal imaging.
4. Paraneoplastic syndromes. Hypercalcemia secondary to parathormone-like production is not uncommon (5%); this may also be due to metastatic bone destruction. Stauffer's syndrome (14%) refers to abnormal liver function studies with hepatomegaly but no metastasis. These values revert to normal in the majority of patients (88%). Recurrent or persistent hepatic dysfunction suggests tumor recurrence or unrelated hepatic disease. Less common syndromes include protein-wasting enteropathy, erythrocytosis, neuromyopathy, and gonadotropin production. Amyloidosis is present in approximately 2% of patients. Thrombocytosis has been associated with worse outcome in some series.

H. Imaging Evaluation

The majority of renal masses (90%) are benign renal cysts. These exist in approximately 5% of all patients older than the age of 55 years. A mass not demonstrating ultrasound criteria for a simple cyst requires a dedicated renal CT scan or MRI with thin cuts. The study should be performed with and without contrast for better definition.

1. Diagnostic Studies

a) Intravenous excretory urography. Traditionally, the intravenous urography (IVU) has been the starting point of the hematuria evaluation to identify parenchymal renal masses as well as calyceal, renal pelvic, and ureteral urothelial abnormalities. Despite the advent of CT urography, a carefully performed limited IVU may provide invaluable anatomic information to plan percutaneous approaches for patients with renal pelvic and calyceal calculi. The scout film evaluates the position, size, and outline of the kidneys and calcifications. Mottled central calcifications indicate a carcinoma with more than 90% specificity. Peripheral or rim calcifications are associated with RCC in 10–20% of cases. After the administration of intravenous contrast media, nephrotomographic views are obtained to evaluate the renal parenchyma. Findings suggestive of a renal mass include renal enlargement, elongation, displacement of the renal pelvis, indistinct or irregular renal borders, or changes in cortical density. Radiographs during contrast excretion are used to evaluate the renal calyces, renal pelvis, and ureters for urothelial lesions.

b) Renal sonography. Ultrasound is used to distinguish cystic from solid renal masses. A classic cyst will be smooth with a definite border of imperceptible thickness, be absent of internal echogenicity, and should display acoustic enhancements beyond the posterior wall. In certain cases, ultrasound may be employed with cyst puncture, cytology, and contrast injection to better define complex lesions. See later for the Bosniak classification of renal masses.

c) CT. A CT scan of the abdomen and pelvis may be performed with or without the injection of intravenous contrast material. CT is also an excellent staging modality and provides superior data on lymph node involvement, perinephric extension, and renal vein or vena caval involvement. CT is probably the single most accurate imaging study for the evaluation of renal masses, especially to identify AMLs (negative Hounsfield units). With the advent of high-resolution spiral CT scanning, CT urography has replaced the IVU as the study of choice for a hematuria evaluation in many centers. This may be performed with three-dimensional (3D) reconstruction of the ureters or by taking several plain film views of the kidneys, ureters, and bladder after intravenous contrast injection and completion of the CT scan sequence. Oral contrast is not used. High-speed spiral CT technology permits 3D renal reconstruction and CT angiography, which may be very useful in preparation for nephron-sparing surgery or laparoscopic renal surgery.

Bosniak classification of cystic masses.

I: Simple cyst, measuring water density and does not enhance. Less than 2% chance of malignancy.

II: Minimally complex cyst. Thin wall (<1 mm) and no enhancement, although may contain several hairline septa. Hyperdense cyst, generally nonsurgical; RCC may be present in 10–15%.

IIF: Indeterminate. Complex cyst with thicker septa requiring further surveillance. No enhancing nodules.

III: Suspicious indeterminate. Thicker, regular, nodular walls with thicker, regular calcifications and septations: RCC in 30–60%. Surgical extirpation recommended.

IV: Malignant. Nodular or solid component: >90% demonstrate RCC. Surgical extirpation recommended.

d) MRI. This imaging modality is most effective in demonstrating the presence and extent of renal vein or vena caval tumor thrombi. In addition, with the use of gadolinium enhancement, it may assist in characterizing cysts that appear hyperdense on CT and are difficult to differentiate from hypovascular tumors. Commonly used in patients with iodinated contrast allergy, renal insufficiency, a nondiagnostic CT scan, or questionable venous invasion. Contraindicated in patients with cardiac pacemakers or metal implants.

e) Angiography. Classic angiography has been replaced by magnetic resonance angiography or 3D CT angiography in the preoperative planning for surgery on solitary kidneys or before partial nephrectomy. Renal angioembolization may be useful before radical nephrectomy especially with very large central tumors or in the presence of bulky hilar adenopathy.

f) Radionuclide imaging. This is most useful in defining "pseudomasses." A normal variant such as a hypertrophied column of Bertin can be distinguished from a tumor by the uniform distribution of radioisotope uptake. Both benign cysts and tumors will appear as photon-deficient areas of uptake.

g) Percutaneous biopsy. Not recommended due to high incidence of false negative biopsies. May be indicated when lymphoma is suspected, in patients with a history of another primary malignancy to rule out metastatic disease, or in complex cysts for cytologic examination. Patients with a history of another primary malignancy (e.g., lung or breast cancer) and a renal mass will rarely harbor a metastasis to the kidney if they are currently disease-free. Therefore, a renal biopsy in these patients may not be necessary.

2. Clinical Staging

Clinical staging consists of a history, physical exam, and:

(1) Chest x-ray (CXR) (chest CT with pulmonary symptoms or abnormal CXR).
(2) CT scan of abdomen and pelvis.
(3) Complete blood count (CBC), liver function tests, alkaline phosphatase, lactate dehydrogenase (LDH), calcium, blood urea nitrogen (BUN), and creatinine.
(4) Bone scan with plain films as indicated (patients with elevated alkaline phosphatase or bone pain).
(5) Brain imaging in patient with neurologic symptoms or extensive metastatic disease.

I. Treatment

1. T1 and T2 Disease

Radical nephrectomy is the gold standard treatment for localized RCC with a normal contralateral kidney. Components of radical nephrectomy include early vascular ligation and en bloc removal of the kidney, surrounding Gerota's fascia, ipsilateral adrenal, upper ureter, and lymph nodes from the crus of the diaphragm to the aortic bifurcation. Although studies have shown that a thorough lymphadenectomy may provide a small (10–15%) benefit in controlling micrometastatic disease, its value remains controversial. Recent data suggest that normal-appearing adrenal glands associated with small renal tumors may be left intact. The most common surgical approaches include an 11th or 12th rib extraperitoneal flank incision, thoracoabdominal (large upper pole tumors), midline transabdominal, or subcostal.

2. Laparoscopic Radical Nephrectomy

Introduced in 1990 by Clayman and colleagues, it is now routinely performed for stages T1 and T2 RCC. It offers the advantages of a smaller incision, shorter length of stay, and shorter convalescence. Approaches include transperitoneal (hand assisted or pure with morcellation) or retroperitoneal. The latter offers expeditious access to the renal pedicle, but with limited working space. The transperitoneal approach may be performed purely laparoscopically or with hand-assistance. No studies have shown a benefit of one approach over the other. The preferred approach is the one that the surgeon feels most comfortable with.

The efficacy and safety of laparoscopic radical nephrectomy have been validated by several large multi-institutional reports. The benefits in convalescence and postoperative pain should not play a role in selecting a laparoscopic radical nephrectomy over open nephron-sparing surgery if the latter is feasible. Refer to the chapter in this manual on minimally invasive approaches for detailed information.

3. Nephron-Sparing Surgery

a) Absolute indications include a solitary kidney, bilateral tumors, and VHL disease (although some believe bilateral nephrectomy is more appropriate). Relative indications include poor bilateral or contralateral renal function.

b) Acceptable option in smaller tumors ($\leq$4 cm) with normal contralateral kidney.

c) Approaches include segmental polar nephrectomy, heminephrectomy, wedge resection, or tumor enucleation (preferred for multiple tumors). This may be done with an open or laparoscopic approach. Refer to the chapter in this manual on minimally invasive approaches for detailed information.

d) Local recurrence is generally less than 10% (nearly zero over 5 years in incidental lesions $\leq$4 cm). In masses measuring less than 4 cm, its safety has been well established even for tumors in the presence of a normal contralateral kidney.

e) The morbidity is similar to radical nephrectomy, but with the potential for slightly greater blood loss or urinary fistula. Although significant urinary fistulas may require prolonged internal ureteral stenting and Foley catheter drainage, the majority will heal with conservative management, avoiding the need for reoperation.

f) Large or central lesions may require renal cooling and complete arterial occlusion to minimize warm ischemic damage. Because ex vivo bench surgery is associated with a high incidence of renal loss and postoperative complications, it should be avoided unless absolutely necessary.

g) Intraoperative ultrasound is paramount for central tumors to ensure adequate margins. Although traditionally a 1-cm margin of normal tissue was thought to be necessary for adequate oncologic efficacy, several studies have demonstrated a negative surgical margin on frozen section is adequate, even if small.

h) Percutaneous or laparoscopic ablation using cryosurgery or radiofrequency. Refer to the chapter in this manual on minimally invasive approaches for detailed information.

4. Stage T3 Tumors

a) Inferior vena cava extension occurs in 4–10% of patients. In the absence of vessel wall invasion or metastasis, nephrectomy with tumor thrombectomy is recommended given a 5-year survival (pT3b or pT3c) of 40–60%. Advanced surgical techniques can be very successful, usually with thoracoabdominal, bilateral subcostal, or midline approaches to ensure complete vascular control above and below the kidneys. Cardiopulmonary bypass with or without hypothermic cardiac arrest can be used in bulky intrahepatic and suprahepatic lesions. Preoperative and intraoperative transesophageal echocardiography is recommended for tumors with cranial extension.

b) Operative mortality ranges from 1.4–14%, with 30–40% postoperative complications such as sepsis, retroperitoneal hemorrhage, or hepatic dysfunction.

c) Tumor subclassification is based on the extent of the thrombus.

5. Metastatic RCC

a) The role for radical nephrectomy in metastatic RCC is limited to those individuals with an excellent performance status who will undergo immunotherapy or who have symptoms of tumor bulk.

b) Management of solitary metastasis. Seen in 1.5–3.5% of patients. Surgical removal recommended given 5-year survival between 30 and 50%. Solitary pulmonary lesions have the best prognosis.

6. Systemic Therapies

a) Chemotherapy. No single agent or combination of chemotherapeutic agents is consistently effective against RCC. Five to 15% response rates have been reported in multiple trials. Very few patients demonstrate a sustained complete response (CR).

b) Cytokine therapy. Interferon alpha provides a 15% partial response rate and 1% complete response rate. Interleukin-2 is approved by the Food and Drug Administration (FDA) specifically for metastatic RCC. A response rate in the 10–20% range has been demonstrated. High-dose interleukin-2 has been associated with durable responses and long-term survival in select patients. A major toxicity of high-dose interleukin-2 is adult respiratory distress syndrome (ARDS) due to the capillary leak syndrome. Because of the significant toxicity associated with high-dose interleukin-2, less toxic continuous infusion or subcutaneous injections have been developed. The benefit of cytokine therapy is limited to clear cell histology.

c) Kinase inhibitors. Sorafenib and sunitinib are FDA approved for the treatment of metastatic RCC. Studies of these agents after cytokine therapy demonstrate response rates as high as 40%. These agents are generally well tolerated. Enrollment of patients in clinical trials evaluating these agents in combination regimens or as first-line therapy is encouraged.

d) Adjuvant systemic therapy. To date, no studies of adjuvant systemic therapy after nephrectomy for high-risk patients have demonstrated a survival advantage.

7. *Management of AML*

This benign lesion can enlarge; therefore, management guidelines are established with regard to initial size and tumor growth.

J. Tumor Stage Is the Most Important Predictor of Prognosis

1. Disease-specific survival after radical nephrectomy (5 and 10 years).
   a) I: 90%, 85%
   b) II: 80%, 70%
   c) IIIA: 58%, 50%
   d) IIIB: 46%, 34%
   e) IIIC: 22%, 16%
   f) IVA: 5%, 3%
2. Extension through the renal capsule and into perinephric fat occurs in 25% of patients.
3. The phenomenon of spontaneous tumor regression is extremely rare and estimated at less than 1%.
4. Metastatic disease presents most commonly to the lung (50%), lymph nodes (35%), liver (30%), bone (30%), and adrenal (5%). Only one third of patients with metastases present with symptoms.

K. Follow-up of RCC After Nephrectomy or Renal-Sparing Surgery

1. Traditionally, most patients with sporadic RCC are followed every 6 months or yearly with a history and physical examination (H+P), liver function studies, serum

chemistry (including alkaline phosphatase, calcium, and LDH), CXR, and abdominal cross-sectional imaging.

2. However, contemporary series from MD Anderson and the Cleveland Clinic suggest that recurrence is generally a rare event for T1 and T2 lesions. In addition, pulmonary metastases are most common and usually diagnosed by chest radiography. Stage-specific follow-up guidelines have been proposed as follows:

- T1: H+P, serum chemistry, and CXR yearly for 5 years.
- T2: H+P, serum chemistry, and CXR every 6 months. Abdominal CT scan at 2 and 5 years for 5 years.
- T3: H+P, serum chemistry, and CXR at 3 months, then every 6 months. Abdominal CT scan at 2 and 5 years.

II. UROTHELIAL TUMORS OF THE RENAL PELVIS AND URETER

A. General Considerations

The urinary system lined by transitional cell epithelium (urothelium) extends from the most proximal calyces to the proximal urethra. In this section attention is given to the tumors of the renal collecting system and the ureter. It is important that they be understood in the broad context of transitional cell carcinoma (TCC), which is discussed in greater detail in the section on bladder cancer.

B. Incidence

1. Account for 7% of all renal tumors.
2. Overall, urothelial tumors are distributed as follows: the bladder (90%), urethra (7%), and ureter or renal pelvis (3%).
3. Patients with a history of bladder cancer have a 2–4% chance of developing upper tract tumors (synchronous or asynchronous). This figure increases up to 25% in patients with bladder carcinoma in situ (CIS).
4. Patients with a history of an upper tract tumor have a 15–50% chance of eventually developing TCC of the bladder. Such patients also have a 2–4% chance of developing a contralateral upper tract lesion.
5. After cystectomy, there is an approximately 7% chance of developing upper tract TCC, regardless of cystectomy specimen ureteral margin. Risk is highest with the presence of CIS in the cystectomy specimen. The highest risk is 3–4 years following cystectomy.

6. Patients with high-grade superficial bladder tumors must undergo routine surveillance of the entire urothelium for the development of cancer once any part has undergone malignant transformation.

C. Pathology

Upper urinary tract tumors include the same pathologic types as those of the bladder. Tumors may be papillary or nodular, muscle invasive or noninvasive. Staging systems are less well defined than for other malignancies but analogous to the bladder TMN system:

1. Stage T0: mucosal lesion without invasion.
2. Stage T1: involvement of the lamina propria.
3. Stage T2: muscularis propria invasion.
4. Stage T3: extension beyond the renal pelvis or ureter.
5. Stage T4: adjacent organ involvement, usually associated with positive lymph nodes.
6. Histologic subtypes.
   a) TCC. Approximately 85% of renal pelvic tumors and almost all ureteral tumors are transitional cell lesions. The male-to-female ratio is 3:1.
   b) Squamous cell carcinoma (10–17% of tumors). Primarily associated with chronic irritation and renal calculi. These lesions are usually of more advanced stage and associated with leukoplakia and metaplastic changes. Large tumors may show a characteristic "bear-claw" appearance on CT.
   c) Adenocarcinoma. This is a very rare (less than 1%) form of upper tract carcinoma. It occurs predominantly in females and is usually associated with chronic infection or irritation and often seen in conjunction with pyelitis cystica or pyelitis glandularis.
   d) Differential diagnosis of upper urinary tract filling defects includes air, papilloma, malakoplakia, sloughed papilla, secondary metastasis, uric acid or matrix calculi, extrinsic compression (vessels, adenopathy, retroperitoneal fibrosis), urinary tuberculosis, ureteritis or pyelitis cystica, inverted papilloma, and sarcoma.

D. Etiology and Natural History

Chemical carcinogenesis is the leading factor in the development of TCC in the upper urinary tract. Probably because of the relative short transit time of urine through the upper tracts, lesions of the upper tract occur much less often than bladder lesions. Tobacco use is associated with at least a twofold increased relative risk for the disease (twofold to six-fold). Two conditions more commonly associated with upper tract lesions are Balkan nephropathy (an inflammatory lesion of the renal interstitium endemic to the Balkan region) and phenacetin abuse (withdrawn by the FDA). In addition, the nephrotoxic Chinese herb *Aristolochia fangchi* has been associated with the development of upper tract urothelial carcinoma.

Papillary tumors of the renal pelvis or ureter tend to be of low grade, whereas nodular or flat lesions tend to be of higher grade. Patients with low-grade lesions (grade 1) have a nearly 100% 5-year disease-specific survival, whereas patients with high-grade lesions (grade 3) display a 20% 5-year survival.

E. Clinical Presentation

Sixty to 90% of patients present with microscopic or gross hematuria. Only 10% are noted serendipitously. Almost one third of patients with a renal pelvic lesion will complain of flank pain, as will one sixth of patients with ureteral tumors. Physical examination is usually unrevealing.

F. Diagnosis

1. Radiologic studies.
   a) Intravenous excretory urography. Either a fixed radiolucent defect or nonvisualization of part or all of the collecting system is noted. Stippled calcifications may also be seen on the plain film.
   b) Retrograde pyelography is indicated to evaluate pyelocalyceal and ureteral segments not adequately visualized on excretory urography, given its greater sensitivity. Upper tract tumors demonstrate filling defects in up to 75% of cases.
   c) CT may help to differentiate a renal parenchymal mass from a renal pelvic mass or a ureteral tumor from a radiolucent calculus. It may evaluate for the presence of hilar or periureteral lymphadenopathy.
   d) Although ultrasonography may delineate nonopaque calculi from a soft tissue density, its use is limited in tumor staging.
2. Brush biopsy/cytology. This is usually performed during pyeloureterography and may be done by a urologist or radiologist. Although the combination of an upper tract filling defect and a positive renal wash cytology in the same side is sufficient evidence for definitive surgical

treatment, ureteroscopy may identify multifocal tumors. However, a renal wash cytology positive for TCC without the presence of urothelial filling defects on urography mandates further evaluation with ureteroscopy.

3. Ureteroscopy allows direct visualization and biopsy of the upper tract urothelium. In addition, laser photocoagulation of the lesion may be performed in patients with small, low-grade lesions, a solitary kidney, or in the setting of compromised renal function. Nephroscopy may also allow direct biopsy, resection, ablation, or fulguration of renal pelvic or ureteral tumors if retrograde access if not feasible.

G. Treatment

1. TCC of the Renal Pelvis

a) Nephroureterectomy. The classic therapy for upper tract TCC is nephroureterectomy with excision of a bladder cuff. The open procedure may be performed via a single thoracoabdominal incision or a two-incision approach (flank and infraumbilical midline). If the ureteral stump is left in place, there is a 30–60% chance for recurrence at a site that is difficult to monitor. Less aggressive surgery has been performed in patients with solitary renal units, bilateral lesions, or compromised renal function. Stage and grade are often stronger predictors of long-term survival than treatment choice. For this reason, more conservative treatments have been advocated. Even with improvements in ureteroscopy, this treatment philosophy requires persistent, often difficult, and perhaps less than adequate active observation of the remaining urothelium. Endoscopic evaluation and treatment can be employed in lower grade lesions.

b) Laparoscopic nephroureterectomy. This procedure has now been popularized and performed routinely in both academic and community settings. Nephroureterectomy may be performed purely laparoscopically via a transperitoneal or retroperitoneal approach. It may also be performed with a hand-assisted transperitoneal laparoscopic technique. The management of the bladder cuff is controversial. Some have advocated that the safest approach includes bladder cuff excision using an open approach via the kidney extraction incision. This may be performed extravesically or through a transvesical approach. Others have recommended a "ureteral pluck" technique by unroofing the ureteral orifice using a Collins knife prior to the laparoscopic procedure. Short-term data have shown that laparoscopic nephroureterectomy operative times and oncologic outcomes are similar to the open technique. However, analgesic requirements and hospital length of stay may be reduced by approximately 60%. There have been no reports to date of trocar site or peritoneal seeding after laparoscopic nephroureterectomy. Refer to the chapter in this manual on minimally invasive approaches for detailed information.

c) Antegrade (percutaneous) or retrograde nephroscopy. Indicated only in patients with a solitary kidney, compromised renal function, or very small low grade lesions. Treatment may involve endoscopic resection with diathermy, cold-knife, or laser tissue destruction.

2. TCC of the Ureter

a) Nephroureterectomy with excision of a bladder cuff remains the classic treatment for this condition given its multifocal nature, especially in tumors of the upper two thirds of the ureter. However, in cases of tumors of the distal third of the ureter or in patients with compromised renal function, distal ureterectomy and ureteroneocystostomy has been proven as effective as a nephroureterectomy.

b) Indications for endoscopic percutaneous or retrograde treatment include a single low-grade ureteral lesion, high-risk surgical candidates, solitary kidney, bilateral disease, and renal insufficiency. Strict compliance with follow-up is paramount in these patients.

c) A less-favored option includes ureteral resection with ileal interposition.

3. Chemotherapy

a) Topical therapy. Not standard of care, but indicated for patients with compromised renal function, a solitary kidney, high-risk surgical candidates, or patients with CIS of the ureter or the renal pelvis. Refer to the section on superficial bladder cancer for commonly used agents (bacille Calmette-Guérin [BCG], thiotepa, mitomycin, doxorubicin, and interferon); their indications; and side effect profiles.

b) Systemic chemotherapy. Although the historic standard of care for management of metastatic TCC is methotrexate, vincristine, Adriamycin (doxorubicin), cisplatin (MVAC) chemotherapy, combination chemotherapy with cisplatin and gemcitabine has proven to be very effective. Chemotherapy with paclitaxel and carboplatin may be better tolerated by patients with compromised renal or cardiac function. Although the neoadjuvant chemotherapy paradigm used in locally advanced bladder cancer has been applied to bulky upper urinary tract tumors, it has not been studied in a prospective fashion. Prospective trials are ongoing to evaluate the long-term efficacy of adjuvant chemotherapy in patients with positive lymph nodes or unfavorable pathology.

4. Surveillance After Definitive Treatment

No strict guidelines exist for follow-up after nephroureterectomy or distal ureterectomy. At our institution, we follow these patients with a history, physical examination, cystoscopy, urinalysis, and cytology every 3 months for a year, then every 6 months for 2 years, then yearly. We obtain a CXR, intravenous urogram, and abdominal cross-sectional imaging yearly or as indicated based on pathologic stage or clinical symptoms.

III. URETHRAL CANCER

A. Carcinoma of the Female Urethra

1. Anatomy

The female urethra measures 2.5–4 cm in length and is lined with transitional epithelium in its proximal third and stratified squamous epithelium in its distal portion. However, boundaries between these types are not discrete, and areas of pseudostratified and stratified columnar epithelium may also be present. The wall of the urethra also contains glands and smooth muscle bundles. The lymphatics of the proximal urethral segment primarily drain to the internal and external iliac nodes, whereas distal lymphatics drain to the inguinal and subinguinal lymph nodes.

2. Epidemiology

Carcinoma of the urethra is a rare tumor. It is more common in older, Caucasian women, with most cases occurring in patients older than 50 years. Urethral strictures and diverticula are thought to have some association with urethral carcinoma.

3. Pathology

Squamous cell carcinoma is the most prevalent histologic pattern, accounting for 60–70% of cases. TCC may be present in up to 20% of cases as a direct continuation of a bladder cancer or as part of a multifocal process. Adenocarcinoma (10–18% of cases) may be seen in association with urethral diverticula or in the rare occurrence of prostate cancer of the female urethra. Melanomas and lymphomas may occur in less than 1% of cases.

4. Presentation

Urethral bleeding or spotting is the most common symptom. Other symptoms may include urinary frequency, dysuria, and obstruction. The possibility of malignancy should at least be considered with any urethral mass or stricture.

5. Diagnosis

Physical examination, urinalysis, and urine cytology, endoscopy, and biopsy are usually sufficient to make the diagnosis. Differential diagnosis includes caruncle, urethral prolapse, leukoplakia, structure, fistulas, erosion, and, rarely, nephrogenic adenoma. Spread is by local infiltration followed by lymphatic spread.

6. Management

Caruncles of the female urethra may mimic carcinoma but are best managed conservatively given their benign nature. Only caruncles that develop erosion or bleeding should be biopsied. Distal third carcinomas may be managed by distal urethrectomy and/or radiation therapy (external beam or brachytherapy) with excellent results. Proximal or advanced lesions exhibit a poor prognosis and are best managed by anterior exenteration with adjuvant radiation therapy. The rare case of a urethral melanoma warrants radical cystourethrectomy. Due to its rarity, the management of the inguinal region with or without intraoperative lymphatic mapping remains controversial.

7. Urethral Diverticula

Less than 50 cases of carcinoma arising in female urethral diverticula have been reported. Five of these cases were associated with a calculus within a urethral diverticulum. The association with urethral diverticula must be considered rare given the relatively high rate of urethral diverticula in the general population. Any filling defect within a diverticulum, however, demands exploration. The most common histology in this setting is adenocarcinoma.

B. Carcinoma of the Male Urethra

1. Anatomy

The male urethra is approximately 20 cm in length and is divided into prostatic, bulbomembranous, and penile segments. The prostatic segment is lined by transitional epithelium. The remaining urethra is covered by pseudostratified columnar epithelium, and the meatus is lined by stratified squamous epithelium. The lymphatics of the prostate and posterior urethra are drained by the internal and external iliac nodes.

2. Epidemiology

The incidence of urethral carcinoma in males is only one third to one half of that in females. Chronic inflammation may have an etiologic role. Patients are generally older than 50 years.

3. Pathology

As many as two thirds of these tumors originate in the bulbar or bulbomembranous urethra. Most anterior lesions are at the fossa navicularis. The most common histologic type is squamous cell carcinoma, followed by TCC. Adenocarcinoma is rare and usually found in the bulbomembranous urethra.

4. Presentation

This carcinoma is usually a locally invasive lesion. Symptoms include urethral obstruction, stricture, bloody discharge, perineal mass, abscess or fistula, perineal pain, or adenopathy. Distant metastases are rare at initial presentation.

5. Diagnosis

Endoscopic biopsy under anesthesia is the mainstay of diagnosis. Urinary or urethral cytology may also be useful. Imaging modalities include retrograde urography, CT, and MRI. The differential diagnosis includes benign stricture disease, periurethral abscess, and inflammatory phlegmon.

6. Management

Therapy is dependent on tumor location. Low-grade lesions in any part of the urethra may be managed by transurethral resection, whereas higher-grade distal urethral tumors may require a partial or total penectomy. Invasive proximal lesions require an aggressive en bloc resection of the urethra and rim of the pubis and an anterior exenteration. There may be a role for adjuvant radiation therapy. Similar treatment is recommended for cases of melanoma. Although the role of prophylactic inguinal lymphadenectomy is controversial, most would agree that an inguinal node dissection is indicated in patients with adenopathy despite antibiotics and in patients with poorly differentiated tumors.

IV. PENILE AND SCROTAL CANCER

A. General Considerations

The incidence of penile cancer in the United States is approximately 1 per 100,000 males per year. Of an estimated 1530 penile cancers estimated for 2006, approximately 280 patients will die of the disease. However, in underdeveloped countries or in areas where circumcision is not practiced, it may account for up to 20% of all tumors in men and up to 45% of genitourinary tumors. The disease is almost nonexistent in populations practicing infant circumcision. Because of its rarity, there are few controlled trials to direct therapy. Therapeutic decisions can also be difficult because surgery can be disfiguring or cause significant morbidity.

B. Penile Cancer

1. Premalignant Lesions

Condylomata acuminata (genital warts). These lesions are caused by human papillomavirus (HPV) infection and may involve the glans, prepuce, or shaft of the penis. Five percent of patients have urethral involvement. The virus types most commonly associated with genital cancer are HPV 16, 18, 31, 33, 35, and 39. It is believed that tumor virus transforming proteins E6 and E7 may target tumor-suppressor gene products pRb and p53, leading to oncogenesis. Although local recurrences are common, the risk of malignant transformation in the most common types (associated with HPV 6 and 11) is negligible, and routine tumor typing is not warranted. There is also a 10–30% rate of spontaneous regression due to cell-mediated immunity. Initial therapy of genital warts may be home or office based. The preferred initial approach includes the use of topical agents at home. Although topical therapies such as 0.5% podophyllin, 5% 5-fluorouracil (Efudex cream), trichloroacetic acid, and bichloroacetic acid are effective, the most enduring responses have been associated with the immune modulator imiquimod. Imiquimod (5%) cream enhances natural killer cell activity and is currently the only topical treatment with the potential to eradicate the virus. Topical podophyllin, which is also indicated for home use, may offer up to 50% clearance if used for 8 weeks. Patients who desire immediate wart removal or those with refractory lesions are candidates for cryoablation, local excision, or laser ablation. Laser ablation is most effectively achieved with the CO_2 and neodynium:yttrium-aluminum-garnet (Nd:YAG) lasers.

Classic series have shown that up to 5% of patients may also have urethral involvement, underscoring the need for a careful examination of the urethra. Distal urethral lesions may be managed with topical 5-fluorouracil cream alone, although large lesions may require tumor debulking with the Nd:YAG laser followed by topical therapy. Prevention should be stressed for all patients with condyloma, given its risk of transmission through sexual contact as well as its higher association with cervical neoplasia in women. Although HPV vaccines have recently become available for female use, their role in men has not been defined.

Although the risk of malignant transformation of penile condyloma in human immunodeficiency virus (HIV) patients is unclear, several studies have established an association between anal and vulvar intraepithelial neoplasia and HPV infection in patients with HIV. Until the natural history of condylomata acuminatum in immunosuppressed patients is better understood, these patients should undergo more intensive surveillance, perhaps with biopsy and HPV typing of recurrent genital lesions. In addition, patients with rapidly recurring lesions despite standard therapy should be counseled for HIV testing.

a) Buschke-Löwenstein's tumor. This lesion is also known as giant condyloma acuminatum. It does not metastasize but may cause local tissue destruction as it enlarges. It may be treated by wide local excision or partial penile amputation.

b) Leukoplakia. This term describes a white cutaneous plaque that may be hypertrophic or atrophic. It may co-exist with or precede the development of squamous cell carcinoma. It is usually secondary to chronic irritation. Circumcision, surgical excision, and irradiation have all been used in treatment. Close follow-up to detect malignant degeneration is essential.

c) Balanitis xerotica obliterans (BXO). A subcategory of lichen sclerosus et atrophicus limited to the male genitalia associated with destructive inflammation, phimosis, urethral stenosis, and squamous cell carcinoma. These hypopigmented, papular, or atrophic lesions typically involve the glans and urethral meatus in uncircumcised men. Initial management of BXO should include biopsy to exclude the presence of carcinoma, followed by topical steroids. Meatoplasty may be required in advanced cases of meatal stenosis. Although the risk of malignant transformation is probably low, close follow-up and self-examination are recommended, given the unknown natural history of BXO.

d) Bowenoid papulosis. Uncommon genital dysplasia now considered to be a sexually transmitted disease caused by human papillomavirus type 16. Clinically, it usually resembles persistent warts, but histologically it resembles squamous cell CIS. Unlike Bowen's disease, it does not progress to invasive squamous cell carcinoma. Female sexual partners should be screened given the association of bowenoid papulosis with sexual transmission and cervical neoplasia. Given the benign course of this disease, less morbid strategies such as excision, cryoablation, topical 5-fluorouracil, or laser photocoagulation should be employed.

2. CIS and Other Malignant Lesions

a) Queyrat's erythroplasia and Bowen's disease. Histologically, these conditions are CIS of the skin of the penis. The former presents as a localized, velvety red lesion on the glans or prepuce. The latter can develop on the skin anywhere on the penis and may be associated with internal carcinomas. Circumcision and biopsy will confirm the diagnosis. Penile CIS represents approximately 10% of all diagnosed cases of squamous carcinoma of the penis but rarely results in regional metastatic disease; in fact, only two cases of metastasis in association with penile CIS have been reported. Although the standard of care for management of CIS remains local excision with a 5-mm margin to exclude invasive carcinoma, newer alternatives such as laser ablation and Mohs' microsurgery have been shown to achieve acceptable local control with organ preservation.

b) Kaposi sarcoma. Penile or genital involvement of Kaposi sarcoma as painless, raised, bluish lesions may be an early manifestation of the acquired immunodeficiency syndrome. In patients who have failed systemic chemotherapy, radiation therapy offers the best chance for palliative control.

3. Invasive Squamous Cell Carcinoma

a. Pathology

Various types of penile carcinomas have been identified, including:

i) Verrucous carcinoma. Comprises approximately 10% of all penile carcinomas. Typically present as large, well-differentiated, fungating lesions that have a tendency for local extension and recurrence but low metastatic potential. Although verrucous carcinoma in other anatomic sites such as the larynx has been reported to metastasize, this has not been shown in tumors of the genital region. Nevertheless, close surveillance is warranted, given that microscopic foci of infiltrating carcinoma may be present in up to 23% of cases, and degeneration into frankly invasive carcinoma has been reported. Phallus-sparing strategies such as local excision and laser ablation should be employed whenever feasible. The propensity of verrucous carcinoma to recur locally and result in local tissue destruction warrants close surveillance in conjunction with patient self-examination. If detected early, recurrences can usually be managed with minimally invasive strategies, given that this tumor rarely invades beyond the subepithelial connective tissue. If neglected, however, these lesions can become quite extensive, producing complete local destruction of the penis. In such cases, amputation is the best alternative.

ii) Basaloid carcinoma. Poorly differentiated variant usually presenting with advanced disease.

iii) Spindle cell (sarcomatoid) carcinoma. Very rare but associated with a better prognosis than conventional squamous cell carcinoma.

iv) Penile malignant melanoma. Less than 1% of penile carcinomas. Depth of invasion important.

b. Etiology

The development of penile carcinoma has long been associated with poor hygiene and exposure to irritants, carcinogens, or possible viral pathogens. In particular, the organism *Mycobacterium smegmatis* has been shown to convert sterols present in smegma to substances that have been shown to be carcinogenic in mice. In addition, infection with HPV 16 or

HPV 18 has been associated with up to 60% of penile and cervical carcinomas, suggesting a venereal basis for both malignancies. Penile and urethral condyloma has been identified in up to 55% of sexual partners of women with cervical carcinoma. On the other hand, sexual partners of men with penile carcinoma have a threefold higher incidence of cervical carcinoma. Malignant transformation of HPV-infected cells is thought to result from the inactivation of tumor suppressor gene proteins (p53 and Rb) by viral gene products E6 and E7.

c. Natural History

Carcinoma of the penis usually begins as a small lesion on the glans or prepuce, which may be exophytic or ulcerative and accompanied by secondary infection. Invasion is usually direct and capable of destroying surrounding tissue. Exophytic lesions tend to be better differentiated than ulcerative lesions, which may also exhibit spindle cell morphology and tend to metastasize earlier. Regional inguinal and iliac nodes are the earliest sites of dissemination, in that order. The right and left lymphatic drainage systems are interconnected. The lymphatic drainage of the prepuce terminates in the upper inner group of superficial inguinal lymphatics. In the glans, however, lymphatics divide to follow the femoral canal and drain to superficial inguinal nodes, the nodes of Cloquet (or Rosenmueller), and retrofemoral nodes. Distant metastases may involve the abdominal lymph nodes, liver, and lungs. Death is usually secondary to involvement of regional nodes, which results in skin necrosis, chronic infection, sepsis, or hemorrhage secondary to erosion into the femoral vessels.

d. Clinical Features

Carcinoma of the penis generally begins as a painless nodule, wart-like growth, ulceration, or vesicle. Phimosis is present in as many as 50% of patients. Because the patient usually ignores the lesion until it reaches a considerable size, the mean time lag for diagnosis is 1 year after initial recognition. Lymph nodes are palpably enlarged in almost 50% of patients, but in many cases the adenopathy is secondary to infection.

e. Diagnosis and Staging

Diagnosis depends on tissue biopsy. Tumor size, location, fixation, and involvement of the corporal bodies should be assessed. Careful bilateral palpation of the inguinal areas is of extreme importance. The Jackson and American Joint Commission on Cancer (AJCC) staging systems are commonly employed (Table 16-3a, b). Metastatic evaluation should include a CXR, CBC, and comprehensive metabolic panel including an alkaline phosphatase and calcium level. Patients with prior inguinal surgery or obese patients should undergo CT or MRI of the groin. A bone scan may be ordered based on the patient's symptoms and alkaline phosphatase.

4. *Treatment*

a. Primary Lesion

All penile lesions present for more that 3 weeks should undergo biopsy with a deep margin to ensure proper staging. Lesions confined to the prepuce may be treated by simple circumcision.

Penile salvage strategies:

i) **Laser ablation:** The four most widely used laser energy sources include the CO_2, argon, Nd:YAG, and potassium titanyl phosphate (KTP) lasers. The superficial depth of penetration of the CO_2 laser (limited to 0.1 mm) makes it suboptimal for the treatment of penile CIS or small T1 tumors, with recurrence rates as high as 50%. Conversely, the Nd:YAG laser results in protein denaturation at a depth of up to 6 mm by emitting at a wavelength of 1060 nm. Although overall recurrence rates after laser ablation have been reported around 8% for penile Tis and have ranged from 10–25% for T1 lesions, results from more contemporary series using the Nd:YAG laser with tumor base biopsies have been more encouraging. In this setting, recurrence rates have remained below 7%. Close surveillance and patient self-examination are paramount after this modality. Recurrences are best treated with wide local excision or partial amputation.

ii) **Mohs' microsurgery** has had a positive impact on the management of penile CIS and small superficially invasive tumors. As originally described by Mohs, it involves layer-by-layer complete excision of the penile lesion in multiple sessions (fixed tissue technique), with microscopic examination of the undersurface of each layer. Its sequential microscopic guidance offers improved precision and control of the negative margin while maximizing organ preservation. Although results with Mohs' microsurgery are likely equivalent to those for partial amputation for CIS or for small, distal, superficially

Table 16-3a:—Jackson Classification for Squamous Penile Carcinoma

Stage I	Tumor confined to glans or prepuce
Stage II	Invasion into shaft or corpora; no nodal or distant metastases
Stage III	Tumor confined to penis; operable inguinal nodal metastases
Stage IV	Tumor involves adjacent structures; inoperable inguinal nodes and/or distant metastasis(es)

Table 16-3b:—AJCC Staging System for Penile Carcinoma

Primary tumor (T)	
TX	Tumor stage cannot be assessed
T0	No evidence of primary tumor
Tis	Carcinoma in situ
Ta	Noninvasive verrucous carcinoma
T1	Tumor invades subepithelial connective tissue
T2	Tumor invades corpus spongiosum or cavernosum
T3	Tumor invades urethral or prostate
T4	Tumor invades other adjacent structures
Regional lymph nodes (N)	
NX	Regional lymph nodes cannot be assessed
N0	No regional lymph node metastasis
N1	Metastasis in a single, superficial, inguinal lymph node
N2	Metastasis in multiple or bilateral superficial inguinal lymph nodes
N3	Metastasis in deep inguinal or pelvic lymph nodes
Distant metastasis (M)	
MX	Presence of distant metastasis cannot be assessed
M1	No distant metastasis
M1	Distant metastasis

invasive tumors, the use of this technique in higher stage tumors (corpora cavernosum or urethral involvement) or in those larger than 3 cm should be discouraged.

iii) **Brachytherapy:** Interstitial radiation has been used successfully to treat penile carcinoma with a variety of radioisotopes, including radium[226], iridium[192], and cesium[137]. Data from a number of centers in Canada, Europe, and India show that penile conservation may be achieved in up to 83% of patients, with 5-year local recurrence rates varying between 24 and 57%. The pathologic variables associated with treatment failure in most studies have been the presence of corporal invasion and tumor size greater than 4 cm. Although some series report 5-year disease-free survival rates as high as 78%, delayed side effects have been reported in up to 53% of patients. The most common complications include urethral stricture disease (45%) and penile necrosis (23%).

iv) **Partial penectomy:** In summary, patients with superficial tumors (stages Tis and T1) may be managed with Mohs' microresection, laser photocoagulation (CO_2 or Nd:YAG), or radiation therapy (external beam or brachytherapy) with approximate recurrence rates of 6%, 25%, and 21%, respectively. Large stage T1 tumors and T2 lesions of the glans or penile shaft should be treated by partial penile amputation, ensuring a 2-cm tissue margin proximal to the tumor, because local wedge resection has a 50% recurrence rate versus 0–8% with partial penectomy. In bulky T3 and T4 tumors or if tumor location is such that amputation would leave a penile stump inadequate for voiding or sexual activity, a total penectomy with perineal urethrostomy is preferred.

b. Inguinal Lymph Nodes

For patients with invasive penile carcinoma, the most important prognostic factors for survival are the presence and extent of inguinal lymph node metastases. It is rational to perform a traditional inguinal lymphadenectomy in those patients with clinically positive lymph nodes, as penile squamous cancer represents one of the few urologic malignancies in which patients with limited inguinal metastases are cured with surgery alone. Unfortunately, if the procedure is applied to all patients with invasive penile cancer and clinically negative inguinal examinations, it would benefit only an average of 20–25% of patients. This is relevant given that, even in recent reports, approximately 58% of patients will develop at least one complication. Therefore, unless a patient presents with an obvious inguinal mass warranting a fine-needle biopsy, patients with inguinal adenopathy should be treated with 6 weeks of oral antibiotics after undergoing penectomy to segregate those patients with true metastases. One quarter of patients without palpable adenopathy will harbor nodes containing metastases.

Patients with palpable inguinal lymphadenopathy despite oral antibiotic therapy should undergo superficial and deep ipsilateral ilioinguinal lymphadenectomy. These patients should also undergo a contralateral superficial inguinal lymphadenectomy because contralateral inguinal node involvement may be present in 50% of patients and iliac node metastases in one third of cases. An exception to performing inguinal routine lymphadenectomy in the presence of a clinically positive lymph node would be in the case where the primary tumor was proven to be CIS or verrucous carcinoma. Given the reportable incidence of metastases in patients with these diagnoses, a course of antibiotic therapy followed by excisional biopsy (if enlargement persists) of the involved node is a rational initial step.

Although approximately 20% of patients with nonpalpable inguinal lymph nodes harbor microscopic metastasis, the performance of a prophylactic inguinal lymphadenectomy is controversial due to its significant morbidity. Nevertheless, recent reports indicate that survival is significantly improved in patients who undergo a prophylactic (5-year survival, 88%) versus delayed (38%) inguinal lymphadenectomy. Although no strict criteria have been established, indications for prophylactic superficial inguinal lymphadenectomy in patients with a normal inguinal physical examination include invasive T1–T3 lesions, lymphovascular invasion, and advanced tumor grade.

The margins of dissection of the inguinal lymphadenectomy include the inguinal ligament, adductor longus, sartorius, and the base of the femoral triangle. The fascia lata separates the superficial from the deep inguinal lymph node compartments. The development of modified dissections involving limited surgical margins and the preservation of the saphenous vein may incur less morbidity. The sartorius muscle may be detached from the anterior superior iliac spine and repositioned more medially to protect the femoral vessels. Alternatively, a gracilis or rectus muscle flap may be used to fill large defects after resecting large masses, thus preventing vessel erosion and skin necrosis.

Because the presence of pelvic node disease portends a very poor outcome, patients with clinically positive lymph nodes should undergo a chest radiograph and cross-sectional imaging (CT or MR) of the abdomen and pelvis before surgery to detect the presence of pelvic or distant metastases. Given the increased risk of treatment failure for those patients with clinically proven pelvic lymph node metastases, bilateral positive inguinal lymph nodes, multiple unilateral nodes, as well as extranodal extension of cancer (correlates with a $\geq$4-cm node or fixed inguinal adenopathy), a fine-needle aspiration of nodal sites is reasonable to document the presence of cancer. Once cancer is confirmed, our preferred approach for these patients includes neoadjuvant chemotherapy followed by surgical consolidation.

Those patients with poor prognostic pathologic features after lymphadenectomy, such as extranodal extension, two or more positive nodes, bilateral inguinal metastases, or positive pelvic nodes, are considered for adjuvant chemotherapy because of the high risk of relapse in this subset of patients. Patients who exhibit minimal microscopic disease may be followed closely.

5. Prognosis

The 5-year survival rate in patients without palpable adenopathy is 65–80%. Patients with positive lymph nodes have 5-year survival rates of 20–50%, with the poorest survival noted in patients with iliac metastases. As many as 90% of patients with pathologically negative inguinal nodes may survive 5 years. Chemotherapy regimens for metastatic disease include single-agent therapy with cisplatin, methotrexate, bleomycin, or cyclophosphamide. Combination therapy regimens include bleomycin, vincristine, and methotrexate; methotrexate, bleomycin, and cisplatin; and cisplatin and 5-fluorouracil. Up to 30% of patients will exhibit a partial response, but complete responses are rare. Chemotherapy with ifosfamide, paclitaxel, and cisplatin has been effective in head and neck squamous cell carcinomas and has shown promising results in phase II trials with penile cancer patients. Radiation therapy may be effective for T1 and T2 lesions but has been traditionally poor for higher stage lesions.

6. Surveillance

In penile carcinoma, surveillance strategies can be tailored to the risks of recurrence, which vary according to the pathologic characteristics of the primary tumor and the modalities employed for local therapy (phallus-sparing or extirpative) and regional therapy (surveillance or lymphadenectomy). Men at a higher risk for local or regional recurrence who should have more rigorous follow-up include those (1) treated with phallus-sparing strategies such as laser ablation, topical therapies, or radiotherapy; (2) patients with clinically negative inguinal lymph nodes who are managed without lymphadenectomy despite high-risk primary tumors (pT2–3, grade 3, vascular invasion); and (3) those with lymph node metastases after lymphadenectomy. Good candidates for less stringent surveillance include patients with low-risk primary tumors (pTis, pTa, pT1, grades 1–2) and those with negative inguinal nodes after lymphadenectomy whose primary tumors were managed with partial or total penectomy.

C. Carcinoma of the Scrotum

Carcinoma of the scrotum, initially identified in chimney sweeps by Sir Percival Pott, was one of the first environmentally related carcinomas described. Mule spinners also suffered from scrotal carcinoma, as their clothes became saturated with lubricating oil from the spinning jenny. Squamous cell carcinoma arose from exposure to the aromatic hydrocarbons in soot, tars, and petroleum products. These tumors are exceedingly rare. They present as ulcerated or exophytic growths. Wide local excision with or without ipsilateral ilioinguinal lymphadenectomy is the treatment of choice. Nonoccupational tumors of the scrotum include reticulum cell carcinoma, rhabdomyosarcoma, leiomyosarcoma, liposarcoma, and melanoma.

D. The Pigmented Penile Lesion

Primary malignant melanoma of the penis, male urethra, or scrotum is rare. Since initially described in 1859, fewer than 150 cases of penile melanoma have been reported. This accounts for approximately 1.4% of all primary penile carcinomas and 0.1–0.2% of all extraorbital melanomas. Reports of male urethral and scrotal melanoma are even less common, with approximately 50 cases of male urethral melanoma since the initial report by Tyrell in 1871. Only 17 cases of scrotal melanoma have been reported. The differential diagnosis of penile melanoma is broad, including melanocytic nevi, penile melanosis, genital lentiginosis (also referred to as atypical pigmented penile macules), pigmented squamous cell carcinoma, sarcomas, spindle cell carcinoma, hemangiomas, and extramammary Paget's disease. Any lesion changing in size, shape, or consistency should be biopsied. The treatment of penile melanoma is similar to penile squamous carcinoma and is beyond the scope of this chapter.

V. TESTICULAR TUMORS

A. General Comments

Testicular tumors are uncommon but are the most curable form of urologic cancers. More than 95% of lesions are derived from germinal tissue, whereas the rest arise from nongerminal or stromal cells. Germ cell tumors (GCTs) of the testicle are classified as pure seminoma or as nonseminomatous. Seminomas are exquisitely sensitive to radiation therapy, whereas both seminoma and nonseminomatous germ cell tumors (NSGCT) are very responsive to platinum-based combination chemotherapy. Retroperitoneal lymphadenectomy plays a very important role in the treatment of NSGCT. The tumor markers beta-human chorionic gonadotropin (beta-HCG) and alpha-fetoprotein (AFP) are extremely useful in diagnosing and monitoring the disease.

B. Incidence

The general incidence of testicular cancers (2.3 per 100,000 per year) appears to be slowly rising; 8250 new cases of testicular cancer are estimated per year. Only 370 deaths from this disease are expected. This mortality statistic is almost 10-fold lower than it was 15 years ago due to the ability of platinum-based chemotherapy to cure this disease.

C. Etiology

No definitive cause of testicular cancer has been identified. Testicular maldescent has been associated with the disease, and a 5- to 15-fold relative risk for developing a testicular tumor exists if this condition is present. Of patients with testicular cancer, 7–12% have a prior history of cryptorchidism. In patients with unilateral cryptorchidism and testicular cancer, the tumor occurs in the contralateral testicle in 5–15% of cases. There is a slight predilection for testis tumors on the right side. This coincides with the slightly greater involvement of the right testis with cryptorchidism.

D. Epidemiology

Testicular cancer occurs most frequently in young men and is the most common solid tumor in men between the ages of 20 and 34. Smaller peak incidences exist for men older than 60 years. The cumulative lifetime risk of developing testicular cancer is 1 in 500. The incidence of testicular cancer in black Americans is approximately one fourth to one third of that in whites, although a slight rise in incidence has been recently reported among African-Americans. A higher incidence of disease has been noted in Scandinavia.

E. Natural History

Intratubular germ cell neoplasia in situ initially grows beyond the basement membrane to eventually replace some or all of the testicular parenchyma. Because 50% of patients with testicular CIS will progress to a GCT, patients with this finding on testis biopsy (usually performed as part of an infertility evaluation) should undergo radical orchiectomy. Epididymal and cord involvement is hindered by the tunica albuginea.

1. Although pure seminoma is confined to the testis at initial presentation in two thirds to three fourths of cases, up to two thirds of patients with NSGCT may present with metastasis. Lymphatic spread may occur early and usually precedes vascular invasion. Early vascular invasion is noted frequently in pure choriocarcinoma. Sites of hematogenous spread include the lungs, liver, and bone.

2. In patients with organ-confined NSGCT after orchiectomy (stage I or A), distant failure will occur in about 30% of patients (80% retroperitoneal; 20% distant). If a retroperitoneal lymph node dissection (RPLND) is performed for stage I disease, the risk of recurrence depends on the number and size of involved nodes. These recurrences are almost exclusively at an extraretroperitoneal site, usually in the chest.

3. All germinal cell testis tumors in adults should be treated as malignant. Spontaneous regression of this disease is extremely rare. The majority of patients who die from testicular cancer do so within 3 years of diagnosis. Delay in diagnosis has been associated with a worse outcome.

F. Pathology

1. Germinal Neoplasms

a. Seminoma

i) Classic. Pure or "classic" seminoma accounts for approximately 85% of seminomas and 30% of all testicular GCTs. Approximately 15% will also contain syncytiotrophoblastic elements, which may produce HCG. Peak incidence is seen in the fourth and fifth decades of life, one decade later than NSGCT. Grossly, seminomas appear as well-defined, yellow-tan tumors.

ii) Anaplastic. Account for approximately 10% of seminomas. Characterized by increased mitotic activity. Although they usually present at higher stages than classic seminoma, stage for stage, these tumors carry the same prognosis. These tumors account for 30% of mortalities due to seminoma.

iii) Spermatocytic. Classically seen in an older age group (50% are older than 50 years), it accounts for 1–2% of all testicular tumors. Only one case of metastasis has been reported, so inguinal orchiectomy is sufficient treatment.

b. Embryonal Carcinoma

Represent approximately 3% of pure GCTs but may be a component of up to 25% of mixed GCTs.

c. Teratoma (With or Without Malignant Transformation)

These tumors may be composed of endodermal, mesodermal, or ectodermal elements. It is the second most common testicular tumor in children after yolk sac tumor. Treatment is surgical because response to radiotherapy and chemotherapy is poor. Many arise from transformation of NSGCT after chemotherapy.

i) Mature.
ii) Immature.
iii) Malignant non-germ cell.

d. Choriocarcinoma

Represent less than 1% of all NSGCT. Usually present with advanced clinical stage and very high serum levels of HCG.

e. Yolk Sac Tumor

Also referred to as endodermal sinus tumor, it is the most common NSGCT in children. It accounts for roughly 2% of all GCTs in its pure form but may be present in up to 25% of mixed GCTs. Cells produce AFP, which may be measured in serum.

2. Nongerminal Neoplasms

a. Specialized Gonadal Stromal Tumors

i) Leydig cell tumor. May be associated with gynecomastia.
ii) Sertoli cell tumor.

iii) Gonadoblastoma.
iv) Miscellaneous neoplasms.

b. Carcinoid

c. Adrenal Rests

d. Mesenchymal Neoplasms

G. Staging

1. Different systems for staging testicular tumors are not uniform but are based on the basic subdivisions proposed by Boden and Gibb: stage A (I): confined to the testicle; stage B (II): retroperitoneal node involvement; stage C (III): extranodal metastasis.
2. Stage II disease has been subdivided by Skinner and others to more accurately express its clinical manifestations.
   IIa: Less than six positive nodes, none more than 2 cm in any dimension.
   IIb: More than six positive nodes, any more than 2 cm in any dimension.
   IIc: Massive retroperitoneal disease (>5 cm).
3. Seminoma. There is a wide variance in the representative staging systems. Stage 1: limited to the testis; stage 2A: positive retroperitoneal nodes on imaging examination; stage 2B: palpable abdominal mass; stage 3: supradiaphragmatic adenopathy, mediastinal, and/or cervical; stage 4: visceral metastases.
4. The AJCC staging system includes a separate category for tumor marker status to aid in identifying patients with high risk for relapse (Table 16-5).

H. Clinical Presentation

1. Because this disease affects a younger age group not generally aware of the possible diagnosis, a 4- to 6-month delay in diagnosis is not uncommon. The most common symptom is a painless testicular mass. In some series, however, pain has been associated with almost one half of the presentations.
2. Between 5 and 25% of patients may be initially misdiagnosed and treated for epididymitis.
3. Gynecomastia may be present and is secondary to elevation of HCG in GCT or the effect of tumor estradiol synthesis with Leydig cell tumors. Cough, abdominal mass, back pain, and supraclavicular or other lymphadenopathy may present in cases of advanced disease.

Table 16-4:—Definitions of Clinical Stages for Testis Cancer	
I or A	Tumor confined to the testicle or cord structure
II_A or B_1	Microscopic regional lymph node involvement in <6 nodes
II_B or B_2	Microscopic involvement in >6 regional lymph nodes or gross nodal involvement <6 cm
II_C or B_2	Gross nodal involvement >6 cm in one lymph node or as an aggregate of lymph nodes
III or C	Disease above the diaphragm or involving abdominal organs
(Regional Nodes) Clinical	
NX	Regional lymph nodes cannot be assessed
N0	No regional lymph node metastasis
N1	Metastasis with a lymph node mass 2 cm or less in greatest dimension; or multiple lymph nodes, none more than 2 cm in greatest dimension
N2	Metastasis with a lymph node mass, more than 2 cm but not more than 5 cm in greatest dimension; or multiple lymph nodes any one mass greater than 2 cm but not more than 5 cm in greatest dimension
N3	Metastasis with a lymph node mass more than 5 cm in greatest dimension

I. Diagnosis

1. Transcrotal ultrasound can confirm the presence of an intraparenchymal testicular mass, rule out benign processes such as a hydrocele or epididymitis, and effectively evaluate the contralateral gonad.

2. Inguinal (radical) orchiectomy. The primary lesion is best handled by early clamping of the spermatic cord near the

Table 16-5:—Staging for Testis Carcinoma

Primary tumor T stage (pT)

pT0	No evidence of tumor in testis (scar may be present)
pTis	Intratubular germ cell neoplasia (CIS)
pT1	Tumor limited to the testis/epididymis without vascular or lymphatic invasion. Tumor may invade the tunica albuginea but not the tunica vaginalis
pT2	Tumor limited to the testis/epididymis with vascular or lymphatic invasion or tumor extending to and involving the tunica vaginalis
pT3	Tumor invading the spermatic core ± vascular or lymphatic invasion
pT4	Tumor invading the scrotum ± vascular or lymphatic invasion

Regional nodes (N)

pNX	Regional lymph nodes cannot be assessed
pN0	No regional lymph node metastasis
pN1	Metastasis with a lymph node mass, 2 cm or less in greatest dimension and less than or equal to 5 nodes positive, none more than 2 cm in greatest dimension
pN2	Metastasis with a lymph node mass, more than 2 cm but not more than 5 cm in greatest dimension; or more than 5 nodes positive, none more than 5 cm; or evidence of extranodal extension of tumor
pN3	Metastasis with a lymph node mass more than 5 cm in greatest dimension

Distant metastasis (M)

MX	Distant metastasis cannot be assessed
M0	No distant metastasis
M1	Distant metastasis
M1a	Nonregional nodal or pulmonary metastasis
M1b	Distant metastasis other than to nonregional lymph node and lungs

Serum tumor markers (S)

SX	Marker studies not available
S0	Markers within normal limits
S1	LDH $<1.5 \times$ normal AND HCG <5000 mIu/mL AND AFP <1000 ng/mL

| S2 | LDH 1.5–10 × normal OR HCG 5000–50,000 mIu/mL OR AFP 1000–10,000 ng/mL |
| S3 | LDH >10 × normal OR HCG >50,000 mIu/mL OR AFP >10,000 ng/mL |

CIS, carcinoma in situ; LDH, lactate dehydrogenase; HCG, human chorionic gonadotropin; AFP, alpha-fetoprotein.

internal ring and complete removal of the gonad. Only in very rare circumstances are exploration and frozen biopsy performed. Children with teratomas may be managed with partial orchiectomy. The extent of local involvement by the tumor, tumor size, presence of vascular invasion, and tumor histology will dictate the need for adjuvant therapy. A scrotal approach should not be employed because this may theoretically increase the risk of inguinal nodal metastasis and recurrence. Nevertheless, there is no need for a hemi-scrotectomy or prophylactic inguinal lymph node dissection in the rare patient who has undergone a scrotal orchiectomy for testicular cancer.

3. Imaging is best conducted with a standard CXR and a CT scan of the abdomen/pelvis. There is a 20–30% chance of understaging lesions by this method. Chest CT detects many small nodules, which are usually benign. Pedal lymphangiography is no longer performed on a regular basis.

4. Tumor markers.

   a) HCG. HCG is a heterodimeric protein with immunologically distinct chains. Circulating levels are extremely low (1 ng/mL) in normal males. The syncytiotrophoblastic tissue of some GCTs produces this substance. It can therefore be detected in almost all choriocarcinomas, 40–60% of embryonal cell carcinomas, and 5–10% of pure seminomas. The half-life for this substance is roughly 24 hours, but the beta subunit alone has a half-life of 1 hour. Because beta-HCG shares structural homology with luteinizing hormone (LH), spurious elevations may occur in patients with inadequate testosterone production from the contralateral testis (thus higher LH).

   b) AFP. AFP is an oncofetal protein detected in testis and liver tumors. It is produced by yolk sac elements that may or may not be histologically recognized. This substance is not produced in pure choriocarcinoma or pure seminoma. The presence of elevated AFP in a patient with histologic seminoma precludes the diagnosis of pure seminoma. The half-life of AFP is 5–7 days.

c) LDH. This general cellular enzyme is not particularly specific for testicular lesions but provides a correlation to tumor bulk. It may have some role in monitoring patients with advanced seminoma and in marker-negative patients with NSGCT and persistent disease.

d) Over all stages, 90% of patients with nonseminomatous tumors will have an elevation of one or both markers. Fifty to 70% will display an elevation of AFP and 40–60% will have an elevation of beta-HCG. In stage I lesions, two thirds of patients will have an elevation of one or both major markers. After therapy, tumor markers should display a logarithmic pattern of decrease in accordance with their half-lives. Sustained elevation of markers or slower decrease after orchiectomy or RPLND suggests residual disease. Normalization of markers is not definite evidence of complete surgical cure.

J. Treatment (After Orchiectomy)

1. Seminoma

Patients with stage I tumors may exhibit a 15% risk of retroperitoneal recurrence, depending on the tumor size, local stage, and presence of vascular invasion. In this setting, the most conservative approach consists of prophylactic retroperitoneal radiotherapy. In the era of platinum-based chemotherapy, prophylactic mediastinal radiotherapy is no longer recommended due to its toxicity. The 5-year actuarial cure rates approach 97% in low-stage disease. In Europe, randomized trials have shown that single dose carboplatin may be as effective as radiotherapy in preventing recurrence, but long-term follow-up has not been reported.

Patients with small primary tumors and no vascular invasion and no invasion of the rete testis may elect to forego radiotherapy and choose close surveillance. The benefits of surveillance include a decreased risk of gastrointestinal complications and secondary malignancies. These patients should be committed to intense follow-up, with either radiation therapy or chemotherapy initiated at the time of progression. Some debate exists with regard to treatment for intermediate stage disease, whereas most agree that chemotherapy should be employed in bulky or advanced disease (stage IIb and III). Although anaplastic seminoma usually presents at a higher stage than classic seminoma, it carries the same prognosis stage for stage and should be treated as such. The use of RPLND in the treatment of post-chemotherapy residual disease is controversial. Due to the significant desmoplastic reaction of the mass to the retroperitoneum, most centers choose to observe masses that are smaller than 3 cm in size. Recently, fluorodeoxyglucose positron emission tomography (FDG-PET) has demonstrated the ability to identify which seminoma patients with a residual mass have viable tumor.

2. *Nonseminomatous Germ Cell Tumors*

Stage I. Clinical stage I NSGCTs are best treated with RPLND or careful surveillance, depending on the pathologic characteristics of the primary tumor. RPLND may be performed by a transabdominal or thoracoabdominal approach. Only 10% of patients treated this way will relapse, and virtually all recurrences will occur in the chest, which is easily monitored and treated. The cure rate for this approach is roughly 99%. If a patient decides against surgery and undergoes intensive surveillance after orchiectomy, relapse may occur in up to 30% of cases (chest and retroperitoneum), even decades after the primary tumor. Lymphovascular invasion in the orchiectomy specimen increases the risk of metastatic progression. Some investigators have reported on adjuvant chemotherapy in this setting.

The major long-term complication of RPLND is disruption of ejaculatory function as a result of damage to the sympathetic nerve fibers to the pelvis. Decreased morbidity has been obtained by mapping the metastatic deposits of NSGCT and developing surgical templates specific for the involved testicle. Lymphatics from the right testicle drain primarily to retroperitoneal nodes in the interaortocaval region. In addition, metastatic disease from right-sided tumors may cross over to the left side. For this reason, a modified right-sided template RPLND should include a complete dissection above the level of the inferior mesenteric artery (IMA) up to the renal vessels, laterally up to both ureters, and caudally (below the IMA) down to the aortic bifurcation on the ipsilateral side. Left-sided tumors, however, primarily metastasize to the para-aortic lymph nodes and rarely cross over to the right side. A modified left-sided RPLND is the mirror image of a modified right-sided template, except that the right-sided border only extends near the right margin of the inferior vena cava and not the ureter. Using a nerve-sparing technique, ejaculation is preserved in 75–90% of patients with little potential compromise of

surgical cure. Oral sympathomimetics may aid in decreasing
the incidence of ejaculatory dysfunction.

3. Early Stage 2 Disease May Be Treated With Surgery or Chemotherapy

Although this is controversial, most would agree that the presence of teratoma in the primary specimen favors surgery over
chemotherapy in this setting. Advanced stage 2 and 3 disease is
best treated by chemotherapy first, followed by a postchemotherapy RPLND for suspected residual disease. Postchemotherapy
tumor histology may show only necrotic tumor (40%), mature
teratoma (40%), or residual carcinoma (20%).

4. Chemotherapy

Platinum-based combination chemotherapy has revolutionized the treatment of this disease. Patients with metastatic
disease are risk stratified according to the International
Germ Cell Consensus Classification into good-, intermedi-
ate-, and poor-risk categories (Table 16-6). Patients with
good-risk disease are treated with three cycles of the bleomy-
cin/etoposide/cisplatin (BEP) regimen or four cycles of the
etoposide/cisplatin (EP) regimen. Patients with intermedi-
ate- and high-risk disease are treated with BEP for four
cycles. For patients who are intolerant of bleomycin, etopo-
side/ifosfamide/cisplatin (VIP) for four cycles can be substituted but is associated with more toxicity. Present clinical
research efforts are now being directed at salvage chemotherapy and the combined use of chemotherapy and
stem cell transplant in patients with advanced disease.
Patients who have a residual retroperitoneal mass after chemotherapy for metastatic NSGCT with normalization of
serum tumor markers should be considered for retroperitoneal lymphadenectomy, given that histology will demonstrate fibrosis (50%), teratoma (40%), or residual
carcinoma (10%). Consideration should be given to resection of all sites of residual disease if possible. Resection of
the entire mass is required because teratomas are not radio-
sensitive or chemosensitive and if left untreated can invade
structures or transform into malignant tumor. Patients with
residual viable GCT should undergo two additional cycles of
EP chemotherapy. Patients with residual masses after treatment for seminoma should undergo PET. If the PET scan
is negative, these patients can be observed. Patients with
metastatic disease who do not normalize their markers or
who relapse after having attained a remission are generally
treated with salvage chemotherapy, which may include an

Table 16-6:—International Germ Cell Consensus Risk Classification for Metastatic Germ Cell Tumor

	Seminoma	NSGCT
Good	Any primary; normal AFP, any HCG or LDH; nonpulmonary visceral mets absent	Testis/retroperitoneal primary; AFP <1000 ng/mL, HCG <5000 mIU/mL, LDH <1.5× ULN; and, nonpulmonary visceral mets absent
Intermediate	Any primary; normal AFP, any HCG or LDH; nonpulmonary visceral mets present	Testis/retroperitoneal primary; AFP 1000–10,000 ng/mL, HCG 5000–50,000 mIU/mL, LDH 1.5–10× ULN; and nonpulmonary visceral mets absent
Poor		Mediastinal primary; or AFP >10,000 ng/mL, HCG >50,000 mIU/mL, LDH >10× ULN; or nonpulmonary visceral mets present

NSGCT, nonseminomatous germ cell tumor; AFP, alpha-fetoprotein; HCG, human chorionic gonadotropin; LDH, lactate dehydrogenase; ULN, upper limits of normal.

ifosfamide-based regimen or high-dose chemotherapy with stem cell transplant.

5. Patient Surveillance

For detailed guidelines concerning various surveillance protocols, the reader is referred to the National Comprehensive Cancer Network Clinical Practice Guidelines in Oncology—v.1.2006 (www.nccn.org).

K. Other Testis Neoplasms

1. Leydig Cell Tumors

a) Constitute 1–3% of testis tumors.
b) Ten percent are malignant. They are never malignant in prepubertal patients.

c) Malignancy is diagnosed by presence of metastases.
d) Histologic determination of malignancy unreliable.

2. Sertoli Cell Tumors

a) Less than 1% of testis tumors.
b) Ten percent are malignant (determined by presence of metastases).

SELF-ASSESSMENT QUESTIONS

1. What is von Hippel-Lindau disease? What nonurologic abnormalities are part of the condition? What genetic abnormalities are associated with it?
2. What are the advantages and disadvantages of a laparoscopic radical nephrectomy when compared to open nephrectomy?
3. What paraneoplastic syndromes are associated with renal cell carcinoma?
4. What are the anatomic boundaries of the inguinal lymphadenectomy for penile cancer?
5. What are the indications for inguinal lymphadenectomy in penile cancer?
6. What occupational risk is classically associated with scrotal cancer?
7. A 35-year-old man with stage I embryonal carcinoma elects watchful waiting over retroperitoneal lymph node dissection. What is his risk of relapse? If he does relapse, what is his chance of cure with chemotherapy?
8. A 30-year-old male undergoes primary chemotherapy for a NSGCT metastatic to the retroperitoneum (6 cm) with a reduction in size of 40%. His tumor markers are negative and he undergoes RPLND. What is the pathology likely to show?
9. What are possible complications after retroperitoneal lymph node dissection?
10. How should patients with seminoma be followed? Is this different from patients with nonseminomatous germ cell tumor?

SUGGESTED READINGS

1. Cadeddu JA, Ono Y, Clayman RV, et al: Laparoscopic nephrectomy for renal cell cancer: evaluation of efficacy and safety: a multicenter experience. *Urology* 52:773–777, 1998.

2. Catalona WJ: Modified inguinal lymphadenectomy for carcinoma of the penis with preservation of saphenous vein: technique and preliminary results. *J Urol* 140:306–310, 1988.

3. Donohue JP, Thornhill JA, Foster RS, et al: Retroperitoneal lymphadenectomy for clinical stage A testis cancer (1965 to 1989): modifications of technique and impact on ejaculation. *J Urol* 149:237–243, 1993.

4. Flanigan RC, Salmon SE, Blumenstein BA, et al: Nephrectomy followed by interferon alfa-2b compared with interferon alfa-2b alone for metastatic renal-cell cancer. *N Engl J Med* 345:1655–1659, 2001.

5. Levy DA, Slaton JW, Swanson DA, Dinney CP: Stage specific guidelines for surveillance after radical nephrectomy for local renal cell carcinoma. *J Urol* 159:1163–1167, 1998.

6. Novick AC, Derweesh I: Open partial nephrectomy for renal tumours: current status. *BJU Int* 95(Suppl 2):35–40, 2005.

7. Sánchez-Ortiz RF, Pettaway CA: Natural history, management, and surveillance of recurrent squamous cell penile carcinoma: a risk-based approach. *Urol Clin North Am* 30:853–867, 2003.

8. Williams SD, Birch R, Einhorn LH, et al: Treatment of disseminated germ cell tumors with cisplatinum, bleomycin and either vinblastine or etopide. *N Engl J Med* 316:1435, 1987.

9. Zbar B, Brauch H, Talmadge C, Linehan M: Loss of alleles of loci on the short arm of chromosome 3 in renal cell carcinoma. *Nature* 327:721, 1987.

Radiation Therapy

Pinaki R. Dutta, MD, PhD and
Richard Whittington, MD

Because of the high success rates of disease control with different treatment modalities, the role of radiation in the management of genitourinary malignancy is one of the more controversial topics in clinical oncology. Radiation may be used alone in the curative management of some tumors or in combination with other therapies as an adjuvant to surgery or chemotherapy. It also may be used as a salvage therapy after failure of surgical therapy or as a palliative therapy to alleviate symptoms in patients with advanced disease. Appropriate utilization of radiation requires knowledge of its mechanisms and techniques to understand the potential and the limitations of this modality.

X-rays and **gamma** rays, the two types of electromagnetic energy used to treat cancer, were discovered during the last decade of the 19th century, and the effects on tumors and normal tissues were quickly described. The first use of external beam radiation was reported by Pratt in 1896. In 1904, Alexander Graham Bell suggested that radioactive sources should be planted "directly into the heart of the tumor" and was brought to reality in 1912 when the first patient was treated with interstitial brachytherapy. Other modalities such as electrons, protons, neutrons, and π-mesons have been investigated. Thus far, only protons have shown potential utility in managing prostate cancer.

PHYSICS

Both x-rays and gamma rays are electromagnetic radiation. Gamma rays are radiation produced by the decay of radioactive isotopes, either natural or man-made, whereas x-rays, or **photons,** are artificially produced when charged particles strike a target. Gamma rays have well-defined energies characteristic of the isotope that emits them, whereas x-rays have a broader spectrum that is determined by the energy of the machine that produced them. Radiation dose delivered to the body is expressed in Gray (**Gy**). The energy of the electromagnetic radiation determines the ability of the radiation to penetrate tissue, with higher energy allowing deeper penetration. Higher energies scatter their energy in a more forward direction, so that with high-energy machines, the maximum energy is deposited below the skin surface. For this reason, a low-energy machine operating at a peak energy of 140,000 volts (140 kVp) would be preferable in treating superficial tumors such as skin cancer because the maximum dose is deposited in the skin, and the dose decreases exponentially to less than 25% of the maximum dose at a depth of 4 cm. For tumors deeper in the body, a more penetrating beam such as one operating at a peak energy of 10–15 million volts (10–15 MV) is preferable. A 15-MV beam deposits its maximum energy at a depth of 2.8 cm and is still able to deliver 50% of its maximum dose at a depth of 20 cm. Unlike the higher energy photons, electrons deposit their maximum dose at or near the surface, penetrate to a predictable depth with a relatively constant dose, and then decrease rapidly.

In some situations, it is preferable to deliver radiation to the tumor from an internal source. Radiation dose is determined by the ability of the radiation to penetrate tissue and the distance from the source of the radiation. Like visible light, the intensity of the radiation decreases in proportion to the square of the distance from the source ($1/d^2$). Because doubling the distance from the source of radiation will decrease the intensity by 75% and tripling the distance will decrease the intensity by 89%, it is reasonable to consider placing the source of radiation within the tumor to minimize the dose that would be delivered to the surrounding tissue.

Radioactive **isotopes** produce radiation with a decreasing dose rate as time passes, a process known as radioactive decay. Every isotope has a **half-life,** defined as the time required for the dose rate to decrease by 50%. However, there are situations in which a constant dose of radiation is desired, and therefore a long-lived isotope is inserted and then removed after a prescribed dose is delivered. In other cases it may be difficult to remove radioactive sources, and a permanent implant is used.

RADIOBIOLOGY

Radiation causes its effects in tissue by producing ionizations within the cell. The target in cells is the DNA molecule, and the ionizations will produce breaks in the DNA strand. Cells can repair this damage if it is confined to a single strand because the opposite strand serves as a template for repair. However, if two strand breaks occur on opposite chains in close proximity, the two ends of the chromosome may drift apart. These fragmented chromosomes may adhere to other chromosomes or they may sort out randomly when the cell divides, resulting in the daughter cells to be missing critical segments of DNA or have excess and unregulated copies of other genes, either of which may be fatal to the cell. Thus the damaged cells are observed to die a mitotic death; the lethal effect of radiation is not expressed until the cell dies.

Radiobiologic research is ongoing in identifying factors that affect the survival of cells and methods to selectively increase these effects on tumor cells. The easiest method to assay the effect of radiation is to deliver a dose of radiation to a suspension of single cells and then measure the percentage of surviving cells. The technique uses a suspension with a known concentration of cells. A sample is placed on a culture plate and the colonies are counted. At the same time a similar sized sample is radiated and plated and the number of colonies counted. The ratio of number of colonies developing on the two plates is the surviving fraction.

Because a Gy represents a specific amount of energy transferred to tissue, each Gy in theory should have an equal physical effect on the cell. However, the biologic effect is less for the first Gy than it is for the 101st Gy, suggesting that cells are capable of accumulating a certain amount of damage that is not lethal. Interestingly, if the radiation dose is split up and delivered over several **fractions** with time between fractions for cells to repair the damage, each fraction of radiation will kill the same proportion of the surviving cells. If the cells are allowed to completely repair the damage from the first dose, the second dose of radiation will have the same effect on the surviving cells as it would have if they had never been radiated the first time. This effect demonstrates the importance of uninterrupted radiation treatments. In vitro studies have shown normal cells to repair radiation-induced damage more efficiently than tumor cells, and attempts to deliver two doses of radiation per day, known as **hyperfractionation,** may increase the efficacy of treatment.

Oxygen is known to enhance the effects of radiation both in vivo and in vitro. Cells are more sensitive when radiated under oxygenated conditions than when they are hypoxic. Normal tissues are always oxygenated, but experimental measurements in tumors have shown that these cells will pile up around a capillary and consume the available oxygen, limiting diffusion into the tissues. This scenario results in well-oxygenated, relatively sensitive cells adjacent to the capillary and necrotic material at a distance from the capillary. Between these two areas is a region of viable but hypoxic cells that are more resistant to radiation. All in vitro studies thus far show that hypoxic cells require 1.5–3.0 times as much radiation to achieve the same cell kill.

Current efforts are being taken to develop substances that act like oxygen in cells but are not metabolized like oxygen. Ideally, these substances will help to deal with the problem of hypoxic tumor cells without affecting the sensitivity of normal cells. In vitro work showed that these compounds, known as **radiosensitizers,** sensitized hypoxic tumor cells to the effects of radiation. However, clinical trials were limited by toxicity. Similarly, efforts to develop drugs that protect normal cells from the effects of radiation are under way. Although, these trials have also have failed to show in vivo benefit, efforts continue to develop a new generation of sensitizers and protectors. More importantly, chemotherapy and hormonal therapies have been observed to affect tumor sensitivity in vivo and these agents form the basis of many current combined modality trials.

TREATMENT PLANNING

The delivery of radiation to a tumor requires a physician to perform five functions: (1) identify and locate the structures to be treated, (2) identify those adjacent structures that need to be protected, (3) prescribe the appropriate dose of radiation for the tumor based on its size and histology, (4) consider the tolerance of tissue within the target that may be affected by treatment, and (5) consider the tolerance of tissues between the skin and the target (transit volume). Although a complex but solvable problem, most clinical situations require some compromise on one or more issues. The clinician must select those compromises that will minimize effects on normal tissue while maximizing tumor control.

Modern equipment allows for sophisticated **three-dimensional conformal radiation treatment** (3D-CRT) planning and is becoming the standard in modern radiation oncology centers. Patients undergo computed tomography (CT)-based treatment planning in which a series of axial images is obtained of the target as well as the adjacent critical structures. The target or targets, depending on other areas at risk for tumor involvement, bony structures, and sensitive normal tissues, are defined on each CT slice. With computer assistance, a reconstruction of the target and the critical structures is obtained. Today's treatment machines are able to deliver radiation from a wide range of angles, no longer restricting the plane for treatment delivery. In addition, the system can calculate the dose to many small volumes within the target and to adjacent normal tissues.

For example, in the treatment of prostate cancer, the target consists of the prostate and a margin of tissue to account for day to day variation in setup, beam edges where the dose is not uniform, and organ motion. Newer techniques for consistent localization and patient positioning allow for tighter margins. Figure 17-1 shows the **dose volume histogram** for the prostate, bladder, and rectum of a patient being treated for prostate cancer. The dose through the prostate is homogenous with a minimum dose that is less than 5% less than the maximum dose. As a small volume of rec-

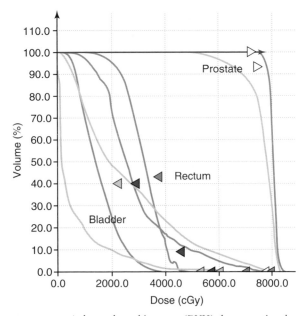

FIGURE 17-1. A dose volume histogram (DVH) demonstrating the dose delivered to the target organ (prostate) and organs at risk (bladder and rectum) is shown here. The goal in evaluating radiation treatment plans is to maximize the dose to the maximum volume of the target while minimizing the dose to normal structures.

tum will tolerate high doses of radiation, this figure shows that most of the rectum receives a much lower dose. In this histogram only 10% of the rectum received more than 50% of the total dose, but 50% of the rectum received less than 30% of the total dose. Older methods using anterior-posterior and lateral fields delivered at least 60% of the dose to the entire rectum and 40% of the rectum received more than 80% of the dose. Newer techniques using **intensity-modulated radiation treatment** (IMRT) have been able to reduce the dose exposure to normal tissues, and allow for higher doses to be delivered to the prostate without increased complications.

IMRT is a technique that has been recently developed that allows higher doses to be delivered to the target while minimizing radiation exposure to normal tissues. Again, CT images are obtained to identify the target and surrounding normal organs. Computers are used to plan the delivery of radiation to the 3D shape of the tumor and the radiation intensity is controlled using several smaller radiation fields, known as **beamlets,** from different beam directions. Each beamlet treats only a portion of the prostate, but when the dose from all of the beamlets are added together, the entire prostate receives the full dose with acceptable homogeneity, while reducing the volume of normal tissue receiving a high dose. Although the target receives the maximal dose, a larger volume of normal tissue is exposed to a small amount of radiation. Because of the decreased exposure to normal tissues, much higher and more effective doses can be delivered to the target with patients experiencing fewer side effects. As with conventional radiation delivery techniques, patient positioning is extremely critical in the delivery of IMRT. However, drawbacks from this technique include longer treatment times on the treatment machine and the technique requires advanced software capable of IMRT planning.

Once a plan has been developed by the dosimetrist and approved by the physician, the patient is taken to a **conventional simulator.** Alternatively, a CT machine can be adapted to function for both image acquisition and for simulation. If a **CT simulator** is not available, the conventional simulator uses the same projection and localization system as the treatment machine but produces a low-energy beam to produce diagnostic quality films. These machines are useful because the radiation machine produces a rectangular beam, and the diagnostic films are used to draw blocks. The film is used as a template to cut a **block** out of a low-melting-point lead alloy, which can be hung on a plate from the head of the machine. Blocks allow the field to be shaped to conform to the shape of the target. Modern machines use a **multileaf collimator** (MLC), instead of the metal alloy, to block and conform the radiation fields. The MLC is a series of 80–120 "leaves," each mounted with individual motors, that allows a computer system to set each leaf's position quickly. This technique approximates the shape of a customized block. Because the collimator only approximates an individual customized block, the field edges are not as sharp as the individual blocks.

Examples of simulation films for a whole pelvis field are shown in Figure 17-2. With the CT simulator, a **digitally**

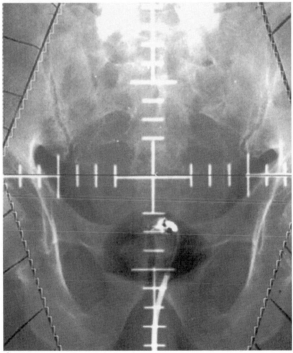

A

FIGURE 17-2. Conventional simulator film of a whole pelvis field. **A.** The anterior-posterior view. A rectal tube filled with contrast material is inserted to visualize the rectum. **B.** The same field from a lateral view. Blocks are drawn in black to protect normal tissues when possible. Treatment of the whole pelvis allows radiation dose to be delivered to the associated lymph nodes.

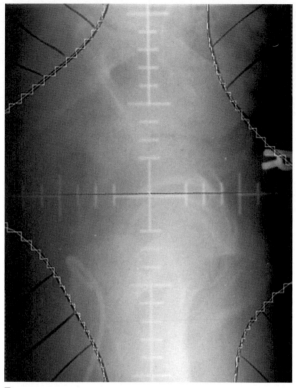

B

FIGURE 17-2. (Continued)

reconstructed radiograph (DRR) (Figure 17-3) is created that reproduces the beam's projection. This DRR takes the place of the diagnostic film produced by the conventional simulator and can be compared directly with the port film to verify beam angles and position. Along with bony structures, target volumes and normal structures can be outlined on the CT slices and can be visualized on the DRR. The final fields are then confirmed on the treatment machine with a high-energy low-resolution film, known as a **port film,** which is obtained with the treatment beam.

Fixed fields may be used when blocks are critical, but when they are not needed rotational fields may be used. In this method the tumor is placed on the central axis of rotation of the machine. Radiation is delivered as the machine rotates around the patients in either a full circle or one or

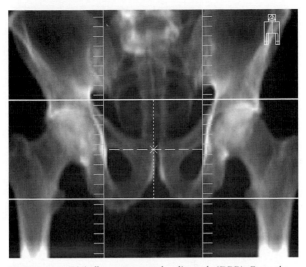

FIGURE 17-3. Digitally reconstructed radiograph (DRR). From the CT scan, the computer generates this image for treatment planning purposes. Structures drawn on the CT slices can be superimposed on this field to give their relation to bony landmarks. The resolution in the DRR is much less compared with the conventional simulator film.

more limited arcs. Because the contour of the target and the patient change as the patient rotates, rotational techniques may not be feasible. In treating prostate cancer, the fixed fields treat a smaller volume of normal tissue but deliver a higher dose to that volume, while the rotational technique treats a substantially larger volume of tissue to a substantially lower dose. The use of MLC has decreased the need to use rotational arcs in radiation therapy.

An alternative method is to deliver the radiation from within the tumor using interstitial radiation, or **brachytherapy.** Permanent implants using radioactive seeds made of iodine or palladium isotopes are usually used to treat the prostate. The patient is taken to the operating room, hollow needles are placed through the perineum into the prostate, and the radioactive seeds are deposited interstitially. The needles are removed after the procedure. Seed positions within the prostate are determined prior to the procedure using reconstructed images from sophisticated CT and ultrasound planning equipment. After the procedure, reimaging confirms seed placement, and the quality of the implant can be judged. Figure 17-4A shows axial slices through the

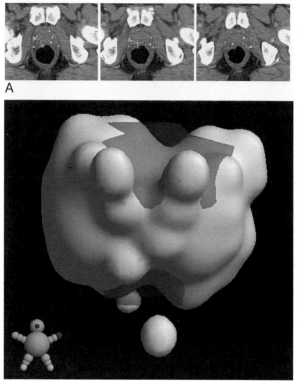

FIGURE 17-4. A. Transaxial slices through the prostate. The radioactive seeds appear as high density spots that can be counted. The prostate is contoured in black, and the relation of seed positions to the prostate gland is used to analyze the dose delivered. **B.** Dose delivery calculation in a 3D reconstructed image. The prostate gland is shown in the darker grey, and the dose contribution from each seed is shown as the light grey spheres. The conglomeration of spheres results in a dose cloud that ideally envelopes the prostate.

prostate demonstrating the placement of seeds in the prostate. Figure 17-4B shows a 3D reconstruction of the prostate obtained from the post implant CT scan demonstrating radioactive dose clouds from the seeds within the prostate. Although the implant delivers lower doses to the periprostatic tissues, substantially higher doses are delivered to the interior of the prostate. Because many tumors have some degree of extracapsular extension, the reduced periprostatic dose may not effectively treat the tumor volume. Furthermore, facility with the implant procedure allows experienced users to deliver a more homogenous dose to the prostate while minimizing the dose to adjacent structures. This skill increases with increased experience. Alternatively, intraoperative planning can be accomplished with the assistance of a physicist in the operating room allowing for real-time modification of the treatment plan at the time of the procedure.

Other recent developments have improved the staging and treatment planning for prostate cancer. Magnetic resonance imaging (MRI) has allowed the detection of clinically occult extracapsular extension and seminal vesicle extension. This has reduced the risk of local recurrence in clinical T2 tumors by filtering out the occult T3 tumors that are then sent for radiation and hormones. Similarly, the use of CT-based treatment planning allows the clinician to precisely determine the border of the prostate and to treat the necessary volume with tighter margins. Open table tops (the belly board), body casting, and other immobilization techniques allow better immobilization of the prostate and the more accurate treatment setup. Tightening of the margins with better definition of the treatment volume reduces the dose to the bladder and rectum. The end result of these modifications is the ability to increase the dose delivered to bladder tumors from 50–60 Gy to 63–67 Gy, and for prostate cancer from 65–66 Gy to 77–85 Gy. However, it remains to be determined whether this increase in dose will translate into an improved long-term survival.

CLINICAL RADIATION ONCOLOGY

There is no role for radiation (alone or with chemotherapy) in the treatment of unresected renal cell carcinoma. However, the use of radiation in the treatment of patients following resection remains controversial. Among patients with tumor transgressing the renal capsule, the risk of local recurrence is higher and radiation can reduce the risk of local recurrence. Rafla reviewed his experience and found an apparent benefit to the use of adjuvant radiation therapy for patients with involvement of the renal capsule (T3). Among patients receiving adjuvant radiation, the 5-year survival was 57% compared to 28% for patients treated with surgery alone. It is presumed that the improved survival was related to the reduced incidence of local recurrence, although this finding could not be documented as these patients were treated in the pre-CT era. In contrast, subsequent trials reported by Finney et al. and Kjaer et al. found no benefit to treating these patients with adjuvant radiation. The results of the Finney trial are limited by the small number of patients and the 8% treatment related mortality due to liver injury in the radiation arm. The results reported by Kjaer are clouded by the registration of node-positive patients in whom Rafla demonstrated no benefit. This study also was complicated by the fact that 16% of the patients randomized to radiation did not receive radiation and those patients who were treated experienced a 44% incidence of major toxicity. Kao has reported that this toxicity can be avoided by using CT-based treatment planning. Both Finney and Kjaer used anterior and posterior fields, and the toxicity occurred in patients with right-sided tumors. In such cases, large parts of the liver were treated to 45 Gy, which is well above liver tolerance. Because many tumors today are found incidentally at the time of a diagnostic CT scan for other reasons, it is not clear that these patients have the same prognosis after surgery as patients in these older studies who presented with hematuria, mass, or other more ominous findings.

Radiation can be used for metastatic renal cell carcinoma to palliate bleeding, pain, or neurologic symptoms related to spinal or central nervous system (CNS) involvement. These tumors have traditionally been thought to be radioresistant, arguing for surgical excision of limited metastatic disease. In a review of their experiences, Onufrey and Halpern reported that, although these tumors tended to respond slowly and did not seem to respond to higher doses of radiation, they achieved good palliation of symptoms in most cases. There are still experts that favor surgical excision as it removes the tumor focus immediately and allows the patient to begin rehabilitation more rapidly than following radiation. Therefore, the clinician must compare the relative risks and benefits of radiation against the functional deficits and more rapid rehabilitation after surgery in selecting the appropriate treatment for individual patients.

The one area of active radiation research is in the management of CNS metastases. Previous problems with control of the tumor frustrated both the radiation oncologist and the neurosurgeon. It is difficult to deliver an adequate dose of radiation to the tumor to produce durable local control because of the toxicity to normal CNS tissues with high doses. Similarly, the neurosurgeon cannot get a margin around the tumor because the residual neurologic effects are related to the manipulation of the normal tissues at the margin of the tumor. Many tumors are not accessible to the neurosurgeon because of the deep location of some metastases. Patients also need whole brain radiation after resection because most patients with a clinically isolated metastasis will have other microscopically occult metastases, as the most common site of recurrence of tumor following neurosurgical excision without radiation is the CNS.

Because of the problems managing brain metastases, many patients were managed with combined surgery and postoperative radiation. Recently, the development of stereotactic radiosurgery has allowed the delivery of a single large dose of radiation to a small volume encompassing the tumor without a margin. The purpose of this radiation is to produce areas of necrosis within the gross tumor. This is used for deep-seated lesions or tumor adjacent to critical structures that are surgically inaccessible. Whether this will lead to improved local control and improved quality of survival is being studied in prospective trials.

RENAL PELVIC AND URETERAL CARCINOMA

There are very limited data on the use of radiation to manage tumors in the renal pelvis and ureter. The rationale that supports the use of radiation is based on the anatomy of the retroperitoneum as it affects the surgical resection. Tumors of the renal pelvis and ureter are resected with wide proximal and distal margins. Because these tumors are frequently multifocal and can spread along the urothelium, the resection includes the kidney and a generous bladder cuff. The radial margin is more problematic and radiation may be indicated to sterilize any tumor in this region. The thin wall of the ureter is the only barrier to lateral spread of the tumor and the surgeon is limited in the ability to laterally extend the dissection. There are no additional barriers to tumor spread in the retroperitoneum. There have been no recent reports of the use of radiation in the postoperative setting, but an older report from MD Anderson described 8 patients out of 58 patients who underwent nephroureterectomy for transitional cell carcinoma who were thought to have a high risk for local recurrence. The proximal and distal margins of resection were negative, but because of the thin wall of the ureter and the transmural extension of the tumor, there was concern that the radial margin may not have been adequate. These 8 patients received 40–60 Gy of radiation to the ureteral bed with no major morbidity reported, although most of the patients did develop anorexia, nausea, and diarrhea. Four of the 8 patients died with tumor, but only one of these patients had a recurrence of tumor in the retroperitoneum. Extrapolating these findings to tumors in the renal pelvis would suggest that patients with transitional cell carcinomas lower in the pelvis or extending into perinephric fat may benefit from adjuvant radiation.

The fields that have been used in patients with renal pelvis tumors are the same as those used in the adjuvant radiation of renal cell carcinomas to encompass the renal bed and the renal hilar structures. Although there is no proven benefit to adjunctive radiation in patients with lymph node metastases, these nodes are frequently sampled in conjunction with the nephrectomy so there is concern about possible contamination of the medial structures. Therefore, including the preaortic, para-aortic, and paracaval lymph nodes in the treatment field is reasonable. Ureteral tumors are generally treated with fields that extend proximally and distally to encompass the preoperative tumor volume with a 5- to 7-cm margin. The medial and lateral margins are determined by the surgical resection and the gross lateral extent of the tumor, although the prevertebral structures are generally not included. The decision regarding the use of radiation must be individualized so that an assessment is made of the potential risks of recurrence and benefits of adjunctive radiation so that an appropriate recommendation can be reached.

BLADDER CARCINOMA

The application of radiation in the management of transitional cell carcinoma of the bladder (TCCB) is very controversial. Radiation was initially used prior to cystectomy to increase the probability of successful cystectomy. At Memorial Sloan-Kettering Cancer Center (MSKCC) a substantial number of patients, mostly with T3b and T4 tumors or poorly differentiated tumors, were taken to cystectomy but did not complete the procedure because of the presence of extravesical extension or lymphadenopathy. They developed a policy in which these patients initially received a dose of 40 Gy in 4 weeks with a 4-week break prior to resection. Intraoperatively, many of these patients were found to have substantial regression of tumor and were able to have a greater probability of complete resection and a reduction in the risk of pelvic recurrence. However, the surgical procedure was more difficult because radiation-induced fibrosis limited the amount of ureter that could be used in the urinary reconstruction. As many of these patients had such dramatic responses, they attempted definitive treatment of bladder carcinoma with radiation alone. They received further radiation to a total dose of 60 Gy with the intent of achieving tumor control, although the 4-week break did reduce the efficacy of radiation compared to 60-Gy continuous radiation over 6 weeks.

Subsequently, with a dose of 20 Gy in 1 week during the week prior to surgery, there was less fibrosis, but no change in the complication rate. Subsequent to the MSKCC report, Montie et al. at the Cleveland Clinic, and Skinner and Lieskovsky at the University of Southern California, reviewed their experience and found that survival and pelvic failure in their patients treated with surgery alone had the same survival and pelvic recurrence rates as patients treated with preoperative radiation. Montie did select a significant number of patients who were thought to be marginally resectable or thought to be at high risk for local recurrence and referred them to receive adjuvant radiation and excluded them from the analysis. This may bias the analysis by excluding patients thought to have a poorer prognosis. Many of the patients reported by Skinner received adjuvant chemotherapy, and it is not clear whether the results are due to the fact that there is no benefit from adjuvant radiation or whether a similar effect can be achieved with adjuvant chemotherapy. The INT-0080 trial demonstrated a survival benefit with neoadjuvant chemotherapy in patients with T2–4a bladder tumors that is comparable to that achieved with adjuvant irradiation.

Although a large meta-analysis by Parsons et al. showed a survival benefit with preoperative radiation in patients with clinical T3 tumors, this analysis has been criticized. The trials that did not meet the criteria for inclusion generally supported the use of surgery alone; most of them were not randomized or critical parameters were not reported. In the absence of a randomized trial, there is no role for radiation today except in unusual circumstances. The reports of neoadjuvant chemotherapy show a clear benefit to the use of chemotherapy in marginally resectable lesions by increasing the rate of resection, although there is no evidence to support or disprove an effect on survival. The response rates reported with methotrexate, vinblastine, and cisplatin, and doxorubicin (Adriamycin) (methotrexate, cisplatin, and vinblastine [MCV] or methotrexate, vinblastine, Adriamycin, and cisplatin [MVAC]) approach 80%. More recent results suggest that paclitaxel (Taxol) and carboplatin have similar efficacy and may have reduced toxicity.

In Europe and Canada, the initial focus of treatment was to use radiation as the primary modality and to deliver high-dose external beam radiation in an attempt to preserve the bladder and sterilize the tumor. These experiences showed that the local control rates are only 35–45% in T2 tumors and even poorer for patients with T3–4 tumors. Compared to patients undergoing cystectomy, in whom survival rates are approximately 75% in T2 tumors and 50–65% for patients with T3 tumors, radiation appears to be inferior. To further improve these results, radiation sensitizers or particles such as neutrons and π mesons have been tried. Although some improvement in the rates of local control and survival were achieved, there was a 15–30% risk of major complications, including small bowel or rectal injury, severe bladder contracture, or bleeding, thus precluding the general recommendation for these treatments.

Interstitial radiation has been used by a number of centers to treat bladder tumors and deliver a higher dose to a small portion of the bladder with relative sparing of the rectum and the rest of the bladder. Van der Werf-Messing treated patients with three fractions of 3.5 Gy to reduce the risk of intraoperative tumor dissemination and then carried out a cystotomy to perform a radium needle implant under direct vision. The sources were attached to suture material that was brought out through a stab wound adjacent to the incision. The sources were left in place to deliver a dose of 70 Gy in 7–8 days, following which they were removed through the stab wound. This reduced the risk of local recurrence in T1 or T2 tumors from 75 to 18% and reduced the need for cystectomy from 65 to 20%. A similar reduction was seen in the 10-year risk of metastatic tumor from 50 to 18%. For more extensive low-grade tumors, including larger T2 tumors and small T3 tumors, a preimplant dose of 30 Gy was delivered in 3 weeks to the pelvis and then an additional 45 Gy with the implant. This treated any subclinical disease that may have extended beyond the high-dose implant volume and also delivered a higher dose to the larger gross tumor. The local control in this group was 92% with an actuarial disease-free survival of 74%.

In the United States there has been an interest in chemosensitized radiation in treating a number of tumors based on the theories advanced by Steele and Peckham. Chemotherapy can reduce the tumor burden so that radiation may deal more effectively with the residual tumor. Similarly, there may be spatial cooperation allowing the radiation to deal effectively with the bladder tumor, whereas systemic chemotherapy may treat subclinical metastatic tumor.

Chemotherapy may also be beneficial in the adjuvant setting, with the final mechanism being the effect of chemosensitization, which is still under investigation. Soloway et al. evaluated the response of a bladder cell line and found that a dose of chemotherapy that produced a 1 log cell kill and in vitro without a growth delay in nude mice could be given in conjunction with a dose of radiation that would produce a 3 log cell kill and a 5-week growth delay. The result was a 4 to 5 log cell kill with a 9-week growth delay suggesting a three- to sevenfold enhancement of the individual effects due to a synergistic interaction between the radiation and cisplatin.

The National Bladder Cancer Cooperative Group (NBCCG) in the United States and the group in Innsbruck, Austria, sponsored trials delivering cisplatin on days 1, 22, and 43 of radiation following transurethral resection of bladder tumor (TURBT) with re-evaluation after 40 Gy had been delivered. Patients with less than visual complete responses after 40 Gy were sent to cystectomy, as they found it was unlikely that these patients would achieve a complete response with an additional 20–25 Gy. Among patients with complete responses or only positive cytology who received an additional 20–25 Gy, the 2-year relapse-free survivals were 68% and 53% in the Innsbruck and NBCCG, respectively. In an effort to improve the results with conservative surgery and chemosensitized radiation, the NBCCG and Radiation Therapy Oncology Group (RTOG) began a joint trial delivering two cycles of MVC prior to radiation-cisplatin therapy. The 4-year survival with bladder conservation was 44% and the overall survival was 62%. A subsequent trial randomized patients to neoadjuvant chemotherapy prior to chemosensitized radiation versus immediate chemosensitized radiation; no benefit to the neoadjuvant therapy was observed.

The current role for neoadjuvant chemotherapy is restricted to patients who decline cystectomy and have no other curative option. In this setting a trial of chemotherapy may allow the identification of patients with chemoradiation-sensitive disease that may be controlled with radiation and cisplatin. Patients with clearly unresectable tumors should proceed directly to radiation-cisplatin. The availability of continent diversions has sharply reduced the utility of bladder conservation because continent diversion has been shown to preserve normal voiding function in men with the chance of preserving potency. Women and some men will intermittently catheterize an internal reservoir, which is much easier than maintaining an external appliance. Other risks of radiation include rectal ulcers (7%), bladder contracture (10%), impotence in men (>50%), and bowel injury (3%). In institutions with the availability of continent diversions, chemosensitized radiation is generally reserved for patients with unresectable tumors or patients unable or unwilling to undergo cystectomy.

PROSTATE CANCER

As controversial as the treatment decisions may appear in patients with bladder cancer, the disagreements surrounding the management of prostate cancer are that much greater. With the advent of prostate-specific antigen (PSA) screening, the incidence of prostate cancer has skyrocketed from 120,000 new cases annually to more than 230,000 new cases in 2005. Many of these tumors are probably not clinically significant as there is a high prevalence of occult prostate cancer found incidentally in autopsy series. Although, it is difficult to distinguish these men with incidental tumors from those with clinically significant tumors, the annual number of deaths from prostate cancer in the United States has fallen to 30,500 in 2005.

The critical elements in evaluating a man with prostate cancer require that the clinician estimate the annual risk of tumor dissemination and tumor related mortality as well as the annual non-prostate cancer related mortality for the individual. The 2002 census reports suggest that a 70-year-old man has an average life expectancy of 13.3 years for Caucasians and 11.8 years for African-Americans. At age 80 the median survival falls to 7.7 years and 7.5 years, respectively. This estimate must be adjusted downward for comorbid conditions such as diabetes, atherosclerotic disease, renal insufficiency, and chronic lung disease, and adjusted upward for men who are in good health with no comorbid conditions. In completing an ad hoc risk benefit analysis it is also necessary to factor into the equation any conditions that may increase the risk of radiation-related morbidity including prior abdominal surgeries, any history of peritonitis or pelvic inflammatory conditions including Crohn's disease or ulcerative colitis, or a history of diverticulitis.

It is necessary to have the proper equipment to deliver radiation for prostate cancer, and the Patterns of Care studies were inaugurated in 1976 to identify treatment factors associated with better outcomes in radiation oncology. One of the first sites studied was prostate cancer, and the factors associated with better control and/or less morbidity are (1) treatment simulation, (2) customized blocking to shape fields, (3) computerized treatment planning, (4) treatment with machines with beam energies >10 million volts (MV), and

(5) a dose >66 Gy for T2 tumors and 70 Gy for T3 tumors to a point 4 cm lateral to the center of the prostate.

Recent developments suggest that newer methods that may further improve the results in managing prostate cancer include CT-based treatment planning, 3D-CRT and IMRT, and escalation of the dose to the prostate past 70 Gy. CT treatment planning is available in most institutions today and allows the treatment of larger fields with less morbidity. Previously, clinical judgment was used to set the field location and size based on diagnostic CT images and bladder and rectal contrast placed at the time of simulation. The potential for errors in translation from CT to radiographs requires the clinician to use wider margins to be confident that the tumor is adequately covered.

Current CT-based treatment planning uses a CT scan directed by the radiation oncologist to define the pelvic anatomy with techniques that are better adapted for translation to a plain film or, as previously mentioned, a DRR. The diagnostic study maximizes the resolution of structures to identify any abnormality and determine its extent. The treatment planning study is done to define the location of the organs in the region of the tumor. It is possible on the CT scan to outline the prostate, the bladder and the rectum as well as the bony structures to locate in three dimensions the edges of each of the organs. This information can then be translated onto the beam's eye view projection DRR of the treatment field with relation to bony structures, the bladder, and rectum. Bladder and rectal contrast may be used in this technique to register the beam's eye view projection onto the simulator film using multiple reference points. From the beam's eye view projection, blocks are drawn to shield areas not at risk for cancer spread from the radiation. Because machines only produce rectangular treatment fields, it is necessary to customize the shape of the field to the shape of the irregularly shaped target. Modern CT simulators allow for computer assistance in drawing blocks.

The plan that is produced is still a two-dimensional (2D) plan of a cross-section through the center of the tumor along the common axis of all the beams. This 2D view is useful for simple plans, but as the isodose lines will be more round shaped at the edges of the field, the effect on isodose lines will be most pronounced at the corners of the treatment volume. This scenario results in a point being technically in the field but not receiving the full dose (Figure 17-5). To determine the extent of this **inhomogeneity,** it is necessary to look at a 3D plan. 3D-CRT or IMRT can render dose distributions in any plane and also will produce a dose volume histogram,

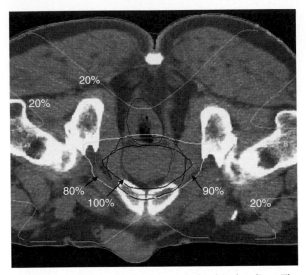

FIGURE 17-5. CT slice with the drawn calculated isodose lines. The radiation oncologist chooses an isodose line to prescribe to, such that the entire volume receives a minimum of that dose. The 100% isodose line covers the majority of the prostate, with the dose falling off farther away.

which will visually demonstrate how much of the target receives excess of any specified dose. A sample histogram for a patient treated with external beam radiation for prostate cancer was shown in Figure 17-1. In that example, when a dose of 75.6 Gy was delivered to the point where the beams intersect, the entire target volume receives a minimum dose of 75.6 Gy, but a small fraction of the prostate received higher doses. Likewise, similar histograms for the rectum and bladder demonstrate the maximum and minimum doses delivered to each organ, respectively. Furthermore, with multiple and non-coplanar beams, it is possible to use a tetrahedral or pyramidal field arrangement to minimize the overlap of entrance and exit beams outside of the target volume.

The maximum radiation dose tolerated by the prostate continues to be defined. Although some centers currently use doses of 74–81 Gy, others such as Memorial Sloan Kettering and the University of Michigan are exploring doses of 84–91 Gy, utilizing the concept of dose escalation. Between October 1988 and December 1998, Zelefsky et al. treated more than 1000 patients with clinical stages T1c–T3 prostate cancer with either 64.8–70.2 Gy or 75.6–86.4 Gy. Five-year actuarial PSA relapse-free survival was significantly improved with the higher dose. However, the question that remained was whether PSA control had affected overall survival, and did the improved PSA control outweigh the higher toxicity observed with the higher doses.

The use of higher doses has necessitated tighter margins that do not compromise adequate coverage of the tumor. This combination requires precise prostate localization, and to further improve the precision of treatment these centers and many others adopted individualized immobilization devices such as body casts as well as specialized techniques to reduce organ motion. As previously mentioned, daily ultrasound or placement of fiducial markers was implemented as part of radiation treatments.

With the advent of IMRT techniques, radiation doses were further escalated. This advanced form of 3D-CRT allows dose distribution to be tailored to a complex and irregular target volume using nonuniform beam and beamlet intensities, often with the underlying goal to escalate doses to the target, and to reduce complications from irradiation of surrounding normal tissue, especially the rectum. Using this technique for whole pelvis radiation to 45 Gy, rectal volume irradiation was reduced from 50% in 3D-CRT to 6% with IMRT, and the bladder from 52% to 7%. Although Zelefsky et al. reported significant reduction in toxicity with IMRT compared to 3D-CRT, long-term tumor control has yet to be reported beyond 5 years; 3-year actuarial PSA relapse-free survival ranges from 81–92%.

In comparing the results from different series, it is necessary to compare the definitions of tumor control and treatment-related morbidity. There is no universally accepted definition of biochemical control after radiation as there is after surgery. Following surgery, PSA should be undetectable, as all prostatic tissue has been theoretically removed. However, following radiation the residual normal prostate epithelium will produce PSA. Some investigators have argued that the PSA should be less than 0.5, or 1.0, or 1.5 ng/mL, whereas others argue that it only needs to be stable and does not rise during the follow-up period. These definitions are problematic because radiation oncologists who use higher doses of radiation report that follow-up PSA levels are lower. It is not clear whether this biochemical response reflects better tumor control or possibly more fibrosis of the normal residual prostate. Similarly, many studies have used concurrent hormones and radiation. Hormones cause the normal prostate to involute, and when hormones are withdrawn, the prostate function may return to normal, and the PSA will rise to its baseline level. If the clinician is too sensitive to the results of the serum PSA, the risk of recurrence may be overestimated.

Grading of radiation-induced side effects is also subject to a lack of uniformity. Individuals who have had radiation may develop painless rectal bleeding, and proctoscopy often reveals mucosal atrophy and telangiectasias. Many physicians would score this effect as a minimal or grade I toxicity, whereas others would score it as a grade II toxicity because they may have a lower threshold to recommend symptomatic treatment. Some studies have also considered rectal hemorrhage requiring transfusion or laser ablation of the anterior rectal wall as grade II toxicity, whereas others consider it grade IV (life-threatening) toxicity. Similarly, men who advise their physicians they are able to obtain partial erections may be considered by some physicians to be potent, although they are not able to complete vaginal intromission. Others require that men be able to sustain an erection and reach orgasm.

Furthermore, controversy in the treatment of prostate cancer exists over the definition of the target volume. Many institutions will deliver a dose of 45 Gy to the obturator, hypogastric, external iliac, and common iliac lymph nodes and boost the prostate to the final total dose. Others will treat the prostate only, with or without the seminal vesicles. One of the major contradictions in the literature arises out of retrospective reviews of several hundred men at both Stanford and the Cross Clinic in Alberta. Both institutions had an experience that had evolved over the years, initially treating the lymph nodes as well as the prostate and subsequently only the prostate. Each found that the risk of distant metastases was higher in patients treated to the prostate only when compared to patients who received prophylactic pelvic irradiation. The RTOG carried out a subsequent randomized trial that sampled lymph nodes in men with prostate cancer. Men with negative lymph nodes were randomized to either prostate radiation alone or to prophylactic pelvic radiation plus prostate radiation. There was no difference in the survival of these men following surgical lymph node staging.

In a contemporaneous series of men with involved lymph nodes, Sause et al. and the group at MSKCC found that the clinical disease-free survival curves in node-positive patients continued to deteriorate for more than 15 years and that there was no evidence of cure. In a review of RTOG studies of men with involved lymph nodes from prostate cancer, only 2 of 90 men were biochemically without evidence of progression at 10 years. The 10-year overall survival was 29% and the clinical no evidence of disease (NED) survival was 7%. It appears contradictory but true that men with negative lymph nodes do not benefit from prophylactic nodal irradiation, whereas men with positive nodes cannot be cured. Yet, when the nodal status is unknown there is a benefit to prophylactic lymph node irradiation. The explanation may lie in the fact that all of the studies were conducted before the general availability of CT scanning. It is possible that the fields used for prostate radiation may not have included the superior-lateral prostate gland, which was included in the pelvic lymph node field.

The beam arrangements to treat the pelvic lymph nodes can be accomplished with opposed anterior-posterior, posterior-anterior, and right and left lateral fields; this technique is known as a **four-field box.** These fields are shown in Figure 17-2A and 17-2B. Alternatively, IMRT can be used to treat the pelvic nodes and spare bowel toxicity. The large field is designed to include the common, external, and internal iliac lymph nodes as well as the obturator and presacral nodes because these are the most common sites of lymph node metastases. It also includes the entire prostate and the proximal pendulous urethra. To include these structures and nodes, the field extends from the middle of L5 to the bottom of the ischial tuberosity and laterally goes at least 1 cm lateral to the pelvic brim. Laterally, the fields extend 1 cm anterior to the symphysis and to at least the S3–4 interspace. With IMRT for pelvic irradiation, a volume of 1–2 cm around the iliac vessels is expanded during the simulation and is targeted during the radiation session. Typical dose to the pelvic lymph nodes is around 45 Gy.

Treatment to only the prostate gland, for low-risk disease or **conedown** after pelvic irradiation, is shown in Figure 17-6. The prostate field is designed to encompass the prostate as defined by treatment planning CT scan. The CT-rendered images are registered to the simulation film using the bladder, rectum, and bony structures as landmarks. Often, an urethrogram is performed at the time of treatment planning CT scan to identify the proximal prostatic urethra. Some clinicians will include the seminal vesicles in the treatment volume, whereas others will not, and still others will include them in selected patients. The concern in this area is related to the fact that seminal vesicle involvement occurs in 20–30% of men with stage T2 prostate cancer and in approximately 50–70% of men with T3–4 prostate cancer. If this portion of the tumor is not treated, then the tumor cannot be cured, but when the seminal vesicles are included the amount of rectum in the treatment field will sharply increase. Roach has developed

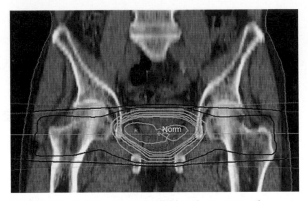

FIGURE 17-6. Radiation treatment field to the prostate only.

an algorithm that allows the clinician to predict the risk of nodal involvement based on the Gleason score and the PSA, and D'Amico has demonstrated that MRI with an endorectal coil is extremely sensitive in detecting actual involvement. Algorithm 17-1 is presented to risk stratify patients to treatment regimens.

Although node-positive prostate cancer has become less frequent in this era of community screening, there is still controversy over the treatment of node-positive disease. Because these patients have such a high rate of distant metastases, many oncologists do not recommend local therapy. A review of the results in patients with conservatively treated prostate cancer shows that there is a significant risk of bladder outlet obstruction, bladder invasion, hemorrhage, and pain, which may be prevented with radiation. Furthermore, radiation may offer the opportunity to "debulk" the tumor, leaving a smaller tumor burden to be treated by the hormones. There is a spectrum of androgen sensitivity in prostate tumors at diagnosis, and hormonal therapy will select the androgen-independent population to proliferate while the more androgen-dependent population involutes entering an extended G_0 state or undergoes apoptosis. In men with locally advanced nonmetastatic prostate cancer treated with deferred therapy and androgen ablation at the time of symptomatic progression, the median time to develop hormone-resistant tumor was 48 months, whereas men treated with immediate androgen ablation did not develop hormone-independent tumor until a median of 84 months after diagnosis. These findings argue for earlier intervention at the time of diagnosis. The most common

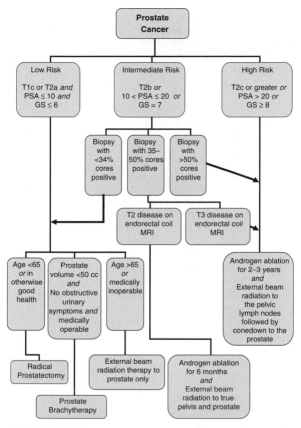

ALGORITHM 17-1.

sites of progression when androgen resistance develops are at sites of previous disease. Therefore, at the University of Pennsylvania, these men are treated with concurrent hormones and radiation to address both the pelvic tumor and occult distant metastatic disease. In a series of 80 patients with a median follow-up of 5 years, the 12-year cancer-specific survival was 90% and the biochemical relapse-free survival was 57%.

For men with earlier stage prostate cancer, there are three accepted treatments from which men can choose: radical prostatectomy, external beam radiation, or interstitial therapy. In reviewing a large series of men, most physicians divide patients into three groups. The group with a low risk of recurrence within 5 years consists of men with tumors confined to less than one half of one lobe of the gland, PSA <10.0 ng/mL, and a Gleason score <6. The intermediate-risk group has tumors greater than one half of one lobe of the gland but not involving the other lobe, PSA between 10.0 and 20.0 ng/mL, or a Gleason score of 7. The high-risk group has tumors involving both lobes of the gland or extracapsular extension, a PSA >20.0 ng/mL, or a Gleason score >8. In one analysis comparing these three treatments in the three risk groups, D'Amico found no difference in the relative risk of recurrence between the treatments in the low-risk population. Among intermediate- and high-risk patients there was a three-fold higher risk of recurrence among men undergoing interstitial therapy when compared to external beam or surgery, although the difference disappeared in the intermediate-risk group when men were treated with 6 months of androgen ablation therapy in addition to the implant. Among men with high-risk cancers, the risk of recurrence was greater than 65% in all of the treatment groups, but the recurrences occurred earlier after interstitial therapy than with surgery or external radiation. The inference from these results is that new treatment approaches are needed possibly combining current therapies with androgen ablation or introducing new therapies such as cytotoxic chemotherapy, higher radiation doses, or more extensive surgery.

A number of centers have reported that men in the intermediate-risk group appear to have a longer biochemical disease-free survival with higher doses of radiation, but the follow-up thus far is less than 5 years in these series and further follow-up is necessary to determine whether the difference will translate into a longer overall survival and whether the morbidity is acceptable. Hanks initially reported in a retrospective review that the biochemical no evidence of disease (bNED) survival was better with doses greater than 76 Gy than with doses less than 70 Gy. A preliminary report at a median of 30 months of follow-up of a randomized trial of 70 Gy versus 78 Gy carried out at MD Anderson show that the bNED survival is 47% with 70 Gy and 68% with 78 Gy. Zelefsky reported intermediate-risk patients treated to 81–86.4 Gy as having 3-year actuarial PSA relapse-free survival of 86%. Again, it is important to note that biochemical failure has not yet been shown to correlate with overall survival.

The use of combined hormonal and radiation therapy has been prospectively studied in four studies. The earliest study from MD Anderson demonstrated comparable 10-year survivals among men with T3 tumors treated with radiation including the pelvic lymph nodes with or without lifelong adjuvant diethylstilbestrol (DES) 5 mg/day. In reviewing these results, it was found that there was an excess of cardiovascular deaths in the hormone group and an excess of cancer-related deaths in the control group. Two subsequent RTOG trials randomized men to radiation with or without hormone therapy and found that the hormones prolonged disease-free survival, although they have yet to show a benefit in overall survival. One study treated men with 4 months of androgen deprivation therapy using a luteinizing hormone releasing hormone (LHRH) agonist delivering 2 months of therapy before starting radiation and completing treatment with the end of radiation. The second study began radiation concurrently with the LHRH agonist and continued the therapy indefinitely. The median duration of hormone therapy in this group was 24 months. In a recent analysis of the results of these two trials, there appeared to be a small advantage favoring the longer course of therapy, although the results are not conclusive because there were slight differences in the eligibility for the two studies. Most of the patients in both studies had T3 N0 tumors, but patients with involved lymph nodes, positive margins following radical prostatectomy, and high-grade tumors were eligible for the study with indefinite hormones. There is currently a randomized trial being conducted by the RTOG to compare these two regimens.

The final study was reported by Bolla who reported a European randomized trial comparing radiation and 3 years of hormonal therapy to radiation alone. His report is the only one thus far to find a clear survival benefit with a 5-year overall survival of 79% in the patients receiving radiation and hormones versus 62% in men treated with hormones alone. Most of these men had T3 N0 disease based on CT scan, lymphangiogram, or node sampling, although approximately 10% of the patients on each arm had T3 WHO grade 3 tumors. One concern here is that men treated with radiation alone ended treatment within 2 months after registration, whereas the hormone group had 3 years of treatment after registration, so the follow-up after treatment is significantly shorter in the latter group. There is also the problem that many men will develop permanent hypogonadism after prolonged androgen deprivation, although the exact incidence of testicular failure is unknown.

Current trends for the use of androgen ablation are most often used in the intermediate- and high-risk patients. Patients with low-risk disease who have large prostates may benefit from androgen ablation to shrink the size of the gland. If the gland can be decreased in size to less than 50 cm^3, brachytherapy may be a suitable alternative to external beam in some patients. For patients in the intermediate-risk group, a course of 6 months of androgen ablation is usually given. Longer courses of androgen ablation of 2–3 years are generally prescribed for patients falling in the high-risk categories. Side effects from androgen ablation, which include impotence, hot flashes, and/or anemia, should be discussed with patients before patients are placed on long-term androgen ablation.

There are still challenges remaining in managing a man with prostate cancer. The first is to assess each man as an individual and specifically address the potential of each treatment to render the patient free of tumor and simultaneously to weigh the effects of treatment on quality of life including the effect of and on associated conditions such as bladder outlet obstruction and bladder and rectal dysfunction and the effect of comorbid conditions such as diabetes, vascular disease, and intra-abdominal processes. The second is to develop a treatment plan within the abilities of the institution, which should include, but is not limited to, CT-based treatment planning and simulation, customized treatment planning and blocks, and development of a treatment plan that allows the delivery of an adequate dose to control the tumor. Therefore, in high-risk patients with extracapsular disease, PSAs greater than 20.0 ng/mL, Gleason scores >8, or metastatic lymphadenopathy, consideration should be given to adjuvant hormones with or without pelvic irradiation or higher doses of radiation.

For patients with rising PSA after prostatectomy, radiation has been shown to salvage approximately 50% of these patients. Recent studies by Jones et al. have demonstrated that early intervention with radiation directed to the prostatic fossa after the first detectable PSA has better results compared to deferred treatment. Toxicity from salvage radiation is substantially increased compared to patients treated with radiation alone. Therefore, it is suggested to wait until postprostatectomy incontinence has resolved or stabilized before starting radiation.

TESTICULAR CANCER

The role of radiation in managing testicular tumors is limited to the management of seminoma. There are data showing efficacy for radiation in clinical stage I nonseminomatous germ cell tumors, but the necessary dose and the associated toxicity suggest that these patients are better treated with more extensive staging and close observation or chemotherapy if indicated. Radiation is a standard treatment for seminoma because of the unique sensitivity of these germ cell tumors to radiation. Almost all cells need to divide to express the lethal effects of radiation; seminoma cells undergo an intermitotic death because of their inability to accumulate and repair sublethal damage. Because of this characteristic, there is no shoulder on the cell survival curve.

Staging of seminomas requires chest roentgenography to rule out metastatic disease, serum α-fetoprotein and β-human chorionic gonadotropin, and abdominal CT scan or lymphangiography. Men who have not completed their family should consider a semen analysis, because 10% of newly diagnosed seminoma patients are infertile, and an estimate of fertility is needed to counsel a patient concerning the effects of treatment on fertility. The use of chest CT is limited to patients with disease beyond the testicle, because the incidence of distant metastases in patients with stage I disease is small, as evidenced by the <5% relapse rate among patients treated with adjuvant radiation.

The treatment of seminoma has evolved over the last 10 years with the reports by Duchesne and Thomas that in patients followed without adjuvant therapy the risk of recurrence is less than 20%. For men willing to undergo close follow-up with CT scanning and chest x-ray every 3 months for 2 years, observation may be an option with the understanding that they may need higher doses of salvage radiation or chemotherapy if they relapse. Because younger men are the largest group with this tumor, preservation of fertility is an issue and many steps are taken to minimize the scattered radiation to the opposite testicle, but many men elect surveillance and avoid radiation entirely. In an effort to further reduce the dose to the testicle, Fossa et al. have reported the results of a randomized trial with treatment to the para-aortic lymph nodes and renal hilum versus the same field as well as the common and external iliac nodes as well. Figure 17-7 shows radiation treatment fields for treatment of the para-aortic lymph nodes. Because most of the scattered dose to the testicle comes from the pelvic portion of the field, eliminating this part of the field substantially reduces the dose to the testicle and the risks of treatment-related infertility. Doses between 24 and 30 Gy are used to treat these tumors as that will reduce the risk

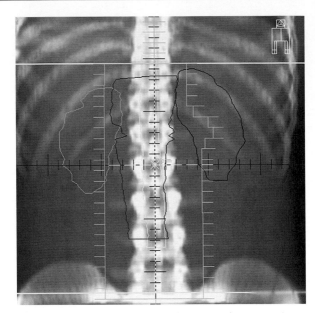

FIGURE 17-7. Radiation treatment fields to treat the para-aortic lymph nodes. The left and right kidneys are outlined to block excess dose to these structures.

of retroperitoneal recurrence from 15% to less than 1% in both groups. The incidence of azospermia was reduced from 30% in the group treated to the iliac region to 11% in the group treated to the para-aortic nodes only. The 11% figure is identical to the risk of primary infertility with no adjuvant therapy in men with a history of seminoma.

Stage II tumors are a heterogenous group including patients with retroperitoneal nodes between 1 and 20 cm. Patients with nodes smaller than 5 cm are generally treated with radiation portals similar to those used to treat a stage I tumor with the inclusion of the external and common iliac nodes. After a dose of 25–30 Gy is delivered, the initially involved nodes are boosted to a dose of 35–40 Gy. Relapse-free survival rates are about 90%. Some experts argue that this can be further reduced by prophylactic radiation to the mediastinum, although this is a matter of institutional policy and has not been studied in a prospective trial. In general, most centers in the United States will not treat the mediastinum when the lymph nodes are smaller than 5 cm, although most will treat to a dose of 25 Gy when nodes are larger.

Stage II tumors with lymph nodes larger than 5 cm are rare and the management is more controversial. In the United States, these tumors may be treated with combination chemotherapy, whereas in Canada and Europe many of these patients are treated with radiation. The difficulty in carrying out primary radiation in patients with bulky adenopathy is that the lateral extent of the retroperitoneal lymph node mass is difficult to define without a treatment planning CT scan and CT-based treatment planning. Despite this limitation, the rate of control of infradiaphragmatic tumor is high and long-term disease-free survivals are between 50 and 60%. The most common site of recurrence is in the mediastinum; thus, many institutions recommend prophylactic mediastinal radiation. Review of the major series that provided mediastinal radiation demonstrated the 5-year relapse-free survival to be 76%, which is not significantly different from the disease-free survival rates reported with chemotherapy.

Acute and long-term toxicity is the limiting factor with radiation therapy. Abdominal radiation to a dose of 40 Gy will cause some scarring, increasing the risk of peptic ulcer, and complicating any future surgery that might be necessary in these relatively young patients. Prophylactic mediastinal radiation will substantially increase the cure rate but would complicate the delivery of any salvage chemotherapy that might be necessary, given the pulmonary effects of bleomycin and the higher risk of infertility associated with chemotherapy. There are also reports of an increased risk of Raynaud's phenomena and a possible increased risk of cerebrovascular disease in men treated with cisplatin, vinblastine, and bleomycin. It would appear that neither treatment offers a survival, or disease-free survival, benefit and therefore treatment should be individualized. There is little modern experience with radiation for stage III and IV seminoma, and the results that are available suggest that these patients are better treated with chemotherapy.

PENILE CANCER

Squamous cell carcinoma of the penis is rare in the United States and is more prevalent in other countries. Most patients are treated with initial surgery, but some patients are not candidates for surgery or refuse surgery. Superficial lesions can be treated with either external radiation or interstitial radiation using radium needles or iridium seeds in catheters. It is frequently necessary to treat the superficial inguinal nodes, because 50% of men will have palpable adenopathy and the risk of occult involvement of nodes is high in men with poorly differentiated tumors or tumors of the glans. If a patient is treated with external radiation, he may most easily be treated with an en face electron beam to treat the penis and the lymph nodes (which can lie at a depth of 5 cm below the skin), within one field. In this situation, a Lucite block is placed behind the penis to spare the scrotum. A dose of 45–50 Gy is sufficient to treat clinically uninvolved skin and lymph nodes, but the primary tumor needs to be treated to a dose of 65–70 Gy. Morbidity of radiation to this area includes moist desquamation of the penis and scrotum with accompanying edema, often lasting 8–12 weeks after radiation. Nodal dissection increases the frequency and severity of edema. For small low-grade tumors (<2 cm) of the shaft of the penis, the risk of nodal involvement is low and these patients may be treated with interstitial radiation.

Most of the series of definitive radiation are small but as a group they suggest that radiation is effective in controlling the tumor, but the morbidity is substantial. Haile and Delclos reported that in 8 patients treated with external radiation, 7 were controlled, but 1 patient required surgical amputation due to necrosis, whereas 11 of 12 patients treated with brachytherapy were controlled with 1 patient requiring amputation for necrosis. In older series, Knudsen and Brennhovd and Lederman described a lower control rate (38 and 30%, respectively), and 6% of the patients required amputation of the penis for necrosis. Duncan and Jackson reported the experience of the Holt Radium Institute initially with brachytherapy and subsequently with external beam radiation. They found that the control rates improved from 46 to 90% as they emphasized external radiation because of the ability to treat larger volumes with a more homogenous dose and adequately cover the tumor. At the same time, these authors found that the risk of urethral stricture or penile necrosis rose from 4 to 10%. Although radiation may be used to treat this disease, there is significant morbidity and the treatment requires adequate equipment and a commitment on the part of the patient and physician to persist in treatment in the face of the acute reactions. It remains to be determined whether radiation and chemotherapy may be combined to reduce the risk of distant metastases and to allow lower doses of radiation to be used to minimize the morbidity.

SUMMARY

There is extensive experience with radiation in the treatment of genitourinary tumors that demonstrates that it is an effective adjuvant treatment for selected patients with renal cell carcinoma, stage I seminoma, and selected patients with biochemical recurrences after radical prostatectomy. External and interstitial radiation, possibly with hormones, may be an effective alternative to radical prostatectomy or to penectomy or emasculation procedures. Radiation with chemotherapy may be an alternative to radical cystectomy in patients with comorbid medical conditions or extensive nonmetastatic tumors that preclude surgery.

Treatment decisions must be individualized based on the clinical findings and the experience, resources, and capabilities of the institution providing treatment. Although the incidence of incontinence following radical prostatectomy may vary from 1–30%, the incidence of both local and proctitis following radiation may vary from 3–20% following radiation. In facilities with state of the art equipment and physicians with specialized skills, there may be little to recommend one treatment over another, whereas in other facilities, one department may have special abilities that would suggest that there may be a treatment preference based on the institutional experience.

It is likewise necessary to consider the working relationship between the departments of urology and radiation oncology within each institution. Even though chemosensitized radiation may be equivalent to radical cystectomy, it may not be desirable to pursue a course of bladder conservation if the urologist does not believe that a salvage cystectomy is possible after radiation.

Because there may be alternatives that are similarly effective, it is important to avoid confusing patients with conflicting claims of superior results. Patients may be presented with alternative treatments and select the treatment that will produce the most desirable results and the most acceptable morbidity risks. The current directions of radiation research include exploring combinations of hormones and radiation and higher doses of radiation in the management of prostate cancer. Photodynamic therapy is an evolving type of radiation that may play a role in future initial management of malignancies and/or salvage treatment after radiation. Radiation oncologists are also looking at new radiation and chemotherapy schedules in bladder carcinoma to improve the chances for organ preservation.

SELF-ASSESSMENT QUESTIONS

1. What factors need to be assessed in deciding treatment options for patients with prostate cancer?
2. Compare and contrast the risks and benefits of prostate brachytherapy and external beam radiation for the management of prostate cancer.
3. Which groups of patients would benefit from androgen ablation in management of prostate cancer?
4. What are possible options for a patient who does not want to undergo cystectomy for management of bladder cancer?
5. What are the risks and benefits of irradiation for patients with seminoma?

SUGGESTED READINGS

1. D'Amico AV: Radiation and hormonal therapy for locally advanced and clinically localized prostate cancer. *Urology* 60(3 Suppl 1): 32–37; discussion 37–38, 2002.
2. D'Amico AV, Moul J, Carroll PR, Sun L, et al: Cancer-specific mortality after surgery or radiation for patients with clinically localized prostate cancer managed during the prostate-specific antigen era. *J Clin Oncol* 21:2163–2172, 2003.
3. D'Amico AV, Whittington R, Malkowicz SB, et al: Biochemical outcome after radical prostatectomy, external beam radiation therapy, or interstitial radiation therapy for clinically localized prostate cancer. *JAMA* 280:969–974, 1998.
4. Fossa SD, Horwich JM, Russell JP, et al: Optimal field size in adjuvant radiotherapy (XRT) of stage I seminoma—A randomised trial. *Proc Am Soc Clin Oncol* 15:595, 1997.
5. Jani AB, Su A, Milano MT: Intensity-modulated versus conventional pelvic radiotherapy for prostate cancer: analysis of acute toxicity. *Urology* 67:147–151, 2006.
6. Kao GD, Malkowicz SB, Whittington R, et al: Locally advanced renal cell carcinoma: low complication rate and efficacy with post-nephrectomy irradiation during the computed tomography (CT)-era. *Radiology* 193:725–730, 1994.
7. Nguyen PL, Whittington R, Koo S, et al: Quantifying the impact of seminal vesicle invasion identified using endorectal magnetic resonance imaging on PSA outcome after radiation therapy for patients with clinically localized prostate cancer. *Int J Radiat Oncol Biol Phys* 59:400–405, 2004.

8. Pollack A, Kuban DA, Zagars GK: Impact of androgen deprivation therapy on survival in men treated with radiation for prostate cancer. *Urology* 60(3 Suppl 1): 22–30, 2002.

9. Pollack A, Zagars GK: Androgen ablation in addition to radiation therapy for prostate cancer: is there true benefit? *Semin Radiat Oncol* 8:95–106, 1998.

10. Pollack A, Zagars GK, Smith LG, et al: I. Preliminary results of a randomized dose-escalation study comparing 70 Gy to 78 Gy for the treatment of prostate cancer. *Int J Rad Oncol Biol Phys* 45(Suppl 1):146–147, 1999.

11. Shipley WU, Kaufman DS, Tester WJ, et al: Overview of bladder cancer trials in Radiation Therapy Oncology Group. *Cancer* 97(8 Suppl):2115–2119, 2003.

C H A P T E R 18

Retroperitoneal Diseases

Thomas J. Guzzo, MD and
S. Bruce Malkowicz, MD

RETROPERITONEAL ANATOMY

Retroperitoneal anatomy is a topic in which all practicing urologists should be well versed. Multiple disease entities, both urologic in origin and not, can occur in the retroperitoneum and are treated by urologists. The retroperitoneal space is bounded anteriorly by the posterior parietal peritoneum, superiorly by the diaphragmatic reflection, inferiorly by the pelvic diaphragm, and posteriorly by the muscles of the body wall.

Anatomic structures from virtually every organ system lie within or traverse the retroperitoneum. This includes major vascular structures such as the aorta and inferior vena cava and many of their respective branches. Large nerve plexuses associated with the great vessels including the celiac, hypogastric, and sacral plexuses can all be found in the retroperitoneum. Portions of the gastrointestinal tract including the pancreas and portions of the duodenum and colon lie within the retroperitoneum. Finally, multiple structures specific to the practice of urology are found in the retroperitoneum including the kidneys, adrenal glands, and ureters.

BENIGN LESIONS OF THE RETROPERITONEUM

Retroperitoneal Fibrosis

Idiopathic retroperitoneal fibrosis is an uncommon entity that generally affects adults between 40 and 60 years of age. Men have a two to three times higher incidence than women. Children and adolescents are rarely afflicted. Classically, idiopathic retroperitoneal fibrosis appears as a dense mass in the center of the retroperitoneum, usually at the L4–5 vertebral level. It can envelope the great vessels and extend from the aortic bifurcation superiorly to the renal pedicles and laterally beyond the psoas muscle. The inflammatory process can involve almost

653

any retroperitoneal structure, and involvement outside of the retroperitoneum has occasionally been observed.

There are many well-documented causes of retroperitoneal fibrosis (Table 18-1) and a thorough evaluation must be completed before the diagnosis of idiopathic retroperitoneal fibrosis can be made. It is paramount to exclude a primary or metastatic malignancy as the cause of retroperitoneal fibrosis.

Retroperitoneal fibrosis can present with a variety of clinical signs and symptoms depending on the organs affected and the degree of fibrosis. Symptoms generally begin insidiously, often starting out as vague complaints. Patients can present with abdominal and flank pain, malaise, anorexia, weight loss, nausea, or vomiting. Patients may initially present in renal failure secondary to ureteral obstruction. With such a variety of symptoms and presentations, a high index of suspicion is needed to not overlook the diagnosis of retroperitoneal fibrosis.

Multiple imaging modalities are useful in the diagnosis of retroperitoneal fibrosis. Classically, the triad of proximal

Table 18-1: Causes of Retroperitoneal Fibrosis

Drugs	Malignancies	Infections
Methysergide	Primary retroperitoneal tumors	Chronic UTI
B-Blockers		Tuberculosis
Ergot alkaloids	Metastatic retroperitoneal tumors	Gonorrhea
Haloperidol		Syphilis
Reserpine	Carcinoid retroperitoneal tumors	
Phenacetin		
Methyldopa		**Inflammatory Processes**
LSD	**Chemicals**	Endometriosis
Amphetamines	Asbestos	Sarcoidosis
	Talcum powder	Collagen vascular disease
	Avitene	
Traumatic	**Iatrogenic**	
Hemorrhage	Radiation	
Urinary extravasation		
Postsurgical		

LSD, lysergic acid diethylamide; UTI, urinary tract infection.

hydroureteronephrosis, medial ureteral deviation, and extrinsic compression of the ureters was noted on intravenous pyelography. Patients presenting with an elevated creatinine are often initially evaluated with ultrasonography or with a noncontrast computed tomography (CT) scan. CT of the abdomen and pelvis allows for visualization of the extent of fibrosis. In patients with normal creatinine levels, CT scanning with intravenous contrast permits further evaluation of lymphadenopathy, fibrosis, and possible malignancy. Laboratory tests are nonspecific for the diagnosis of retroperitoneal fibrosis. As in many inflammatory conditions, erythrocyte sedimentation rates and gamma globulin levels are often elevated.

In patients presenting with acute renal failure and bilateral obstruction, decompression of the urinary tract and restoration of metabolic homeostasis are a must prior to definitive treatment of the retroperitoneal fibrosis. This can usually be done with ureteral stenting, but in cases in which stent placement fails or it is unsafe to give a general anesthetic, percutaneous nephrostomy tubes should be placed. Once an acute obstruction has been relieved or in the patient presenting without acute renal failure, care must be taken to rule out a primary or metastatic malignancy as the cause of retroperitoneal fibrosis prior to instituting definitive therapy. Should any ambiguity of diagnosis remain following a complete workup, a percutaneous or open biopsy should be performed to definitively rule out malignancy.

First-line treatment for idiopathic retroperitoneal fibrosis can be either medical or surgical depending both on physician and patient preference. Medical therapies for retroperitoneal fibrosis include glucocorticoids and immunosuppressive therapies. Glucocorticoids have been used with a variable success in the literature. There is no standardized dosing schedule, but treatment should not be abandoned early because regression of the fibrotic plaque can be seen up to 20 months after steroid therapy.

Typically, patients are treated with 1–2 months of high-dose steroids and then slowly tapered down over the remaining treatment time. Immunosuppressant therapy has been reported both in combination with glucocorticoid treatment and as a single-line therapy. There are published reports of success with azathioprine, cyclophosphamide, penicillamine, and mycophenolate mofetil.

Should medical therapies fail or the patient does not want medical therapy, surgical exploration with ureterolysis can be performed. Preoperative ureteral stent placement greatly aids in ureteral dissection. At the time of open exploration, deep biopsies should be performed to rule out an undiagnosed malignancy. Once the ureters are completely freed of the fibrotic plaque they can be intraperitonealized or wrapped with omentum to ensure surgical success. Regardless of whether the disease process is unilateral or bilateral, a bilateral ureterolysis should be performed. Postoperative steroid therapy is often used in an attempt to prevent recurrence. Laparoscopic ureterolysis is also a surgical option at centers with laparoscopic expertise.

Retroperitoneal Hemorrhage

Spontaneous retroperitoneal hemorrhage is a rare event and can occur in a wide variety of age groups depending on etiology. When the bleeding is renal in origin it is classically referred to as Wunderlich's syndrome. The causes of retroperitoneal hemorrhage are numerous (Table 18-2). The most common cause of spontaneous retroperitoneal hemorrhage in most series are angiomyolipomas. Patients can present with a variety of symptoms including abdominal, hip, and upper thigh pain. Acute onset of flank pain is not uncommon. Physical examination may be significant for flank ecchymosis, hypotension, or hypovolemic shock, and

Table 18-2: Causes of Spontaneous Retroperitoneal Hemorrhage

Retroperitoneal Tumors	
Benign	Malignant
Angiomyolipoma	Renal cell carcinoma
Lipoma	Sarcoma
Adenoma	Wilms' tumor
Fibroma	Granulosa cell tumors
Hamartoma	
Papilloma	
Hemorrhagic renal cyst	
Vascular	**Hematologic**
Panarteritis nodosa	Anticoagulant therapy
Renal artery arteriosclerosis	Hemophilia
Renal artery aneurysm rupture	Blood dyscrasia
Aortic aneurysm rupture	

gross hematuria can be present. Cross-sectional radiographic imaging (usually CT) is most useful in documenting the possible cause and extent of the bleed.

Patients should be resuscitated with intravenous fluids and/or blood transfusions as needed. Any anticoagulant medications should be discontinued in the acute setting and any specific coagulopathies be treated and reversed. Patients can be monitored with serial imaging to evaluate for resolution of the hematoma and bleeding. In cases in which conservative therapy fails to stabilize the patient, angiography with selective embolization of active bleeding can be performed. Retroperitoneal exploration should be approached with caution as it can result in massive blood loss and often results in nephrectomy. Repeat imaging should be obtained after complete resolution of the hematoma to rule out malignancy as a cause of the spontaneous bleeding.

Pelvic Lipomatosis

Pelvic lipomatosis is a benign condition in which there is an excessive deposition of mature unencapsulated fat in the pelvic retroperitoneum. The etiology of pelvic lipomatosis is unknown. It is most common in the 20–50 year age range and occurs predominantly in men.

Fifty percent of patients with pelvic lipomatosis will present with voiding dysfunction. Symptoms can include frequency, dysuria, nocturia, and suprapubic tenderness. Constipation can also be a presenting feature. Physical exam is nonspecific, but a suprapubic mass may be palpated. Hypertension is present in a significant proportion of these patients as well as azotemia due to extrinsic compression of the ureters. Cystitis glandularis, cystitis cystica, and cystitis follicularis have been observed in association with pelvic lipomatosis in as high as 75% of patients in some series. This situation should merit special attention from urologists as cystitis glandularis is a potential premalignant lesion of bladder adenocarcinoma. Pelvic lipomatosis has a classic "pear-shaped" or "teardrop-shaped" bladder on intravenous urogram. The upper tracts can range from normal to severely dilated and the distal ureters are typically deviated medially. CT scan can be useful in the diagnosis of pelvic lipomatosis given its ability to identify fat.

Conservative management of pelvic lipomatosis includes weight reduction and routine radiographic evaluation to monitor for upper tract deterioration. In patients who develop worsening hydronephrosis or progressive azotemia, urinary tract decompression should be performed. Ureteral stenting, nephrostomy tube placement, ureteral reimplantation into the bladder dome, and urinary diversion have all been employed in this setting. Debulking of pelvic fatty tissue has also been reported with success but is technically difficult and not without potential significant complications including large blood loss and bowel and urinary tract injury.

Myelolipoma

Myelolipomas most commonly occur in the adrenal gland but can be seen as an isolated lesion in the retroperitoneal pelvis. As their name implies, myelolipomas are tumor-like growths of mature fat and bone marrow elements. These lesions are generally seen in patients older than 40 years and are typically smaller than 5 cm. Myelolipomas are typically found as incidental lesions during abdominal imaging.

Leiomyoma

Leiomyoma are benign tumors of smooth muscle origin. They are most commonly found in the female genital tract, but they can also be found in the retroperitoneum and the urinary bladder. Leiomyomas of the retroperitoneum have been found in women following hysterectomy leading to the conclusion that they are not as hormonally responsive as their uterine counterparts. When found in the retroperitoneum, they can grow to be quite large. Leiomyomas are difficult to distinguish from malignant lesions based on imaging alone and are generally surgically excised for this reason. Leiomyomas can be distinguished from malignant leiomyosarcoma histologically because they stain positive for desmin.

MALIGNANT LESIONS OF THE RETROPERITONEUM

Primary Retroperitoneal Sarcoma

Retroperitoneal sarcomas are rare tumors accounting for 0.1–0.2% of all malignancies and 10–20% of all soft tissue sarcomas. Five hundred to 1000 new cases of retroperitoneal sarcoma are diagnosed each year. One third of all malignant tumors arising in the retroperitoneum are sarcomas. They are most common in the fifth to sixth decade of life but can affect almost any age group. They are slightly more common in men but have not documented racial or ethnic predilection.

Information with regard to risk factors for retroperitoneal sarcomas is sparse, but prior radiation, trauma, and environmental exposure to dioxin and asbestos have all been documented. Malignant fibrous histiocytoma is the most common radiation-induced retroperitoneal sarcoma.

Sarcomas are thought to develop from mesenchymal stem cells residing in muscle, fat, and connective tissues. Retroperitoneal sarcomas arise primarily from soft tissues of fibrous and adipose origin. Histologically, liposarcoma is the most common followed by leiomyosarcoma and fibrosarcoma. Specific chromosomal transformations have been found for many of these tumors resulting in the production of tumor specific transcription factors. Abnormalities on chromosome 12 resulting in amplification of certain gene products involved in p53 inactivation have also been cited in the carcinogenesis of retroperitoneal sarcomas.

Pathology

Liposarcomas are the most common primary retroperitoneal tumor. They comprise 10–15% of all soft tissue sarcomas. They are most commonly seen during the fifth to sixth decade of life and can grow to be quite large in size. Grossly, liposarcomas have a "fish flesh" appearance and tend to be encapsulated. Well-differentiated liposarcomas can closely resemble lipomas and are classified as low grade. Higher grade liposarcomas tend to bear little resemblance histologically to fat-filled structures. Even though higher grade lesions still tend to be encapsulated, they tend to be locally invasive and recur after local excision.

Although leiomyosarcoma accounts for less than 10% of all soft tissue sarcomas, when they do occur, 50% of the time it is in the retroperitoneum. They occur more frequently in women with a 2:1 female-to-male predilection and are found most commonly in the sixth decade of life. Low-grade lesions can be distinguished from leiomyomas by the increased number of mitoses seen with high-power microscopy (>5 mitoses per high-power field). There is no definitive evidence that these sarcomas arise from malignant degeneration of leiomyomas.

Malignant fibrous histiocytoma (MFH) was first described in 1963 and is now the most common contemporary reported soft tissue sarcoma. These lesions are most frequently seen on the extremities, less commonly occurring in the retroperitoneum. There are several subtypes of MFH including storiform-pleomorphic, myxoid, giant cell, and inflammatory. Several histologic subtypes can occur in the same lesion. The storiform-pleomorphic pattern is most common (40–60% of all MFH) and is histologically identified by its collagen pattern of curling fascicles of cells. Fibrosarcomas, as their name implies, are malignant tumors of fibroblast origin. They are less frequently reported than in past series because they are now often classified as MFH.

Although, rhabdomyosarcoma is a common lesion in pediatric urologic oncology patients, it is rarely seen in the adult population as a primary retroperitoneal tumor. Several subtypes exist including embryonal, botryoid, alveolar, and spindle cell, with embryonal being the most common.

Diagnosis

Although retroperitoneal sarcomas can present in a broad spectrum of age groups, they are most commonly diagnosed in the sixth decade of life. Due to their relatively slow growth and retroperitoneal location, they are generally quite large at the time of diagnosis. Symptoms are generally due to tumor mass effect or local invasion. The vast majority of patients will present with abdominal pain or an abdominal mass (60–80%). Twenty to 30% will have accompanying nausea, vomiting, early satiety, and weight loss. Urinary symptoms tend to be infrequent. On physical exam, a protuberant abdomen is often easily identifiable. Lymphadenopathy is an uncommon finding, found in approximately 5% of presenting patients. Lower extremity edema can be seen in approximately 20% of patients, usually due to compression of the inferior vena cava.

Cross-sectional imaging with either CT or magnetic resonance imaging (MRI) is essential in the workup of patients suspected of having a retroperitoneal mass. The size of the mass, its relationship to other important anatomic structures, the presence of lymphadenopathy, and visceral metastases can all be assessed with these modalities. CT is also excellent for the detection of bony invasion. If there is a question of vascular involvement after initial imaging, it is often advisable to obtain magnetic resonance angiography (MRA) images to more precisely delineate the relationship of important vascular structures to the retroperitoneal mass.

If imaging does not provide a diagnosis with reasonable certainty, CT or ultrasound (US)-guided biopsy has been advocated at some centers to obtain a tissue diagnosis. Due to the infrequency of these lesions and the low sensitivity and specificity of diagnostic biopsy of these lesions in inexperienced hands, if a biopsy is warranted, it is recommended that it be performed at a center experienced in dealing with masses of this nature. In specific cases in which the diagnosis may be in question, open biopsy can be performed. Care must be taken during biopsy to avoid tumor spillage.

Staging

Tumor grade plays is an integral aspect of the staging of primary retroperitoneal tumors. Tumor grading is determined by the number of atypical mitoses, cytoplasmic and nuclear pleomorphism, and the presence of necrosis. Tumor grades range from G1 to G4 with G1 being well differentiated and G4 being undifferentiated (Table 18-3). The TNM system is combined with tumor grading for the complete clinical staging of these tumors (see Table 18-3).

Clinical staging should include a thorough physical examination, bone scan, and CT of the chest, abdomen, and pelvis. It is important to obtain information on bilateral renal function prior to exploration in case nephrectomy is warranted intraoperatively.

Table 18-3: American Joint Commission on Cancer GTNM Classification of Soft Tissue Sarcomas

Tumor Grade

G1 Well differentiated
G2 Moderately differentiated
G3 Poorly differentiated
G4 Undifferentiated

Primary Tumor

T1 Tumor ≤5 cm in greatest diameter
T1a Superficial tumor
T1b Deep tumor
T2 Tumor >5 cm in greatest diameter
T2a Superficial tumor
T2b Deep tumor

Regional Lymph Node Involvement

NX Regional lymph nodes cannot be assessed
N0 No known metastasis
N1 Confirmed lymph node metastasis

Distant Metastasis

MX Distant metastasis cannot be assessed
M0 No known distant metastasis
M1 Confirmed distant metastasis

Surgery

Extirpative surgery is the most effective form of therapy for patients with primary retroperitoneal tumors. Complete resection, with negative margins, has proven to be the most important predictor of outcome in this patient population. It is essential to be aware of the extent of the disease preoperatively and organs that potentially may need to be sacrificed to optimize the chances of obtaining a negative margin.

The surgical approach is generally through a large midline incision, chevron incision, or thoracoabdominal approach. Regardless of approach, it is of paramount importance to gain wide exposure to the retroperitoneum to access resectability and safely resect tumor. En bloc removal of all tumor and affected organs is essential to patient outcome. It is more often the rule than not for at least one adjacent organ to be removed to obtain negative margins. Major vascular structures, kidney, portions of the diaphragm, liver, stomach, gallbladder, spleen, pancreas, and bowel can be involved. The most frequently resected organ is the ipsilateral kidney followed by a portion of the colon, adrenal gland, pancreas, and spleen.

Surgical morbidity and mortality in contemporary surgical series range from 6–25% and 2–7%, respectively. Hemorrhage, intra-abdominal abscess, and enterocutaneous fistula formation are commonly described complications.

Outcomes

Classically the overall survival for patients with primary retroperitoneal sarcomas is poor. Two-, 5-, and 10-year survivals have been cited at 56%, 34%, and 18% for all outcomes. In patients without metastatic disease, 2- and 5-year survivals can be as high as 70% and 50–60%, respectively.

Patients receiving a complete surgical resection with negative margins achieve superior survival compared to patients in which complete surgical resection is incomplete. Five-year survival for patients with complete surgical resection averages 54% compared to 17% for those with incomplete resections. Unfortunately, tumor recurrence, even after complete surgical resection, is the rule rather than the exception. Tumor recurrence can be as high as 70% at 5 years and up to 90% at 10 years. In the absence of metastatic disease, surgery is the mainstay of treatment for recurrent local disease. Studies support that a significant number of patients can experience prolonged disease-free survival when all recurrent tumor can be resected.

Tumor grade has a significant impact on patient survival. Low-grade lesions demonstrate approximately a 50% survival advantage compared to intermediate and high-grade lesions. This survival advantage is maintained regardless of margin status.

Given the fact that the vast majority of failures occur in the abdomen, with an additional 20–30% of recurrences in the lungs, a surveillance regimen including physical examination, combined with CT of the chest, abdomen, and pelvis, appears to be a reasonable approach. The current guidelines from the National Comprehensive Cancer Network for the surveillance of retroperitoneal sarcomas includes physical examination with chest, abdomen, and pelvic CT every 3–6 months for 2–3 years then annually for low-grade disease and every 3–4 months for 3 years, then every 6 months for 2 years and annually thereafter for patients with high-grade disease.

Radiation and Chemotherapy for Retroperitoneal Sarcoma

The use and timing of radiotherapy in patients with retroperitoneal sarcoma are controversial. Retrospective studies on the benefit of postoperative adjuvant radiotherapy have yielded mixed results, but a decrease in local recurrences has been cited in some studies. Postoperative radiation doses in the range of 50 Gy have been associated with significant gastrointestinal toxicities. Intraoperative radiotherapy has been used in a small amount of patients at specialized centers. Intraoperative radiotherapy allows for the ability to directly target the resection bed while sparing nearby radio-sensitive tissue. The potential advantage of preoperative radiation therapy is unknown, but a multicenter phase III trial set to answer this question is ongoing.

The exact role and benefit of chemotherapy in the treatment of retroperitoneal sarcomas are also controversial. Modest benefits have been noted using adjuvant doxorubicin chemotherapy in patients with extremity sarcomas, but these benefits are difficult to extrapolate to patients with retroperitoneal sarcomas. For patients with advanced or metastatic disease doxorubicin is the principle chemotherapeutic agent. A response rate of 20–25% has been noted, but complete or sustained responses are rare. Combination agents have been employed but have not demonstrated superior responses compared to single-agent treatment and have shown significant increased toxicities.

SELF-ASSESSMENT QUESTIONS

1. What are the potential treatments, both surgical and nonsurgical, for retroperitoneal fibrosis?
2. What are the possible etiologies of a spontaneous retroperitoneal hematoma?
3. What are the radiographic manifestations of pelvic lipomatosis and what is the clinical significance of cystitis glandularis in the setting of pelvic lipomatosis?
4. What is the most important predictor of outcome in patients with retroperitoneal sarcomas?
5. What is the role of radiation and chemotherapy in patients with retroperitoneal sarcomas?

SUGGESTED READINGS

1. Albi G, Del Campo L, Tagarro D: Wunderlich's syndrome: causes, diagnosis radiological management. *Clin Radiol* 57:840, 2002.
2. Kabalin JL: Surgical anatomy of the retroperitoneum, kidneys, and ureters. *Campbell's Urology*, 8th ed. Philadelphia, Saunders, 2002.
3. Malkowicz SB, Ferlise V: Retroperitoneal tumors: Diagnosis, staging, surgery, management, and prognosis. *Urologic Oncology*. St. Louis, Elsevier, 2005.
4. Porter GA, Baxter NN, Pisters PW: Retroperitoneal sarcoma: a population based analysis of epidemiology, surgery and radiotherapy. *Cancer* 106:1610, 2006.
5. Sozen S, Gurocak S, Nukhet U, et al: The importance of re-evaluation of patients with cystitis glandularis associated with pelvic lipomatosis: a case report. *Urol Oncol* 22:428, 2004.
6. Varkarakis IM, Jarret TW: Retroperitoneal fibrosis. *AUA Update Series* 24:17, 2005.

C H A P T E R 19

Male Sexual Dysfunction

Ariana L. Smith, MD and
Andrew C. Axilrod, MD

I. INTRODUCTION

Sexuality is a complex bio-psycho-social process. Sexual problems are highly prevalent in men and women yet frequently unrecognized and underdiagnosed in clinical practice.

Sexual dysfunction includes a variety of sexual disorders with erectile dysfunction (ED) being the most common. ED is defined as the persistent inability to attain and maintain a penile erection adequate for satisfactory sexual performance. This condition has been estimated to affect greater than 150 million men across the world.

In the United States, it has been estimated that more than 50% of men 40–70 years of age have at least mild ED with more than 10% having complete ED (Figure 19-1). Moreover, it has been shown that ED prevalence increases as men age (Figure 19-2).

The introduction of sildenafil as the first effective oral therapy for ED in 1998 has increased the public's awareness about sexual dysfunction as a medical condition. Yet, even among clinicians who acknowledge the relevance of addressing sexual issues in their patients, there is a general lack of understanding of the optimal approach for identification and evaluation. It is clear, however, that treatment is beneficial for both patient and partner quality of life.

ED is more than just about sex. It is increasingly recognized as a public health problem with organic etiologies and associations with clinical comorbidities. The condition greatly affects patient quality of life, self-esteem, and ability to maintain intimate relationships. The concept of reciprocity of disease is particularly relevant to sexual dysfunction because concomitant disease processes can cause greater morbidity and mortality than the sexual dysfunction itself. Studies have shown that men with ED are more likely to have hypertension, hypercholesterolemia, cardiac disease, angina, diabetes mellitus, prostate disease, and depression than men without ED (Figure 19-3). The converse has also been shown; men

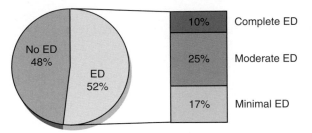

FIGURE 19-1. Erectile dysfunction prevalence in men 40–70 years of age is 52%; complete dysfunction is present in 10% of men. (From Feldman HA, Goldstein I, Hatzichristou DG, et al: Impotence and its medical and psychosocial correlates: results of the Massachusetts Male Aging Study. *J Urol* 151:54–61, 1994.)

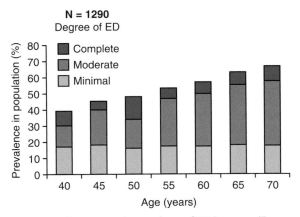

FIGURE 19-2. As men age the prevalence of ED increases. (From Feldman HA, Goldstein I, Hatzichristou DG, et al: Impotence and its medical and psychosocial correlates: results of the Massachusetts Male Aging Study. *J Urol* 151:54–61, 1994.)

with other medical disease are more likely to have ED than those with no comorbid condition (Figure 19-4).

Vasculogenic ED is believed to share a common etiology with other disease processes including coronary artery disease (CAD), hypertension, diabetes, and lipid abnormalities. It is thought that the common link is endothelial dysfunction secondary to oxidative stress. The recognition of ED as a warning sign of silent vascular disease has led to the concept that a man with ED and no cardiac symptoms is a cardiac patient until proven otherwise (Figure 19-5).

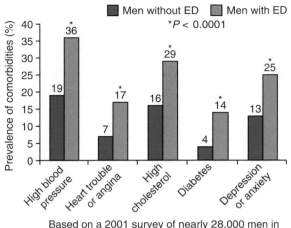

FIGURE 19-3. Prevalence of comorbidities in men with ED compared to those without ED. (From Rosen RC, Fischer WA, Eardley I, et al: The Multinational Men's Attitudes to Life Events and Sexuality [MALES] Study: I. Prevalence of erectile dysfunction and related health concerns in the general population. *Curr Med Res Opin* 20:607–617, 2004.)

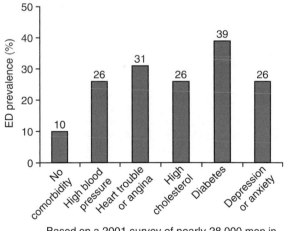

FIGURE 19-4. Prevalence of ED in men with other medical conditions. (From Rosen RC, Fischer WA, Eardley I, et al: The Multinational Men's Attitudes to Life Events and Sexuality [MALES] Study: I. Prevalence of erectile dysfunction and related health concerns in the general population. *Curr Med Res Opin* 20:607–617, 2004.)

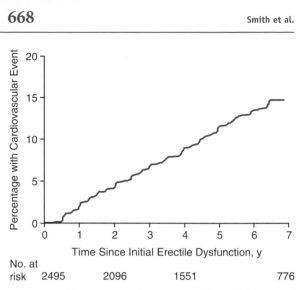

FIGURE 19-5. Time to any cardiovascular event from initial report of ED. (From Thompson IM, Tangen CM, Goodman PJ, et al: Erectile dysfunction and subsequent cardiovascular disease. *JAMA* 294 [23]:2996–3002, 2005.)

II. PHYSIOLOGY OF SEXUAL FUNCTION

A. Erection

Complex interactions between physiologic, neuroendocrine, and vascular mechanisms as well as psychogenic interplay produce penile erection. Sexual stimulation triggers a cascade of events. In essence, erections are neurovascular phenomena combining neurotransmission and vascular biologic responses. There is a release of neurotransmitters that result in smooth muscle relaxation in both penile erectile tissue and the penile arterial walls. This transforms the penile vasculature and erectile tissues from a contracted, minimally perfused state to a relaxed, blood engorged state.

1. Functional Anatomy of the Penis

a. Corporal Bodies

The penis is composed of three cylindrical units, the paired corpus cavernosum dorsally and the corpus spongiosum ventrally. Each corpora cavernosum is a network of endothelial-lined sinusoids within a trabecula of smooth muscle. The paired corpora cavernosum are supported by a fibrous skeleton and exhibit compliance characteristics similar to arterial vasculature. There is an incomplete septum between them, which allows passage of blood from one side to the other. With inflow of blood, these sinusoids expand and fill, producing an increase in pressure and a firm erection. Disease processes that produce corporal fibrosis create resistance to inflow of blood and diminished compliance of the sinusoidal space. Many diseases including diabetes, hypercholesterolemia, vascular disease, and penile injury are associated with deposition of collagen and decreased elastic fibers in the corpora. The corpus cavernosum is covered in two layers of tunica albuginea, which provide flexibility, rigidity, and tissue strength to the penis. Between these layers of tunica run the emissary veins, which are compressed during erection, ensuring high pressure rigidity. In the ventral groove of the tunica albuginea (between the 5- and 7-o'clock position), the outer layer is absent leaving this area most vulnerable to penile prostheses extrusion.

The corpus spongiosum covers the urethra and expands distally to form the glans penis. The spongiosum is covered with only one layer of tunica albuginea, allowing low pressure during erection. The glans penis has a high concentration of nerve receptors to provide sensory input to facilitate erection and enhance pleasure.

b. Neurophysiology and Pharmacology of Erection

The limbic system, part of the cerebral cortex, appears to contain the centers from which stimulation can elicit erection. The medial preoptic area and the paraventricular nucleus of the hypothalamus are known to be higher integration centers for sexual drive and erection. These centers have a close relationship to areas involved in emotional function such as fear, rage, olfaction, and vision, which may be the link to psychogenic impotence. Both dopaminergic and adrenergic receptors appear to promote sexual drive, whereas serotonin receptors and prolactin suppress sexual function.

Both the autonomic (sympathetic and parasympathetic) and somatic (sensory and motor) nervous systems play a role in the erectile process. The sympathetic nerves originate in the spinal segments of T11 to L2 and after passing through the sympathetic chain ganglia travel in the hypogastric nerves to the pelvic plexus. The parasympathetic nerves originate in the S2 to S4 segments and travel as preganglionic fibers in the pelvic nerves to the pelvic plexus. Together the fibers of the pelvic plexus form the cavernous nerves. These nerves supply the corpus cavernosum and spongiosum with parasympathetic innervation for erection and sympathetic innervation for ejaculation. The somatic nerves also originate at the level of the S2 to S4 spinal segment in Onuf's nucleus. These nerves travel in the sacral nerves to the pudendal nerve. The sensory center receives pain, temperature, and tactile sensation, whereas the motor center is responsible for contraction of the ischiocavernosus and bulbocavernosus muscles, which aid in ejaculation.

Neurally mediated erections can be reflexogenic, psychogenic, or nocturnal. Psychogenic erections are the result of audiovisual stimuli or fantasies that produce an impulse from the brain to the spinal erection centers. Psychogenic erections are usually lost in patients with spinal cord lesions above T9. Reflexogenic erections are the result of genital stimulation via a complex process involving ascending sensory afferent pathways to the brain and descending parasympathetic efferent nerves to the penis. Injury to the sacral spinal cord or the pudendal nerves abolishes reflexogenic erections. Nocturnal erections occur during rapid eye movement (REM) sleep by an unknown mechanism.

In corporal cavernosal tissue, nitric oxide (NO) is accepted as the principal neurotransmitter responsible for erectile response (Figure 19-6). With sexual arousal, NO synthase converts L-arginine and oxygen to NO. NO is also released from nonadrenergic-noncholinergic nerves as well as endothelial cells to cause an increase in the production of cyclic guanosine monophosphate (cGMP), a second messenger, which activates protein kinase G. NO enters into the target cell and binds to guanylate cyclase launching a signaling pathway. This leads to opening of potassium channels and closing of calcium channels, which ultimately leads to a drop in cytosolic free calcium. This drop in calcium is the direct cause of arterial and cavernous smooth muscle relaxation culminating in increased

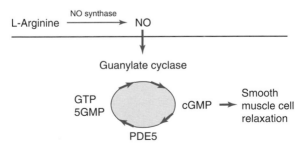

FIGURE 19-6. Nitric oxide-cGMP mechanism of action in corpus cavernosal smooth muscle relaxation and penile erection.

penile blood flow. Thus, the cyclic nucleotide signaling pathway mediates the smooth muscle relaxing effects of NO necessary for normal erectile function (EF). Down-regulation of this pathway is thought to be central to the pathophysiology of many forms of ED.

Cyclic nucleotide levels are determined by both synthesis, through the activities of guanylate cyclase on GTP, and enzymatic degradation, through the activity of phosphodiesterases (PDEs). Penile detumescence is in part the result of phosphodiesterase inhibitor type 5 (PDE-5), which breaks down cGMP. The smooth muscle regains its tone when cGMP is degraded by PDE-5. Competitive inhibition of the action of PDE-5 with inhibitors enhances erection.

c. Vasculature

The arterial supply of the penis is via the internal pudendal artery, a branch of the internal iliac artery. The internal pudendal becomes the penile artery, which gives off the dorsal, bulbourethral, and the cavernous arteries. The cavernous artery is responsible for tumescence of the corpora, whereas the dorsal artery supplies the glans during erection. The bulbourethral artery supplies the spongiosum and bulb. Occasionally, accessory arteries exist arising from the external iliac, obturator, vesical, and femoral arteries and can be the dominant or the only arterial supply to the corpora. Damage to these arteries can cause vasculogenic ED.

The venous drainage originates from the sinusoids via tiny venules to form the emissary veins (Figure 19-7). After piercing the tunica albuginea, the emissary veins drain into four structures: the circumferential veins, the deep dorsal veins, the superficial dorsal veins, and the periurethral veins. These ultimately terminate in the saphenous and internal pudendal veins.

d. Hemodynamics

In the flaccid penis, the smooth muscles of the arterial walls and the corpus cavernosum are tonically contracted allowing only a small amount of arterial flow. Tonic contraction of the flaccid penis is facilitated by adrenergic neurotransmission and endothelium derived contracting factors including prostaglandin F2. Sexual stimulation triggers release of neurotransmitters from the cavernous nerve terminals resulting in smooth muscle relaxation in both the corporal sinusoids and the arterial walls. The inflow of blood via the internal pudendal artery allows penile elongation and expansion of erectile tissues. The incoming blood is then trapped in the

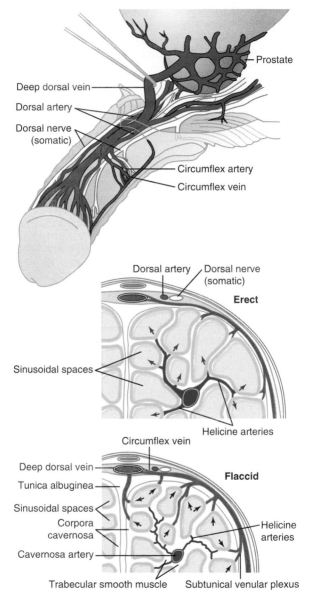

FIGURE 19-7. Penile vascular anatomy showing compression of venous outflow with erection.

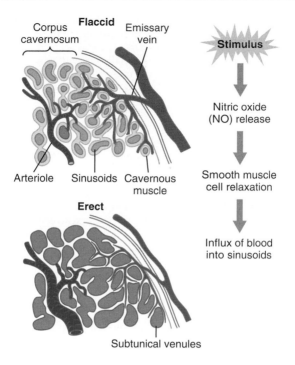

FIGURE 19-8. Physiology of erection showing smooth muscle relaxation and arterial inflow with erection.

cavernous tissue by the tunica albuginea. Compression of the emissary veins between the two layers of tunica albuginea as it is stretched to capacity further reduces venous outflow (Figure 19-8). As blood is retained within the penis by this veno-occlusive mechanism, intercavernous pressure rises to approximately 100 mm Hg, which allows the penis to rise from the dependent position to the fully erect phase. The rigid erectile phase is augmented by contraction of the ischiocavernosus and bulbocavernosus muscles.

During erection, the pressure in the corpus spongiosum and the glans is only one third of that in the corpora due to the thin tunical covering allowing only minimal venous occlusion. In the rigid erectile phase, the ischiocavernosus and bulbocavernosus muscles forcibly compress the veins allowing further engorgement of the spongiosum and glans.

Detumescence, a sympathetically derived return to flaccidity, is initiated by smooth muscle contraction followed by reopening of venous outflow channels and return to basal level of intracorporeal pressure.

B. Emission

Emission and ejaculation are temporally related events occurring at the culmination of sexual excitement. They are reflexogenic events and appear to involve both sensory stimuli from the genitalia and cerebral stimuli. Cerebral control over emission can be halted voluntarily to a point, but once the sensation of inevitability occurs with the filling of the posterior urethra it can no longer be delayed. Glandular secretions from periurethral glands, prostate, seminal vesicles, and the vas deferens are deposited into the posterior urethra during emission. Sympathectomy and adrenergic blockade can eliminate emission.

C. Ejaculation

The afferent stimulus for ejaculation seems to be the passage of semen from the posterior to the bulbous urethra. At this point, rhythmic contraction of the pelvic floor musculature with compression of the urethra produces antegrade expulsion of semen via the urethral meatus. Stimulation of serotonin receptors facilitates seminal emission and ejaculation, thus providing the mechanism for the effect of selective serotonin reuptake inhibitors (SSRIs) on sexual function. The bladder neck, which is under sympathetic control, under normal conditions remains tightly closed; if it does not, retrograde ejaculation into the bladder will occur. Retrograde ejaculation is commonly seen in patients status post transurethral resection of the prostate (TURP) and non-nerve sparing retroperitoneal lymph node dissection (RPLND) and in some with diabetic neuropathy. Coordination between sympathetic and somatic nervous systems allows ejaculation with rhythmic contractions of the bulbocavernosus and ischiocavernosus muscles to facilitate expulsion.

D. Orgasm

Orgasm is described as an intense and satisfying whole body sensation occurring at the time of neurotransmitter release. Following orgasm, detumescence takes place and a refractory period in which the male is unable to achieve full erection or repeat orgasm.

III. SEXUAL DYSFUNCTION IN THE MALE

Sexual dysfunction is a highly prevalent health problem with considerable impact on quality of life of middle-aged men. Sexual dysfunction includes not only ED but also premature ejaculation (PE), priapism, Peyronie's disease, ejaculatory incompetence, and decreased libido. These topics are discussed in a separate section at the end of this chapter.

A. Erectile Dysfunction

ED is defined as the persistent inability to attain and maintain a penile erection adequate for satisfactory sexual performance. Primary ED, ED present since puberty, is rare and when present demands a full diagnostic workup to rule out an organic etiology. Secondary ED implies adequate EF was present at some point and is much more common. It is suggested that a minimum duration of 3 months be present for establishment of the disease except in instances of trauma or surgically induced ED. ED has many causes, with most (75–80%) cases being attributed to vascular or neural disorders.

Many male sexual function questionnaires have been developed to attempt to quantify sexual function or dysfunction. These questionnaires not only provide quantifiable efficacy endpoints for drug trials as they attempt to measure sexual interest, performance, and satisfaction but also aid in the ability to assess patient response to therapy. The most commonly used and referenced questionnaire is the International Index of Erectile Function (IIEF), which is statistically validated in many languages. It contains 15 items that quantify five domains: EF, orgasmic function, sexual desire, intercourse satisfaction, and overall satisfaction. An abridged 5-item version (IIEF-5) has been developed to allow a quick office setting evaluation. ED severity can be classified into five categories based on the IIEF-5, which assigns a numeric value of 0, 1–5 for each of the five questions. Severe ED is classified as a score of 5–7, moderate ED a score of 8–11, mild to moderate ED a score of 12–16, mild ED a score of 17–21, and no ED a score of 22–25. Another commonly used, however not validated, questionnaire is the Sexual Encounter Profile (SEP). Of the five questions, SEP 2, which assesses penetration, and SEP 3, which assesses completion, are particularly important in clinical evaluation.

The obvious drawback of sexual inventories is their reliance on self-assessment. This clearly does not differentiate among the various causes of ED and diagnostic tests may be necessary in patients with complex ED. Therefore, in clinical evaluation, a good case history, preferably taken from both partners, physical examination, and proper laboratory studies still form the cornerstone in the evaluation of ED.

1. Vasculogenic

Thromboembolic occlusion, fibrosis, calcification, obliteration, scarring, and aneurysmal dilations decrease the blood flow through the penile arteries and result in arterial ED. Additionally, the process of aging causes progressive obliteration of the cavernosal arteries and atherosclerotic narrowing of the aortoiliac and pudendal vessels. The increase in blood flow required for erection is comparable to that required by the heart for vigorous exercise. ED may be analogous to CAD arising from progressive blockage of small vessels and reduced arterial compliance. It would follow that ED and CAD share the modifiable risk factors leading to arteriosclerosis such as cigarette smoking, diabetes, high fat diet, elevated serum lipids, hypertension, physical inactivity, and obesity. Many studies have suggested that ED is predictive of other disease processes and reciprocity of disease exists. The implications for preventative medicine are significant because many are behaviorally modifiable. Further extrapolation of this data would suggest that the onset of ED, to the degree that it reflects systemic arterial compromise, could be interpretable as a sentinel event of subclinical coronary disease. This has obvious public health implications in that erectile problems can call attention to coronary risk and contribute to prevention of morbidity and mortality from coronary disease.

Diabetic vasculopathy can also contribute. Other risk factors include hypertension, cardiovascular disease, smoking, hyperlipidemia, and pelvic/perineal trauma. Pelvic steal syndrome is seen in large vessel arteriosclerosis in which there is shunting of the blood to the pelvic and gluteal muscles resulting in detumescence.

Veno-occlusive dysfunction is caused by presence of large abnormal channels, plaques in the tunica albuginea (Peyronie's disease), structural alteration in fibroelastic components, insufficient smooth muscle relaxation, and acquired shunts as seen after the treatment of priapism.

2. Neurogenic

Neurogenic impotence can be secondary to a cerebral lesion, a spinal cord lesion, or a peripheral neuropathy. Central nervous system (CNS) disorders associated with ED include Parkinson's disease, Alzheimer's disease, Huntington's chorea, stroke, multiple sclerosis, head trauma, brain tumor, temporal lobe epilepsy, and major depressive disorder.

Spinal cord injury, tabes dorsalis, spina bifida, syringomyelia, amyotrophic lateral sclerosis, compression due to herniated disks and tumors, lateral chordotomy for intractable pain, and Shy-Drager syndrome may cause sexual dysfunction.

Diabetes, uremia, amyloidosis, chronic alcoholism, scleroderma, vitamin B deficiency, systemic lupus erythematosus, acquired immunodeficiency syndrome (AIDS), and pelvic surgery are known to involve the peripheral autonomic nerves and are associated with ED. Sensory penile thresholds often increase significantly as a result of peripheral nervous system disorders. These thresholds are critical in achieving and maintaining erections.

3. Endocrine

Diabetes is the single most frequent cause of ED in the United States. In diabetic men, impotence is more common than retinopathy or neuropathy with approximately half of diabetic men complaining of ED. Impotence does not correlate with severity of diabetes or the adequacy of its control. Although diabetes itself is an endocrinologic disorder, it causes ED through its vascular, neurologic, endothelial, and psychogenic complications rather than through hormonal deficiency. The prevalence of ED is three times higher in diabetic men (28% vs. 9.6%), occurs at an earlier age, and increases in prevalence with disease duration. In 12% of diabetic men, deterioration of sexual function can be the first symptom. In animal models, it has been shown that diabetes causes endothelial cell dysfunction, which results in an increased prevalence of vascular disease. Particularly important effects are reduced activity of NO synthase as well as a diminished effect of the released NO. This has important effects on EF.

Hypogonadism is also a frequent cause of ED with an estimated 5 million affected men in the United States. Interestingly, only about 5% receive treatment. Testosterone is necessary for normal libido, ejaculation, and spontaneous erection. There is a threshold with individual variation, below which sexual function is impaired. The World Health Organization (WHO) recommends that testosterone be assayed in men with low sexual desire and in those with atrophic testis (<19 mL) because hypogonadism is treatable.

Primary testicular failure (hypergonadotropic hypogonadism) causes ED as a result of decreased testosterone. Various causes include Klinefelter's syndrome, chemotherapy, radiation therapy, and congenital defects. Hypogonadotropic hypogonadism causes ED as a result of diminished luteinizing hormone (LH) production from the anterior pituitary and can be associated with Kallmann's, Prader-Willi, and Laurence-Moon-Biedl syndromes.

There is a significant increase in hypogonadism with age. A significant interrelationship among hypogonadism, depression, and ED underscores the importance of the endocrine evaluation. Alterations in androgen production in aging men have been recognized for some time and may be referred to as andropause. Aging is associated with a progressive decline in the production of several hormones including testosterone, dehydroepiandrosterone, thyroxine, melatonin, and growth hormone. Hypogonadism is associated with a decrease in sexual interest and a deterioration in the quality of EF, both of which can be improved with androgen supplementation. Other symptoms may include depression, irritability, cognition, insomnia, decreased strength, and diminished endurance.

Initial biochemical studies should include bioavailable testosterone and/or calculated free testosterone measured between 8:00 and 11:00 AM. A morning testosterone value below 350 ng/dL in a young man with chronically elevated gonadotropins makes a clear diagnosis of hypogonadism. In older men, the diagnostic value is not so clearly defined. If the value is below the lower limit of normal, a repeat value along with an assessment of LH and prolactin should be performed. Sex hormone binding globulin (SHBG) also increases with age and causes decreased free testosterone.

Hyperprolactinemia, drug induced or from a prolactin secreting pituitary tumor, is rarely the cause of ED. However, when biochemical hypogonadism has been documented with associated diminished libido, gynecomastia, or galactorrhea, determination of prolactin level is recommended and a space-occupying pituitary lesion must be excluded.

Hyperprolactinemia impairs the pulsatile LH secretion, which in turn produces a decline in serum testosterone production by the gonads. The resulting hypogonadism is thought to be the main cause of ED. Treatment of hyperprolactinemia is with the dopamine agonist bromocriptine, and sexual improvement correlates better with the decrease of serum prolactin than with the increase in testosterone level.

Thyroid disorders, both hyper- and hypothyroidism, are known to cause sexual dysfunction. Hyperthyroidism is commonly associated with diminished libido more so than ED. It is believed that this may be caused by the increased circulating estrogen levels. Hypothyroidism is associated with low testosterone secretion and elevated prolactin levels, which contribute to ED.

Patients with chronic renal failure have a 20–50% risk of sexual dysfunction, and 45% of men on hemodialysis report severe ED. Persistent uremia can contribute to ED via disturbance of the hypothalamic-pituitary-testis sex hormone axis, hyperprolactinemia, accelerated atheromatous disease, and psychologic factors. Following renal transplant, up to 50% of patients regain potency.

4. Psychogenic

Most cases of psychogenic ED are actually mixed. Until recently it was thought that 80–90% of impotence was psychogenic. Contemporary studies have demonstrated that 70–80% of ED has an organic cause with less than one third being purely psychogenic. Normal sexual function requires self-confidence, absence of anxiety, presence of arousing mental and/or physical stimuli, and the ability to focus on the sexual activity. Psychogenic dysfunction can produce exaggerated suprasacral inhibition of spinal erection centers as well as excessive sympathetic outflow. Both mechanisms will lead to a decreased erection. Many psychologic components can produce ED including depression, anxiety, stress, general unhappiness, financial burdens, fear of failure, marital or relationship conflict, ignorance, religious beliefs, and personality disorders (obsessive-compulsive, anhedonia). Medication treatment for these disorders can also cause ED.

In general, psychogenic and organic categories of ED differ in presentation, severity, and association with certain environmental variables. Psychogenic ED is often characterized by sudden onset with complete and immediate loss of sexual function, although this may vary with the partner and circumstance. The patient tends to display erection on awakening. Organic ED typically is more gradual in onset with incremental progression of dysfunction.

5. End-Organ Failure

Penile deformity, whether congenital, acquired, or secondary to trauma, can adversely affect penile hemodynamics. Congenital abnormalities of the penis that may preclude sexual dysfunction include extrophy/epispadias complex, micropenis, fusiform megalourethra, and severe penile chordee.

Direct trauma to the genital area including the perineum either as a single or repeated event, such as that caused by excessive bicycle riding, which exerts compressive effects on the pudendal vasculature, is also an offender.

6. Iatrogenic/Drug Induced

Vascular surgical procedures, radical pelvic surgery, transplant, surgery for priapism, pelvic irradiation, and trauma to the lower urinary tract are known to cause ED. The prevalence of ED after radical prostatectomy is estimated at 20–70%, after abdominoperineal resection 20–60%, after aorto-iliac vascular bypass 30%, and after TURP 4%. Brain and spinal cord surgery may also lead to ED. Habitual bicycling for long distances can impair EF, possibly via perineal nerve entrapment or penile arterial injury. Many drugs are known to cause impotence including alcohol, recreational drugs, antihypertensives, and psychotropics. The incidence of drug-induced impotence is about 25%. However, the compounding factor is that these drugs tend to be taken by older men with conditions that are themselves risk factors for ED. The underlying disorder may be more relevant to the ED than the medication.

Most of the antihypertensive drugs in use have ED listed as a potential side effect; however, clinical trials give conflicting results. Beta-blockers and thiazide diuretics seem to be associated with higher rates of ED, whereas alpha-adrenergic blockers and angiotensin-converting enzyme (ACE) inhibitors tend to improve EF. Alpha-adrenergic blockers may cause retrograde ejaculation or possibly an ejaculation, which can be concerning to some men. Although nonselective beta-blockers have been associated with a high prevalence of ED, newer selective agents have shown no difference in ED compared with placebo.

Psychotropic medications including antipsychotics, antidepressants, and anxiolytics tend to exert their effect by acting centrally on CNS receptors that also affect sexual function. Cocaine abuse can also elicit ED through effects on endogenous dopamine, as well as through increased alpha-adrenergic activity and endothelial dysfunction. Antiandrogens, which are often used in the treatment of advanced prostate cancer or symptomatic benign prostatic hypertrophy, can cause decreased sexual desire as well as ED.

Many other drugs have been implicated as having sexual side effects, but these data are not supported by controlled trials.

IV. EVALUATION OF SEXUAL DYSFUNCTION

A. History

Many sexual function profiles and questionnaires, as mentioned previously, have been developed to attempt to quantify sexual interest, performance, and satisfaction. These questionnaires are a good start but should not be used as a substitute for a careful history (Figure 19-9).

1. Medical History

The underlying health status of the patient needs to be established first. It is important to identify patients at cardiovascular risk with initiation of sexual activity as these patients should be referred to a cardiologist prior to treatment of ED (Figure 19-10). Low-risk patients are those with less than three cardiac risk factors, and in these patients ED treatment may be initiated without a full cardiac evaluation (Figure 19-11a). Patients experiencing cardiac symptoms when initiating sexual activity should be counseled to seek medical attention immediately and abstain from further sexual activity. Intermediate-risk patients have three or more risk factors, stable angina, recent myocardial infarction, congestive heart failure, a history of stroke, or peripheral vascular disease. These patients need further evaluation prior to initiation of sex (Figure 19-11b). High-risk patients must defer sexual activity until cardiovascular intervention is completed (Figure 19-11c). It is also important to obtain a list of daily medications as these may be implicated in the etiology of the ED. Lifestyle choices including smoking, moderate alcohol use, and long-distance bicycle riding may predispose to ED.

2. Sexual History

This is essential to confirm the diagnosis and differentiate from the normal physiologic changes of aging. It is impor-

ALGORITHM FOR DIAGNOSTIC EVALUATION OF ED

Diagnostic Evaluation

Patient complaining of Erectile Dysfunction

Basic Evaluation

- Findings Necessitate Further Evaluation
- Findings Support Initiation of Treatment

Optional and/or Specialized Testing

Review Diagnostic Findings and Discuss Treatment Options

Sexual, Psychosocial and Medical Assessment

Sexual Function Assessment → Problem with Orgasm, Ejaculation, Genital Pain or Libido → Further Evaluation of other Sexual Dysfunctions

Medical History → Reversible Risk Factors → Review and Manage Accordingly

Medical History → Unstable C.V. Condition → Further C.V. Workup and Management

Pelvic Perineal Trauma? → Specific Imaging and Vascular Testing in Young Patients

Psychosocial Assessment → Psychosocial Distress Including Partner Conflict → In Depth Psychosocial Evaluation and Management

Focused Physical Examination → Penile Abnormality e.g. Peyronie's • Prostatic Disease • Signs Suggestive of Hypogonadism → Evaluate Further and Manage as Needed

Basic Lab Tests → Undiagnosed • Diabetes • Hyperlipidemia • Low Testosterone → Further Endocrine Evaluation and Management if Needed

Specific Indications for Referral to Specialized Management

1. Patient requests referral for specific testing or treatment.
2. Patient requiring vascular, neurological or cardiologic evaluation.
3. Young patient with pelvic, perineal or penile surgery or trauma who may be a candidate for reconstructive vascular surgery.
4. Patient with Peyronie's disease and/or a significant penile bend or deformity that might require surgical correction.
5. Patient with refractory depression, bipolar disorder, psychosis or history of sexual abuse or trauma and those patients with complicated psychiatric or psychosexual disorder as well as those with complex relationship issues.
6. Patient with a complicated endocrinopathy including complicated diabetes mellitus.
7. Patient with treatment failures who may be a candidate for intracavernosal injection therapy or penile implant surgery.

FIGURE 19-9. Algorithm for diagnostic evaluation of ED. (From Lue TF, Giuliano F, Montorsi F, et al: Summary of the recommendations on sexual dysfunction in men. *J Sex Med* 1[1]:6–23, 2004.)

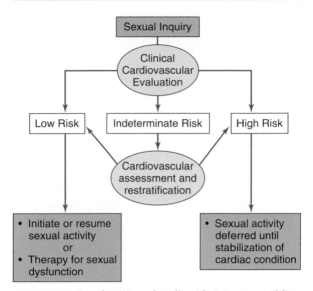

FIGURE 19-10. Sexual activity and cardiac risk: Princeton guidelines algorithm. (From Jackson G, Rosen RC, Kloner RA, et al: The Second Princeton Consensus on Sexual Dysfunction and Cardiac Risk: new guidelines for sexual medicine. *J Sex Med* 3[1]:28–36, 2006.)

tant to address the severity, onset, and duration of symptoms that are present as well as the exact nature of the complaint (lack of desire, difficulty obtaining/maintaining erection, PE, lack of orgasm). With organic impotence, there is usually a gradual deterioration in sexual function, whereas with psychogenic impotence the onset may be acute.

3. Psychosocial History

Questions relevant to other aspects of the patient's life including interpersonal relationships, occupational status, financial security, family life, and social support should be asked as these can affect sexual functioning. Performance anxiety can be the primary cause of ED. Depression is an important etiology of decreased libido. In many cases, organic and psychogenic factors coexist. Psychometric instruments to assess personality, depression, and relationship factors can be extremely useful in determining the psychologic component to sexual dysfunction. It is important for urologists to recognize red flags and refer patients for psychologic evaluation when necessary.

Low Risk: Sexual activity may be initiated without need for additional cardiac evaluation. Asymptomatic patients with less than 3 cardiac risk factors

- Controlled hypertension
- Mild stable angina
- Post successful CABG
- Uncomplicated old MI
- Mild valvular disease
- Class I NYHA CHF

A

Intermediate/indeterminate Risk: Cardiac condition is uncertain or risk profile requires further evaluation before sexual activity is resumed

- >3 CHD risk factors
- Moderate stable angina
- Recent MI (2–6 wks)
- CHF (NYHA II)
- Non-cardiac sequelae of atherosclerotic disease (stroke, PVD)

B

High Risk: Cardiac condition is severe or unstable and sexual activity poses significant risk. Sexual activity to be deferred pending further evaluation

- Unstable angina
- Uncontrolled hypertension
- CHF (NYHA III/IV)
- High risk arrhythmias
- Cardiomyopathies
- Moderate to severe heart disease

C

FIGURE 19-11. Stratification of patients with cardiac disease into low risk (a), intermediate risk (b), and high risk (c). CABG, Coronary artery bypass graft; MI, myocardial infarction; NYHA, New York Heart Association; CHF, congestive heart failure; CHD, coronary heart disease; PVD, peripheral vascular disease.

B. Physical Exam

The physical exam is essential in the evaluation of sexual dysfunction, although it rarely identifies the underlying cause.

An assessment of body habitus including secondary sexual characteristics and the genitalia may occasionally reveal an obvious cause (micropenis; chordee; Peyronie's disease; endocrine disease [i.e., gynecomastia]; or genetic syndromes [i.e., Klinefelter's/Kallmann's]). The size and texture of the testicles also provide important information. General screening of the neurologic and cardiovascular systems may identify potentially more dangerous medical conditions. Evaluation of anal sphincter tone and bulbocavernosus reflex as well as perineal and genital sensation is important. An examination of peripheral pulses and bruits can provide important information.

C. Laboratory Data

Recommended tests include fasting glucose, lipids, and hormonal profiles including testosterone, prolactin, and LH. Additional tests including thyroid-stimulating hormone (TSH) and prostate-specific antigen (PSA) should be performed at the clinician's discretion. A PSA should be obtained prior to considering hormonal replacement therapy.

D. Special Studies

As treatment options have become less invasive, further evaluation of ED has become less common. Indications for further evaluation include failure of initial treatment, Peyronie's disease, primary ED, history of pelvic or perineal trauma, vascular or neurologic disease, and medicolegal concerns.

1. Vascular Evaluation

This is aimed at the diagnosis of arterial and veno-occlusive disorders. The most commonly used test involves intracavernous injection of a vasodilator and sexual stimulation with assessment of the erection. This allows assessment of the vascular status of the penis directly by bypassing the neurologic and hormonal systems. A normal response predicts normal venous occlusion of the corpora but may miss borderline arterial inflow insufficiency. The patient should be monitored until the penis becomes flaccid as iatrogenic priapism rarely may result. If spontaneous detumescence does not occur, treatment with diluted phenylephrine intracavernously can produce flaccidity.

Duplex ultrasonography can be performed at the time of intercavernous injection to assess blood flow velocities and arterial diameters. In a normal subject, intracavernosal injection produces an increase in penile arterial blood flow velocity and arterial diameter with a peak systolic velocity of greater than 25 cm/sec and an arterial diameter increase of greater than 25%. Values less than 25 cm/sec are predictive of arterial insufficiency. Patients with veno-occlusive dysfunction tend to have normal peak systolic velocities greater than 25 cm/sec but have diminished vascular resistance or resistive index (RI). It has been found that an RI less than 0.75 was associated with venous leakage in 95% of cases, whereas an RI greater than 0.9 predicted adequate venous occlusion. Some people have used a criterion of end diastolic velocity of more than 5 cm/sec to represent venous leak.

Arteriography evaluates penile blood flow and is performed after injection of a vasodilating agent. Radiographic contrast is then injected via the internal pudendal artery to allow visualization of the penile and cavernous arteries. There is significant variation in penile arterial anatomy, and this study is more useful in providing anatomic rather than functional information. This is most commonly used in young men with a traumatic arterial injury to the penis in preparation for surgical revascularization.

Dynamic infusion cavernometry and cavernosonography (DICC) can be performed following the injection of a vasodilating agent into the penis. Cavernosometry evaluates intercavernous pressure during saline infusion to assess venous outflow dysfunction. After injection of a high-dose vasodilating agent, saline infusion should raise the intercavernous pressure to the level of mean systolic pressure. If this does not occur or there is a rapid drop in intercavernous pressure with cessation of saline infusion, veno-occlusive disorder is suggested. These patients may be candidates for dorsal vein ligation. These results, however, may be misleading in that fear, anxiety, and lack of privacy can all minimize the erection, confusing it with venous leak.

Cavernosography involves infusion of radiographic contrast in the corpora to visualize the site of venous leakage.

2. Neurologic Evaluation

The effect of a neurologic deficit on EF is complicated. Although neurologic testing should assess peripheral, spinal, and supraspinal centers and both autonomic and somatic pathways, rarely do these results change the management of the patient. Also, the neurologic tests currently available lack sensitivity and reliability in clinical diagnosis. Therefore, neurologic testing is only recommended in research protocols and medicolegal investigations.

Perineal electromyography and bulbocavernous reflex latency testing can evaluate the somatic pudendal nerve. The pudendal nerves (S2-4) supply sensation from the penile skin and provide motor innervation to the bulbocavernosus, ischiocavernosus, and the external urethral sphincter muscles. The sensory aspect is important for erections, whereas the motor aspect is necessary for ejaculation. Dorsal penile nerve conduction velocity can be measured to assess function.

3. Nocturnal Penile Tumescence

The measurement of nocturnal penile tumescence (NPT) uses a device that measures the number of episodes and duration of erections during sleep as well as penile girth and rigidity. The presence of a full erection during sleep, with both corporal expansion and rigidity, confirms that the neurovascular axis is intact and that the cause of ED is most likely psychogenic. NPT usually occurs in conjunction with REM sleep. Normally there are 3–5 erectile episodes per night each lasting 10–25 minutes.

V. NONSURGICAL TREATMENT OF ERECTILE DYSFUNCTION

Although penile prosthesis remains the most effective treatment for all types of ED, the vast majority of patients choose nonsurgical management of their ED.

A. Time

Most men will experience an episode of erection failure at some time in their life. Many of these cases have no organic etiology. It may be the result of fatigue, stresses of daily living, relationship issues, financial issues, and psychologic problems. Many psychologically based sexual problems will disappear with reassurance by the physician and the passage of time.

B. Lifestyle Changes

Lifestyle modifications may be advised for patients who smoke, abuse alcohol, use recreational drugs, or lead sedentary lives. Physical activity is associated with ED, with the highest risk among men who remain sedentary. Of all lifestyle modifications, only increased physical activity has been associated with the reversal of ED. In a recent clinical study, weight loss improved EF in about one third of obese patients. Early investigation has shown that lowering cholesterol in men with hypercholesterolemia improves erectile capacity. Medication changes may be beneficial especially in men taking older antihypertensive drugs.

C. Psychotherapy and Sexual Counseling

Masters and Johnson are credited with describing the most innovative format of psychosexual therapy in the 1970s. Although often effective, the treatment method was impractical because it was therapist intensive and expensive. Most recent approaches to sex therapy have included cognitive-behavioral interventions focused on correcting maladaptive behavior. Exploration of past developmental experiences and their impact on present behavior can be helpful. Addressing performance anxiety with desensitization techniques is a common focus.

D. Hormonal Therapy

Testosterone supplementation is indicated in men who have signs and symptoms of hypogonadism accompanied by subnormal serum testosterone levels.

Testosterone supplementation seems to have its major effect on libido rather than EF. Injectable depot preparations of testosterone are the least expensive form of androgen supplementation. However, this does not replicate normal circadian rhythm. In fact, after initial injection, supraphysiologic levels of testosterone are noted for 72 hours, then a steady exponential decline to subphysiologic levels occurs by 10–12 days. These drastic fluctuations may produce emotional lability and psychologic instability. Transdermal patches most closely mimic circadian rhythms. The most common side effect is local skin irritation. Other forms including gels, pellets, buccal tablets, and oral preparations are all available.

Animal models have shown that normal androgen levels are a prerequisite for PDE-5 inhibitors to work optimally.

Androgen therapy does have potential adverse effects. Suppression of follicle-stimulating hormone (FSH) and LH resulting in infertility can occur with supraphysiologic levels of testosterone. Erythrocytosis, increased platelet aggregation, and increased low-density lipoprotein (LDL) and decreased high-density lipoprotein (HDL) may result from testosterone therapy. These have obvious cardiovascular risks associated with them.

E. Pharmacologic Therapy

1. Oral Agents

The PDE-5 inhibitor sildenafil (Viagra) was approved in 1998 followed by vardenafil (Levitra) in 2003 and tadalafil (Cialis) in 2004. Practice patterns in the treatment of ED changed with the introduction of these drugs. Prior to the release of sildenafil, oral ED therapy was confined to largely ineffective treatments, including off-label trazodone and the herbal product yohimbine. In the United States, presentation rates for ED more than doubled after the regulatory approval of sildenafil.

As mentioned earlier, penile erection is initiated by sexual arousal, which stimulates the release of NO at nerve endings in the penis. NO activates guanylyl cyclase to cyclic GMP thus producing smooth muscle relaxation in the vascular and smooth muscle cells of the corpus cavernosum. This relaxation allows arterial inflow or tumescence. Detumescence is initiated by the breakdown of cGMP by PDEs. The mechanism of action of PDE-5 inhibitors is blockage of this step thus potentiating the erectile phase. Sexual stimulation is vital because PDE-5 inhibitors potentiate NO mediated vasorelaxation only in the presence of adequate sexual arousal.

Eleven types of PDE exist (PDE-1 to PDE-11) with a range of cellular functions. PDE-5 is present in smooth muscle of the corpora cavernosa. Cross reactivity of the PDE-5 inhibitors with PDE-6, PDE-11, and nonpenile PDE-5 produces the majority of side effects with use of these medication. Sildenafil, and to a lesser degree vardenafil, cross react with PDE-6 causing some visual side effects, including sensitivity to light and color changes. The most concerning side effect is the development of nonarteritic anterior ischemic optic neuropathy (NAION). This presents with sudden loss of vision and optic nerve swelling. There is no known etiology and no treatment. In the United States, this has been reported with all three drugs in a total of 43 patients among 30 million users. It is unknown whether this is the result of PDE-5 inhibitor use, underlying disease process, or a combination of the two. Imbalances in cGMP levels can interfere with visual signaling and culminate in photoreceptor cell death and retinal degeneration. Insufficient numbers of patients with retinitis pigmentosa have been studied to safely recommend administration of any PDE-5 inhibitors to patients with this condition. Tadalafil cross reacts with PDE-11, but the effects of this are unknown.

Other side effects of these medications, including headache, facial flushing, sinusitis, and dyspepsia, are caused by PDE-5 inhibition in vascular and gastrointestinal (GI) smooth muscle. Acute postural hypotension has been reported when sildenafil is administered together with the alpha-adrenergic blocker, doxazosin. Prescribing information recommends that sildenafil at doses greater than 25 mg not be administered within 4 hours after a patient takes an alpha-blocker.

For vardenafil and tadalafil, coadministration of alpha-blockers is listed as a precaution. Other antihypertensive drugs seem to be well tolerated in patients taking a PDE-5 inhibitor.

Although no direct comparative study exists, the three PDE-5 inhibitors are effective in the treatment of ED. All three compounds have been proven effective in several patient populations including diabetics and postsurgical patients and have shown to demonstrate dose response. The three drugs do have pharmacologic differences especially with respect to onset of action and half life. Peak serum concentrations for these drugs are achieved at approximately 1 hour with sildenafil and vardenafil and at 2 hours with tadalafil. High fat meal intake influences the absorption of both sildenafil and vardenafil but has no effect on tadalafil.

All three drugs are contraindicated with nitrates, including amyl nitrate. Because PDE-5 inhibitors potentiate the vasodilator and hypotensive effects of NO donors, treatment with any PDE-5 inhibitor is contraindicated in patients taking any form of NO donor. If chest pain develops after use of these drugs, patients are advised to avoid nitrates for 24 hours after use of sildenafil and vardenafil and for 48 hours after use of tadalafil.

Based on a limited study that was presented at the American Urologic Association (AUA) meeting in 2003, early or prophylactic treatment of ED may promote normalization of EF after nerve-sparing radical prostatectomy. This improvement may be attributable to neuronal regeneration secondary to enhanced nocturnal erection oxygenation, although further studies are required to test this hypothesis.

The package inserts for all three drugs warn against the use in the following patients:

- Myocardial infarction in the previous 90 days
- Unstable angina or angina occurring during sexual intercourse
- New York Heart Association class II or greater heart failure in the previous 6 months
- Uncontrolled arrhythmias, hypotension (<90/50 mm Hg), or uncontrolled hypertension (>170/100 mm Hg)
- Stroke within the previous 6 months
- Known hereditary degenerative retinal disorders, including retinitis pigmentosa
- Tendency to develop priapism (sickle cell anemia, leukemia)

Certain drugs, such as ketoconazole and itraconazole, and protease inhibitors can impair breakdown of PDE-5 inhibitors potentiating the effects. Rifampin enhances breakdown of PDE-5 inhibitors diminishing effects. Severe kidney or hepatic dysfunction may require dose adjustment.

Yohimbine is an α_2-adrenergic antagonist that acts centrally to promote sexual behavior. It appears to affect dopamine and serotonin transmission. Clinical studies have not supported the efficacy of yohimbine for ED.

Apomorphine is a dopaminergic agonist with proerectile properties. It acts within the paraventricular nucleus, the sexual drive center in mammals. Clinical trials with the sublingual formulation have shown success over placebo. Side effects include nausea, dizziness, and yawning.

2. Intraurethral Agents

Alprostadil, a synthetic formulate of prostaglandin E1 (PGE_1) can be inserted in pellet form into the urethra for local absorption. Resultant smooth muscle relaxation and vasodilation in the corpora cavernosum occur. Side effects include vaginal discomfort by female partners and penile pain.

3. Intracavernous Injection Therapy

Intracavernous injection of vasoactive drugs was introduced in the early 1980s and dramatically changed the practice of diagnosis and treatment of ED. Many agents and combinations of agents have been used and remain available for use today.

Papaverine was the first inhibitor of PDE developed for treating ED. It inhibits both PDE-5 and PDE-3 leading to increased levels of cGMP and cyclic adenosine monophosphate (cAMP), respectively, with resultant smooth muscle relaxation in the penile vasculature and corporal tissue. Papaverine also blocks voltage-dependent calcium channels impairing calcium influx, further promoting smooth muscle relaxation. Starting dosage is 20 mg and can be titrated up to 80 mg. Side effects include priapism, which may occur in up to 35% of users, and corporal fibrosis, which is seen in 1–33% of users. It is believed that corporal fibrosis is the result of poor technique and can be minimized by compression of the injection site and use of only 1 mL of injectable volume. Its general efficacy as monotherapy is approximately 55%. Although papaverine was the first agent available for intracavernous injection, it has never been approved by the Food and Drug Administration (FDA) for that use.

Phentolamine mesylate is a competitive alpha-adrenergic blocker. It is hypothesized that, by blocking prejunctional α_2 receptors, phentolamine inadvertently increases intracavernous norepinephrine preventing sinusoidal relaxation. Side effects include hypotension, reflex tachycardia, nasal congestion, and GI upset.

Alprostadil (PGE1) causes smooth muscle relaxation and vasodilation by elevation of intracellular cAMP. Available doses range from 2 to 40 μg. Advantages include high response rate and low incidence of priapism and fibrosis. The disadvantages of this drug include higher incidence of painful erection and high cost.

Forskolin directly activates the catalytic domain of adenylate cyclase and increases intracellular cAMP.

Two, three, and four drug mixtures have been formulated to attempt to minimize side effects and maximize therapeutic success. Trimix is comprised of papaverine 30 mg/mL, phentolamine 2 mg/mL, and PGE1 20 μg/mL. This combination has a lower incidence of painful erections than with PGE1 alone. Quadmix adds forskolin 1000 μg/mL to salvage 20% of those who fail trimix. Theoretically because each drug has a different mechanism of action, the combinations should demonstrate synergy and permit use of a lower dose of each.

F. Vacuum Constriction Device

This device consists of a cylindrical tube connected to a vacuum pump and a constricting ring. Negative pressure is produced within the cylinder mechanically drawing blood into the penis, thus causing engorgement. The constricting ring is applied to the base of the penis to maintain the erection. The majority of men report an increase in penile length, rigidity, and circumference. This method is highly effective and is less expensive in the long term than most other treatments. Side effects include penile pain and numbness, difficulty with ejaculation, ecchymosis, and petechiae.

G. Other Therapeutic Options

Acupuncture and herbal supplements have been suggested therapeutic options for ED; however, no randomized clinical trials have proven their efficacy.

VI. SURGICAL TREATMENT

A. History

Penile prostheses were introduced as the first effective organic treatment of ED over three decades ago. They remain an important option for patients when other less invasive methods have proven unsatisfactory. This treatment option provides the highest satisfaction rate of all available ED treatment options. The current devices show excellent operability with low risk of malfunction, infection, or need for revision.

There are two main classes of penile prostheses: hydraulic or inflatable and semirigid. In the hydraulic class, there are two main types, the three-piece inflatable, which requires reservoir placement in the abdominal cavity, and the two-piece inflatable. In the semirigid class, there are also two types, the malleable and the mechanical.

The three-piece inflatable implants are somewhat more complex to insert; however, they provide the best rigidity and best flaccidity. Cylinders are placed through the center of each corpora, which can fill and deflate fully to mimic a true erection. Manual dexterity is required to pump the device. The two-piece device avoids placement of a reservoir in the pelvis, which may be advisable in patients with prior complex abdominal surgeries such as kidney transplant or neobladder. These devices can give good rigidity and fair flaccidity or good flaccidity and fair rigidity but rarely both.

B. Indications

Most patients are advised to consider a vacuum device before a penile implant. The patient should be advised that the length of the penis will likely be shorter than the original erection was. Sensitivity, ejaculatory abilities, and sexual drive are usually unchanged after the procedure. It is also important to inform the patient that, if the prosthesis is removed, the corpora will fill with scar tissue that will not respond adequately to other treatments such as medication or a vacuum device.

C. Prosthetic Surgery

Prior to surgery, any open sores on the penis or comedones should be treated to avoid these being a source of infection during or after surgery. Diabetic patients should demonstrate good glucose control for a period of time preoperatively as manifest by a normal hemoglobin A1C. A urine culture should be negative. Perioperative broad-spectrum antibiotics should be given 1 hour before incision and maintained at least 48 hours postoperatively. Shaving of the area should be performed in the operating room to minimize the chance of nicks in the skin being colonized with bacteria by prior shaving. A 10-minute povidone-iodine (Betadine) scrub should be performed prior to incision.

1. Semirigid

Semirigid prostheses are usually placed via a subcoronal, penoscrotal, or ventral penile incision. If a subcoronal incision is made, simultaneous circumcision is usually recommended. These devices are paired flexible rods composed of medical-grade silicone elastomer, polytetrafluoroethylene, or an intertwined spiral metallic core. After implantation they provide a permanent degree of penile rigidity suitable for vaginal penetration and sexual intercourse.

2. Hydraulic

Inflatable prostheses are usually placed through an infrapubic or a penoscrotal incision. The advantage of the infrapubic incision is the ease of placement of the reservoir in the prepubic space. It is important to avoid damage to the neurovascular bundles, which run between the 11-o'clock and 1-o'clock positions on the corporal bodies.

With the penoscrotal approach, the reservoir is placed blindly through the inguinal canal. It is important to stay medial to avoid the iliac vessels and decompress the bladder to avoid perforation. An adequate reservoir cavity should be created to minimize the chance of autoinflation. This can cause a chronic partial erection, which may be embarrassing and cause discomfort. This is caused by abdominal pressure or a tight reservoir cavity. Fluid placed in the reservoir should be slightly less than the capacity but at least 10 mL more than the volume of the inflated penile cylinders. The prosthesis pump should be placed freely in the scrotum after an adequate subcutaneous pocket has been made.

To place any prosthesis, the normal erectile tissue must be hollowed out to make room for the device. Therefore, if the device is ever removed, the patient will never be able to attain a normal erection. For both types of prostheses, appropriate cylinder sizing is critical. If the cylinder is too large, the patient may have persistent pain, protrusion into the glans, or curvature when the penis is erect. With semirigid rods, the size should be approximately 0.5 cm less than the measured length of the corporal body. With inflatable cylinders, the size should be the same as the measured length of the corporal body. The optimal width of an inflatable cylinder is one that fills the corpora in a finger in glove-like fashion. For narrow corpora, it is important to use narrower cylinders as this will give equally good support with less potential for problem.

During placement of a penile prosthesis, copious irrigation with antibiotic fluid is important. At the conclusion of the procedure, two layers of subcutaneous and a layer of skin closure are recommended over any prosthetic parts.

Repair rates in the range of 10–20% within the first 5 years are to be expected, and when counseling patients pre-operatively it is important to relay this information. When approaching a patient who needs repair of the prosthesis, it is important to consider the number of years it has been in place. If the prosthesis has been in place 2 years or more, strong consideration should be given to replacing the entire device. If the prosthesis malfunctions in the first few months, parts that are not defective can be left in place.

Approximately 1% of patients will suffer persistent pain after prosthesis insertion and will require removal. Notably, the prosthesis can usually be replaced at another time.

ED with concomitant Peyronie's disease can provide a challenge to the urologist. Placement of a penile prosthesis most commonly straightens the area of curvature correcting both problems simultaneously.

Infection of a prosthetic device is catastrophic, necessitating removal. With the use of sterile technique, intravenous antibiotics, and antibiotic irrigation, the current rates of infection are 1–3%. Pain persisting greater than 2 months after surgery can be an indication of underlying infection. The presence of fever, erythema in the wound, or purulence from the incision can also be an indicator of infection. When these symptoms are present, it is rare for intravenous antibiotics to take care of the problem and explanation of the device is necessary. Following explanation, scar tissue will develop in the corpora making placement of another penile prosthesis down the road more difficult. For this reason, a salvage protocol has been gaining popularity. This entails removing all prosthetic parts and foreign material; copiously irrigating the wound with antiseptic solution; changing surgical gowns, gloves, drapes, and instruments; and replacing the prosthesis in the same procedure. Contraindications to salvage include corporal necrosis, patients who are severely ill, and patients with bilateral urethral erosion of the cylinders. Some penile prostheses have been impregnated with a formulation of minocycline and rifampin, which may further reduce infection rates.

D. Vascular Procedures

A complete vascular evaluation is necessary before any vascular procedure is undertaken. Isolated proximal arterial lesions (aortoiliac occlusive diseases) are rare and small vessel lesions frequently co-exist. Occasionally they are associated with the failure of veno-occlusive mechanisms. Various techniques to improve blood flow have been described. These include direct iliac to hypogastric artery graft, hypogastric endarterectomy, and transluminal balloon angioplasty.

Occlusions of the internal pudendal, common penile, and cavernosal arteries can be congenital, atherosclerotic, traumatic, or idiopathic. In general, the revascularization procedures include either a neoartery to cavernosal anastomosis or a neoartery to dorsal artery or dorsal vein anastomosis. The neoarterial source is either the saphenous vein or the inferior epigastric artery, which is considered superior. These procedures seem to be most successful in young patients with trauma related vascular occlusion.

Venous procedures to improve veno-occlusive mechanisms have been described. Ligation of the deep dorsal vein with or without ligation of the circumflex/crural vein is the most commonly performed procedure. Precise location of the venous leak is an important step in planning therapy. Poor patient selection and the generalized nature of this disease are major causes of therapeutic failure. These procedures are rarely performed due to the very high recurrence rates and the generalized nature of this disease.

VII. PREMATURE EJACULATION

Numerous definitions for PE exist. The definition adopted by the AUA is ejaculation that occurs sooner then desired, either before or shortly after penetration, causing distress to one or both partners. Three key elements must exist in any description of premature ejaculatory dysfunction: lack of voluntary control, dissatisfaction or distress, and a diminished intravaginal ejaculatory latency time (IELT). IELT is a measurement of the time between vaginal penetration and ejaculation averaged over a number of sexual encounters and can be used to quantify this problem. There are important exclusionary factors that include PE mediated by alcohol, substance use, or medication; a context that leads to very high levels of arousal because of novelty of partner or situation; and a low frequency of sexual activity.

The real questions is what is a normal IELT. No absolute criteria exist, and there is great variability reported in different countries and cultures. IELT is different when recorded by men compared to that which is reported by their partners. That being said, most people agree that the normal IELT is 5–7 minutes or more, and premature IELT is less than 3 minutes, with the vast majority of patients with PE reporting IELT of less than 1 minute.

The prevalence of PE is in the range of 20–30% of all men. Based on U.S. Census estimates, there are 22–33 million American men in the United States who have PE. The percentage of those men who report that PE is bothersome varies between 25 and 50%.

Three different organic theories have been proposed to explain PE. These include penile hypersensitivity, hyperexcitable ejaculatory reflex, and low serotonin (5-HT) transmission in the CNS. There is conflicting evidence that hypersensitivity and/or hyperexcitability of the ejaculatory reflex is the cause of PE.

Seminal emission, ejaculation, and orgasm are integrated within the CNS by several different structures. They include the medial pre-optic area (MPOA), paraventricular nuclei (PVN) in the hypothalamus, and the nucleus paragigantocellularis (nPGI) in the brain stem. From the nPGI and other centers, there are projections to the lumbosacral spinal cord, which are thought to exert control over ejaculatory activity. Multiple regulatory neurotransmitters have been identified. These include 5-HT, dopamine, oxytocin, γ-aminobutyric acid (GABA), and norepinephrine. It is thought that serotonin has an inhibitory role in sexual behavior in the male and that projections from the brain stem, particularly the nPGi, exert atonic inhibition of ejaculatory activity. Fourteen different classes of 5-HT receptors have been identified, and it has been suggested that PE may be due to hyposensitivity of 5-HT_{2c} receptors or hypersensitivity of 5-HT_{1a} receptors. Men with low CNS 5-HT and/or abnormal 5-HT receptor sensitivity may have their ejaculatory threshold determined at a lower set point and ejaculate quickly, whereas men with a high set point may experience delayed or even absent ejaculatory activity.

PE is either lifelong (primary) or acquired (secondary) and may be limited to specific situations or partners or may be global. Primary PE is thought to be more biologically based and most likely due to abnormalities in serotonin regulation, whereas secondary PE is more likely to involve psychologic components or be associated with ED.

A careful sexual history is needed to establish PE. Diagnosis can be made by history alone. Evaluation should also include a psychosocial history, a general medical history, and a physical examination. It is important to identify the onset and duration of PE, specifically whether it is lifelong or acquired, and if there is any association with ED. It is important to assess the stress level of the patient as well as his partner, the perceived degree of ejaculatory control, and an estimation of the IELT. The impact of PE on the patient and partner's sexual activity and any effect it may have on their relationship or quality of life need to be understood.

Other questions that should be asked include:

- What is the proportion of sexual attempts that are associated with PE?
- Is PE ever related to specific partners?
- What might be aggravating or alleviating factors?
- Is there any evidence of drug use and/or abuse?
- What psychologic or biologic factors might be involved?

Numerous treatment options exist. These include nonmedical treatment, psychobehavioral therapy, topical treatment, PDE-5 inhibitors, and SSRI therapy.

Nonmedical treatments include multiple condoms, masturbatory activity prior to intercourse, and the use of distracting mental exercise during sexual activity.

Psychobehavioral therapies are based on the concept that responses to sexual excitement can be controlled and that ejaculatory reflex can be modified or managed by the patient and/ or his partner. Behavioral therapy focuses on "stop-start" and "squeeze" techniques. Psychologic therapy attempts to analyze and modify individual and relationship problems. There are limitations to psychobehavioral therapy. Oftentimes, it requires the assistance of an unwilling partner, it may be time consuming and costly, therapy takes time to become effective, and efficacy is unclear and may decline over time.

Topical therapy for treatment of PE involves desensitizing creams or ointments, which use either lidocaine or lidocaine with prilocaine applied to the penis 20–30 minutes prior to attempts at sexual activity. Topical application lessens penile sensitivity during foreplay and intercourse and has been shown to be effective if used properly. Topical therapy, however, can lead to penile numbness, which can promote anorgasmia as well as local skin irritation. Should there be transvaginal absorption of cream, there can be vaginal numbness or anorgasmia experienced by the patient's partner. It is recommended that a condom be used and that patients be instructed to wash off any topical cream prior to initiation of sexual activity. Unfortunately, although it is proven to be effective in some patients, there are few studies reported in the literature and most studies involve a small number of patients.

The use of PDE-5 inhibitors for the treatment of PE has been advocated. Mechanism by which PDE-5 inhibition may offer benefit is unclear, although it has been speculated there may be a central effect involving increased NO and reduced sympathetic tone. PDE-5 inhibitors may work, however, by reducing patients' fear of losing an erection, relieving anxiety, and thus eliminating the rush to orgasm. The effect on IELT is questionable. PDE-5 inhibition does decrease refractory period and thus shortens the time when the patient next can achieve an erection satisfactory for sexual activity.

SSRIs have been used off-label in the use of treatment of PE for some time. Delayed ejaculation is an often observed side effect of SSRI use in the treatment of depression. Numerous agents have been investigated including clomipramine, fluoxetine, paroxetine, and sertraline. Both on-demand and chronic dosing have been suggested in the treatment of PE. Chronic dosing may offer more efficacy than on-demand use. A long half-life of these compounds may cause drug accumulation and side effects. If taken on demand, it needs to be given 3 hours or more prior to attempts at sexual activity. Side effects are not insignificant and include dry mouth, nervousness, GI upset, headache, drowsiness, cognitive impairment, decreased libido, and ED with chronic dosing as well as suicidal ideation.

Other inhibitors of serotonin uptake transport have been studied. These are orally absorbed and reach plasma concentrations quickly. These drugs are designed to be taken on demand. Nausea and vomiting is the most common reported side effect. Unfortunately, at this time, no compound is commercially available.

VIII. PRIAPISM

Priapism is defined as an abnormally persistent erection, not associated with sexual desire or stimulation lasting more than 4 hours. There are two types, low flow or ischemic priapism and high flow or nonischemic priapism (Figure 19-12). The vast majority of cases are ischemic and require emergent treatment.

Ischemic priapism is a compartment syndrome with significant pain and tenderness resulting in tissue injury. The persistence of the erection is secondary to occlusion of venous outflow and consequent cessation of arterial inflow. This is associated with increasing organ anoxia, a rising pCO_2, and acidosis. The underlying cause, although somewhat variable, is failure of detumescence. This may occur for a number of reasons including obstruction of venous outflow from the penis, prolonged cavernosal smooth muscle relaxation, or failure of the detumescence mechanism.

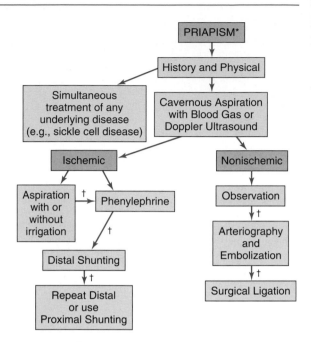

FIGURE 19-12. Management of priapism. (From AUA Clinical Guidelines. Management of Priapism, 2003.)

Treatment must be undertaken within 12–24 hours to avoid damage to the cavernous tissues with necrosis and resultant fibrosis, which can lead to severe ED.

Although approximately 50% of all episodes of priapism are thought to be idiopathic, there are a number of known causes of this disorder. A thorough history to define causative factors and duration of ischemia is vital. Severity of pain, rigidity of the penis, and lack of involvement of the glans penis and the corpus spongiosum must be assessed. Exclusion of a penile tumor by palpation and inspection of the penis as well as palpation of the inguinal area for lymphadenopathy are important. A corporal blood gas should be obtained to establish acid base status and confirm ischemic (pH <7.25, PO_2 <30, PCO_2 >60) versus nonischemic priapism (pH >7.3, PO_2 >50, PCO_2 <40). A blood sample should also be analyzed to exclude sickle cell disease (SCD), thalassemia major, and leukemia. Analgesics should be given promptly as the patient may be in severe pain.

In adults the most common etiology of ischemic priapism is intracavernous therapy with papaverine, phentolamine, or alprostadil. Several other medications including antipsychotics, the antidepressant trazodone, and a few antihypertensives have been implicated. Recreational drugs including cocaine and alcohol have been reported as culprits. Testosterone has also been noted to result in priapism episodes. The high fat content of total parenteral nutrition is believed to cause priapism. Hematologic diseases including SCD or trait and leukemia produce a hyperviscosity syndrome and are the most common causes of priapism in children. Adult malignancies including bladder and prostate cancer and metastatic disease to the corpora cavernosa may infiltrate and obstruct venous drainage leading to ischemic priapism.

It is important to counsel men even in the early phase of priapism about the potential loss of EF. Despite treatment, overall impotency rates are as high as 50%.

Treatment is aimed at the primary cause of the priapism if it can be identified. An important first step is pain control. The first line of treatment is irrigation and evacuation of old blood from the corpora cavernosa. A local anesthetic should be given prior to injection of the penis. The aspirated blood in cases of ischemic priapism is usually very dark, almost black, and blood gas will confirm the hypoxic conditions. Often, the blood needs to be milked out of the corporal bodies until fresh blood is seen. If this alone does not cause detumescence, the next step is injection of an alpha-adrenergic agonist into the corpora. Phenylephrine, which has minimal cardiac side effects, is the drug of choice; however, epinephrine, norepinephrine, and norepinephrine with lidocaine (Xylocaine) have all been used. Phenylephrine is dispensed as 10 mg/mL and this should be diluted in 19 mL of normal saline prior to injection; 0.5-mg increments can be used every 3–5 minutes until detumescence occurs. Especially in patients with underlying heart disease, monitoring of blood pressure and heart rate during treatment is recommended.

Pseudoephedrine and terbutaline can be given orally; however, these drugs have produced inconsistent results and are not recommended for acute ischemic priapism. They can be used as suppressive agents in patients with recurrent priapism.

Patients with SCD have an incidence of priapism as high as 35%. The treatment of these patients should start with analgesia, oxygenation, hydration, and exchange transfusion. Intracorporal therapy should follow if conservative measures do not cause detumescence promptly.

In persistent cases, glans-cavernosal or cavernosal-spongiosal shunting may be required to provide an alternative draining system. Essentially, a fistula is created between the corpora and the glans or spongiosum with the hope that it will close spontaneously after the priapism resolves. If these shunts fail, corporal-venous shunts to the dorsal vein or the saphenous vein can be performed. Both the disease and the shunt procedure can lead to impotence, and closure of the shunt rarely restores potency.

Patients with high flow or nonischemic priapism present differently. Pain is not present, the erection is not as rigid, and intervention is not urgent and often is unnecessary. High arterial inflow into the cavernosal sinusoids produces the persistent erection. This may result from pelvic, perineal, or penile trauma when the cavernosal artery is damaged or may be iatrogenic secondary to shunting procedures for ischemic priapism. Other etiologies include congenital arterial malformation, iatrogenic from prior revascularization procedures directly to the tunica, or idiopathic.

The onset of a post-traumatic high flow priapism may occur up to 72 hours after the injury. Diagnosis can be confirmed by blood gas parameters indicating arterial blood and confirmed by Doppler examination. Selective pudendal arteriography should demonstrate the site of arterial injury when present. Most often a branch of the cavernosal artery can be identified. High flow priapism may resolve spontaneously. Ice packing or compression may cause sufficient vasospasm and thrombosis of the ruptured artery to effect closure of the fistula. However, in most cases closure does not spontaneously occur. Treatment options include embolization of the involved artery (cavernosal or internal pudendal) with Gelfoam, metallic coils, or autologous clot. Impotence rates approach 20%.

Recurrent or stuttering priapism can be difficult to manage as they may be ischemic or nonischemic in the same patient. Many of these patients have SCD and may present at a very young age. If SCD is present, it does require hematologic management. Oral medications can be tried as well as self intracavernosal injections. Androgen suppression with leuprolide (Lupron), for example, is the most effective treatment in suppressing nocturnal penile erection but may cause testicular atrophy with resultant hypogonadism and infertility. It is not appropriate to administer a hormonal agent to a patient who has not reached full sexual maturity and adult stature. Oral baclofen and sildenafil have shown some utility. It has been speculated that priapism is the result of disruption in regulation of NO synthase. It has been proposed that a PDE-5 inhibitor could be efficacious in regulating this pathway and thus treating and preventing recurrent priapism.

IX. PEYRONIE'S DISEASE

Peyronie's disease is an acquired disorder of the tunica albuginea characterized by fibrous plaques. These plaques impair the elasticity of the tunica, which is associated with pain and curvature on erection. There may be difficulty in penetration as a result of the curvature. The inelastic tunic prevents compression of the emissary veins, which impairs the veno-occlusive mechanism leading to ED.

A myriad of oral therapies for Peyronie's disease has been suggested, but there have been few clinical trials. Vitamin E is widely used, free of side effects, and inexpensive but has no evidence as to the effectiveness. Para-aminobenzoate (Potaba) has shown little benefit. Colchicine, which has anti-inflammatory activity, has shown benefit in combination with vitamin E with regard to curvature and plaque size.

Intraplaque injection therapy with steroids, collagenase, and verapamil has been used with variable results. Surgery for Peyronie's disease must take into account the quality of erection present. If erections are poor even with the help of PDE-5 inhibitors, penile prosthesis should be considered as the results are excellent. For patients who maintain EF, Nesbit plication has given consistently good results. This is done by shortening the tunical albuginea opposite the site of plaque to produce a straight erection. The major complaint following this operation is shortening of the penis. To prevent shortening, plaque incision or excision followed by grafting using temporalis fascial graft can be done. Postoperative ED can be a problem. This operation tends to be limited to men with marked foreshortening of the penis, obesity, and good EF. Prior to consideration of surgery, symptoms should be stable for at least 3 months and preferably 6 months. Recurrence of the deformity after surgery may be due to operative failure or to progression of disease. PDE-5 may help, but this is an off-label use.

X. EJACULATORY INCOMPETENCE

This is defined as an inability to ejaculate during orgasm. It is relatively rare and usually psychogenic in nature. Potential etiologies include drug use, recreational or prescribed, and sympathetic nerve injury secondary to trauma, radiation, or surgery. In treating these patients, drugs that delay ejaculatory function (e.g., SSRIs) should be eliminated and substitutions made. In the absence of associated drug use, effective therapy focuses on prolonged foreplay, visual stimulation (e.g., pornography), and vibratory stimulation.

XI. DECREASED LIBIDO

Decreased libido is defined as diminished or absent feelings of sexual interest or desire, absent sexual thoughts or fantasies, and a lack of responsive desire. There is some lessening of sexual interest with age and duration of relationship, but this goes beyond the normally expected decrease. This is very difficult to measure, and hormonal and psychologic issues may need to be addressed.

XII. CONCLUSION

The availability of safe and effective oral agents to treat most cases of ED has revolutionized the field of male sexual dysfunction. The scientific study of sexual dysfunction and its treatment is one of the most rapidly expanding frontiers of urology.

SELF-ASSESSMENT QUESTIONS

1. What is the principal neurotransmitter responsible for erection?
2. Erectile dysfunction may be the first presenting symptom of what more serious condition?
3. Where does the parasympathetic innervation of the penis originate?
4. Which laboratory studies should be included in the evaluation of ED?
5. How does sildenafil work?

SUGGESTED READINGS

1. Chiurlia E, D'Amico R, Ratti C, et al: Subclinical coronary artery atherosclerosis in patients with erectile dysfunction. *J Am Coll Cardiol* 46:1503–1506, 2005.
2. Esposito K, Giugliano F, Di Palo C, et al: Effect of lifestyle changes on erectile dysfunction in obese men: a randomized controlled trial. *JAMA* 291:2978–2984, 2004.

3. Feldman HA, Goldstein I, Hatzichristou DG, et al: Impotence and its medical and psychosocial correlates: results of the Massachusetts Male Aging Study. *J Urol* 151:54–61, 1994.

4. Feldman HA, Johannes CB, Derby CA, et al: Erectile dysfunction and coronary risk factors: prospective results from the Massachusetts Male Aging Study. *Prev Med* 30:328–338, 2003.

5. Fugl-Meyer AR, Fugle-Meyer KS: Sexual disabilities are not singularities. *Int J Imp Res* 14:422–432, 2002.

6. Hatzichristou D, Rosen RC, Broderick G, et al: Clinical evaluation and management strategy for sexual dysfunction in men and women. *J Sex Med* 1:49–55, 2004.

7. Johannes CB, Araujo AB, Felman HA, et al: Incidence of erectile dysfunction in men 40 to 69 years old: longitudinal results from the Massachusetts Male Aging Study. *J Urol* 163:460–463, 2000.

8. Juenemann KP, Lue TF, Fournier GR, Tanagho EA: Hemodynamics of papaverine- and phentolamine-induced penile erection. *J Urol* 136:158–161; 1986.

9. Lewis RW, Fugl-Meyer KS, Bosch R, et al: Epidemiology/risk factors of sexual dysfunction. *J Sex Med* 1:35–39, 2004.

10. Lockmann A, Gallmetzer J: Erectile dysfunction of arterial origin as a possible primary manifestation of atherosclerosis. *Minerva Cardioangiol* 44:243–246, 1996.

11. Lue TF, Broderick GA: Evaluation and nonsurgical management of erectile dysfunction and priapism. In Walsh PC, Retik AB, Vaughan ED, Wein AJ (eds): *Campbell's Urology*, 8th ed. Philadelphia, WB Saunders, 2002, pp 1619–1663.

12. McMahon CG, Abdo C, Incrocci L, et al: Disorders of orgasm and ejaculation in men. *J Sex Med* 1:58–63, 2004.

13. Mercer CH, Fenton KA, Johnson AM, et al: Sexual function problems and help seeking behavior in Britain: national probability sample survey. *BMJ* 327:426–427, 2003.

14. Morales A, Buvat J, Gooren L, et al: Endocrine aspects of sexual dysfunction in men. *J Sex Med* 1:69–79, 2004.

15. Mulcahy JJ, Austoni E, Barada JH, et al: The penile implant for erectile dysfunction. *J Sex Med* 1:98–108, 2004.

16. Pomeranz HD, Bhavsar AR: Nonarteritic ischemic optic neuropathy developing soon after use of sildenafil (Viagra): a report of seven new cases. *J Neuroophthalmol* 9–13, 2005.

17. Pryor J, Akkus E, Atler G, et al: Priapism. *J Sex Med* 1:116–120, 2004.

18. Pryor J, Emre A, Alter G, et al: Peyronie's disease. *J Sex Med* 1:110–113, 2004.

19. Saltzman EA, Guay AT, Jacobson J: Improvement in erectile function in men with organic erectile dysfunction by correction of elevated cholesterol levels: a clinical observation. *J Urol* 172:255–258, 2004.

20. Waldinger MD, Zwinderman AH, Schweitzer DH, Olivier B: Relevance of methodological design for the interpretation of efficacy of drug treatment of premature ejaculation: a systematic review and meta-analysis. *Int J Impotence Res* 16:369–381, 2004.

C H A P T E R 20

Male Fertility and Sterility

Paul J. Turek, MD

I. BACKGROUND

A. The Problem

1. Approximately 25% of couples will become pregnant after 1 month of trying to conceive. However, only **85% of couples will be pregnant after 1 year.**
2. Approximately 15% of couples will therefore have difficulty achieving pregnancy.
3. During the evaluation of these couples, **a male factor alone may be found in approximately 30% of couples,** that a male factor may be involved in the infertility problem in approximately 50% cases.

B. Chapter Plan: Topics to Be Considered

1. Reproductive anatomy and physiology
2. Evaluation of the infertile male
3. Classification of male infertility problems
4. Treatment modalities

II. REPRODUCTIVE ANATOMY AND PHYSIOLOGY

A. Embryology

1. Genital organs are observed during the fifth gestational week and include an indifferent gonad, a mesonephric duct, and the mullerian ducts.
2. The indifferent gonad forms from a thickening in the urogenital ridge near the mesonephros; germ cells migrate from the yolk sac and populate the urogenital ridge. These cells are **primordial germ cells** and are very closely related to **embryonic stem cells.**
3. Sexual differentiation of the embryo stems from the presence or absence of **testis determining factor (TDF)** located on the Y chromosome. This determines gonadal sex, which then forms the basis for gender specific phenotypic development (Figure 20-1).

707

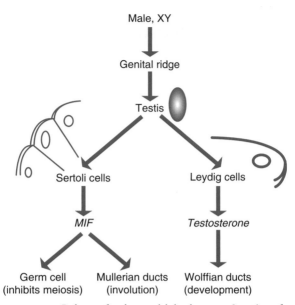

FIGURE 20-1. Pathway of male gonadal development. Secretion of mullerian inhibiting factor (MIF) from Sertoli cells within the early male gonad governs germ cell allocation and mullerian duct inhibition. Testosterone leads to wolffian duct development.

4. Induced to form a testis, the gonad develops clustered cords of germ cells that converge to form the rete testis at the hilum of the testis. These are testis stem cells and serve as the renewing source of germ cells for spermatogenesis throughout life. Interestingly, to further underscore the relatedness of stem cells, testicular stem cells (at least in mice) have been "coaxed" into developing into cells identical to embryonic stem cells.

5. During the eighth week of gestation, testosterone is made by differentiating **Leydig cells** and then declines in production after the 12th week during which external genital development occurs.

6. The **mesonephric duct** forms the ureter in both sexes and regionally specializes to form the vas deferens and epididymis in the male, joining with the testis in the form of ductuli efferentes testis.

7. The **mullerian duct** develops into fallopian tubes, the uterus, and the upper portion of the vagina in the female; in the male this development is inhibited by a mullerian

inhibiting substance produced by the primitive testis. Except for the **appendix testis** and **prostatic utricle,** regression is otherwise complete.

8. Late in gestation, the testis descends caudally along the posterior abdominal wall as a result of differential growth and through the gubernaculum testis pulling toward the scrotum under endocrine control. Descent into the scrotum is usually completed by birth, although descent can still occur during the first year of life.

B. Gross Anatomy

1. The male reproductive system includes the following components: the testes and seminiferous tubules, efferent ductules and rete testis, epididymides, vasa deferentia, ejaculatory ducts, seminal vesicles, prostate, penis, and urethra.
2. From the standpoint of infertility, any consideration of anatomy must also include the hypothalamic/pituitary/gonadal axis.

C. Reproductive Hormonal Axis (Figure 20-2)

1. Components
   a) Extrahypothalamic central nervous system
   b) Hypothalamus
   c) Pituitary

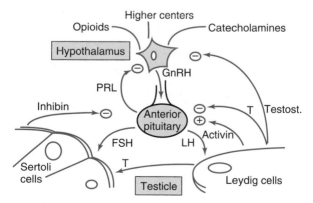

FIGURE 20-2. The hypothalamic-pituitary-gonadal hormone axis. Both inhibitory and stimulatory feedback loops within the axis. Testosterone balance occurs in a negative feedback loop. GnRH, gonadotropin releasing hormone; PRL, prolactin; Testost., testosterone; LH, luteinizing hormone; FSH, follicle-stimulating hormone.

    d) Testes
    e) Steroid sensitive organs
2. Functions
    a) Normal male sexual development
    b) Maintenance of secondary sexual characteristics
    c) Male sexual behavior
    d) Sperm production and maturation

D. Extrahypothalamic Central Nervous System

1. The extrahypothalamic central nervous system is responsible for a variety of stimulatory and inhibitory influences on fertility.
2. In humans, the effects of **stress** of both a physical and/or emotional nature are probably mediated through this system, but the mechanisms are unknown.

E. Hypothalamus—Gonadotropin Releasing Hormone (GnRH)

1. The hypothalamus is the center of integration for neuronal and humoral messages in the brain. The anterior and ventromedial nuclei are most important for male fertility.
2. The hypothalamus is responsible for production of **GnRH,** which is the **primary releasing substance involved in male sexual function.**

F. Pituitary-Luteinizing Hormone (LH) and Follicle-Stimulating Hormone (FSH)

1. The effect of GnRH is the production and release of LH and FSH from the anterior pituitary gland.
2. Both LH and FSH are glycopeptides with two molecular chains. They share a common alpha chain; specificity is determined by a unique beta chain.
3. LH and FSH are both secreted episodically. LH is rapidly metabolized, causing wide swings in its concentration within the bloodstream when determined by radioimmunoassay techniques. Occasionally, more accurate LH levels are needed; this is done with pooled blood samples. FSH is more slowly metabolized, resulting in a more constant level within the bloodstream.
4. The testes are the primary target for LH and FSH. No other target organs for these hormones have been found.

G. The Testes

1. Microscopic Anatomy

a) **Seminiferous tubules comprise the bulk (80%) of the testis** and are responsible for sperm production. Thus, testis atrophy generally suggests a low sperm count.

b) The **interstitium** between the seminiferous tubules contains blood vessels, lymphatics, and **Leydig cells.**

2. Seminiferous Tubule Structural Organization

a) The tubules consist of long ducts lined by **Sertoli cells** that engulf and nurture the developing germ cells.

b) Sertoli cells contain membrane receptors that bind FSH, resulting in increased intracellular cyclic adenosine monophosphate (cAMP) and subsequent cytoskeletal reorganization for protein synthesis.

c) The primary secretion products from Sertoli cells include mullerian inhibiting substance in the fetus, androgen binding protein (ABP), transferrin, and inhibin (a nonsteroidal glycoprotein) in the adult.

d) Sertoli cells appear responsible for regulation of the tubule microenvironment. They govern fluid secretions into the lumen of the seminiferous tubules, phagocytosis, steroid metabolism (in part), sperm production, and sperm movement through their development.

e) Sertoli cells are also mainly responsible for the **"blood-testis barrier."** This anatomic barrier is surrounded by myoid cells, and consists of the basement membrane and Sertoli cell tight junctions. In addition, a selective physiologic barrier is created by active transport processes across Sertoli cells. Further compartmentalization is established as Sertoli cells divide developing germ cells into two areas, the **basal compartment** for immature germ cells and stem cells and the **adluminal compartment** for germ cells undergoing differentiation and maturation. This complex "blood-testis barrier" provides an **immunologically privileged site for mature spermatozoa,** as these haploid cells harbor unique and specific antigens that are not otherwise recognized as "self" by the body's immune system.

3. Seminiferous Tubules—Spermatogenesis

a) LH, FSH, and testosterone are all required for normal spermatogenesis.

b) Sertoli cells, lining 250 m of seminiferous tubules in the average testis, regulate the complex process of spermatogenesis.

c) A variety of germ cell types exist, including spermatogonia, primary spermatocytes, secondary spermatocytes, spermatids, and spermatozoa. Actually, 14 germinal cell subtypes are recognized histologically and are associated with six distinct stages of spermatogenesis. Certain early stage spermatogonia are actually adult testis stem cells and are the source of the constantly self-renewal germ cell lineage. Spermatids and spermatozoa have a haploid complement of chromosomes.

d) The process of spermatogenesis takes about 60 days to complete. The average daily output is 125 million spermatozoa, which declines with age. A normal man makes 1200 sperm for every heartbeat.

e) **Spermiogenesis** is the maturation process of a spermatid to a spermatozoan. This includes nuclear condensation and a programmed repackaging of DNA from histones to protamines, acrosome formation, residual body separation from the sperm, and tail formation. It is one of the most complex series of morphologic changes undertaken by any mammalian cell.

4. Interstitium—Leydig Cells

a) Leydig cells contain membrane receptors that bind LH, resulting again in cAMP production, protein kinase activation, and protein phosphorylation.

b) LH stimulation results in the conversion of cholesterol to testosterone in a steroidogenic pathway.

c) Testosterone diffuses into the plasma (**endocrine** function) or into the seminiferous tubule lumen (**paracrine** function). In the plasma, **testosterone is bound (98%) to sex hormone binding globulin (SHBG) or albumin**. Within the seminiferous tubules, testosterone is bound to ABP.

d) Depending on the target tissue, testosterone may be active itself or may be reduced to **dihydrotestosterone (DHT)** by the enzyme 5-alpha reductase.

e) Testosterone is responsible in part for sexual differentiation, spermatogenesis, gonadotropin regulation, sexual maturation, and behavior.

H. Feedback Mechanisms (see Figure 20-2)

1. GnRH, LH, and FSH are generally thought to be responsible for driving the production of testosterone and spermatozoa as noted previously. There are also feedback mechanisms that regulate the production and release of these substances.

2. LH regulation.
   a) Testosterone and estradiol are the major **negative feedback** substances that control the formation and release of LH.
   b) **Testosterone therefore regulates its own production** and release by acting on the pituitary and in the hypothalamus. This has implications for clinical care: Exogenous testosterone supplements will suppress both endogenous testosterone (through decreased LH) and sperm production (through decreased FSH).
   c) **Estradiol is produced within the testicle and the liver on conversion from testosterone (5-alpha reductase).** It is found in smaller amounts within the bloodstream (testosterone:estrogen ratio is typically 10:1) but is potent in action. The site of regulation is also at the level of the pituitary and hypothalamus.
3. FSH regulation.
   a) Testosterone and estradiol are the major modulators of pituitary FSH secretion. This is why exogenous testosterone supplements suppress spermatogenesis.
   b) In man, Sertoli cells produce **inhibin,** a two-subunit hormone in the transforming growth factor family, which has an inhibitory effect on pituitary FSH output. In contrast, **activin,** a glycoprotein formed as a homodimer of either inhibin chain, has a stimulatory effect on pituitary FSH. Neither inhibin nor activin affects pituitary LH release.
4. There are also a variety of "short feedback loops" and other modulating substances that more finely tune this system.

I. Testicular Transport

1. As noted previously, movement of developing germ cells from the basement membrane to the lumen and release into the lumen of the seminiferous tubules are controlled by Sertoli cells. Unlike most mammalian species, **the stages of spermatogenesis occur in a patchwork pattern** and not in a wave-like manner within the seminiferous tubules. This, in combination with constantly renewing cycles of spermatogenesis, **ensures that sperm production is continuous in nature.**
2. The movement of the spermatozoa from the testis to the epididymis is controlled by four factors:
   a) Fluid pressure generated within the seminiferous tubule.

    b) Myoepithelial contractions of the seminiferous tubules.
    c) Contraction of the tunica albuginea of the testis.
    d) Cilia within and contraction of the wall of the efferent ductules.
3. The spermatozoa enter the epididymis in an immature state.

J. Epididymal Functions

1. Transport and Storage

a) The spermatozoa traverse the length of the epididymis in approximately **12 days.** This process is governed by regular slow contractions of the muscular wall in a fashion similar to intestinal peristalsis.

b) Approximately **700 million sperm are stored within the epididymides and vasa deferentia.** Approximately 60% of these are stored within the tail (cauda) of the epididymides. Sperm become progressively more motile as they traverse the epididymal tubules, knowledge of which is important in harvesting sperm from the epididymis for in vitro fertilization (IVF) with intracytoplasmic sperm injection (ICSI).

c) At the time of **emission,** regular coordinated contractions of the tails of the epididymides and the vasa deferentia occur, mediated by the sympathetic nervous system, propelling sperm into the prostatic urethra. During **ejaculation,** somatic nervous system stimulated rhythmic contractions of periurethral and pelvic floor muscles propel the sperm through the urethra.

2. Sperm Maturation

a) The chemical composition of the intraluminal fluid and spermatozoa changes significantly as one traverses the three anatomic portions of the epididymis.

b) A variety of membrane changes in permeability and antigenicity also occur.

c) Motility and fertilizing capacity are gained during transport through the epididymis.

d) The final process of maturation, **sperm capacitation,** actually takes place after the sperm have been ejaculated and come in contact with the female reproductive tract. **Fertilizing capacity** lasts approximately **48 hours** within the female internal genitalia, an important finding for counseling patients on the optimal frequency of sexual intercourse around the time of ovulation.

K. Semen Composition

1. The bulk of seminal fluid originates from the accessory ducts, with the spermatozoa adding a small (<10%) amount to the total volume.
2. Prostatic fluid.
   a) The **prostatic fluid** is usually found in the first part of the ejaculate and contributes approximately **one quarter of the total volume. This fluid is acidic (pH <6.5).**
   b) Specific prostate products include liquefaction factors such as prostate-specific antigen (PSA), zinc, citric acid, acid, phosphatase, and spermine. The latter substance, when oxidized to aldehydes, produces the characteristic odor of semen.
   c) **PSA, a 33-kd molecular weight serum protease in the family of glandular kallikreins, serves to liquefy the coagulum** of human semen after 5–20 minutes following ejaculation.
3. Seminal vesicle fluid.
   a) The **seminal vesicle fluid** is usually found in the second part of the ejaculate and contributes approximately **two-thirds of the total volume. This fluid is basic (pH >7.0).**
   b) Specific substances secreted by the seminal vesicles include coagulation factors, prostaglandins, and fructose. **Fructose** is measured on a semen analysis to investigate the diagnosis of ejaculatory duct obstruction.

III. CLINICAL EVALUATION OF THE SUBFERTILE MALE (FIGURE 20-3)

A. Fertility History

1. Present Marital History

a) Duration of infertility.
b) Contraceptive methods and length of time used.
c) Length of time trying to conceive.
d) Number of pregnancies including miscarriages and therapeutic abortions, which gives an indication of the potential to conceive.

2. Previous Marital History and Relationships

a) If the patient has attempted to conceive in the past, the duration and number of **pregnancies** achieved should be determined.

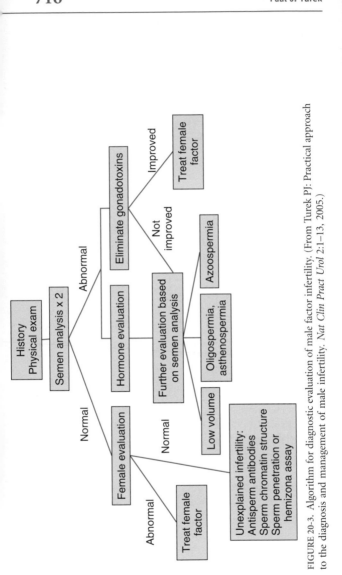

FIGURE 20-3. Algorithm for diagnostic evaluation of male factor infertility. (From Turek PJ: Practical approach to the diagnosis and management of male infertility. *Nat Clin Pract Urol* 2:1–13, 2005.)

b) The duration and number of pregnancies attempted or conceived by the wife or partner should also be determined.

c) Previous marriages are common. Potential fertility problems may be suspected if one partner has previously attempted to conceive without success. However, one must remember that the ability to conceive is a phenomenon involving both partners and therefore is ultimately determined by the current couple.

3. Sexual History

a) Frequency of intercourse and masturbation. Overly frequent (daily) or infrequent (>48 hours apart around the time of ovulation) can adversely affect the couple's ability to conceive.

b) Libido, potency, and sexual technique. A normal desire and ability to have intercourse are critical and problems in these areas are often overlooked by clinicians. **Situational erectile dysfunction** due to stress is common among couples trying to conceive and is easily treated with **phosphodiesterase inhibitors.**

c) Ejaculation. Ejaculation needs to occur deep within the vagina. Severe problems with **premature ejaculation, chordee, or severe hypospadias** may prevent proper deposition of sperm.

d) **Dyspareunia** and the use of lubrication. Problems with adequate natural vaginal lubrication can result in painful intercourse for either partner. Most lubricants are spermicidal. The use of vegetable oil based substances is safe for sperm viability.

e) Understanding of the **ovulatory cycle.** It is important that the couple understand when ovulation occurs and have timed intercourse regularly during this time. There is evidence that "front loading" sexual intercourse, having more before rather than after ovulation, might improve pregnancy rates.

4. Genitourinary History

a) Testicular descent. Bilateral **cryptorchidism** is associated with impaired spermatogenesis and fertility. With unilateral maldescent, there is a slight decrease in fertility potential.

b) Sexual development and onset of puberty. **Delayed puberty** can indicate syndromes (e.g., Kallmann's) or chromosomal issues (e.g., XXY).

c) Infections. Venereal, nonvenereal, mumps (at the time of puberty or later), recent febrile illness, or other infectious problems that directly involve the genitalia or urogenital duct system may be associated with a significant scarring and subsequent fertility problems. Viral infections and other febrile illnesses not specifically involving the genitalia may also cause decreased spermatogenesis and temporarily lower sperm counts.

d) **Trauma or torsion.** Either condition may injure the duct system or result in ischemic damage to the seminiferous tubules.

e) Exposure to chemicals. A variety of drugs and industrial compounds may be associated with abnormal semen analyses. **Industrial solvents** are the most concerning.

f) Exposure to heat. Prolonged exposure to high temperatures may adversely affect spermatogenesis. **Hot tubs, hot baths, saunas, or steam rooms on a regular basis may have significance in this regard.**

g) Exposure to radiation. Even small amounts of ionizing radiation, particularly that used for medical radiation therapy, may destroy sperm forming cells. **Spermatogonia are particularly radiosensitive.**

5. Previous Infertility Evaluation

a) Patient. A history of previous semen analyses and medical or surgical treatment is certainly important for prognosis and the diagnosis of infertility etiology.

b) Wife/partner. It is wise to understand the fertility potential of the female partner (see Figure 20-3). Obviously, conception involves two people and if for some physiologic or anatomic reason, an irreversible problem exists in the female partner, pregnancy is not likely. The evaluation of each partner should be carried out simultaneously, and the male evaluation should be completed prior to any invasive procedures on the female partner. **At least 1 year of maternal reproductive potential should exist for the best outcomes after male infertility treatment.**

B. General Medical History

1. Although most conditions causing male infertility do not lead to long-term medical consequences, 1–2% of men undergoing evaluation for infertility will have a significant underlying medical condition.

a) Medical illnesses. Medical problems such as **diabetes** and **hypertension** or their pharmacologic treatments may adversely affect erectile and ejaculatory function and hence fertility.

b) Abnormal metabolism of sex steroids may be associated with various liver and renal diseases and interfere with the regulatory mechanisms of spermatogenesis. Rare medical illnesses such as **Young syndrome** (immotile cilia syndrome) and **Kartagener syndrome** (ciliary defect with situs inversus) can adversely affect fertility.

2. Surgical history.

a) Inguinal herniorrhaphy, particularly when performed on a young child and when performed bilaterally, may be associated with injury to the vas deferens in 1–2% of patients.

b) Surgery on the ureter, bladder, bladder neck, or urethra may result in problems with emission and/or ejaculation.

c) Retroperitoneal surgery and other major pelvic procedures may result in failure of emission and/or problems with retrograde ejaculation. Young males with testis cancer are now being cured with great success. Many with nonseminomatous tumors are treated with retroperitoneal lymphadenectomy and subsequently have fertility problems due to absent ejaculation from either failure of emission or from retrograde ejaculation. It appears that the adjuvant 2–3 cycles of chemotherapy often given in lieu of retroperitoneal lymphadenectomy do not have a significant effect on male fertility.

3. Current and past medications.
A variety of drugs and chemotherapeutic agents may adversely affect sperm production and/or function. The adverse affects are usually reversible on discontinuation of the medication (Table 20-1).

4. Occupation and habits.

a) Occupation and stress. The effects of daily stress on fertility are poorly quantified. **Severe, acute stress has been associated with decreases in ejaculate volume and sperm count.** Although most patients inquire about stress, it is unlikely that they would change their job or style of living, making this problem difficult to treat. Encouraging regular exercise, yoga, or acupuncture may help with this.

b) The active ingredients in **cigarettes, marijuana, coffee, tea, alcohol,** and some naturopathic herbs have all been demonstrated in laboratory studies to be potentially gonadotoxic. The susceptibility of individuals to these substances varies widely and is difficult to quantify.

Table 20-1: Drugs and Chemicals with Potential Adverse Fertility Effects
Alcohol
Alkylating agents (e.g., cyclophosphamide)
Arsenic
Aspirin (large doses)
Caffeine
Cimetidine
Colchicine
Dibromochloropropane (pesticide)
Diethylstilbestrol (DES)
Lead
Monoamine oxidase inhibitors
Marijuana
Medroxyprogesterone
Nicotine
Nitrofurantoins
Phenytoin
Spironolactone
Sulfasalazine
Testosterone

5. Family history.
   a) Sibling fertility status may help to identify familial conditions such as cystic fibrosis, genetic infertility due to Y chromosome deletions, and congenital adrenal hyperplasia.
   b) In utero exposure to **diethylstilbestrol (DES)** may result in testicular, epididymal, and penile anatomic abnormalities. Despite the finding of impaired semen quality in DES-exposed men, proof of decreased fertility is not obvious in extensive follow-up studies.

C. Physical Examination

1. General examination. The general examination evaluates the patient's **body habitus** and secondary sexual characteristics. In particular, the pattern of hair distribution and **gynecomastia** are evidence of general endocrine disorders.
2. Examination of the genitalia. The genitalia are the most important aspect of the examination. This should be performed in a systematic fashion, taking care to evaluate the areas listed in the following:
   a) Penis. The size of the penis and location of the meatus are important in ensuring the delivery of spermatozoa deep within the vagina at ejaculation.

b) Testes. The **location, size, and consistency** of the testes should be noted. The testes should be in a dependent part of the scrotum. Testicular size is particularly important, as the bulk of the testicle (80%) relates to sperm production. The size of each testis can be compared to the other testis as well as to normal values by noting the length and width of the testicle or by attempting to quantify the volume by comparison to plastic models of known volumes. The normal testicle in the adult is greater than **4 cm in length** and greater than **2.5 cm in width (20 mL).** Each testicle should have a firm consistency. Ethnic variations in testis size are well described.

c) Epididymides. The epididymides should be examined for size and consistency. The **obstructed epididymis feels enlarged and firm.** The epididymis that is scarred from either trauma or chronic infection may be hard and irregular. Part of the epididymis may be missing in association with congenital absence of the vas deferens.

d) Vasa deferentia. Each vas deferens should be palpable as a distinct, firm, cord-like structure in the scrotum. In **1–2% of infertile men, one or both vasa are not palpable in the scrotum, a condition termed congenital absence of the vas deferens (CAVD).**

e) Spermatic cords. Each spermatic cord should be evaluated for size and consistency with the patient in both the upright and supine positions. The patient should be asked to perform a Valsalva maneuver while standing to accentuate differences in blood volume within the cord, characteristic of a **varicocele.** The internal spermatic veins fill while standing and this filling may be increased when the Valsalva maneuver is performed. In the supine position, these veins drain more easily and hence the varicocele is not as easily palpable. Persistent fullness in the spermatic cord on reclining is suggestive of **cord lipoma** and not varicocele. Other abnormalities involving the spermatic cord include **hydrocele and spermatocele,** both of which may be detected during this examination.

f) Inguinal region. The inguinal canals are palpated for evidence of inguinal hernias. In addition, the inguinal regions should be inspected to assess if previous surgery in this area may have injured the vasa deferentia or testicular blood supply.

3. Rectal examination. A general rectal examination should be performed to detect lower gastrointestinal pathology and to palpate the prostate and seminal vesicles. The

prostate should be small and benign in consistency without tenderness or evidence of inflammation. The seminal vesicles are generally not palpable under normal conditions but may be palpable with obstruction of the ejaculatory ducts.

D. Semen Analyses

1. Collection. Generally at least **two semen analyses** are needed to establish a baseline for a patient. If a discrepancy exists, a third or perhaps even a fourth specimen may be required. Each semen analysis is collected after **2–3 days of abstinence.** The specimen is generally collected by masturbation into a clean, dry container and examined within 1 hour. If the specimen is collected at home, it should be kept near body temperature during transportation to the laboratory (shirt pocket). The patient should avoid lubricants during specimen collection. If needed, silicone condom devices are available.
2. Minimal standards of adequacy. Although there is no absolute measure of fertility on semen analysis, minimal standards of semen adequacy have been defined by the World Health Organization (Table 20-2).
3. Additional physical parameters. Other properties examined at the time of a routine semen analysis include:
   a) Color. The semen is generally grayish in color with an opalescent character. It may also appear lumpy.
   b) Coagulation. This occurs immediately after ejaculation.
   c) Liquefaction. This occurs 5–30 minutes following eja-

Table 20-2:   Semen Analysis: Minimal Standards of Adequacy

Seen on at least two occasions:	
Ejaculate volume	1.5–5.0 mL
Sperm density	>20 million/mL
Motility	>50% motile
Forward progression	>2.0 (scale 0–4)
Morphology (WHO)	>30% normal morphology
(Strict)	>14% normal morphology
And:	
No significant sperm agglutination	
No significant pyospermia	
No hyperviscosity	

culation. **PSA** is the serine protease responsible for this process.

d) Viscosity. This parameter refers to the fluid consistency of the semen after coagulation and liquefaction have occurred. Viscosity is normal if it is possible to pour the semen in a drop-by-drop fashion.

e) pH. The pH of semen is normally in the range of 7.2 to 8.0. A low pH implies absence or blockage of the seminal vesicles, as the ejaculate consists entirely of acidic prostatic fluid.

f) Fructose. As noted previously, fructose is produced by the seminal vesicles. It is important to check the semen fructose in cases of azoospermia and when the ejaculate volume is less than 1.5 mL. Absence of fructose in semen suggests absence of the vasa deferentia and seminal vesicles, ejaculatory duct obstruction, or dysfunction of the seminal vesicles.

E. Other Laboratory Tests

1. Urinalysis. This test is useful to rule out infection of the lower genitourinary tract and associated glandular structures.

2. Endocrine evaluation. Although a complete hormonal evaluation includes measurement of serum LH, FSH, testosterone and prolactin, **99% of endocrine conditions can be detected through the initial measurement of serum FSH and testosterone.** Hormonal testing can differentiate between hypogonadism due to hypothalamic or pituitary disease and that due to primary testicular failure.

3. Other tests regularly recommended in the past now appear to be unnecessary on a routine basis. These include tests of **thyroid** and **adrenal function** (<0.5% of cases). **Prolactin** levels should be determined if a low testosterone is found or if the patient has gynecomastia, severe headaches, or visual disturbances. Prolactin secreting pituitary tumors produce high levels of circulating prolactin, and these lesions tend to reduce LH and FSH levels by pituitary compression within the sella turcica.

4. Genetic testing. **Karyotype analysis is critical for all men with azoospermia and severe oligospermia (<10 million sperm/mL) who are planning IVF/ICSI.** In addition, it is now known that specific deletions in the Y chromosome are found in approximately 15% of men with azoospermia and 5–8% of men with severe oligospermia. Several regions of the long arm of the Y chromosome have been classified as **azoospermic factor (AZF) regions** (Figure 20-4). **Most deletions**

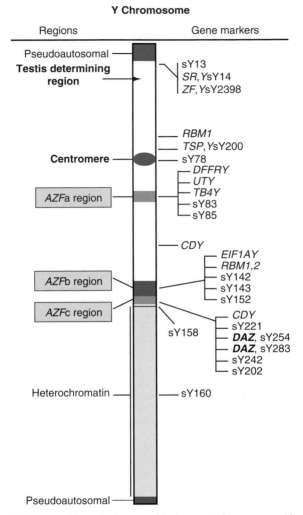

FIGURE 20-4. Schematic diagram of the human Y chromosome with known regions and genes listed. The testis determining region (SRY) is shown on the short arm (Yp) of the chromosome. AZF a,b,c denote the azoospermia regions of the chromosome that are associated with infertility.

are found in the AZFc region in a specific gene complex termed *DAZ* (deleted in azoospermia). **Deletions in these regions appear specific for infertility.** Deletions of AZFa and AZFb have a much poorer prognosis for sperm retrieval from the testis than patients with AZFc deletions.

5. Tests of sperm function.

a) **Sperm morphology.** Sperm cytology is another measure of semen quality. By assessing the exact dimensions and shape characteristics of the sperm head, midpiece, and tail, sperm can be classified as "normal" or not. In the strictest classification system (Kruger morphology), only 14% of sperm in the ejaculate are normal. In fact, this number correlates with the success of egg fertilization in vitro (IVF) and thus is ascribed clinical significance. In addition, **sperm morphology is an indicator of testicular health,** because shape characteristics are determined during spermatogenesis. Sperm morphology complements other information to better estimate the chances of fertility.

b) **Sperm chromatin assay.** The structure of sperm chromatin (the DNA-associated proteins) is independent of semen quality and can be measured by COMET and TUNNEL assays and by flow cytometry after acid treatment and staining of sperm with acridine orange. These tests assess the degree of DNA fragmentation that occurs after chemically stressing the sperm DNA-chromatin complex and can indirectly reflect the quality of sperm DNA integrity. **Abnormally fragmented sperm DNA rarely occurs in fertile men but can be found in 5% of infertile men with normal semen analyses and 25% of infertile men with abnormal semen analyses.** This test can detect infertility that is missed on a conventional semen analysis. Often reversible, causes of DNA fragmentation include tobacco use, medical disease, hyperthermia, air pollution, infections, and varicocele.

c) **Hamster egg penetration test.** This is a cross-species assay that assesses the ability of human spermatozoa to penetrate zona pellucida-free hamster eggs. The zona pellucida is digested from the hamster egg, because it is this layer that determines the species-specific penetration ability of sperm. Although not commonly used, this test can assess several steps necessary for sperm capacitation.

6. Antisperm antibodies. A link between infertility and antisperm antibodies has been recognized for years. The effect of antibodies is to disturb either of two processes: sperm transport through the female reproductive tract or sperm-egg interaction. Enzyme-linked immunosorbent assay (ELISA) and immunobead binding assay are

two commonly used tests to detect the presence of antibodies on sperm.

7. **White blood cells.** Reproductive tract infections are a treatable cause of infertility and are often heralded by the presence of excessive white blood cells in the ejaculate. Special stains are needed to distinguish white cells from immature germ cells; the latter are not pathologic.

F. Radiologic Procedures

1. Transrectal ultrasound (TRUS). TRUS is indicated in infertile men with low volume ejaculates (<1.5 mL). **Ejaculatory duct obstruction** (EDO) may be identified by seminal vesicle dilation (>1.5 cm in diameter); seminal vesicle hypoplasia or absence is also easily diagnosed. Often the causes of EDO, including stones, scar, cysts, or a persistent utricle, can also be diagnosed by TRUS. Seminal vesicle fluid can be sampled to confirm the presence of sperm in patients with suspected obstruction or **seminal vesiculography** or **chromotubation** (antegrade injection of diluted indigo carmine monitored by flexible cystoscopy) can be done to demonstrate obstruction.

2. **Vasography.** Classically, intraoperative, trans-scrotal vasography is used to detect abdominal vas deferens, seminal vesicle, and ejaculatory duct patency prior to definitive surgery for obstruction.

3. **Scrotal ultrasound.** A scrotal ultrasound is indicated when the testes are not easily palpable due to co-existent hydrocele, to confirm the origin and character (solid vs. cystic) of intrascrotal masses, and for confirming the presence of a clinically suspicious varicocele. There is Level I evidence to suggest that finding and treating subclinical varicoceles will not improve male fertility.

IV. CLASSIFICATION OF ABNORMALITIES

A. General Information

1. A variety of classification schemes exist to categorize fertility problems. One of the most useful is based on the findings on semen analyses with initial classification of problems into one of four categories: (1) all parameters normal, (2) azoospermia, (3) a single abnormal parameter, and (4) multiple abnormal parameters. The decision to treat a semen abnormality to improve fertility depends in part on maternal reproductive potential and also on how correctable the problem is, as outlined in Figure 20-5.

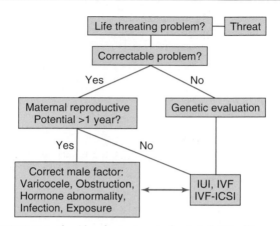

FIGURE 20-5. Algorithm for treatment of male infertility. (From Turek PJ: Practical approach to the diagnosis and management of male infertility. *Nat Clin Pract Urol* 2:1–13, 2005.)

2. Distribution of semen abnormalities among infertile men:

Azoospermia	8%
Single abnormal parameter	37%
Multiple abnormal parameters	55%

Among the single abnormal parameters, isolated abnormalities in motility account for the majority of cases.

B. All Parameters Normal

1. When two semen analyses are normal and the history and physical examination are not suggestive of a specific fertility problem in the male, further evaluation of the female partner is recommended.
2. If the evaluation of the female partner is also found to be normal, and the couple still have not conceived, then sperm function tests noted previously, that is, sperm chromatin assay, sperm morphology, and hamster egg penetration tests, may be useful. Most couples with unexplained infertility will go on to be treated with **intrauterine insemination (IUI) or IVF.**

C. Azoospermia (Figure 20-6)

1. When no sperm are found on semen analysis, the specimen should be centrifuged to confirm the absence of any

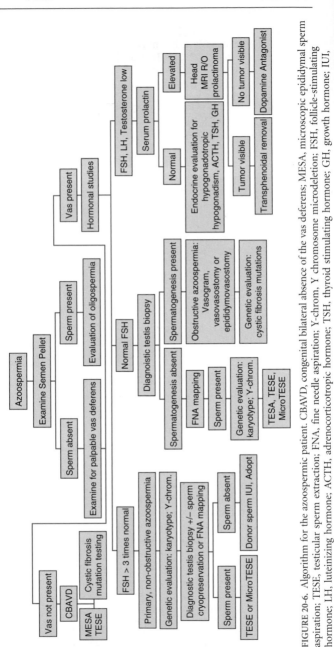

FIGURE 20-6. Algorithm for the azoospermic patient. CBAVD, congenital bilateral absence of the vas deferens; MESA, microscopic epididymal sperm aspiration; TESE, testicular sperm extraction; FNA, fine needle aspiration; Y-chrom, Y chromosome microdeletion; FSH, follicle-stimulating hormone; LH, luteinizing hormone; ACTH, adrenocorticotropic hormone; TSH, thyroid stimulating hormone; GH, growth hormone; IUI, intrauterine insemination.

sperm in the specimen. In addition, a **collection error** and/or retrograde ejaculation must be ruled out as causes of azoospermia. If **retrograde ejaculation** is identified by the finding of sperm in the urine (>10–15 sperm per high-power field [HPF]), treatment can be initiated with oral alkalization and sympathomimetic agents to promote antegrade ejaculation. Alternatively, sperm can be retrieved from the bladder, processed, and used for IUI.

2. The results of the fructose test and gonadotropin levels determine what additional evaluation and treatment are necessary.

   a) The LH, FSH, and testosterone levels can differentiate **primary testicular failure** from secondary testicular failure caused by either pituitary or hypothalamic dysfunction.

   b) A serum **FSH >3 times normal** along with atrophic testicles on physical examination is essentially equivalent to a **"medical biopsy"** of the testis and indicates severe testicular failure. **This does not mean that there is no sperm in the testis, as fully one half of men can have low numbers of sperm on more extensive evaluation.** However, this finding obviates the need for a surgical biopsy to rule out obstructive conditions. Sperm found in these men can be used with IVF/ICSI by testicular sperm extraction techniques (TESE).

3. After ruling out a major endocrine abnormality, the major differential diagnosis is **ductal obstruction** or testicular failure.

   a) Negative fructose test. Three possibilities exist in the azoospermic patient with normal hormone studies and a negative fructose test. These include congenital bilateral absence of the vas deferens (CAVD) and seminal vesicles, bilateral ejaculatory duct obstruction, and, rarely, **seminal vesicle dysfunction** similar to bladder myopathy. The treatment of CAVD is direct sperm aspiration from the epididymis. The sperm are then processed and used in combination with IVF and ICSI techniques. Ejaculatory duct obstruction is managed by transurethral resection of the ejaculatory ducts or unroofing midline cysts.

   b) Positive fructose test. A positive fructose test usually rules out complete obstruction of the ejaculatory ducts and severe dysfunction of the seminal vesicles but does not give an indication of the patency of the ductal system from the level of the testis to the ejaculatory ducts. Therefore, a positive fructose test in azoospermia does not differentiate between proximal ductal obstruction and testicular failure.

c) Testicular biopsy. A testicular biopsy is necessary in the azoospermic patient with normal hormones and normal-sized testes with fructose in the ejaculate. The microscopic examination of the biopsy will indicate whether spermatogenesis is progressing normally. With the advent of IVF and ICSI, sperm found on testicular biopsy can be cryopreserved for future use.

d) If the testicular biopsy indicates active and complete spermatogenesis, scrotal exploration and vasography are indicated. A **vasogram** is performed by injecting contrast material through one vas deferens to determine patency. If patency is demonstrated, then exploration of the epididymis is undertaken to localize the site of obstruction. Fluid within the vas deferens lumen at **vasotomy** should also be examined microscopically to determine if sperm are present or absent. A microscopic **vasoepididymostomy** is necessary to correct epididymal obstruction. If no spermatozoa are detected in the tubules of the epididymis during this exploration, then intratesticular ductal obstruction may be the cause of azoospermia. Because these cases are difficult to correct, IVF and ICSI with testicular sperm is recommended.

4. Vasectomy is one cause of azoospermia amenable to surgical repair with microsurgery (Figure 20-7). It is well established that (1) surgeon experience and (2) use of optical magnification improve outcomes after vasectomy reversal. In experienced hands, **a return of sperm to the ejaculate should be possible in 90–95% of cases of vasovasostomy, with pregnancy rates from 35–60% depending on partner fertility potential.** In older vasectomies, it is often necessary to perform a **vasoepididymostomy** for secondary epididymal obstruction that is acquired due to prolonged obstruction after vasectomy.

D. Multiple Abnormal Parameters on the Semen Analysis

1. Diffuse abnormalities of all or many of the seminal parameters are the most common pathologic pattern identified (55%). Determination of the LH, FSH, and testosterone levels can rule out an endocrine abnormality.

2. Stress, infections, and other environmental factors such as wet heat, drugs, and toxin exposures may produce a transient abnormality of all seminal parameters. Therefore,

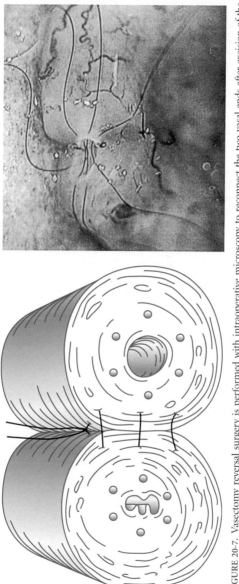

FIGURE 20-7. Vasectomy reversal surgery is performed with intraoperative microscopy to reconnect the two vasal ends after excision of the blocked vasal segment. It is generally reconnected in two layers.

when other specific factors cannot be identified by the history or physical examination, it may be beneficial to follow these patients for 3–6 months to determine if there is self-correction of the abnormality. If spontaneous correction has not occurred, nonspecific therapy can be instituted as discussed later, or, more commonly, couples can be offered assisted reproductive technology (ART) (IUI, IVF).

3. Varicoceles.

a) **A varicocele** is defined as **dilated, varicose internal spermatic veins** producing fullness, dilation, and **poor drainage of the pampiniform plexus.** A varicocele is found in **15%** of males in the general population but is found in **35–40% of men presenting with infertility** problems and results in abnormal semen parameters.

b) Varicoceles are **classified according to size as either large (grade III), medium (grade II), or small (grade I).** Large varicoceles can be seen as a "bag of worms" under the scrotal skin. Medium varicoceles are readily detected by palpation, especially on standing. Small varicoceles can only be identified by feeling an impulse in the scrotum with the Valsalva maneuver or a difference in the size and fullness of the spermatic cord when the patient moves from the standing to the supine position. The majority (90%) of varicoceles occur on the left side, but bilateral varicoceles are more common than previously believed.

c) The exact mechanism through which the varicocele exerts a detrimental effect is not completely clear; the leading theory is that it leads to **increased intrascrotal temperature** through retrograde venous blood flow. It characteristically causes a decrease in normal sperm morphology, with an increase in immature and tapered sperm. There may also be decreased sperm motility and varying degrees of oligospermia.

d) Treatment of varicocele involves surgical ligation or transvenous angiographic identification and embolization of the involved internal spermatic veins. The usual surgical approach is **retroperitoneal, inguinal, or subinguinal ligation** of the internal spermatic and collateral veins. Laparoscopy may be useful in cases of bilateral varicoceles. Newer interventional **angiographic techniques** and catheters allow for selective catheterization of the internal spermatic veins. For venous occlusion, a variety of techniques are used, including sclerosing solutions, balloons and stainless-steel coils.

e) Results of varicocele ligation from a large number of series indicate approximately a **70% improvement in semen quality** associated with a **40% pregnancy rate.** With initial sperm counts greater than 10 million sperm per milliliter, the improvement in pregnancy rates is significantly better than if the initial counts are less than 10 million sperm per milliliter. Both surgical and angiographic techniques for occlusion of varicoceles have a small failure rate with persistence and/ or recurrence of the varicocele noted during follow-up. **Pregnancies, when they occur, generally are noted in a mean of 7–8 months following varicocelectomy.**

E. Isolated Abnormal Parameter on Semen Analysis (Figure 20-8)

1. Abnormal semen volume.
   a) Large ejaculate volume. A volume greater than 5.5 mL may result in dilution of the spermatozoa and poor cervical placement of seminal fluid during intercourse. Mechanical concentration of the spermatozoa and intrauterine insemination may be employed if necessary.
   b) Absent or low ejaculate volume (Figure 20-9). Once a collection abnormality has been ruled out, it is essential to consider **retrograde ejaculation, infection of the accessory sex glands, or endocrine dysfunction (low testosterone).** The presence of retrograde ejaculation is confirmed by the finding of large quantities of spermatozoa in the postejaculatory urine sample (>15 sperm per HPF). Sympathomimetic drugs with alpha-adrenergic activity can reverse this problem in one third of patients, generally those without scar tissue at the bladder neck from prior surgery. In others, it may be necessary to obtain, wash, and inseminate (IUI) sperm collected from the postejaculate urine sample. Endocrine abnormalities and infections are treated with the appropriate hormones and antibiotics.
2. Hyperviscosity. Problems with hyperviscous semen are rare and may reflect enzymatic imbalance in the semen. Mechanical disruption of the sample in the laboratory to decrease viscosity, followed by IUI is useful in this situation.
3. Decreased motility and forward progression (asthenospermia).
   a) This is the most common isolated abnormality found on analysis of semen and can be due to endocrine dysfunction, infection of accessory glands, varicocele, epididymal dysfunction, genetics, reactive oxygen

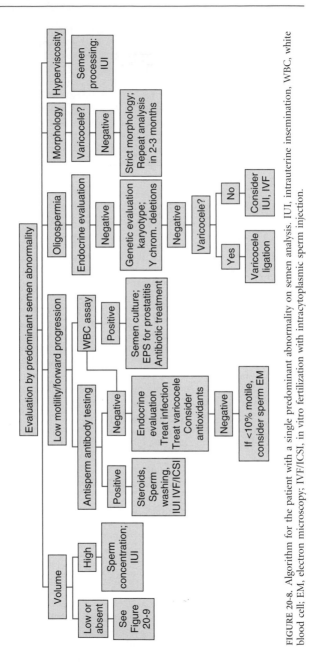

FIGURE 20-8. Algorithm for the patient with a single predominant abnormality on semen analysis. IUI, intrauterine insemination; WBC, white blood cell; EM, electron microscopy; IVF/ICSI, in vitro fertilization with intracytoplasmic sperm injection.

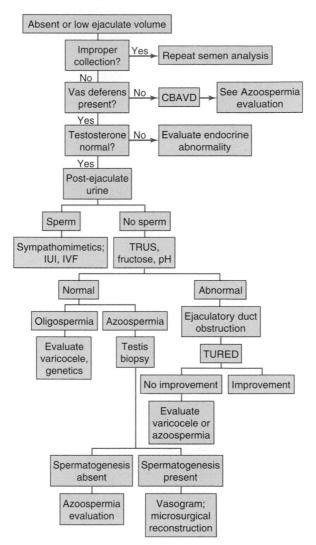

FIGURE 20-9. Algorithm for patients with absent or low volume (<1.5 mL) ejaculate. CBAVD, congenital bilateral absence of the vas deferens; IUI, intrauterine insemination; IVF, in vitro fertilization; TRUS, transrectal ultrasound; TURED, transurethral resection of the ejaculatory ducts.

species (oxidants), or environmental exposures. Specific therapy is available for some of these problems. Empirical treatment with antioxidants (vitamins A, C, and E, zinc, and folate) may also be tried.

b) Sperm motility and forward progression may also be adversely affected by the presence of **antisperm antibodies** that agglutinate or immobilize the spermatozoa. Special sperm tests are available to determine the levels of antisperm antibodies in semen. Several treatments are available for antibodies, including IUI, IVF, and ICSI and treatment of the male with systemic steroids for 6–9 months. The latter treatment has been associated with decreased antibody levels but not necessarily increased natural pregnancy rates.

4. Oligospermia.

a) Decreased sperm numbers as an isolated problem may be secondary to endocrine dysfunction or genetic or idiopathic conditions. Occasionally the absolute number of sperm is relatively normal, but the number of sperm per milliliter may appear to be low due to a large ejaculate volume. **With sperm densities less than 10×10^6 /mL, a karyotype analysis and specific deletions in the Y chromosome should be evaluated** (see Figure 20-4).

b) In general, there are two treatments for oligospermia. One attempts to stimulate the testes with a variety of drugs to increase the output of spermatozoa (see section on idiopathic infertility). Alternatively, with advances in assisted reproduction, spermatozoa can be concentrated for use with IUI. In addition, IVF and ICSI are available when simpler approaches fail.

5. Abnormal morphology. An isolated problem with morphology is unusual. This may result from gonadotoxic exposures (e.g., tobacco), systemic illness, fevers, varicocele, or idiopathic causes.

F. Empirical Treatment of Idiopathic Infertility

1. Second only to the large proportion of patients with varicoceles, **idiopathic infertility** is the next largest group of infertility patients. In fact, nonresponders to varicocele ligation may belong in this category. Essentially, idiopathic infertility refers to men who have an abnormal parameter or parameters on the semen analyses with a normal history, physical examination, and screening hormone analysis. The etiology of the abnormal semen quality is unclear and probably reflects our incomplete

knowledge regarding the genetics of spermatogenesis. Many of these cases are likely to have genetic etiologies, as our knowledge of genetic infertility grows.

2. Nonpharmacologic treatments. A variety of nonpharmacologic treatments have been suggested, but their efficacy has not been rigorously demonstrated. These include:

   a) Vitamins/diet. Specific vitamins and changes in dietary habits have not been associated with improved semen quality and fertility. Antioxidant therapy has been shown to increase motility of in vitro isolated sperm, but treatment of men with unexplained severe asthenospermia with high-dose vitamin E and C did not improve motility in a large, randomized study. However, this therapy is likely to specifically help tobacco smokers to reduce the oxidative effects on sperm.

   b) Changing from jockey shorts to **boxer shorts.** A recent study has refuted the idiom that a switch from jockey to boxer shorts improves spermatogenesis and semen parameters.

   c) Prostatic massage.

   d) Antibiotics for "occult infection."

   e) Varicocelectomy for the "occult" or **subclinical varicocele.** There are three randomized, controlled clinical trials suggesting that there is no benefit to varicocelectomy in cases of nonpalpable, ultrasound-detected varicoceles.

3. Drug therapy for idiopathic infertility.

   a) The use of **human menopausal gonadotropin (hMG)** or **recombinant FSH, human chorionic gonadotropin (hCG**, essentially LH), or the combination of FSH and hCG has not resulted in significant improvements in sperm counts or fertility with idiopathic infertility. GnRH therapy, when given in a pulsatile fashion, has the potential to raise LH and FSH levels, but its administration is complex and costly.

   b) **Clomiphene citrate** is an antiestrogen that has been used nonspecifically for idiopathic infertility for 30 years. As a **selective estrogen receptor modulator (SERM),** this medication blocks the negative feedback of estradiol on the hypothalamic-pituitary axis, resulting in increased LH and FSH levels. Overall improvement in the semen analysis is noted in approximately 50% of patients, and pregnancies occur in 25–30% of patients in uncontrolled studies. Men with low-normal testosterone and FSH levels, indicative of mild central hypogonadism, may respond best to this therapy.

c) Tamoxifen is also an antiestrogen. This agent, how-ever, lacks the estrogenic activities of clomiphene and may provide equal efficacy.

d) Aromatase inhibitors block the conversion of testos-terone to estrogens in men. They may be useful in oli-gospermic or azoospermic men with a **testosterone: estrogen ratio of less than 10:1** to increase sperm yield from the ejaculate or from testis sperm extraction procedures.

e) **L-Carnitine** is found in high concentrations in the normal epididymis and is postulated to be important for sperm motility. Oral L-carnitine is currently avail-able from several popular fertility supplements and there is early evidence that some men with low moti-lity will show improvement, especially those with varicoceles.

G. Assisted Reproductive Technology

1. ART attempts to improve the conception by bypassing many or all of the barriers associated with normal fertili-zation. The simplest techniques involve sperm processing and insemination of the female; the more sophisticated ones involve manipulation of the sperm and ova extra-corporeally. Fertilization with these procedures can occur in vitro or in vivo.

2. Semen processing is used as an isolated procedure or in conjunction with oocyte processing. **Sperm washing, swim-ups, sedimentations, and gradient centrifuga-tions** are commonly employed to remove seminal plasma and leukocytes and to select for and concentrate highly motile sperm. Theoretically, with these procedures, fewer sperm than normal are needed because at least initially, they are placed higher within the female reproductive tract than is an ejaculate during intercourse.

3. **IUI** is used to treat male factor infertility. In this techni-que, a small catheter is used to inject processed sperm through the cervix and into the uterine cavity. By bypass-ing the cervical mucus, more motile sperm can progress to the fallopian tubes where normal fertilization occurs. Indications for IUI include male factor infertility due to mechanical or anatomic problems (e.g., erectile dysfunc-tion, hypospadias) or low semen quality and cervical mucus problems. **Usually, more than 5 million motile sperm are required for IUI. Pregnancy rates are vari-able with these techniques, but average 30–35% in couples who try 3–4 times.**

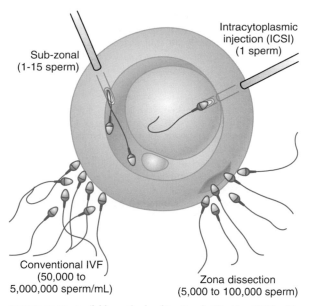

Intracytoplasmic
injection (ICSI)
(1 sperm)

Sub-zonal
(1-15 sperm)

Conventional IVF
(50,000 to
5,000,000 sperm/mL)

Zona dissection
(5,000 to 100,000 sperm)

FIGURE 20-10. Available methods of in vitro fertilization (IVF) with micromanipulation of gametes. Among the techniques illustrated, IVF and intracytoplasmic sperm injection (ICSI) are currently the most commonly used.

4. **IVF,** first introduced in 1978, was developed to manage fallopian tube obstruction. It is now used routinely for male factor infertility (Figure 20-10). Female partners undergo ovarian hyperstimulation to induce the maturation of multiple oocytes, which are then harvested ultrasonographically just prior to ovulation. Processed semen and recovered oocytes are mixed in vitro. If fertilization occurs, embryos are placed back into the uterus transcervically. Usually only 20–30% of replaced embryos survive and become clinical pregnancies. Of those couples who fail the first IVF attempt, 10–18% will fertilize on the second cycle. Depending on the cause of infertility, and the number of embryos replaced, pregnancy rates can approach 40–50% per IVF attempt.

5. In gamete intrafallopian transfer (**GIFT**), sperm and oocytes are placed into the fallopian tubes prior to fertilization. This is done in lieu of uterine placement with the hope that higher pregnancy rates will be achieved with more physiologic placement of gametes. As GIFT

does not improve the fertilizing capacity of sperm, it has no benefit over IVF in male factor infertility. If zygote stage early embryos are transferred, then the technique is called zygote intrafallopian transfer (**ZIFT**) or pronuclear stage tubal transfer (**PROUST**). Given the recent success of IVF and ICSI, tubal transfers are currently used in fewer than 2% of ART cases.

6. Micromanipulation (see Figure 20-10). Sperm and oocyte micromanipulation by **ICSI has become the mainstay of addressing the poor fertilizing capacity of sperm often seen in male infertility.** By injecting a single sperm directly into an oocyte, multiple barriers of fertilization are bypassed and success rates (when compared to standard IVF) are greatly improved. Pregnancy rates of 40–50% have been obtained using this technique even in the most severe cases of male infertility. In addition, not only ejaculated sperm but sperm retrieved from the male reproductive tract are capable of producing pregnancies with ICSI. **Vasal, epididymal, and even testicular sperm, from both obstructed and nonobstructed men, are now routinely used with IVF and ICSI.**

7. **IVF with ICSI** should not be performed without **karyotype analysis on both partners.** Despite its great success, there remain concerns with ICSI.

   a) **Multiple gestations occur in 35% of pregnancies compared to 1–2% of naturally conceived pregnancies.** Multiple gestations are associated with lower birth weights, higher overall complication rates, and increased learning disabilities relative to singletons. In addition, the **delivery costs** associated with managing multiple, often premature, gestations are at least **10–20 times higher** than that associated with the singleton deliveries. There is also strong evidence to suggest that the incidence of low birth weight singletons is also increased after ICSI. Among respectable ART programs, there is a trend to transfer as few embryos back as possible to reduce the multiple gestation rate.

   b) **ICSI bypasses many mechanisms of natural selection such that many men who would not be able to conceive under normal circumstances are now able to father children.** Although overall rates of **major birth defects (3.3%)** associated with IVF and ICSI may be similar to intercourse, there is concern about elevated risks of specific malformations, including **hypospadias**, with this technology. In addition, there are concerns regarding possible **developmental issues.** There is a significant **increase in sex chromosomal abnormalities** among ICSI offspring (**0.8% vs. 0.2% naturally**) that is likely attributable to the chromosomal status of the fathers rather than to the technique itself. As previously mentioned, from 5–8% of men with severe oligospermia have deletions in the AZF region of the Y chromosome. It has been shown conclusively that these genetic deletions are passed to the male offspring produced by these fathers through IVF/ICSI.

c) More recently, concerns have arisen regarding whether **rare imprinting diseases such as Beckwith-Wiedemann syndrome and Angelman syndrome** are increased in children conceived with ICSI. For these reasons, genetic counseling is recommended for all couples considering IVF-ICSI.

8. Preimplantation genetic diagnosis (**PGD**) is now possible by sampling a single cell from an eight-cell developing embryo in vitro and performing either fluorescent in situ hybridization (FISH) or single-cell polymerase chain reaction (PCR) to **examine for aneuploidy, chromosomal translocations, or even specific diseases caused by point mutations.** Current indications for PGD include lethal disease prevention and aneuploidy screening in advanced maternal age couples.

V. CONCLUSION

Our knowledge of testis development, the properties of testis stem cells, sperm production, maturation, and transport is rapidly evolving. Many chromosomal and molecular mechanisms important for normal sperm production are being elucidated. Thus, fewer male patients with infertility now have an undefined etiology. Clearly, more genes such as those assessed on Y chromosome will relate to male infertility; the X chromosome is particularly interesting in this regard. Concurrently, ART has outstripped our understanding of sperm development and allows us to bypass what were in the past natural barriers that prevented the inheritance of genetic defects. As a consequence, the study of human reproduction is particularly relevant for clinical care.

Despite high technology advances, the evaluation and use of classical treatments for male infertility remain cost-effective. The male evaluation is centered on a careful history, physical examination, and hormonal and semen analysis. This process helps to define pathologic and otherwise treatable conditions and identifies ways to correct, and not bypass, the infertility problem.

SELF-ASSESSMENT QUESTIONS

1. Embryologically, what anatomic structures in the male reproductive system develop from the mesonephric ducts?
2. The male ejaculate is derived from what organs?
3. What is the most common and correctable identifiable problem causing male infertility?
4. A 25-year-old bodybuilder eschews the merits of "natural" bodybuilding and cycles and stacks injectable anabolic steroids regularly to maximize muscle bulk. During this period of steroid use, describe what happens to his hormone balance and fertility potential. What happens when he stops using steroids?
5. What is the role of PSA in the ejaculate?

SUGGESTED READINGS

1. Goldstein M (ed): *Surgery of Male Infertility.* Philadelphia, WB Saunders, 1995.
2. Jarow JP, Sharlip ID, Belker AM, et al: Male Infertility Best Practice Policy Committee of the American Urological Association Inc. *J Urol* 167:2138–2144, 2002.
3. Schlegel PN, Chang TSK: Physiology of male reproduction. In Walsh PC, Retik A, Vaughan ED Jr, Wein A (eds): *Campbell's Urology,* 7th ed. Philadelphia, WB Saunders, 1998, pp 1254–1286.
4. Sigman M, Howards SS: Male infertility. In Walsh PC, Retik A, Vaughan ED Jr, Wein A (eds): *Campbell's Urology,* 7th ed. Philadelphia, WB Saunders, 1998, pp 1287–1330.
5. Sigman M, Jarow JP: Endocrine evaluation of infertile men. *Urology* 50:659–664, 1997.
6. Turek PJ: Male infertility. In Tanagho EA, McAninch JC (eds): *Smith's Urology,* 15th ed. Stamford, CT, Appleton and Lange, 2000, Chapter 46, pp 750–787.
7. Turek PJ: Practical approach to the diagnosis and management of male infertility. *Nat Clin Pract Urol* 2:1–13, 2005.
8. Turek PJ, Reijo Pera RA: Current and future genetic screening for male infertility. *Urol Clin North Am* 29:767–792, 2002.

C H A P T E R 21

Sexually Transmitted Disease

Edward Zoltan, MD

INTRODUCTION

Sexually transmitted diseases (STDs) remain a major public health challenge in the United States, affecting more than 19 million men and women annually, nearly half of whom are young people aged 15–24 years. In addition to the physical and psychologic consequences of STDs, these diseases exact a tremendous economic toll. Direct medical costs associated with STDs in the United States are estimated at $13 billion annually.

The curable STDs include gonorrhea, chlamydia, mycoplasma, ureaplasmal infections, syphilis, trichomoniasis, chancroid, lymphogranuloma venereum (LGV), and donovanosis. STDs can be caused by yeast or protozoa and are also curable. Viral STDs include human immunodeficiency virus (HIV), human papillomavirus (HPV), hepatitis B/C virus (HBV, HCV), cytomegalovirus (CMV), and herpes simplex virus (HSV). Although preventable, they are not curable.

URETHRITIS

The scientific foundation for the diagnosis of urethral inflammation dates from 1879 when Neisser demonstrated the bacterium, now known as *Neisseria gonorrhoeae*, in stained smears of urethral, vaginal, and conjunctival exudates. His discovery made possible the distinction between gonococcal (GC) urethritis and nongonococcal urethritis (NGU).

Symptoms of urethritis include **urethral discharge accompanied by burning on urination or an itching sensation.** Urethral discharge is the characteristic finding on physical examination. The principal bacterial pathogens of proven clinical importance in men who have urethritis are *N. gonorrhoeae* and *Chlamydia trachomatis*. Determination of the specific etiology is recommended as such diagnosis may improve treatment compliance, should prompt partner notification, and is reportable to state health departments.

The pathognomonic laboratory finding is an increased number of leukocytes on Gram stain of the urethral smear or first-voided urine specimen. GC urethritis is diagnosed if intracellular gram-negative diplococci are observed. NGU is more likely if they are not present.

Urethritis can be documented on the basis of any of the following signs:

1. Mucopurulent or purulent discharge.
2. Gram stain of urethral secretions demonstrating 5 white blood cells (WBCs) per oil immersion field. The Gram stain is the preferred rapid diagnostic test for evaluating urethritis. It is highly sensitive and specific for documenting both urethritis and/or the presence gonococcal infection. Gonococcal infection is established by documenting the presence of WBCs containing intracellular gram-negative diplococci.
3. Positive leukocyte esterase test on first-void urine or microscopic examination of first-void urine demonstrating 10 WBCs per high power field.

Gonococcal Urethritis

Gonorrhea is the second most commonly reported infectious disease in the United States, with 330,132 cases reported in 2004. Gonorrhea is substantially underdiagnosed and under-reported. Approximately twice as many new infections are estimated to occur each year as are reported.

Diagnosis

A direct Gram stain may be performed as soon as the specimen is collected. Urethral smears from men who have symptomatic gonorrhea usually contain intracellular gram-negative diplococci in polymorphonuclear leukocytes. Endocervical smears from women and rectal specimens require careful interpretation because of colonization with other gram-negative coccobacillary organisms.

The isolation and identification of *N. gonorrhoeae* are still the currently accepted gold standard for the diagnosis of gonococcal infections. It is the recommended method for medicolegal investigations of sexual abuse. Specimens should be inoculated onto selective media, such as modified Thayer-Martin, Martin-Lewis, or New York City.

Current testing for *N. gonorrhoeae* also includes nucleic acid molecular amplification tests (NAATs) that measure DNA and RNA rather than live organisms. Polymerase chain reaction (PCR) (Amplicor, Roche Molecular Diagnostics,

Branchburg, NJ) has been used with sensitivity well above 90% for the detection of *N. gonorrhoeae* in cervical specimens. It is highly accurate with male urine.

Strand displacement amplification (SDA) (ProbeTec, Becton Dickinson, Sparks, MD) is approved for detection of gonorrhea in cervical, male urethral, and female and male urine samples and has achieved widespread use in clinical laboratories throughout the United States and Europe. The BD ProbeTec ET system demonstrated a sensitivity of 97.9% for the detection of *N. gonorrhoeae* in urine from 680 male patients.

Because NAATs measure DNA or RNA rather than live organisms, caution should be used in using DNA amplification tests for test-of-cure assays. Residual nucleic acid from cells rendered noninfective by antibiotics may give a positive amplified test for up to 3 weeks after therapy, although the patient may actually be cured of viable organisms.

Treatment of Uncomplicated Gonococcal Urethritis

Recommended Regimens

Cefixime 400 mg orally in a single dose, **or ceftriaxone** 125 mg IM in a single dose, **or ciprofloxacin** 500 mg orally in a single dose, **or ofloxacin** 400 mg orally in a single dose, **or levofloxacin** 250 mg orally in a single dose, *plus, if chlamydial infection is not ruled out* **azithromycin** 1 gm orally in a single dose **or doxycycline** 100 mg orally twice a day for 7 days.

Quinolones should not be used for infections acquired in Asia or the Pacific, including Hawaii. In addition, use of quinolones is inadvisable for treating infections acquired in California and in other areas with increased prevalence of quinolone resistance.

Pregnancy

Pregnant women should not be treated with quinolones or tetracyclines. Those infected with *N. gonorrhoeae* should be treated with a recommended or alternative cephalosporin. Women who cannot tolerate a cephalosporin should be administered a single, 2-gm dose of spectinomycin IM. Either **erythromycin or amoxicillin is recommended for treatment of presumptive or diagnosed *C. trachomatis* infection during pregnancy.**

Follow-Up

Patients who have uncomplicated gonorrhea and who are treated with any of the recommended regimens need not return for a test to confirm that they are cured. Patients who have symptoms that persist after treatment should be evaluated by culture for *N. gonorrhoeae,* and any gonococci isolated should be tested for antimicrobial susceptibility. Infections identified after treatment with one of the recommended regimens usually result from reinfection rather than treatment failure, indicating a need for improved patient education and referral of sex partners. Persistent urethritis, cervicitis, or proctitis may indicate infection by another organism including *C. trachomatis.*

Complications

Complications of *N. gonorrhoeae* may be local or systemic. Locally, male GC urethritis may spread to the posterior urethra, seminal vesicles, and epididymis. This can lead to epididymitis, urethral stricture disease, and even sterility. In women, gonorrhea is a major cause of pelvic inflammatory disease (PID). PID results from the ascent of infection from the endocervix into the fallopian tubes. **Symptoms include vaginal discharge, abdominal pain, dyspareunia, menorrhagia, fever, and cervical motion or adnexal tenderness.** This may lead to scarring of the adnexal structures and fallopian tubes resulting in chronic pelvic pain, ectopic pregnancy, and infertility.

N. gonorrhoeae can also lead to systemic diseases. Gonococcal perihepatitis (Fitz-Hugh-Curtis syndrome) is manifested by sharp supraumbilical pain and right upper quadrant pain. It results from ascending infection from the pelvis into the paracolic gutters and subphrenic spaces in females. "Violin string" adhesions may be noted between the liver and anterior abdominal wall and diaphragm. Disseminated gonococcal infection can occur in up to 3% of mucosal cases and may include arthritis, tenosynovitis, dermatitis, meningitis, myopericarditis, and/or sepsis.

Nongonococcal Urethritis

Chlamydia Trachomatis

Among the more than 20 STDs that have now been identified, chlamydia is the most frequently reported, with an estimated 4 million new cases each year. In 2004, 929,462 chlamydia diagnoses were reported, up from 877,478 in 2003. Even so, most chlamydia cases go undiagnosed. The increases in reported cases and rates likely reflect the continued expansion of screening efforts and increased use of more sensitive diagnostic tests, rather than an actual increase in new infections. The availability of urine tests for chlamydia may be contributing to the increased detection of the disease in men and consequently the rising rates of reported chlamydia in men in recent years.

The Centers for Disease Control and Prevention (CDC) recommends annual chlamydia screening for sexually active women under age 26, as well as older women with risk factors such as new or multiple sex partners. Screening efforts are critical to preventing the serious health consequences of this infection, particularly infertility.

C. trachomatis is an intracellular bacterium with multiple serotypes. Types L1–3 cause LGV. Types D, E, F, G, H, I, J, and K cause urethritis and cervicitis. It is transmitted during vaginal, oral, or anal sexual contact with an infected partner. *C. trachomatis* **accounts for 30–50% of cases of NGU.**

Common clinical manifestations of chlamydial infection in men include urethritis, epididymitis, and proctitis. The urethritis presents 1–3 weeks after infection with a mild to moderate clear urethral discharge and dysuria. Chlamydial urethritis may present as persistent dysuria and discharge following a course of treatment for gonorrhea, as 15–35% of patients with known gonococcal infections are also infected with chlamydia.

Chlamydial epididymitis tends to run a more protracted course than epididymitis due to other organisms; it is also often less severe. Chlamydial proctitis presents with rectal pain and bleeding, but it is often asymptomatic.

Chlamydial infection may disseminate systemically in 1–3% of patients. Classically know as Reiter's syndrome, it presents with the classic triad of reactive arthritis, urethritis, and conjunctivitis. The Fitz-Hugh-Curtis syndrome may also be seen in about 20% of women with PID secondary to chlamydial infection.

C. trachomatis was the first organism for which there was a commercially available PCR assay. Now there are many published studies using several different types of NAATs and new technologies that are commercially available for detecting *Chlamydia* in urine and urethral, cervical, or vaginal secretions.

Treatment

Treatment should be initiated as soon as possible after diagnosis. Single-dose regimens have the advantage of improved compliance.

Recommended Regimens

Azithromycin 1 gm orally in a single dose **or doxycycline** 100 mg orally twice a day for 7 days.

Alternative Regimens

Erythromycin base 500 mg orally four times a day for 7 days, **or erythromycin ethylsuccinate** 800 mg orally four times a day for 7 days, **or ofloxacin** 300 mg twice a day for 7 days, **or levofloxacin** 500 mg once daily for 7 days.

Recurrent and Persistent Urethritis

Patients who have persistent or recurrent urethritis should be re-treated with the initial regimen if they did not comply with the treatment regimen or if they were re-exposed to an untreated sex partner. Otherwise, a culture of an intraurethral swab specimen and a first-void urine specimen for *Trichomonas vaginalis* should be performed. Some cases of recurrent urethritis following doxycycline treatment may be caused by tetracycline-resistant *Ureaplasma urealyticum*. If the patient was compliant with the initial regimen and re-exposure can be excluded, the following regimen is recommended:

Metronidazole 2 gm orally in a single dose *PLUS* **erythromycin base** 500 mg orally four times a day for 7 days **or erythromycin ethylsuccinate** 800 mg orally four times a day for 7 days.

Patients who have NGU and also are infected with HIV should receive the same treatment regimen as those who are HIV negative.

Nonchlamydial NGU

The etiology of most cases of nonchlamydial NGU is unknown. *U. urealyticum* and *Mycoplasma genitalium* have been implicated as causes of NGU. Specific diagnostic tests for these organisms are not indicated because the detection of these organisms is often difficult and would not alter therapy.

T. vaginalis and HSV sometimes cause NGU. Diagnostic and treatment procedures for these organisms are reserved for situations in which these infections are suspected (e.g., contact with trichomoniasis and genital lesions suggestive of genital herpes) or when NGU is not responsive to therapy.

GENITAL WARTS

Condyloma Acuminata

Human papillomavirus (HPV) is a small, nonenveloped virus containing double-stranded DNA. HPV infects basal epithelial cells and multiplies in the cell nucleus, causing cell death and perinuclear cavitation or **koilocytosis, a histologic feature specific to HPV.** More than 30 types of HPV can infect the genital tract. Most HPV infections are asymptomatic, unrecognized, or subclinical. **Visible genital warts usually are caused by HPV type 6 or 11.** Other HPV types in the anogenital region (e.g., types 16, 18, 31, 33, and 35) have been strongly associated with cervical neoplasia.

Biopsy is recommended under certain clinical conditions:

1. Diagnosis is uncertain.
2. Lesions do not respond to standard therapy.
3. Disease worsens during therapy.
4. Patient is immunocompromised.
5. Warts are pigmented, indurated, fixed, and ulcerated **(suggestive of Buschke-Lowenstein tumor).**

No data support the use of type-specific HPV nucleic acid tests in the routine diagnosis or management of visible genital warts.

In addition to the external genitalia (i.e., the penis, vulva, scrotum, perineum, and perianal skin), genital warts can occur on the uterine cervix and in the vagina, urethra, anus, and mouth.

When urethral lesions occur, 80% are located within the distal 3 cm of urethra. Patients present with dysuria, bloody urethral discharge, and changes in urinary stream. **Bladder condyloma are rare.** If meatal condyloma are identified, urethroscopy should be performed to look for other urethral lesions. **To prevent iatrogenic seeding of the prostatic urethra and bladder, a tourniquet should be placed at the peno-pubic junction or urethroscopy should stop at the external sphincter.**

Intra-anal warts are seen predominantly in patients who have had anal receptive intercourse; these warts are distinct from perianal warts, which can occur in men and women who do not have a history of anal sex.

HPV types 6 and 11 have been associated with conjunctival, nasal, oral, and laryngeal warts. HPV types 6 and 11 rarely are associated with invasive squamous cell carcinoma of the external genitalia. Depending on the size and anatomic location, **genital warts can be painful, friable, and pruritic, although they are commonly asymptomatic.**

HPV types 16, 18, 31, 33, and 35 are found occasionally in visible genital warts and have been associated with external genital (i.e., vulvar, penile, and anal) squamous intraepithelial neoplasia (i.e., squamous cell carcinoma in situ, bowenoid papulosis, erythroplasia of Queyrat, or Bowen's disease of the genitalia). These HPV types also have been associated with vaginal, anal, and cervical intraepithelial dysplasia and squamous cell carcinoma. Patients who have visible genital warts can be infected simultaneously with multiple HPV types.

Treatment

The primary goal of treating visible genital warts is the removal of symptomatic warts. In most patients, treatment can induce wart-free periods. If left untreated, visible genital warts may resolve spontaneously, remain unchanged, or increase in size or number. Existing data indicate that currently available therapies for genital warts may reduce, but probably do not eliminate, infectivity.

Most patients have fewer than ten genital warts, with a total wart area of 0.5–1.0 cm^2. These warts respond to most treatment modalities. Factors that may influence the selection of treatment include wart size, wart number, anatomic site of wart, wart morphology, patient preference, cost of treatment, convenience, adverse effects, and provider experience.

Many patients require a course of therapy rather than a single treatment. In general, warts located on moist surfaces and/or in intertriginous areas respond better to topical treatment than do warts on drier surfaces.

Recommended Regimens for External Genital Warts
Patient-Applied

Podofilox 0.5% solution or gel. Patients should apply podofilox solution with a cotton swab or podofilox gel with a finger, to visible genital warts twice a day for 3 days, followed by 4 days of no therapy. This cycle may be repeated, as necessary, for up to four cycles. The total wart area treated should not exceed 10 cm^2, and the total volume of podofilox should be limited to 0.5 mL per day. The safety of podofilox during pregnancy has not been established.

Or Imiquimod 5% cream. Patients should apply imiquimod cream once daily at bedtime, three times a week for up to 16 weeks. The treatment area should be washed with soap and water 6–10 hours after the application. The safety of imiquimod during pregnancy has not been established.

Physician-Administered

Cryotherapy with liquid nitrogen or cryoprobe. Repeat applications every 1–2 weeks.

Or Podophyllin resin 10–25% in a compound tincture of benzoin. A small amount should be applied to each wart and allowed to air dry. The treatment can be repeated weekly, if necessary. To avoid the possibility of complications associated with systemic absorption and toxicity, the application should be limited to less than 0.5 mL of podophyllin or an area of less than 10 cm^2 of warts per session. The preparation should be thoroughly washed off 1–4 hours after application to reduce local irritation. The safety of podophyllin during pregnancy has not been established.

Or Trichloroacetic acid (TCA) or bichloroacetic acid (BCA) 80–90%. A small amount should be applied only to warts and allowed to dry, at which time a white "frosting" develops. If an excess amount of acid is applied, the treated area should be powdered with talc, sodium bicarbonate (i.e., baking soda), or liquid soap preparations to remove unreacted acid. This treatment can be repeated weekly, if necessary. **Or Surgical removal** for very large wart burden. **Or Intralesional interferon.** Intralesional injection of interferon alpha 2b increases success of podofilox but the recurrence rate is the same. **Or Laser surgery.** CO$_2$ laser vaporizes tissue with a shallow depth of penetration. **Must use laser mask and vacuum because viral DNA has been demonstrated in the smoke plume.** Neodymium:yttrium-aluminum-garnet (Nd:YAG) coagulates tissue and causes less plume. Overall success with laser is 88–100%. Recurrence occurs in 2–3 months.

GENITAL ULCERS

In the United States, most young, sexually active patients who have genital ulcers have genital herpes, syphilis, or chancroid. Although genital herpes is the most prevalent of these diseases, the relative frequency of each differs by geographic area and patient population. Patients with genital ulcers may have more than one disease. Conversely, not all genital ulcers are caused by sexually transmitted infections. Each disease has been associated with an increased risk for HIV infection.

A diagnosis based only on the patient's medical history and physical examination often is inaccurate.

Only three ulcer presentations are pathognomonic:

1. A fixed drug eruption is always triggered by the use of one particular medication.
2. A group of vesicles on an erythematous base that does not follow a neural distribution is pathognomonic for herpes simplex infection.
3. A genital ulcer that develops acutely following sexual activity is diagnostic of trauma.

Specific tests for evaluation of genital ulcers include:

1. Serology and either darkfield examination or direct immunofluorescence test for *Treponema pallidum*.
2. Culture or antigen test for HSV.
3. Culture for *Haemophilus ducreyi* (chancroid)

The differential diagnosis of genital ulcers must include premalignant processes (e.g., erythroplasia of Queyrat); malignant processes such as squamous cell carcinoma of the penis; and nonmalignant processes including syphilis, chancroid, LGV, and granuloma inguinale (GI). Biopsy of ulcers may be helpful in identifying the cause of unusual ulcers or ulcers that do not respond to initial therapy.

GENITAL HERPES

Genital herpes is a recurrent, life-long viral infection. Two serotypes of HSV have been identified: HSV-1 (30%) and HSV-2 (70%). Most cases of recurrent genital herpes are caused by HSV-2. At least 50 million persons in the United States have a genital HSV infection; most are undiagnosed.

Herpes virus invades the body via breaks in the skin or moist membranes of the penis, vagina, urethra, anus, vulva, or cervix. **Genital lesions appear 2–20 days after infection.** The lesions are initially papules, which ulcerate and scab before re-epithelializing. Flu-like symptoms may develop with the initial infection and are much worse than subsequent episodes or in patients without history of previous oral herpes. Local lesions may persist an average of 10 days following the initial infection. Recurrent lesions last 5–7 days. Tender inguinal adenopathy can develop in 2–3 weeks. Dysuria is present in 80% of females and 40% of males with genital herpes.

Late complications include mild meningitis (10–30%) and sacral or autonomic dysfunction (1%), which can result in urinary retention, pneumonitis, and hepatitis. The most serious consequence is neonatal transmission, which carries high rates of morbidity and mortality for the infant.

All practices of intercourse may transmit HSV. HSV may be passed on to the baby during birth as well. Most genital herpes infections are transmitted by persons who are either unaware of their status or asymptomatic. Rarely does first-episode genital herpes manifest with severe disease requiring hospitalization.

Recurrences are much less frequent for genital HSV-1 infection than genital HSV-2 infection. Making the distinction between HSV serotypes is important in prognosis and counseling. As such, the clinical diagnosis of genital herpes should be confirmed by laboratory testing.

Cell culturing and type analysis by immunofluorescence tests are standard options for diagnosis. Fluorescence tests can be done without viral amplification in the cell culture but with decreased sensitivity. Polymerase chain reaction (PCR) and ligase chain reaction (LCR) amplification of HSV show much better sensitivity, but the techniques are too expensive for routine use. Cytologic detection of cellular changes of herpes virus infection is insensitive and nonspecific, both in genital lesions (Tzanck preparation) and cervical Pap smears, and should not be relied on for diagnosis of HSV infection.

Treatment

Systemic antiviral drugs partially control the symptoms and signs of herpes episodes when used to treat first clinical episodes and recurrent episodes or when used as daily suppressive therapy. Nonetheless, these drugs neither eradicate latent virus nor affect the risk, frequency, or severity of recurrences after the drug is discontinued.

Randomized trials indicate that **three antiviral medications provide clinical benefit for genital herpes: acyclovir, valacyclovir, and famciclovir.** Valacyclovir is the valine ester of acyclovir and has enhanced absorption after oral administration. Famciclovir, a prodrug of penciclovir, also has high oral bioavailability. Topical therapy with antiviral drugs offers minimal clinical benefit.

First Clinical Episode of Genital Herpes

Many patients with first-episode herpes present with mild clinical manifestations but later develop severe or prolonged symptoms. Therefore, most patients with initial genital herpes should receive antiviral therapy.

Recommended Regimens

Acyclovir 400 mg orally three times a day for 7–10 days, **or acyclovir** 200 mg orally five times a day for 7–10 days, **or famciclovir** 250 mg orally three times a day for 7–10 days, **or valacyclovir** 1 gm orally twice a day for 7–10 days.

Episodic Therapy for Recurrent Genital Herpes

Effective episodic treatment of recurrent herpes requires initiation of therapy within 1 day of lesion onset or during the prodrome that precedes some outbreaks. The patient should be provided with a supply of drug or a prescription for the medication with instructions to self-initiate treatment immediately when symptoms begin.

Recommended Regimens

Acyclovir 400 mg orally three times a day for 5 days, **or acyclovir** 200 mg orally five times a day for 5 days, **or acyclovir** 800 mg orally twice a day for 5 days, **or famciclovir** 125 mg orally twice a day for 5 days, **or valacyclovir** 500 mg orally twice a day for 3–5 days, **or valacyclovir** 1.0 gm orally once a day for 5 days.

Suppressive Therapy for Recurrent Genital Herpes

Suppressive therapy reduces the frequency of genital herpes recurrences by 70–80% among patients who have frequent recurrences (i.e., six recurrences per year), and many patients report no symptomatic outbreaks.

The frequency of recurrent outbreaks diminishes over time; therefore, periodically during suppressive treatment (e.g., once a year), discontinuation of therapy should be discussed with the patient to reassess the need for continued therapy.

Suppressive antiviral therapy reduces but does not eliminate subclinical viral shedding. Therefore, the extent to which suppressive therapy prevents HSV transmission is unknown.

Recommended Regimens

Acyclovir 400 mg orally twice a day, **or famciclovir** 250 mg orally twice a day, **or valacyclovir** 500 mg orally once a day, **or valacyclovir** 1.0 gm orally once a day.

Severe Disease

Intravenous (IV) acyclovir therapy should be provided for patients who have severe disease or complications that necessitate hospitalization, such as disseminated infection, pneumonitis, hepatitis, or complications of the central nervous system (e.g., meningitis or encephalitis). The recommended regimen is acyclovir 5–10 mg/kg body weight IV every 8 hours for 2–7 days or until clinical improvement is observed, followed by oral antiviral therapy to complete at least 10 days of total therapy.

SYPHILIS

Syphilis is a systemic disease caused by *T. pallidum,* a spirochete bacteria. Patients who have syphilis may seek treatment for signs or symptoms of primary infection, secondary infection, or tertiary infection.

The ulcer in primary syphilis is characteristically **firm, hard (due to endarteritis and vascular sclerosis), and painless.** In men, the most common area is on the corona of the penis. In women, the most common locations are the labia majora, labia minora, fourchette, and perineum.

The primary mode of transmission is sexual contact. Ten percent of cases are due to transmission via saliva, transfusion, and accidental inoculation. **The disease is most contagious during the secondary stage due to the increased number of lesions present.** The risk of transmission exists during all stages, except latent syphilis.

Primary Syphilis

The time from transmission to the appearance of primary lesions averages 21 days (the range is 10–90 days). The clinical presentation of syphilis is extremely diverse and may occur decades after initial infection.

The primary chancre appears at the site of initial treponemal invasion of the dermis. It may occur on any skin or mucous membrane surface and is usually situated on the external genitalia. Initial lesions are papular but rapidly ulcerate. They are usually single, but "kissing" lesions may occur on opposing mucocutaneous surfaces. Typically, the ulcers are nontender (unless there is co-existing infection) and indurated and have a clean base and raised edges. There is often surrounding edema, especially with vulval lesions. Nontender, nonsuppurative, rubbery inguinal lymphadenopathy appears 1 week later and usually becomes bilateral after 2 weeks. The chancre usually heals spontaneously within 3–6 weeks but leaves a scar.

Secondary Syphilis

The manifestations of generalized treponemal dissemination first appear about 8 weeks after infection. Constitutional symptoms consist of fever, headache, and bone and joint pains. There is wide diversity in physical features. Skin rashes are the commonest feature. They are initially macular and become papular by 3 months. Lesions appear initially on the upper trunk, the palms and soles, and flexural surfaces of the extremities.

Generalized lymphadenopathy occurs in 50% of cases of secondary syphilis. It has similar characteristics to the localized lymphadenopathy of primary infection. Other systemic features of secondary syphilis include panuveitis, periostitis and joint effusions, glomerulonephritis, hepatitis, gastritis, myocarditis, and aseptic meningitis.

The lesions of secondary syphilis resolve spontaneously in a variable time period and most patients enter the latency stage within the first year of infection. In some, especially the immunocompromised, primary or secondary lesions may recur.

Latent Syphilis

In latent syphilis, there are no clinical stigmata of active disease, although disease remains detectable by positive serologic tests. In early latency, within 2 years of infection, vertical transmission of infection may still occur, but sexual transmission is less likely in the absence of mucocutaneous lesions. The late manifestations of syphilis arise, often decades later, in about 25% of those who have latent syphilis.

Tertiary Gummatous Syphilis

The characteristic lesions of tertiary syphilis appear 3–10 years after infection and consist of granulomas or gummas. The granulomas appear as cutaneous plaques or nodules of irregular shape and outline and are often single lesions on the arms, back, and face. Gummas can cause painless testicular swelling, which may mimic a tumor. The typical lesion of cardiovascular syphilis is aortitis affecting the ascending aorta and appearing 10–30 years after infection. This can result in aortic aneurysms or aortic insufficiency. Symptoms of neurosyphilis include dementia, sensory ataxia, areflexia, paresthesias, auditory abnormalities, and Argyll-Robertson pupils (pupils that have accommodation but no pupil response).

Diagnosis

Darkfield examinations and direct fluorescent antibody tests of lesion exudate or tissue are the definitive methods for diagnosing early syphilis. A presumptive diagnosis is possible with the use of two types of serologic tests for syphilis: (1) nontreponemal tests (e.g., Venereal Disease Research Laboratory [VDRL] and rapid plasma reagin [RPR]) and (2) treponemal tests (e.g., fluorescent treponemal antibody absorbed [FTA-ABS] and T. pallidum particle agglutination [TP-PA]). The use of only one type of serologic test is insufficient for diagnosis, because false-positive nontreponemal test results may occur secondary to various medical conditions.

Nontreponemal test antibody titers usually correlate with disease activity, and results should be reported quantitatively. A fourfold change in titer, equivalent to a change of two dilutions (e.g., from 1:16 to 1:4 or from 1:8 to 1:32), is considered necessary to demonstrate a clinically significant difference between two nontreponemal test results that were obtained using the same serologic test. Nontreponemal tests usually become nonreactive with time after treatment; however, in some patients, nontreponemal antibodies can persist at a low titer for a long period of time, sometimes for the life of the patient. This response is referred to as the "serofast reaction."

Treatment

Penicillin G, administered parenterally, is the preferred drug for treatment of all stages of syphilis. The preparation(s) used (i.e., benzathine, aqueous procaine, or aqueous crystalline), the dosage, and the length of treatment depend on the stage and clinical manifestations of disease. However, neither combinations of benzathine penicillin and procaine penicillin nor oral penicillin preparations are considered appropriate for the treatment of syphilis.

Parenteral penicillin G is the only therapy with documented efficacy for syphilis during pregnancy. Pregnant women with syphilis in any stage who report penicillin allergy should be desensitized and treated with penicillin. Skin testing for penicillin allergy may be useful in pregnant women; such testing also is useful in other patients.

The Jarisch-Herxheimer reaction is an acute febrile reaction frequently accompanied by headache, myalgia, and other symptoms that usually occurs within the first 24 hours after any therapy for syphilis. Patients should be informed about this possible adverse reaction. **It occurs most often among patients who have early syphilis.** Antipyretics may be used, but they have not been proven to prevent this reaction. The Jarisch-Herxheimer reaction may induce early labor or cause fetal distress in pregnant women. This concern should not prevent or delay therapy.

Primary and Secondary Syphilis

Recommended Regimen for Adults

Benzathine penicillin G 2.4 million units intramuscular (IM) in a single dose.

Patients with penicillin allergy can be treated with doxycycline (100 mg orally twice daily for 14 days) or tetracycline (500 mg four times daily for 14 days), or ceftriaxone 1 gm daily either IM or IV for 8–10 days, or azithromycin as a single oral dose of 2 gm. **Patients whose compliance with therapy or follow-up cannot be ensured should be desensitized and treated with benzathine penicillin.**

CHANCROID

Chancroid is a bacterial disease caused by *H. ducreyi*, a gram-negative rod, which is transmitted by direct sexual contact. In the United States, chancroid usually occurs in discrete outbreaks, although the disease is endemic in some areas. Chancroid is a cofactor for HIV transmission; high rates of HIV infection occur among patients who have chancroid in the United States and other countries.

An erythematous papule develops where the bacteria entered the body 3–14 days after contact. The pustule breaks down into the classic dirty, painful, nonindurated ulcer. Fifty percent of patients will have tender inguinal adenopathy, with matting of nodes. The lymph nodes in the groin are pus-filled (buboes).

The combination of a painful ulcer and tender inguinal adenopathy, symptoms occurring in one third of patients, suggests a diagnosis of chancroid; when accompanied by suppurative inguinal adenopathy, these signs are almost pathognomonic.

Diagnosis

A definitive diagnosis of chancroid requires identification of *H. ducreyi* on special culture media (supplemented gonococcal base and Mueller-Hinton agar) that is not widely available from commercial sources; even using these media, sensitivity is 80%. No Food and Drug Administration (FDA)-approved PCR test for *H. ducreyi* is available in the United States.

Treatment

Successful treatment for chancroid cures the infection, resolves the clinical symptoms, and prevents transmission to others. In advanced cases, scarring can result despite successful therapy. Resistance to various antibiotics has been a problem in the treatment of chancroid due to plasmid-mediated phenomenon.

Recommended Regimens

Azithromycin 1 gm orally in a single dose, **or ceftriaxone** 250 mg IM in a single dose, **or ciprofloxacin** 500 mg orally twice a day for 3 days, **or erythromycin** base 500 mg orally three times a day for 7 days.

LYMPHOGRANULUM VENEREUM

LGV is caused by *C. trachomatis* subtype L1, L2, or L3. The disease occurs most commonly in tropical climates and rarely in the United States. The most common clinical manifestation of LGV among heterosexuals is tender inguinal and/or femoral lymphadenopathy that is most commonly unilateral. Women and homosexually active men may have proctocolitis or inflammatory involvement of perirectal or perianal lymphatic tissues resulting in fistulas and strictures, tertiary LGV. A self-limited genital ulcer sometimes occurs at the site of inoculation. The lymphadenopathy occurs 2–6 weeks after inoculation. However, by the time patients seek care, the ulcer usually has disappeared (conversely, patients with chancroid have the ulcer and lymphadenopathy concomitantly.)

The diagnosis of LGV is usually made serologically and by exclusion of other causes of inguinal lymphadenopathy or genital ulcers. The chlamydiae have to be cultured in special cell cultures (McCoy cells) and can be diagnosed by fluorescence antibody tests. Complement fixation titers 1:64 are consistent with the diagnosis of LGV.

Recommended Regimen

Doxycycline 100 mg orally twice a day for 21 days, **or erythromycin** base 500 mg orally four times a day for 21 days.

Pregnant and lactating women should be treated with erythromycin. Azithromycin may prove useful for treatment of LGV in pregnancy, but no published data are available regarding its safety and efficacy. Doxycycline is contraindicated in pregnant women.

GRANULOMA INGUINALE

GI, also known as donovaniasis, is a genital ulcerative disease caused by the intracellular gram-negative bacterium *Calymmatobacterium granulomatis*. The organism is found in vacuolated inclusions within leukocytes known as **Donovan bodies.**

The disease occurs rarely in the United States, although it is endemic in certain tropical and developing areas, including India; Papua, New Guinea; central Australia; and southern Africa. Clinically, the disease commonly presents as painless, progressive ulcerative lesions **without regional lymphadenopathy**. The lesions appear 8 days to 12 weeks after inoculation. They are highly vascular ("beefy red appearance") and bleed easily on contact. However, the clinical presentation can also include hypertrophic, necrotic, or sclerotic variants.

GI is generally diagnosed by visual observation of the external symptoms. Gram-stained samples will show the bacteria, which can be cultured under special conditions only. Donovan bodies are found in macrophages on tissue crush preparation or biopsy.

Treatment

Treatment halts progression of lesions, although prolonged therapy may be required to permit granulation and re-epithelialization of the ulcers. Relapse can occur 6–18 months after apparently effective therapy.

Recommended Regimens

Doxycycline 100 mg orally twice a day for at least 3 weeks **or trimethoprim-sulfamethoxazole** one double-strength (800 mg/160 mg) tablet orally twice a day for at least 3 weeks.

Alternative Regimens

Ciprofloxacin 750 mg orally twice a day for at least 3 weeks, **or erythromycin base** 500 mg orally four times a day for at least 3 weeks, **or azithromycin** 1 gm orally once per week for at least 3 weeks.

IV gentamicin (1 mg/kg IV every 8 hours) can be used if lesions do not respond to initial oral therapy in several days or if the patient is HIV positive.

MOLLUSCA CONTAGIOSUM

Mollusca contagiosum is a benign dermatologic disease caused by a poxvirus that has a sexual mode of transmission. Scratching, picking, or breaking will also spread the virus.

The incubation period is 2–7 weeks. The lesions caused by mollusca contagiosum virus (MCV) typically appear as flesh-colored, pearly pink, umbilicated, raised papules (1–5 mm in diameter) or nodules (6–10 mm), which may be single or multiple. They are often asymptomatic.

The diagnosis can be confirmed by light microscopy or electron microscopy of biopsies taken from a blister. Biopsy shows molluscum body, cytoplasmic inclusions containing viral particles. These intracytoplasmic inclusions are also known as Henderson-Paterson bodies.

Treatment

Blisters will regress spontaneously under the control of the immune system. If not, surgical removal by laser, cryotherapy, electro-surgery, or chemical treatment is recommended.

VAGINITIS

Vaginal infection is usually characterized by a vaginal discharge or vulvar itching and irritation; a vaginal odor may be present. The three diseases most frequently associated with vaginal discharge are trichomoniasis (caused by *T. vaginalis*), bacterial vaginosis (caused by a replacement of the normal vaginal flora by an overgrowth of anaerobic micro-organisms, mycoplasmas, and *Gardnerella vaginalis*), and candidiasis (usually caused by *Candida albicans*). These infections are often diagnosed in women being evaluated for STDs.

The cause of vaginal infection can be diagnosed by pH and microscopic examination of the discharge. The pH of the vaginal secretions can be determined by narrow-range pH paper for the elevated **pH (>4.5) typical of bacterial vaginosis (BV) or trichomoniasis.** Discharge can be examined by diluting one sample in one to two drops of 0.9% normal saline solution on one slide and a second sample in 10% potassium hydroxide (KOH) solution. **An amine odor detected before or immediately after applying KOH suggests BV.** The motile *T. vaginalis* or the clue cells of BV usually are identified easily in the saline specimen. The yeast or pseudohyphae of *Candida* species are more easily identified in the KOH specimen.

Bacterial Vaginosis (BV)

BV is a clinical syndrome resulting from replacement of the normal H_2O_2-producing *Lactobacillus* sp. in the vagina with high concentrations of anaerobic bacteria (e.g., *Prevotella* sp. and *Mobiluncus* sp.), *G. vaginalis*, and *Mycoplasma hominis*. BV is the most prevalent cause of vaginal discharge or malodor; however, up to 50% of women with BV may not report symptoms of BV. BV is associated with having multiple sex partners, douching, and lack of vaginal lactobacilli; it is unclear whether BV results from acquisition of a sexually transmitted pathogen. Women who have never been sexually active are rarely affected. Treatment of the male sex partner has not been beneficial in preventing the recurrence of BV.

BV can be diagnosed by the use of clinical or Gram-stain criteria. Clinical criteria require three of the following symptoms or signs:

1. A homogenous, white, noninflammatory discharge that smoothly coats the vaginal walls.
2. The presence of clue cells on microscopic examination.
3. A pH of vaginal fluid >4.5.
4. A fishy odor of vaginal discharge before or after addition of 10% KOH (i.e., the whiff test).

Recommended Regimens

Metronidazole 500 mg orally twice a day for 7 days, **or metronidazole gel** 0.75%, one full applicator (5 gm) intravaginally, once a day for 5 days, **or clindamycin** cream 2%, one full applicator (5 gm) intravaginally at bedtime for 7 days.

Trichomoniasis

Trichomoniasis is caused by the protozoan *T. vaginalis*. Most men who are infected with *T. vaginalis* do not have symptoms. Many infected women have symptoms characterized by a diffuse, malodorous, yellow-green discharge with vulvar irritation. However, some women have minimal or no symptoms. Diagnosis of vaginal trichomoniasis is usually performed by microscopy of vaginal secretions.

Culture is the most sensitive commercially available method of diagnosis. No FDA-approved PCR test for *T. vaginalis* is available in the United States.

Recommended Regimens

Metronidazole 2 gm orally in a single dose.

Vulvovaginal Candidiasis

Vulvovaginal candidiasis (VVC) usually is caused by *C. albicans* but occasionally is caused by other *Candida* sp. or yeasts. Typical symptoms of VVC include pruritus and vaginal discharge. Other symptoms include vaginal soreness, vulvar burning, dyspareunia, and external dysuria. None of these symptoms is specific for VVC. An estimated 75% of women will have at least one episode of VVC, and 40–45% will have two or more episodes.

Treatment

Short-course topical formulations (i.e., single dose and regimens of 1–3 days) effectively treat uncomplicated VVC. The topically applied azole drugs are more effective than nystatin. Treatment with azoles results in relief of symptoms and negative cultures in 80–90% of patients who complete therapy.

ECTOPARASITES

Phthirus pubis

Phthirus pubis is a tiny insect that infects the pubic hair of its victims and feeds on human blood. They use crab-like claws to grasp the hair of their host and can crawl several centimeters per day. Female lice lay 2–3 eggs daily and affix them to the hairs (nits). During direct sexual contact, the insects can move from one partner to the other. **Itching in the pubic area is a telltale sign.** Microscopic examination of the lice or the nits can confirm this. Treatment involves application of 1% gamma benzene hexachloride ointment or lotion. The scalp is treated with lindane 1% shampoo applied for 4 minutes and then washed off. Patients with pediculosis pubis should be evaluated for other STDs.

HUMAN IMMUNODEFICIENCY VIRUS

HIV is an RNA virus (retrovirus) that binds to the CD4 molecule on T4 lymphocytes and some other cell types. Viral RNA undergoes reverse transcription to DNA, which is incorporated into the host DNA. Viral replication occurs by transcription of proviral DNA into viral mRNA, which is associated with a decline in the CD4 cell count and defeat of the immune system. HIV has been isolated from blood, semen, vaginal secretions, saliva, tears, urine, amniotic fluid, breast milk, and cerebrospinal fluid. However, **evidence has implicated only blood, semen, and vaginal secretions in the transmission of the virus.**

Both viral load (molecules of viral RNA/mL) and CD4 T-cell count are used to monitor and prognosticate disease progression to acquired immunodeficiency syndrome (AIDS). **CD4 counts of fewer than 500/mm³ are associated with a greater risk of opportunistic infections and progression to AIDS.**

Most diagnostic tests for HIV measure anti-HIV antibodies using an enzyme linked immunosorbent assay (ELISA); antibody positive specimens are tested using the Western blot assay, which is more specific. Seroconversion usually occurs 1–3 months after initial exposure, during which tests for antibody to HIV are negative, although the person may transmit the infection.

Treatments include nucleoside analogue reverse-transcriptase inhibitors, non-nucleoside reverse transcriptase inhibitors, and protease inhibitors. Indinavir and nelfinavir are associated with renal stones in up to 4% of cases. These stones are not visualized on x-ray or computed tomography. Patients usually improve with hydration and discontinuation of the drug. If necessary, ureteral stenting will usually suffice.

Epidemiology

According to World Health Organization (WHO) estimates, 40 million people worldwide were infected with HIV by December 2003; more than 80% occurred through sexual intercourse. An estimated 70% of HIV-positive men acquired the virus through vaginal intercourse. HIV is more likely in people who have had STDs, especially genital ulcer disease.

Individuals who are infected with STDs are at least two to five times more likely than uninfected individuals to acquire HIV if they are exposed to the virus through sexual contact. In addition, if an HIV-infected individual is also infected with another STD, that person is more likely to transmit HIV through sexual contact than other HIV-infected persons.

STDs probably increase susceptibility to HIV infection by two mechanisms. Genital ulcers (e.g., syphilis, herpes, or chancroid) result in breaks in the genital tract lining or skin. These breaks create a portal of entry for HIV. Nonulcerative STDs (e.g., chlamydia, gonorrhea, and trichomoniasis) increase the concentration of cells in genital secretions that can serve as targets for HIV (e.g., CD4+ cells).

Studies have shown that when HIV-infected individuals are also infected with other STDs, they are more likely to have HIV in their genital secretions. For example, men who are infected with both gonorrhea and HIV are more than twice as likely to shed HIV in their genital secretions than are those who are infected only with HIV. Moreover, the median concentration of HIV in semen is as much as 10 times higher in men who are infected with both gonorrhea and HIV than in men infected only with HIV.

In the HIV-positive patient, genital ulcers are usually caused by STDs such as genital herpes, syphilis, and chancroid, but they may also be part of a systemic illness such as herpes zoster or CMV or may be related to drug therapy (e.g., with the antiviral agent foscarnet).

Serologic tests for syphilis may be false negative in the HIV-infected patient, with a tendency to delayed appearance of seroreactivity. HIV patients with syphilis are more likely to encounter neurologic complications and have a higher rate of treatment failure. Condyloma acuminatum is very common in HIV-infected patients. Visible genital warts caused by HPV type 6 or 11 are found in 20% of HIV-infected patients, compared with 0.1% of the general population.

MCV infection occurs in 5–18% of HIV-positive patients. HIV-positive patients tend to develop giant (>1 cm) lesions or may have clustering of hundreds of small lesions and are at greater risk for secondary inflammation and bacterial infection. MCV lesions in patients with HIV do not resolve quickly, are spread easily to other locations, and are refractory to common treatments. Differential diagnosis includes condylomata acuminata for small, and squamous carcinoma for large, solitary lesions. Treatment options for MCV are the same as for genital warts.

Malignancies

Kaposi's sarcoma (KS) is a sarcoma of endothelial origin, which prior to 1981 was seen only in elderly men of Mediterranean descent, affecting the feet and lower extremities, rarely the genitalia, and ran an indolent course (now called "classic" Kaposi's sarcoma). Development of KS in the HIV population is from a KS-associated herpes virus that is sexually transmitted. Twenty percent of patients with HIV-associated KS will develop lesions on the genitalia. Lesions are subcutaneous, nonpruritic nodules. They can be pigmented, sometimes appearing blue. Lymphedema is common.

Treatment includes local excision, laser fulguration, or radiation therapy for the small solitary lesion. Larger lesions are treated with radiation therapy with possible side effects of urethral strictures or fistulae. Disseminated KS is treated with chemotherapy and interferon.

Testicular tumors occur in up to 0.2%, or 50 times that of the general population. Seminomatous and nonseminomatous tumors are seen, along with HIV-related non-Hodgkin's lymphoma involving the testes. Testicular lymphoma in HIV patients presents in younger men and with higher grade tumor than in non-HIV men.

Treatment for these tumors follow the standard treatment guidelines provided the patient can tolerate the therapy.

Renal, penile, and cervical cancers are also more common in HIV patients and adopt more aggressive courses.

Impotence

Erectile and ejaculatory dysfunction are common problems in HIV-infected men. It is estimated that 67% and 33% of men with AIDS have decreased libido and impotence, respectively. Typically, these HIV-positive men have low serum testosterone levels, normal luteinizing hormone (LH) but high follicle-stimulating hormone (FSH) levels, and oligoteratospermia. Testicular atrophy results from the direct cytotoxic effect of HIV on the germinal and Sertoli cells and secondary effects of HIV infection such as opportunistic infection of the testes, side effects from medication, and effects of cytokines on the hypothalamic-pituitary-gonadal axis.

They may also suffer from psychologic depression, AIDS-related dementia, and neurogenic dysfunction including peripheral neuropathy from viral myelitis and myelopathy, which occurs in 30–40% of AIDS patients. **Patients can be treated successfully with testosterone supplements, phosphodiesterase-5 (PDE-5) inhibitors, or intracavernosal/intraurethral prostaglandins.**

Voiding Dysfunction

Impaired micturition becomes more common with disease progression and can occur as part of an overall neurologic dysfunction or through infection. In a series of 39 HIV-positive patients presenting with lower urinary tract symptoms (LUTS) and undergoing urodynamics, a urodynamic abnormality, an overactive or underactive detrusor or detrusor sphincter dyssynergia was identified in 87% of patients. Of these, 61% had AIDS-related neurologic problems such as cerebral toxoplasmosis, HIV demyelination disorders, and AIDS-related dementia. This heralded a poor prognosis, as 43% in this group died after 2–24 months (mean 8). Detrusor failure caused by lower motor injury is uncommon and is usually ascribed to malignancy or infection such as herpes. Patients should be taught clean intermittent catheterization (CIC) as **long-term indwelling catheters are best avoided in HIV-infected patients because of their vulnerability to *Staphylococcus aureus* bacterium.**

SELF-ASSESSMENT QUESTIONS

1. What is the histologic feature specific to granuloma inguinale?
2. Which antibiotics can be used in pregnancy?

3. What is the most common cause of genital ulcers in the United States?

4. A 35-year-old man presents with tender unilateral inguinal adenopathy. There is some suppuration of the nodes along with the spread to involve the rectum. He does not recall having a genital lesion at any time. What is the most likely diagnosis?

5. A sexually active 25-year-old woman presents with a 3-day history of dysuria and vaginal discharge. The pH of the discharge is 4.5. There is no amine odor on addition of 10% KOH to the discharge (i.e., a negative whiff test). On microscopy, there are numerous poly-morphonuclears (PMNs) and no clue cells. What is the most likely diagnosis?

SUGGESTED READINGS

1. Centers for Disease Control and Prevention: Sexually transmitted diseases treatment guidelines 2002. *MMWR Morb Mortal Wkly Rep* 51:18, 2002.

2. Coburn M: Urological manifestations of HIV infection. *AIDS Res Hum Retroviruses* 14(Suppl 1):S23, 1998.

3. DiCarlo RP, Martin DH: The clinical diagnosis of genital ulcer disease in men. *Clin Infect Dis* 25:292–298, 1997.

4. Goldmeier D, Guallar C: Syphilis: an update. *Clin Med* 3:2009–2011, 2003.

5. Kane CJ, Bolton DM, Connolly JA, et al: Voiding dysfunction in human immunodeficiency virus infections. *J Urol* 155:523, 1996.

6. Krieger JN: Urological implications of AIDS and related conditions. In Wein AJ, Kavoussi LR, Novick AC, Partin AW, Peters CA (eds): *Campbell-Walsh Urology*, 9th ed. New York, Elesvier, 2006, pp 386–404.

7. Miller KE: Sexually transmitted diseases. *Prim Care Clin* 24:179–193, 1997.

8. Potts J: Sexually transmitted and associated diseases. In Wein AJ, Kavoussi LR, Novick AC, Partin AW, Peters CA (eds): *Campbell-Walsh Urology*, 9th ed. New York, Elsevier, 2006, pp 371–385.

9. Rosen T, Brown TJ: Genital ulcers: evaluation and treatment. *Dermatol Clin* 16:673–685, 1998.

10. Wiley DJ, Beutner K, Cox T, et al: External genital warts: diagnosis, treatment and prevention. *Clin Infect Dis* 35: S210–S224, 2002.

C H A P T E R 22

Disorders of the Adrenal Gland

Alexander Kutikov, MD

Urologists care for patients with adrenal disorders principally from the surgical perspective. In this capacity, it is vital to have a fluent knowledge of adrenal anatomy, pathophysiology, and strategies to evaluate adrenal disorders. This chapter provides an overview of adrenal pathophysiology and addresses tactics used in urologic clinical practice to assess and manage surgical adrenal disease.

I. ADRENAL ANATOMY

A. Overview

1. Adrenals, each weighing approximately 4–5 gm and measuring $5 \times 3 \times 1$ cm, are positioned in the retroperitoneum within Gerota's fascia anterior and superomedial to each kidney.
2. The right adrenal, described as triangular, lies posterior and lateral to the inferior vena cava (IVC) and contacts the liver anteriorly.
3. The smaller left gland tends to be semilunar and is intimately related to the upper pole of the left kidney. Anterior to the left adrenal lies the tail of the pancreas and the splenic artery. The diaphragm borders both adrenals posteriorly.

B. Vasculature

Blood flow through the adrenals is substantial, given the endocrine function of the glands. Understanding adrenal vasculature is critical for safe retroperitoneal surgery. The venous drainage of the right gland differs from that of the left, and the surgeon must be aware of this fact.

1. Arterial Supply

a) No one dominant artery supplies either adrenal.
b) Small vessels enter the glands from three main sources:
   (1) Inferior phrenic artery: superior adrenal arteries, majority of blood supply.

    (2) Aorta at the level of the superior mesenteric artery (SMA): middle adrenal arteries.

    (3) Renal artery: inferior adrenal arteries.

c) Arteries rapidly branch, and as many as 60 separate vessels may penetrate the adrenal capsule in a stellate fashion.

2. Venous Drainage

a) Right adrenal vein.

    (1) Short vessel drains directly into the posterior aspect of the IVC.

    (2) If torn during dissection, can result in life-threatening bleeding and has been called "the vein of death."

    (3) In some patients, joins with a right hepatic vein prior to entering the vena cava.

    (4) Accessory right adrenal vein(s) occasionally may be present.

b) Left adrenal vein.

    (1) The left adrenal vein is substantially longer than the right.

    (2) Drains directly into the left renal vein.

    (3) Usually joins with the inferior phrenic vein at some point in its course.

    (4) As on the right, occasionally accessory veins may be present.

C. Histologic Structure

The adrenal gland, surrounded by a capsule, is composed of a yellowish cortex and a red to grey medulla. The cortex stems from the mesoderm, and the medulla originates from the neuroectoderm. At birth, the adrenal is of adult size. The gland rapidly begins to involute following delivery, losing tissue from a region known as the fetal cortex and weighing only 50% of its weight at birth when the child is 1 month of age.

1. Cortex—the adult cortex is composed of three distinct concentric regions and comprises 80% of total adrenal weight.

    a) Zona glomerulosa: mineralocorticoid production (outer zone).

    b) Zona fasciculata: glucocorticoid production (middle zone).

    c) Zona reticularis: androgen production (inner zone).

2. Medulla—lies in the center of the gland beneath the zona reticularis. Rich in chromaffin cells (named so because precipitate chromium salts), the medulla produces catecholamines such as epinephrine, norepinephrine, and dopamine.

II. ADRENAL PHYSIOLOGY

A. Adrenal Cortex Physiology

Adrenal cortex and the adrenal medulla not only have distinct embryologic origins but also function as independent hormone-producing units. With cholesterol-derivative pregnenolone as substrate, numerous enzymes of the adrenal cortex catalyze synthesis of essential hormonal agents. Each of the three zones of the cortex contains different enzymes along the three major synthetic pathways, resulting in three different classes of steroid hormones produced in each zone (Figure 22-1). Steroid hormones do not bind to receptors on cellular membranes but instead modulate gene transcription by uniting with their receptors within the cell and then binding directly to DNA as the receptor-hormone complex.

1. **Zona glomerulosa** is the site for daily production of up to 150 mg of aldosterone, the major mineralocorticoid in humans. Aldosterone is a pivotal player in the renin-angiotensin system and participates in control of the body's fluid and electrolyte equilibrium. This hormone, through its action on the distal convoluted tubule of the kidney, promotes sodium (and therefore fluid) retention and potassium and proton excretion. Secretion of aldosterone is directly influenced by the body's angiotensin II and potassium levels. It is important to note that the hypothalamic-pituitary-adrenal axis plays little role in aldosterone secretion. Indeed, the zona glomerulosa is the only region of the adrenal cortex that does not atrophy following loss of pituitary function.

2. **Zona fasciculata** is the site of glucocorticoid production and excretes up to 30 mg of cortisol each day. Unless pathology is present, cortisol secretion is under tight control of pituitary adrenocorticotrophic hormone (ACTH) through the hypothalamic-pituitary-adrenal axis. Cortisol, essential for life, modulates numerous complex physiologic pathways that include metabolism, immunity, maintenance of intravascular volume, and regulation of blood pressure (BP).

3. **Zona reticularis,** the innermost zone of the adrenal cortex, is the source of adrenal androgens. The major sex steroid hormone of the adrenal is dehydroepiandrosterone (DHEA). Androstenedione and sulfated form of DHEA (DHEA-S) are also formed and along with DHEA act as weak androgens. In normal physiologic states, these hormones have little influence; however, excess production of these agents can lead to profound consequences (e.g., congenital adrenal hyperplasia [CAH]).

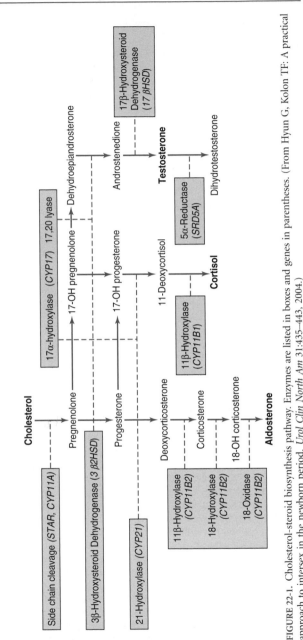

FIGURE 22-1. Cholesterol-steroid biosynthesis pathway. Enzymes are listed in boxes and genes in parentheses. (From Hyun G, Kolon TF: A practical approach to intersex in the newborn period. *Urol Clin North Am* 31:435–443, 2004.)

B. Adrenal Medulla Physiology

The adrenal medulla is an integral part of the autonomic nervous system and the fight and flight response. Chromaffin cells, innervated by preganglionic sympathetic fibers, secrete norepinephrine, epinephrine, and dopamine.

1. Liver rapidly metabolizes catecholamines that are released by the medulla. This breakdown is catalyzed by:
   a) Catechol-O-methyltransferase (COMT).
   b) Monoamine oxidase (MAO).
2. Catecholamine metabolites and small amounts of norepinephrine are excreted in the urine. The major metabolites include:
   a) Metanephrine.
   b) Normetanephrine.
   c) Vanillylmandelic acid (VMA).

III. ADRENAL DISORDERS

A. Increased Adrenal Function

Cushing's syndrome, Conn's syndrome, and pheochromocytoma.

1. **Cushing's syndrome**—condition of excess circulating glucocorticoid.
   a) Signs and symptoms arise from chronic hypercortisolism (Table 22-1).
   b) Causes of excess cortisol: only a minority arise from the adrenal gland.
      (1) Primary adrenal hypercortisolism is a rare cause of Cushing's syndrome.
         (a) Adrenal adenoma and adrenal carcinoma cause approximately the same number of cases of Cushing's syndrome per year ($\sim$10% each).
         (b) Bilateral micronodular hyperplasia is a rare cause of primary adrenal hypercortisolism.
         (c) Bilateral ACTH-independent macronodular hyperplasia—adrenals weigh up to 500 gm each. Extremely rare.
      (2) Nonadrenal causes of Cushing's syndrome.
         (a) Iatrogenic steroid administration is a very common cause of Cushing's syndrome.
         (b) **ACTH-producing pituitary tumors** (Cushing's disease) are responsible for up to 70% of cases of Cushing's syndrome. Adrenal glands are hyperplastic (6–12 gm) but less so than in nonpituitary ectopic ACTH cases.

Table 22-1: Clinical Manifestations of Cushing's Syndrome			
	All[a] (%)	Disease[b] (%)	Adenoma/ Carcinoma[c] (%)
Obesity	90	91	93
Hypertension	80	63	93
Diabetes	80	32	79
Centripetal obesity	80	—	—
Weakness	80	25	82
Muscle atrophy	70	34	—
Hirsutism	70	59	79
Menstrual abnormalities/ sexual dysfunction	70	46	75
Purple striae	70	46	36
Moon facies	60	—	—
Osteoporosis	50	29	54
Early bruising	50	54	57
Acne/pigmentation	50	32	—
Mental changes	50	47	57
Edema	50	15	—
Headache	40	21	46
Poor healing	40	—	—

[a]Hunt and Tyrrell, 1978.
[b]Wilson, 1984.
[c]Scott, 1973.
From Scott HW Jr: In Scott HW, ed. *Surgery of the Adrenal Glands,* Philadelphia, J.B. Lippincott, 1990.

(c) **Ectopic ACTH** is responsible for up to 15% of cases of Cushing's syndrome. Half are caused by paraneoplastic action of small-cell lung cancer. Other malignancies such as carcinoid and pancreatic and thyroid tumors can also be culprits. Adrenal glands become extremely hyperplastic (12–30 gm).

(d) **Ectopic corticotropin-releasing hormone (CRH)** is extremely rare.

c) Comprehensive patient evaluation for Cushing's syndrome is complex and is beyond the scope of this text.

Diagnostic strategies as they relate to urologic practice, however, are discussed later in this chapter (see Evaluation of Adrenal Pathology in Urologic Practice).

2. **Conn's syndrome**—primary hyperaldosteronism.
   a) Signs and symptoms stem from physiologic action of aldosterone to promote renal sodium reabsorption by opening sodium channels in cells of the renal cortical collecting system lumen. Increased urinary potassium secretion results, causing hypokalemia in some patients.
      (1) Hypertension.
         (a) Results from intravascular volume expansion.
         (b) Mean BPs of 180/110 mm Hg in patients with aldosterone-secreting adenomas and 160/100 mm Hg in those with idiopathic bilateral adrenal hyperplasia.
         (c) Renin levels are very low. In cases of secondary hyperaldosteronism (usually due to renal artery stenosis or congestive heart failure [CHF]), renin levels are high.
         (d) Normotensive patients are extremely rare.
      (2) Hypokalemia.
         (a) Not present in all patients.
         (b) Balanced by the renal potassium-sparing effects of hypokalemia itself. Can be exacerbated by sodium loading.
         (c) Can result in polyuria, polydipsia, and muscle weakness.
      (3) Metabolic alkalosis is caused by potassium induced H^+ wasting.
      (4) Lack of edema is due to what has been called the "aldosterone-escape phenomenon." Despite high mineralocorticoid levels, volume urinary fluid loss quickly equilibrates with intake, and volume expansion is only mild.
      (5) Other metabolic abnormalities include mild hypernatremia ($\sim$145 mEq/L) and hypomagnesemia.
      (6) Increased cardiac risks—patients with hyperaldosteronism have higher rates of cardiovascular events independent of hypertension and potassium levels.
   b) Causes of Conn's syndrome.
      (1) Adrenal adenoma.
         (a) Cause of up to 70% of cases of primary hyperaldosteronism.
         (b) Surgical disease.
            (i) BP falls and potassium level return to normal in almost all patients following

adrenalectomy. A lesser degree of hypertension can linger in up to 70% of patients. This may be due to many factors, but the urologist should keep in mind that up to 30% of patients with a solitary adrenal mass actually have bilateral adrenal hyperplasia when adrenal vein sampling is performed.

    (ii) Treatment with preoperative spironolactone has been suggested. Long-term spironolactone or its counterpart eplerenone (lesser binding affinity to androgen and progesterone receptors) is used to treat poor surgical candidates.

  (2) Bilateral adrenal hyperplasia.

    (a) Idiopathic.

      (i) Responsible for 30–40% of Conn's syndrome.

      (ii) Poor response to surgery—a medical disease. Aldosterone receptor blockade is employed.

    (b) Glucocorticoid-suppressible aldosteronism.

      (i) Causes less than 1% of Conn's syndrome.

      (ii) Autosomal dominant.

      (iii) Hyperaldosteronism is ACTH dependent and therefore responds to exogenous glucocorticoid administration.

  (3) Adrenal carcinoma is responsible for less than 1% of primary hyperaldosteronism.

 c) Evaluation of patients with hyperaldosteronism as it relates to urologic practice is addressed later in this chapter (see Evaluation of Adrenal Pathology in Urologic Practice).

3. **Pheochromocytoma** is a tumor of the adrenal medulla that generates, stores, and secretes catecholamines.

 a) Signs and symptoms are a result of epinephrine, norepinephrine, and dopamine release into the bloodstream by neoplastic chromaffin cells.

  (1) Classic symptom triad of headache, palpitations, and diaphoresis.

  (2) Paroxysmal hypertension present in only ~50%, whereas other patients behave identical to those with essential hypertension.

  (3) Orthostatic hypotension (result of hypovolemia), papilledema, weight loss, leukocytosis, polycythemia, hyperglycemia, and cardiovascular

complications have all been associated with pheochromocytoma.

(4) Patients with pheochromocytoma as part of a genetic syndrome (von Hippel-Lindau [VHL], multiple endocrine neoplasia type 2 [MEN2], neurofibromatosis type 1 [NF1]) are often asymptomatic and account for 25% of all patients with pheochromocytomas.

b) Clinical characteristics—the rule of 10s.

(1) Malignant 10%—pathologic documentation of malignancy is problematic as even benign lesions exhibit capsular penetration and vascular invasion. Histologic features are also nonspecific. Malignancy, therefore, is defined as presence of metastasis or invasion of surrounding tissues.

(a) More common in women.

(b) More common in extra-adrenal disease.

(c) Five-year survival 36–60%.

(d) Radiation, resection of metastases, and chemotherapy can be used to treat aggressive cases.

(2) Bilateral 10%—more common with familial disease. Interesting to note that solitary right-sided tumors are ~40% more common than left-sided tumors for unclear reasons and have a three-fold higher risk of recurrence.

(3) Extra-adrenal 10%—known as paragangliomas. Most common extra-adrenal site is the organ of Zuckerkandl (chromaffin bodies at aortic bifurcation). Can also occur in neck, abdomen, and pelvis including the bladder. More common with familial disease. Ten-fold higher risk for recurrence if tumor is extra-adrenal.

(4) Pediatric 10%—common in familial cases.

c) Treatment—sporadic pheochromocytoma is a surgical disease and should be resected. Treatment strategies for familial cases are more controversial as bilateral disease and recurrence rates are high, yet mortality and morbidity of bilateral adrenalectomy are also significant. Partial adrenalectomy has gained popularity in recent years. A multidisciplinary management approach is advised in these patients.

(1) Preoperative catecholamine blockade is paramount, as life-threatening and even lethal catecholamine surges may occur perioperatively. Prior to routine use of prophylactic blockade, surgical mortality was as high as 50%.

(a) Alpha-blockade (or calcium channel blockade) must be initiated 10–14 days preoperatively.

Phenoxybenzamine 10 mg per os (PO) twice a day (b.i.d.) is started and titrated by daily increases of 10–20 mg to a BP of 120/80 mm Hg in a seated position. Mild postural hypotension (systolic blood pressure [SBP] >90 mm Hg in standing position) is tolerated and is a sign of appropriate dosing. In children, 0.2 mg/kg (max 10 mg) daily (QD) dosing should be used with incremental increases by 0.2 mg/kg. Some investigators have shown that calcium channel blockade is just as effective and may be safer than alpha-blockade for preoperative management of pheochromocytoma.

(b) Beta-blockade can be lethal if initiated prior to appropriate alpha-blockade. Used to treat tachycardia, which may result from alpha-blockade and alpha-blockade-induced arrhythmias. Beta-blockade must be administered with great care as CHF, bradycardia, myocardial depression, asystole, and death have all been documented in patients with pheochromocytoma.

(c) α-Methyl-para-tyrosine (metyrosine) administration results in depletion of stored catecholamine, as the agent inhibits tyrosine hydroxylase, the rate-limiting enzyme in biosynthesis of catecholamines. The medication should be used with care as side effects are significant.

(d) Increased salt intake and hydration—after alpha-blockade is initiated the patient should be encouraged to increase salt intake to increase intravascular volume. Admission at least 24 hours prior to surgery is mandatory, so that intravenous (IV) hydration can be administered and appropriate volume status secured.

(e) Intraoperative and postsurgical management—intraoperative hypertension is managed with a nitroprusside drip. Following surgery, a short intensive care unit (ICU) stay is recommended for BP and blood sugar monitoring. Aggressive IV fluids and glucose administration are the postoperative routine.

(2) Prognosis.

(a) Familial, right-sided, and extra-adrenal tumors are more likely to recur.

(b) Recurrence rate for presumed benign lesions is ~15% with 50% of recurrences proving malignant.

(c) Follow-up should be indefinite, because tumors, whether malignant or benign, can recur many years following resection.

(d) Diagnosis of pheochromocytoma demands comprehensive biochemical testing and radiographic evaluation. Diagnostic strategies as they relate to urologic practice are addressed later in this chapter (see Evaluation of Adrenal Pathology in Urologic Practice).

B. Decreased Adrenal Function

Addison's disease (primary adrenal insufficiency), a nonsurgical entity. Etiologies include:

1. Autoimmune/idiopathic.
2. Infectious—tuberculosis, cytomegalovirus (CMV) adrenalitis in human immunodeficiency virus (HIV) patients, fungal infections, syphilis.
3. Infarction/hemorrhage—meningococcemia (Waterhouse-Friderichsen syndrome), pseudomonal and other infections, coagulopathy, trauma.
4. Metastasis—although mets to the adrenals are common, adrenal insufficiency is rare.

C. Abnormal Adrenal Function

CAH is addressed in Chapter 25 of this text.

D. Adrenal Neoplasia

1. **Adrenal carcinoma** is a rare cancer with an abysmal prognosis.
   a) Clinical features.
      (1) Annual incidence is 0.5–2 in 1,000,000 (10 times higher in southern Brazil).
      (2) Occurs in patients 40–50 years of age (most common) and children younger than 5 years of age.
      (3) Linked to MEN1, Beckwith-Wiedemann, and Li-Fraumeni syndromes.
      (4) Left tumors are more common.
      (5) 60% of tumors are functional.
         (a) ~40% Cushing's syndrome.
            (i) Cortisol production per unit volume of tumor is low.
            (ii) Hypercortisolism results from larger masses.

      (b) ~25% Cushing's with virilization—this combination is suggestive of carcinoma, as it is almost never seen with adrenal adenomas.

      (c) 20–30% virilization alone (most common presentation in children).

        (i) Serum testosterone, DHEA, DHEA-S elevated.

        (ii) 17-ketosteroids in 24-hour urine elevated.

      (d) Feminization (~6 %) and hyperaldosteronism (2.5%) are rare.

  (6) Up to 20% of tumors can have vena caval extension.

  (7) 92% of adrenal carcinomas are greater than 6 cm at diagnosis.

  (8) Metastasize to liver, lungs, lymph nodes, and bone.

b) Treatment.

  (1) Surgical resection is the only treatment that impacts survival.

    (a) Local resection is not always curative.

    (b) Debulking is controversial but recommended by most experts.

  (2) Mitotane.

    (a) Drug poisons mitochondria of the adrenal cortical cells.

    (b) Used as primary therapy, adjuvant therapy, and with or without cytotoxic agents for disease recurrence.

    (c) Short-term benefits but not shown to affect survival.

  (3) Cytotoxic agents—cisplatin-based chemotherapy is often used for patients with recurrent adrenal carcinoma in combination with mitotane.

c) Prognosis.

  (1) Children superior prognosis to adults.

  (2) Stage is the most significant prognostic indicator.

    (a) Stage I.

      (i) Tumor ≤5 cm, no local invasion, negative nodes.

      (ii) 5-year survival is up to 50%.

    (b) Stage II.

      (i) Tumor >5 cm, no local invasion, negative nodes.

      (ii) 5-year survival is up to 50%.

    (c) Stage III.

      (i) Local invasion into periadrenal fat or positive nodes without local invasion.

      (ii) 5-year survival is 5%.

    (d) Stage IV.
        (i) Metastatic disease or locally invasive tumor with positive nodes.
        (ii) 5-year survival is 0%.
        (iii) >40% of patients present with stage IV disease.

  d) Diagnosis—diagnostic evaluation of adrenal masses for presence of carcinoma is discussed later in this chapter (see Evaluation of Adrenal Pathology in Urologic Practice).

2. **Neuroblastoma** is addressed in Chapter 26 of this text.

3. **Benign adenoma**—benign tumor of the adrenal cortex.
  a) Prevalence of up to 6% in large autopsy series.
  b) Rich in intracellular lipid, resulting in characteristic imaging features.
  c) No treatment necessary if diagnosis of nonfunctional adenoma can be established with certainty.

4. **Oncocytoma**—benign, nonfunctional cortical tumor.
  a) As is true for renal oncocytoma, adrenal oncocytoma cannot be differentiated from carcinoma on imaging.
  b) Diagnosis is made on pathology following adrenalectomy.

5. **Myelolipoma**—rare, benign, nonfunctional cortical tumor consisting of fat and hematopoietic elements.
  a) Diagnosis easily made on imaging—macroscopic fat is present.
  b) No treatment necessary.
  c) Metabolic workup is suggested as concurrent functional adenomas can occur.

6. **Cysts**—rare adrenal lesions seen in only ~0.2% of autopsies.
  a) Endothelial cysts are most common (~40%).
    (1) Benign.
    (2) Calcifications are common and do not suggest malignancy.
  b) Pseudocysts are second most common adrenal cystic lesion.
    (1) Lack epithelial lining.
    (2) Arise from encapsulation of foci of previous adrenal hemorrhage.
    (3) Can get very large and cause symptoms, otherwise benign.
  c) Cystic lymphangiomas are benign.
  d) Echinococcal cysts can be found in the adrenal.
  e) Epithelial cysts are the most common cystic lesion in the kidney but very rare in the adrenal gland.

7. Metastasis.
   a) Most common primary is the lung.
   b) Fine needle aspiration is helpful in differentiating primary adrenal mass from metastatic disease.

IV. EVALUATION OF ADRENAL PATHOLOGY IN UROLOGIC PRACTICE

Urologists routinely face patients who are referred with an adrenal mass incidentally discovered on imaging (incidentaloma). It is the urologist's responsibility to determine what evaluation is necessary and if intervention is needed.

A. Imaging of Adrenal Masses

Imaging characteristics, size, and interval growth of tumor are used to assess risk of malignancy. Imaging characteristics also afford ability to differentiate between various benign pathologic entities.

1. Imaging characteristics.
   a) Ultrasound is rarely used to evaluate adrenals as normal glands and small nodules are difficult to visualize.
   b) Computed tomography (CT).
      (1) 98% sensitive for adrenal mass (as small as 3 mm).
      (2) Adenoma.
         (a) Homogenous.
         (b) Smooth borders.
         (c) <10 Hounsfield units (HU) on noncontrast CT.
            (i) Up to 100% specific.
            (ii) 70% of adenomas exhibit this finding (remainder of lesions are lipid-poor).
         (d) If >10 HU, assessment with washout imaging can be diagnostic. Adenomas wash out IV contrast much faster (~50% at 5 minutes and ~70% at 15 minutes) than carcinomas and pheochromocytomas.
      (3) Carcinoma.
         (a) Heterogenous contrast enhancement.
         (b) Larger lesions.
         (c) Indistinct margins and irregular contour.
      (4) Myelolipomas: <−30 HU, macroscopic fat, and calcifications.
      (5) Adrenal hemorrhage.
         (a) Acute and subacute: 50–90 HU on unenhanced CT (very specific).

(b) Need to follow bleed to resolution to verify that there is no underlying lesion.

(c) Bilateral hemorrhage is often associated with coagulopathy.

(6) Benign adrenal cysts.

(a) Thin walls (<3 mm).

(b) 50% can have calcifications.

c) Magnetic resonance imaging (MRI).

(1) Fat-suppression and chemical shift analysis can supplement CT imaging. Presence of microscopic fat (intracellular lipid) suggests adenoma.

(2) Adenomas on T2 darker than liver, whereas carcinomas as bright or brighter than liver.

(3) Pheochromocytoma have very high signal intensity on T2 (light bulb sign—not as bright with modern MR techniques). Other lesions can mimic this.

(4) Affords visualization of venous tumor thrombus that is often not possible with CT.

d) [131]I and ^{125}I-metaiodobenzylguanidine (MIBG) isotope scanning is selectively used for pheochromocytoma imaging when possibility of metastatic, extra-adrenal, or recurrent disease must be evaluated.

e) [131]I iodocholesterol (NP-59) scintigraphy.

(1) Early (<5 days) unilateral uptake of tracer suggests functional lesion, whereas no uptake is suggestive of carcinoma.

(2) Currently very limited clinical use.

f) Arteriography—in the past employed to distinguish adrenal tumor from upper pole renal mass. MRI or reformatted CT is able to provide adequate information in current era.

2. Size and growth.

a) Adrenal lesions >4 cm should be resected.

(1) 4 cm cut-off affords ~90% sensitivity.

(2) ~75% of lesions >4 cm are benign on resection.

b) Interval growth.

(1) Current recommendation is to resect all incidentalomas that grow >1 cm on follow-up imaging.

(a) Up to 25% of benign adenomas will have >1 cm increase in size.

(b) Resection of lesions for interval growth seldom uncovers malignancy, especially if growth is sluggish.

(2) Repeat imaging is suggested at 3 and 12 months— can stop if no growth noted.

B. Biopsy of Adrenal Masses

1. Risk of bleeding, hypertension, track seeding, and disruption of surgical planes.
2. Biopsy is unable to differentiate adenoma from carcinoma.
3. Only indicated to assess for adrenal metastasis in the setting of another known malignancy; pheochromocytoma must be biochemically ruled out prior to biopsy.

C. Assessment of Function of Adrenal Masses

1. Up to 18% of incidentalomas harbor metabolic function or malignancy.
   a) 5.3% Cushing's syndrome is subclinical in many patients.
   b) 5.1% pheochromocytoma.
   c) 4.7% adrenocortical carcinoma.
   d) 1% aldosteronoma.
   e) 2.5% metastatic disease.
2. Metabolic workup—all adrenal masses >1 cm in size must be assessed for metabolic function.
   a) **Testing for Cushing's syndrome**—opinions regarding best screening test vary.
      (1) 24-hour urinary cortisol is believed to be most sensitive (up to 100%) and specific (up to 98%) test for diagnosis of Cushing's syndrome.
         (a) Cortisol >20 μg when measured by radioimmunoassay is diagnostic.
         (b) Cortisol >5 μg when measured by high-pressure liquid chromatography is diagnostic.
      (2) Low-dose dexamethasone suppression test (LDDST) is advocated as the initial screening tool by some experts.
         (a) Patient given prescription for 1 mg of dexamethasone (0.3 mg/m^2 in children) and instructed to take the drug at 11 p.m.
         (b) 8 a.m. plasma cortisol level is obtained the following day.
            (i) Cortisol of 5 μg/dL: tumor deemed non-cortisol secreting, but one should be aware that LDDST is at best 95% sensitive at this threshold.
            (ii) Cortisol >5 μg/dL: obtain 24-hour urinary cortisol to confirm.

(3) Other tests—standard 2-day low-dose dexamethasone suppression test, high-dose dexamethasone suppression test (used primarily to test for Cushing's disease), and evening serum and/or salivary cortisol levels can be useful in confirming the diagnosis of Cushing's syndrome.

b) **Testing for pheochromocytoma**—opinions regarding best screening test vary.

  (1) 24-hour urinary metanephrine **and** catecholamine levels (VMA levels not necessary due to low sensitivity).

    (a) Advocated by some experts as the initial screening test in patients with incidentaloma due to high sensitivity and specificity.

    (b) Urinary metanephrine level >1.2 mg/day is indicative of pheochromocytoma.

    (c) Labetalol and buspirone may interfere with some assays and produce false-positive results.

  (2) Plasma fractionated metanephrines (metanephrine and normetanephrine).

    (a) Has gained popularity due to ease of testing and high sensitivity (up to 99%).

    (b) False-positive results are not uncommon (up to 15%) and some believe use of this test is unjustified in patients with incidentalomas (pretest probability too low).

      (i) False positives can arise due to administration of tricyclic antidepressants, phenoxybenzamine, and acetaminophen.

      (ii) Clonidine and/or glucagons suppression tests can help identify false-positive results.

    (c) Test is recommended when clinical suspicion for pheochromocytoma is high, in cases of suspected familial disease, or when a reliable 24-hour urine specimen cannot be obtained (e.g., children).

    (d) Plasma metanephrine level >1.4 pmol/mL or normetanephrine >2.5 pmol/mL indicates a positive test.

c) **Testing for Conn's syndrome.**

  (1) Testing not absolutely indicated in patients without hypertension.

  (2) Morning plasma aldosterone to plasma renin ratio and morning aldosterone level are obtained as a screening test.

(a) Ratio of 20 **and** plasma aldosterone concentration of 15 ng/dL is indicative of Conn's syndrome.
(b) Test can be performed while the patient is taking any antihypertensive medication other than spironolactone (angiotensin-converting enzyme [ACE] inhibitors may give a false-negative result in some patients).
(3) 24-hour urinary aldosterone is the confirmatory test.
   (a) Three days of oral salt loading.
   (b) Daily K^+ level is monitored to avoid hypokalemia (suppresses aldosterone).
   (c) 24-hour urine for aldosterone, Na^+, and creatinine obtained.
   (d) Elevated aldosterone (>14 μg) is diagnostic.
(4) Adrenal vein sampling.
   (a) Some experts believe adrenal vein sampling for aldosterone should be performed in all cases of Conn's syndrome.
   (b) Up to 30% of patients with an adrenal mass and hyperaldosteronism are shown to have bilateral adrenal hyperplasia at the time of adrenal vein sampling, as aldosterone hypersecretion is demonstrated in both glands.
   (c) Adrenal vein sampling in some cases is able to localize mineralocorticoid secretion to one gland or the other when imaging fails to reveal an adrenal nodule.
d) Testing for adrenal sex steroids.
   (1) Routine screening of incidentalomas for androgen/estrogen secretion is not recommended.
   (2) 17-ketosteroid levels can be elevated in 24-hour urine samples of patients with virilizing adrenocortical carcinoma.
e) **Repeat functional testing** is recommended at 12 and 24 months in patients with initially nonfunctional small incidentalomas.

D. Summary of Surgical Indications (Figure 22-2)

1. Functional adrenal mass.
2. Increased risk of malignancy.
   a) Worrisome radiographic findings.
   b) Nonfunctional mass >4 cm.
   c) Nonfunctional mass of 4 cm that is increasing in size.

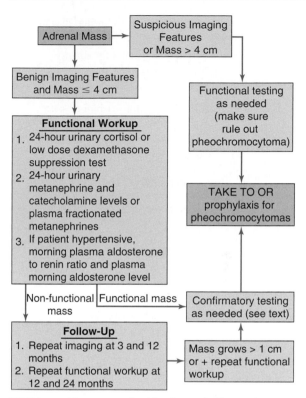

FIGURE 22-2. Management algorithm for newly diagnosed incidental adrenal mass.

SELF-ASSESSMENT QUESTIONS

A 43-year-old man presents to your office following an emergency room visit for left renal colic. Noncontrast CT obtained in the emergency room revealed a 3-mm left distal ureteral stone and a 3.4-cm right adrenal mass measuring 5 HU in attenuation. By the time of the office visit, the patient is pain free and the stone has passed.

1. What is your management?
2. What is your management if the adrenal mass measured 15 HU?

A 25-year-old woman with hypertension, severe headaches, and weight loss is referred to your practice by her family practice physician following diagnosis of pheochromocytoma in the left adrenal gland.

3. How do you prepare this patient for surgery?
4. Intraoperatively, the patient's blood pressure is steadily climbing as you perform the retroperitoneal dissection. As the CRNA pages the attending anesthesiologist, which medication do you instruct him to start?
5. At the postoperative visit, you inform the patient that the pathology report indicates that the lesion is benign. The patient asks you about her chances of recurrence and if any further follow-up is necessary. What do you tell her?

SUGGESTED READINGS

1. Ilias I, Alesci S, Pacak K: Current views on imaging of adrenal tumors. *Hormone Metab Res* 36:430–435, 2004.
2. Ng L, Libertino JM: Adrenocortical carcinoma: diagnosis, evaluation and treatment. *J Urol* 169:5–11, 2003.
3. Pacak K, et al: Recent advances in genetics, diagnosis, localization, and treatment of pheochromocytoma. *Ann Intern Med* 134:315–329, 2001.
4. Thompson GB, Young WF: Adrenal incidentaloma. *Curr Opin Oncol* 15:84–90, 2003.
5. Vaughn ED Jr, Blumenfeld JD, Del Pizzo J, et al: The adrenals. In Walsh PC, Retik AB, Vaughn ED Jr, Wein AJ (eds): *Campbell's Urology*, 8th ed. Saunders, 2002, Philadelphia, pp 3507–3569.

Renal Transplantation

Heidi Yeh, MD,
Kerem H. Bortecen, MD, PhD,
Abraham Shaked, MD, PhD, and
James F. Markmann, MD, PhD

INTRODUCTION

Renal replacement therapy by transplantation is regarded as the treatment of choice for a spectrum of pathology leading to end-stage renal disease. The three diseases most commonly leading to renal failure and treated by kidney transplantation are insulin-dependent diabetes mellitus, glomerulonephritis, and hypertensive nephrosclerosis. Other important causes include polycystic kidney disease, Alport's disease, IgA nephropathy, systemic lupus erythematosus, nephrosclerosis, interstitial nephritis, pyelonephritis, and obstructive uropathy. Although renal transplantation improves survival and quality of life for end-stage renal disease patients, a shortage of donor organs is the major limiting factor; 70,249 are currently on a waiting list for a kidney. In 2005, only 16,478 patients received kidney transplant.

HISTOCOMPATIBILITY CONSIDERATIONS IN LIVING DONOR SELECTION

The transplant between genetically different individuals of the same species is referred to as an allogeneic graft. The exposure to allogeneic grafts stimulates an immune response called alloresponse, which is mediated by alloreactive lymphocytes. The genes that encode key molecules that stimulate rejection of grafts are the major histocompatibility complex (MHC). The human leukocyte antigens (HLAs) are gene products of alleles at a number of closely linked loci on the short arm of chromosome 6 in humans. At least six HLAs (A, B, C, DQ, DP, DR) have been defined, and the existence of several others has been deduced from family studies and immuno-chemical findings. The extreme polymorphism of the HLA system plays a pivotal role in regulation of the immune response as these molecules serve physiologically to bind endogenous and exogenous peptides to allow their presentation to T cells to promote tolerance and immunity.

HLAs are inherited as codominant alleles, and because of the relatively low recombinant frequency, the HLA genes are usually inherited en bloc from each parent. In immediate families, inheritance of the HLA, which significantly impacts transplant outcome, can be determined serologically and falls into four different combinations. Any two siblings have a 25% chance of being HLA identical, that is, of having inherited the same chromosome 6 (haplotype) from each parent, a 50% chance of sharing one haplotype, and a 25% chance of sharing neither haplotype. Parent-to-child donation always involves a one-haplotype identity. The importance of matching HLAs in the selection of living related donors for renal transplantation is well established. Excellent graft survival (>95%) can be expected when a related donor and a recipient are HLA identical. There is a progressively lower graft survival associated with one or zero haplotype matches, although even totally mismatched related living donor grafts have a significantly better outcome than cadaveric grafts.

ALLOGRAFT REJECTION

The clinical manifestations of allograft rejection fall under three categories: hyperacute, acute, and chronic. **Hyperacute rejection** is the classic and most exuberant example of antibody-mediated rejection. Large quantities of preformed antibodies against ABO or MHC antigens bind to these molecules on endothelial cells and activate the classical complement pathway. Early complement components, C3a and C5a, function as anaphylatoxins attracting inflammatory cells and platelets to the target area. The late complement components, C5b-9, form a membrane attack complex (MAC) that, in turn, activates and damages the endothelium. Once the endothelial cells are damaged, the underlying matrix is exposed and tissue factor is released in the circulation. Binding of the tissue factor with factor VIIa activates the extrinsic coagulation cascade, which results in widespread intravascular thrombosis, hemorrhage, and rapid graft loss. With the advance of blood typing and cross-match testing, this type of rejection has become a rare event in the clinical arena. However, hyperacute rejection remains a major barrier to xenotransplantation. Binding of "xenoreactive natural antibodies" to the carbohydrate galactose-a-1,3-galactose expressed in porcine endothelial cells causes the activation of human complement on xenogeneic cells leading to hyperacute rejection. **Acute rejection** is typically viewed as a T cell–mediated process. In several animal models, recipients lacking T cells cannot reject fully mismatched allografts, and reconstitution of these animals with T cells restores the rejection process. Current immunosuppressive protocols directly target T cells and many agents exert their action through the inhibition of T-cell activation. T cells involved in allorecognition can be sensitized against alloantigen via one of two distinct, but not mutually exclusive, pathways: direct and indirect. Direct recognition requires that the recipient T cells recognize intact donor MHC molecules complexed with peptide on donor antigen presenting cells (APCs). In contrast, indirect recognition requires that recipient APCs process donor MHC antigens prior to presentation to recipient T cells in a self-restricted manner. The direct pathway is unique to transplantation. **Chronic allograft rejection** is the major cause of late allograft loss. Although the pathogenesis is not fully understood, it has been suggested that in contrast to acute rejection the indirect pathway may dominate in chronic rejection because the donor-derived APCs that are the primary trigger for the direct pathway are progressively depleted over time. There are data suggesting that antibodies and complement play a key role in chronic rejection. Production of alloantibodies in association with episodes of acute rejection has been long recognized. Recent evidence suggests that the development of anti-MHC class II alloantibodies after transplantation may be a risk factor for chronic rejection, independent of acute rejection. Chronic rejection associated vasculopathy is a poorly understood phenomenon, involving both immune- and nonimmune-mediated damage to the endothelial cells, which leads to endothelial proliferation, a process known as intimal hyperplasia. Immunosuppression itself has been attributed to the development of transplant-associated vasculopathy. Apoptosis might be an important mechanism of antibody-mediated injury during chronic rejection. Although modern immunosuppressive regimens are very effective in reducing episodes of acute rejection, chronic rejection continues to be the major cause of long-term graft loss.

IMMUNOSUPPRESSION

Immunosuppression following kidney transplant can be considered in three phases: (1) induction, a short period of heavy immunosuppression at the time of transplant to enable acceptance of the organ; (2) maintenance therapy, chronic immunosuppression at lower levels to prevent episodes of acute rejection; and (3) treatment of acute rejection, brief periods of high-dose immunosuppression directed toward an activated immune system attacking the organ. Some of the drugs commonly used in renal transplantation include the following.

Steroids (Induction, Rejection, Maintenance)

Corticosteroids complex with intracellular receptors and inhibit transcription of cytokines such as interleukin (IL)-1, IL-2, IL-6, interferon (IFN)-gamma, and tumor necrosis factor (TNF)-alpha. They also prevent lymphocyte margination, decrease chemotaxis, and impair macrophage and granulocyte function. Long-term use of corticosteroids is associated with multiple side effects including hypertension, hyperlipidemia, hyperglycemia, cataracts, osteoporosis, psychosis, pancreatitis, gastrointestinal (GI) bleeding, ulceration and perforation, poor wound healing, and growth retardation. Historically, chronic steroids have been used for all patients as part of a maintenance regimen, with high-dose pulses being given at induction or for treatment of acute rejection. Because of adverse effects, newer protocols for select patients can include steroid withdrawal within a week to months of transplant.

Calcineurin Inhibitors (Maintenance)

The complex of cyclosporine (Neoral/Sandimmune) and cyclophilin binds calcineurin, inhibiting its ability to upregulate IL-2 expression. Cyclosporine is metabolized by the cytochrome p450 system in the liver, and its dosing must be adjusted when given with other drugs that either compete for the p450 system or upregulate its activity. One of the notable side effects accompanying cyclosporine use is nephrotoxicity, with long-term use leading to the development of interstitial fibrosis. Other side effects include tremor, seizures, gingival hyperplasia, hypertension, and hyperkalemia.

Tacrolimus (FK506/Prograf) binds to an intracellular protein named FK-506 binding protein (FKBP). The complex of FK506 and FKBP inhibits calcineurin activity, ultimately inhibiting IL-2 expression. Tacrolimus also inhibits production of IL-3, IL-4, IFN-γ, and expression of the IL-2 receptor. Tacrolimus can cause significant nephrotoxicity, hypertension, hypomagnesemia, and hyperkalemia. Tacrolimus-induced central nervous system (CNS) toxicity can manifest as headaches, tremors, mental status changes, or seizures. Another serious side effect of tacrolimus is diabetes, which seems to be related to inhibition of insulin gene transcription as well as some degree of beta cell damage. Tacrolimus-associated diabetes is sometimes reversible.

Cell Cycle Inhibitors (Maintenance)

Sirolimus (rapamycin/Rapamune) also binds to FKBP but does not exert its immunosuppressive activity via the calcineurin pathway. Rather, the complex of sirolimus and FKBP ultimately inhibits cyclin dependent kinases necessary for T cells to progress from G1 to S phase during the proliferative response to IL-2 and IL-6. Sirolimus exhibits much less nephrotoxicity than calcineurin inhibitors but does cause hyperlipidemia, hypertension, pneumonitis, acne, and rashes. It is not used in the perioperative period because its profound inhibition of fibroblast activity prevents wound healing.

Antimetabolites (Maintenance)

Mycophenolate mofetil or its active form, mycophenolic acid (MPA) (MMF/Cellcept/Myfortic), inhibits the activity of inosine monophosphate dehydrogenase (IMPDH), an enzyme in the de novo guanine synthesis pathway. B and T cells are dependent on de novo guanine synthesis for proliferation, so MPA inhibits leukocyte proliferation without the skin, hair, and GI side effects that other antimetabolites cause. MPA also blocks glycosylation of adhesion molecules, inhibiting leukocyte recruitment. Although MMF has no renal toxicity, it does cause bone marrow suppression and GI symptoms such as nausea, diarrhea, and vague abdominal pain and is contraindicated in pregnancy. MMF has reduced absorption with magnesium and aluminum hydroxide.

Once the first-line antimetabolite, azathioprine (Imuran) is now used only for patients who are intolerant of MMF. It is converted to 6-thioguanine in the liver and has preferential uptake into B and T cells where it is incorporated into DNA and inhibits DNA replication and RNA transcription. Adverse effects include increased risk of malignancy, hepatitis, myelosuppression (especially leukopenia), cholestasis, alopecia, and pancreatitis. Azathioprine is contraindicated in pregnancy and should not be used with angiotensin-converting enzyme (ACE) inhibitors as the combination can result in severe anemia and pancytopenia. Azathioprine doses must be decreased when given with allopurinol, because allopurinol inhibits the degradation of azathioprine to its inactive metabolite.

Anti-T Cell Antibodies (Induction, Rejection)

Thymoglobulin is a polyclonal rabbit antithymocyte antibody preparation, whereas ATGAM is isolated from horses. Once T cells are bound by antibody, they are depleted from the circulation through opsonization and complement-assisted, antibody-dependent cell-mediated cytotoxicity (ADCC). Damaged T cells are cleared by the lymphoreticular system. OKT-3 (muromonab-CD3) is a monoclonal murine IgG2a antibody against the TCR-CD3 complex. Initially, after administration of OKT-3 there is a transient activation of T cells and a massive release of cytokines. This is called the "cytokine release syndrome" and is characterized by fevers, chills, dyspnea, bronchospasm, flash pulmonary edema, and CNS complications. Antibody-bound T cells are then removed from the circulation by opsonization and ADCC. Although T cells will reappear, they are CD3-negative as a result of receptor downregulation and are not able to be activated.

Anti-IL2 Receptor Antibodies (Induction)

Basiliximab (Simulect) and daclizumab (Zenapax) are chimeric murine/human antibodies that bind to the IL-2 receptor alpha chain. Also known as CD25, this component of the high-affinity IL-2 receptor is expressed preferentially on activated T lymphocytes. There are few serious side effects from IL-2 receptor antibodies, but they are less potent than antithymocyte antibodies and are generally reserved for recipients who are at low risk for rejection (receiving HLA identical kidneys) or those with high risk for secondary infections.

Anti-B Cell Antibodies (Rejection, Desensitization)

Rituximab is a human/murine chimeric antibody with the human Fc regions fused to the murine variable regions that recognize CD20, a surface marker found on B cells. Frequently used to treat non-Hodgkin's B cell lymphoma, its use in the transplant arena is mainly for treatment of steroid-resistant antibody-mediated rejection or rejection with evidence of vasculitis, especially those with peritubular C4d-positive immunohistochemical staining as a marker for humoral rejection. Rituximab is sometimes used in conjunction with plasmapheresis and intravenous immunoglobulins (IVIG) to deplete potential recipients of preformed antibodies in an attempt to find compatible kidneys for them. It is also used for treatment of post-transplant lymphoproliferative disorder (PTLD) that does not respond to reduced immunosuppression.

EVALUATION OF KIDNEY DONORS

Living Donors

Transplant outcomes with kidneys from living donors are better than those from cadaveric donors because of a variety of factors including that living donor kidneys are in better condition and have minimal cold ischemia time, the time of transplant may be optimized for the recipient, and the recipient and donor may be better matched for HLA and non HLA encoded minor antigens. The donor must be in good health and have two normal kidneys, as confirmed by standard renal function tests and imaging of the kidneys, collecting system, and vessels. Magnetic resonance angiography (MRA) or computed tomography angiography (CTA) is now substituted for contrast arteriography and intravenous pyelography at many centers. This minimizes the risk of the procedure to the donor, although it has the disadvantage that small accessory renal arteries may not be visualized by this technique. The left kidney is chosen if possible because its longer renal vein facilitates the recipient operation. However, if the arteriogram shows multiple renal arteries on one side, the kidney with a single artery is usually selected. Following nephrectomy, the remaining kidney hypertrophies, resulting in near-normal renal function, and normal life expectancy; some develop proteinuria, hypertension, and renal failure, but at rates similar to the control population.

Deceased Donors

Optimal cadaveric kidneys come from previously healthy, brain dead donors between 2 and 60 years of age who are hemodynamically stable with good urine output and have a normal creatinine and urinalysis. Extended criteria donor (ECD) kidneys are taken from older donors, donors with elevated creatinines, donors with a long history of hypertension, and donors after cardiac death and are additionally evaluated by frozen section for glomerulosclerosis, fibrosis, and tubular necrosis. Suboptimal kidneys may be totally adequate for older recipients who need fewer years of function from the transplant or may be the only option for highly sensitized recipients who have few compatible donors. The use of kidneys from infants is associated with an increased incidence of technical complications because of small vessel size. Active viral infections or history of human immunodeficiency virus (HIV), systemic bacterial and fungal infections, and a history of malignancy with risk of metastasis are usually contraindications to cadaveric kidney donation. Hepatitis B virus (HBV)- and hepatitis C virus (HCV)-positive kidneys are used selectively for HBV-positive/immune and HCV-positive recipients, respectively, and a history of cytomegalovirus (CMV) exposure in the donor is treated with prophylaxis in the recipient.

DONOR OPERATION

Laparoscopic Nephrectomy

The laparoscopic approach is now the preferred technique at most institutions. Its advantages include more rapid recovery and reduced perioperative pain, and it has been proven to be safe and able to recover a kidney with function equivalent to the traditional open approach.

Following the induction of general anesthesia, the patient is positioned in right lateral decubitus position. Pneumoperitoneum is established with a 12-mm port placed in the mid-left upper abdomen and a second port is generally placed just lateral to the rectus at the level of the iliac crest. An 8-cm Pfannenstiel incision is created midway between the umbilicus and the symphysis pubis for placement of a hand-assist device. First, the colon and spleen are mobilized medially along the white line of Toldt to expose the renal hilum. The renal vein is then skeletonized and the adrenal and gonadal branches divided as are a varying number of lumbar branches. The ureter is dissected down to the pelvic brim with care being taken to avoid its devascularization. The artery is then skeletonized to its origin from the aorta. Once the kidney is fully mobilized except for artery, vein, and ureter, the patient is treated with mannitol and furosemide (Lasix) to promote diuresis, and intravenous heparin is administered after the ureter is divided. The artery and vein are then stapled with the endovascular stapler and then divided. Once the kidney is extracted, it is taken to the back table for perfusion with cold heparinized preservation solution and prepared for implantation.

Open Nephrectomy

The "open" technique is a well-proven procedure to safely procure kidneys from live donors. It remains the fallback procedure in patients with complex arterial anatomy and for laparoscopic cases in which difficulties are encountered intraoperatively.

It is performed through an incision made over the eleventh rib, deepened through the subcutaneous tissue, and extended anteriorly toward the rectus muscle. The latissimus dorsi muscle posteriorly and external oblique muscles are divided with the underlying transversalis fascia to expose the retroperitoneal. After the incision of the Gerota's fascia, the perinephric adipose tissue is removed and the renal vein and artery are exposed. Gonadal and adrenal veins and lumbar branches are ligated separately. After transecting the ureter, first the renal artery is ligated and transected at its origin from aorta, then the renal vein is transected. The kidney is taken to the back table for perfusion with cold heparinized preservation solution and prepared for transplantation.

ALLOCATION

United Network for Organ Sharing (UNOS)'s point system for cadaveric kidney allocation emphasizes wait time, which accrues only after the glomerular filtration rate (GFR) is <20 mL/min, and HLA matching. In addition, crossmatching by mixing recipient serum with donor cells in the presence of complement is performed at the time of allocation to detect preformed antibodies that could result in hyperacute rejection. A positive crossmatch, meaning the donor recipient pair is considered incompatible, indicates the presence of antidonor antibodies in the recipient. Periodically, while on the wait list, a panel reactive antibody (PRA) is checked by screening recipient serum with a panel of randomly selected HLA-typed lymphocyte donors. The results are reported as a percentage of donors with which the recipient serum reacts and predicts the likelihood that a recipient will be compatible with a donor. Although the benefits of six antigen-matched (or zero antigen-mismatched) kidney transplants is well established, the importance of lesser degrees of HLA-matching remains controversial. Extra points may also be granted by request for recipients who were previously living kidney donors and patients with intractable dialysis access problems. Children now get preference for cadaveric kidneys from donors younger than 35 years.

EVALUATION OF RECIPIENTS

Recipients undergo a standard medical workup with special attention to cardiovascular status, especially in older patients and diabetics. Efforts are made to eradicate infections prior to immunosuppression. Prior malignancies require varying time periods of disease-free survival to reduce the probability that immunosuppression would promote recurrence. Dialysis should be initiated if necessary to optimize the patient's volume, nutrition, and electrolyte status rather than compromising the recipient's health for the sake of avoiding dialysis prior to transplant. Potential recipients are tested for CMV, syphilis, HIV, HBV, HCV, ABO, and HLA. CMV and syphilis can be treated, and HBV and HCV infection are not contraindications to transplant in the absence of liver damage (in the presence of cirrhosis, patients may be candidates for combined liver/kidney transplant), although there is a risk of disease progression with initiation of immunosuppression. Investigational protocols are now under way for transplanting HIV+ patients who meet strict criteria. Bilateral nephrectomy is performed only for special indications, such as recalcitrant urinary tract infections (especially in the presence of stones, reflux, or obstruction), uncontrollable hypertension, massive proteinuria, bilateral renal tumors, or large polycystic kidneys, for bleeding, infection, or to make space for the new kidney.

RECIPIENT OPERATION

Following general anesthesia, the iliac vessels are exposed retroperitoneally through an oblique incision just above the inguinal ligament. A consideration in selecting the appropriate side should be made to avoid sites of previous transplants, other operations (e.g., appendectomy, herniorrhaphy, or bladder or ureteral operations), or peritoneal dialysis catheters. Lymphatics that must be divided to expose the iliac vessels are ligated to prevent prolonged lymph drainage or lymphocele formation. Exposure of the bladder is facilitated by dividing the inferior epigastric vessels and, in females, the round ligament. Spermatic cord should not be divided to avoid epididymitis, testicular ischemia, and atrophy. Vascular anastomoses are performed in an end-to-side fashion between the renal artery and external iliac artery and donor renal vein to the external iliac vein. If there are multiple donor renal arteries that are not on a common aortic cuff, anastomoses of the end of the smaller renal arteries to the side of the largest renal artery could be performed. Attempts should be made not to sacrifice even small accessory donor renal arteries to avoid renal infarcts. Preservation of accessory arteries to the lower portion of the kidney is especially important because they may constitute the blood supply of a segment of collecting system or ureter and their ligation may lead to necrosis and urinary fistula. Venous collateral circulation is almost always adequate so that, in instances of multiple renal veins (which are even more common than multiple arteries), only one large vein need be saved for anastomosis. If a large adult kidney is to be transplanted into a small child, a transperitoneal approach is used to provide adequate room for the kidney, which is revascularized via the aorta and vena cava. Urinary tract continuity is usually established by ureteroneocystostomy. The ureter should pass beneath the spermatic cord to avoid obstruction. Ureteropyelostomy (anastomosis of the recipient's ureter to the pelvis of the donor kidney) is an alternative procedure, which should be used in instances of donor ureteral devascularization or injury. A few surgeons prefer this procedure to ureteroneocystostomy, but it is associated with a higher incidence of urinary fistula. Meticulous technique and hemostasis are particularly important because of the coagulopathy and susceptibility to infection of uremic immunosuppressed patients. We prefer to close the wound without drains, but if hemostasis is suboptimal, closed suction catheters may be used.

POST-TRANSPLANT MANAGEMENT

In the absence of severe ischemic damage, a brisk diuresis is likely to begin within minutes of revascularization due to osmotic factors secondary to uremia or high glucose concentrations in intravenous fluids, total body fluid and electrolyte overload secondary to chronic uremia, and mild proximal tubular damage resulting from allograft ischemia. Mild diuresis is reassuring and should be encouraged by replacement of urine volumes and, if necessary, by diuretics. Severe dehydration and electrolyte abnormalities can be the outcome of inadequate replacement of losses during a massive diuresis, especially in children. If diuresis continues, fluid replacement should lag behind the urine output, allowing gradual return to normal urine volumes over the next 12–24 hours.

COMPLICATIONS OF RENAL TRANSPLANTATION

Complications occurring in the first few hours or days after transplantation are commonly related to technical problems in establishing vascular and urinary continuity or to damage that occurs during donor nephrectomy or preservation. Because rejection may also be an early event, its differentiation from various other causes of poor function may be difficult.

Acute Tubular Necrosis

Ischemia and reperfusion injury occasionally precipitate acute tubular necrosis (ATN) in a living donor transplant and more frequently in cadaver transplants. Even in transplants from "heart-beating cadavers," some degree of ATN occurs in 5–30%. A kidney may have adequate urine output briefly and then lapse into ATN. Delayed graft function reduces the 5-year graft survival by 10%.

Urinary Tract Complications

Ureteroneocystostomy anastomosis may become occluded by a hematoma at the site of the submucosal tunnel in the bladder or by a technically unsatisfactory anastomosis. An adynamic ureter or edema at the orifice in the bladder can also cause temporary partial obstruction. Devascularization of the ureter during donor nephrectomy is a more serious problem that may lead to ureteral necrosis and fistula within the first few days or weeks. Mild ureteral ischemia is the probable cause of an occasional late distal ureteral stenosis, which may lead to partial or total occlusion. Ultrasound, radioactive scans, and cystograms are helpful. However, ureterography is usually necessary to define the status of the ureter and is best accomplished by percutaneous fine-needle puncture of the kidney and antegrade catheterization of the pelvis and ureter. Treatment must be individualized and may consist either of reconstruction of the ureteroneocystostomy (if it is not ischemic) or of ureteropyelostomy using the patient's own ureter.

Vascular Complications

Arterial obstruction, although less common than ATN or urinary tract complications as a cause of early postoperative oliguria or anuria, should be considered promptly if an established diuresis suddenly ceases. Partial occlusion of the transplant vessels may be caused by kinking from unfortunate positioning of the kidney. Although radioisotopic scanning and arteriography will confirm suspected vascular occlusion, immediate reoperation without delay for diagnostic studies is usually the only chance for salvaging such a graft. Occlusion of the transplant renal vein, although rare, can result from technical anastomotic errors or from kinking or compression.

Hemorrhage

Imperfect operative hemostasis in the setting of uremic coagulopathy or anticoagulation during hemodialysis is the usual cause of early postoperative bleeding. Fracture and frank rupture of the transplanted kidney are unusual causes of bleeding, but these may occur from rapid swelling of the transplant during acute rejection. Rupture is more common in kidneys from infant or child donors, in which the small organ is sometimes unable to tolerate adult levels of blood pressure and flow. Bleeding from the arterial suture line, except in the early hours postoperatively, should bring to mind the strong possibility of infection.

Lymphoceles

Extensive mobilization of the iliac vessels during the transplant operation or failure to ligate lymphatics crossing them may predispose to lymphoceles, which have a variable reported incidence (0.6–18%). Possible manifestations that can occur weeks or months postoperatively are swelling of the wound; edema of the scrotum, labia, and lower extremity; and urinary obstruction from pressure on the collecting system or ureter. Ultrasound to identify a fluid-filled mass is the most useful diagnostic study. Aspiration of the cyst will be of only temporary benefit because lymph rapidly reaccumulates. External drainage should be avoided because this will place the kidney and vascular suture line at risk from infection. The treatment of choice is fenestration of the cyst into the peritoneal cavity. This can be performed by open or laparoscopic technique.

NONTECHNICAL COMPLICATIONS

Opportunistic Infections

The period between 30 and 180 days after transplantation, usually the time of most intense immunosuppression, is the most common time for infection with opportunistic organisms, which in normal individuals rarely cause significant illness.

CMV is the most important viral pathogen. Although in healthy individuals CMV infections are either clinically silent or mild, the presence of the latent virus and seropositivity persists for life. After renal transplantation, previously seropositive patients may have symptomatic illness sometimes (20%) and it is usually mild. However, seronegative recipients who receive a kidney from a seropositive donor are subject to a three times greater incidence of symptomatic illness, and of affected patients 25% have severe disease. CMV "disease" varies in severity from mild fever and malaise to a debilitating syndrome marked by leukopenia, hepatitis, interstitial pneumonia, arthritis, and CNS changes including coma, GI ulceration and bleeding, renal insufficiency, bacterial or fungal infection, and even death.

Polyomavirus nephropathy. Primary infections with the polyomavirus (type BK) are known to occur in up to 90% of the population, typically without specific signs or symptoms. This virus persists in the kidney where reactivation and shedding into the urine may be detected in 0.5–20% of healthy individuals. Progression from an inflammatory stage to a fibrotic stage and finally to sclerosis and irreversible allograft failure has been observed in as many as 45% of affected cases. Current management is based on judicious decreases in immunosuppression to allow clearance of viral replication. In a few instances, the antiviral agent cidofovir has been used with success.

Other opportunistic infections such as aspergillosis, blastomycosis, nocardiosis, toxoplasmosis, and cryptococcosis are particularly likely to occur in transplant patients. The protozoan *Pneumocystis carinii* is a pulmonary pathogen most commonly causing fatal pneumonia in immunodeficient patients. A prompt diagnosis by aggressive measures such as bronchoscopic alveolar lavage and brushing or percutaneous transbronchoscopic or open-lung biopsy is important in cases of *P. carinii* infection because effective treatment exists (trimethoprim and sulfamethoxazole). Prophylaxis with the same agents is warranted in the early postoperative period and also reduces the incidence of bacterial urinary tract infections. Mycobacterial infections are unusual, but their potential lethality mandates constant vigilance.

Hyperparathyroidism

Secondary hyperparathyroidism from chronic renal failure usually subsides after a successful transplant. However, its persistence ("tertiary hyperparathyroidism") has been reported. In cases in which significant hypercalcemia and elevated parathyroid hormone levels persist for more than 12 months after transplant despite normal renal function, total parathyroidectomy and autotransplantation of fragments from a portion of one gland is recommended to avoid the sequelae of hyperparathyroidism, such as renal calculi, bone pain, and muscle weakness.

Malignancy

In renal transplant recipients, the reported incidence of 6% de novo malignant neoplasms represents a risk approximately 100 times greater than that in normal age-matched populations. The increased incidence of tumors appears to be related to the degree and duration of immunosuppression rather than to any particular agent. These tumors often occur in young patients, and their behavior is unusually aggressive. Cancers common in the general population (lung, breast, prostate, and colon) are not increased, but certain uncommon neoplasms are extremely prevalent (lymphomas, lip cancers, renal cancers, various other sarcomas, hepatobiliary carcinomas, Kaposi's sarcoma, and carcinomas of the vulva and perineum). Carcinomas of the uterine cervix are also very common, although most of these are in situ lesions. All transplant recipients have a disproportionately high incidence of lymphomas (350 times normal), known as PTLD, covering a spectrum of lesions ranging from benign hyperplasia to frankly malignant lymphomas. In patients with these tumors, extranodal involvement is common (69%) and the transplanted kidney is often involved (23%). Growing evidence implicates infection with the Epstein-Barr virus as the most important factor in PTLD. These patients often have a syndrome resembling mononucleosis with fever, pharyngitis, and diffuse lymphadenopathy. Treatment is usually the reduction or cessation of immunosuppressive therapy.

RESULTS OF RENAL TRANSPLANTATION

At 5 years, 90% of HLA-identical sibling grafts survive and at 10 years, survival is 65%. Despite striking advances in immunosuppressive therapy, the survival of cadaveric grafts at 5 years is only 65% and at 10 years less than 40% unless they are matched for the recipient's HLA antigens; in this case survival is improved with 5-year survival to about 73%. Many other factors also influence the results of transplantation. Those compromising outcomes include unusually young or old recipients or donors (<5 or >50 years); inter-racial grafts; broadly sensitized recipients as identified by preformed antibodies against a panel of donor lymphocytes; previous failed transplants, especially if lost from early rejection; delayed transplant function, requiring dialysis; poor early function (serum creatinine >3 mg/dL at time of hospital discharge); and certain disease states (e.g., hypertensive nephrosclerosis, oxalosis). Despite improvements in crossmatching and immunosuppression, sensitized recipients of first cadaveric kidneys had a 14% greater incidence of delayed graft function and an 8% lower graft survival at 5 years. Impatience with long waiting times for cadaveric donor kidneys has led to a considerable increase in the use of living donors, which now exceed the number of cadaveric donors in the United States compared with less than 20% a decade ago. Unfortunately, donation of cadaveric kidneys has increased little, and most of this minimal increase has been from suboptimal donors; the percentage of cadaveric kidneys from donors older than 50 years increased from 26% in 1988 to 46% in 2000. The incidence of delayed graft function in kidneys from donor after cardiac death (DCD) was nearly double that of transplantation from heart-beating brain-dead donors (43% vs. 22%).

SELF-ASSESSMENT QUESTIONS

1. What are the indications for kidney transplant and what are the advantages of transplant over dialysis?
2. Who is a candidate to be a living kidney donor? How are laterality and operative approach chosen?
3. Why are living donor kidneys preferable to cadaveric kidneys?
4. What diagnostic tests and maneuvers are available to monitor transplant kidney function?
5. How does immunosuppression alter peri- and post-operative management in the transplant patient?

SUGGESTED READINGS

1. Buell JF, Gross TG, Woodle ES: Malignancy after transplantation. *Transplantation* 80(2 Suppl):S254–264, 2005.
2. Halloran PF: Immunosuppressive drugs for kidney transplantation. *N Engl J Med* 351:2715–2729, 2004.
3. Humar A, Matas AJ: Surgical complications after kidney transplantation. *Semin Dial* 18:505–510, 2005.
4. Scandling JD: Kidney transplant candidate evaluation. *Semin Dial* 18:487–494, 2005.
5. The OPTN/UNOS renal transplant registry: *Clin Transpl* 1:1–16, 2004.

C H A P T E R 24

Renovascular Hypertension

Jagajan Karmacharya, MD,
Shane S. Parmer, MD, and
Jeffrey P. Carpenter, MD

I. OVERVIEW

Renovascular hypertension (RVH) is present in 1–5% of all patients with high blood pressure (BP). Severe hypertension (HTN) particularly in the extremes of age is most likely due to renovascular disease. Clinically significant renal artery disease correlates with age, severity of HTN, and the presence of renal insufficiency and is the most common cause of surgically treatable high BP. Currently, the vast majority of these patients are treated by vascular surgeons using minimally invasive endovascular techniques.

II. HISTORICAL OVERVIEW

Bright from Guys Hospital, London was the first to associate HTN and renal disease in 1836. The classic experiments of Goldblatt in 1934 clearly demonstrated that ischemia localized to the kidneys was sufficient to elevate BP, which, in its early stages, was unaccompanied by decreased renal function. Clinical evidence of the validity of Goldblatt's experiment came in 1938 when Leadbetter and Burkland cured sustained diastolic HTN in a 5-year-old boy by nephrectomy. Pathologic examination of the renal artery from this kidney revealed a lumen severely occluded by a mass of smooth muscle outlined by an elastic lamella representing fibromuscular hyperplasia (FMH). Evidence linking atherosclerotic obstruction of the renal arteries to HTN was described in 1937 by Moritz and Oldt, who described severe vessel obstruction in an autopsy series of chronic hypertensives. These findings set a trend toward many unfortunate nephrectomies over the next several years, until Smith in 1956 published a large series demonstrating only a 26% cure rate and questioned the use of unilateral nephrectomy for RVH. It was the development of translumbar arteriography in the 1950s that opened the door to large-scale investigation, ultimately paving the way for the development of surgical techniques for the correction of RVH. Most recently, with the rapid progress in the use of less invasive endovascular techniques for RAS, open surgical management has become less common.

III. PATHOLOGY

A. General

1. Significant stenosis of the renal artery is necessary to produce RVH.
2. The specific etiology of the narrowing may be related to atherosclerosis, renal artery fibrodysplasia, developmental renal artery stenosis, renal artery thrombosis or embolism, dissecting aortic aneurysm, arteriovenous fistula, trauma, Takayasu's arteritis, transplant renal artery stenosis, or renal artery aneurysm.
3. Most common causes for RVH are atherosclerosis and renal artery fibrodysplasia.

B. Etiology

1. **Atherosclerotic renovascular disease** is by far the most common etiology of renovascular disease. Men are affected twice as often as women, reflecting the prevalence of arteriosclerosis in the male population. The sex difference is less apparent in the elderly. The frequency of renovascular **arteriosclerosis is more common in elderly patients.** In autopsy series, moderate to severe renal artery atherosclerosis is found in 50% of normotensive patients and in 75% of hypertensive patients. **Most renovascular atherosclerotic lesions occur at the renal artery ostium of the aorta or within the first few centimeters of the main renal artery** (Figure 24-1). These lesions often represent "aortic spillover" lesions and are a continuation of the atherosclerotic disease in the aorta as it enters the renal artery ostium. Distal renal artery arteriosclerotic lesions affect less than 5% of patients. Fifty percent of patients have bilateral renal artery disease.
2. **Fibrodysplastic lesions** affect less than 0.5% of the general population. Although uncommon, it is second only to atherosclerosis as the most frequent cause of RVH. These lesions are found in the distal two thirds of the renal artery and may involve segmental branches (Figure 24-2). Fibrodysplastic disease is subdivided into intimal, medial, or perimedial dysplasia.

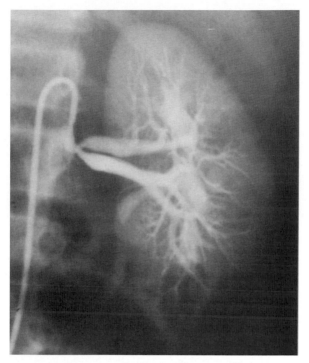

FIGURE 24-1. Aortogram of a 57-year-old woman with severe hypertension that displays a significant proximal left renal artery stenosis consistent with atherosclerotic disease *(arrow).*

a) **Intimal dysplasia.** This process accounts for only 5% of renal artery fibrodysplastic lesions. It is seen more often in infants and younger adults. It is seen with equal frequency in both genders. It appears angiographically as a smooth focal stenosis of the main renal artery and rarely affects the segmental vessels. The etiology of this lesion is unknown, but it may represent focal proliferation of fetal arterial remnants within the vessel resulting in intimal hyperplasia. The media and adventitia are usually normal. Intimal fibroplasia can also be an acquired lesion after trauma or intraluminal injury to the vessel.

b) **Medial fibroplasia.** It is often part of a systemic arterial process involving the renal, carotid, and iliac arteries. This lesion accounts for 85% of renal artery fibrodysplasia and nearly all of these patients are

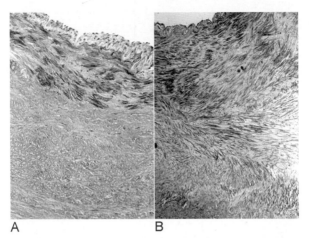

A   B

FIGURE 24-2. **A.** High-power photomicrographs demonstrating the appearance of a normal renal artery and tunica media *(arrow).* **B.** Vessel with fibromuscular hyperplasia of the tunica media demonstrates overgrowth of the fibrous tissue and smooth muscle of that layer *(arrow).*

women. Although the lesion may be solitary, it is more commonly a series of stenoses with intervening aneurysmal dilations appearing as a string of beads on arteriography (Figure 24-3). It is bilateral in 55% of patients. The lesions often extend into the segmental branches of the renal artery.

c) **Perimedial dysplasia.** This lesion accounts for 10% of renal artery fibrodysplasia. Almost all of these patients are women. These lesions affect the main renal artery as focal stenoses or multiple constrictions without mural aneurysms.

3. **Developmental renal artery stenoses.** These failures of complete development of the renal artery account for approximately 40% of childhood RVH.

4. **Renal artery aneurysm.** HTN is the most common clinical presentation of renal artery aneurysm. The etiology of this HTN may be associated arterial stenosis, dissection of the artery, arteriovenous fistula formation, thromboembolism, or compression of arterial branches by the aneurysm.

5. **Renal artery dissection.** Patients with these lesions develop severe HTN as the kidney becomes ischemic. These lesions may be iatrogenic from catheter injuries or associated with trauma. They may occur spontaneously

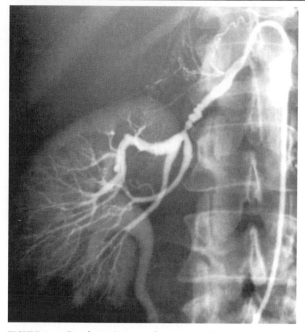

FIGURE 24-3. Renal arteriogram of a 60-year-old woman with hypertension and postprandial pain who was found to have fibromuscular disease of both renal arteries as well as the superior mesenteric artery. The classic "string of beads sign" is demonstrated in the arteriogram.

as a complication of underlying atherosclerotic or fibrodysplastic renovascular disease.

6. **Renal artery embolism.** Embolic occlusion of the renal artery is rare. The most common etiology is embolism from the left heart. These patients present with flank pain, HTN, and hematuria.

7. **Takayasu's arteritis and giant cell arteritis.** Takayasu's disease is common in Asia and affects younger women. Typically, the aorta and its distal branches are affected. Renal artery stenosis and RVH may occur and the initial treatment is with steroid suppression supplemented with cytotoxic agents. Angioplasty and surgical revascularization are reserved for failure of medical therapy.

8. **Transplant renal artery stenosis.** The incidence of this iatrogenic condition is increasing as more renal transplants are carried out. The stenosis is usually anastomotic in most instances; however, atherosclerosis, fibrous stricture, chronic rejection, and kinking may result in significant functional

stenosis. The presentation varies from worsening or refractory HTN, insidious graft dysfunction, and volume overload (pulmonary edema).

IV. PATHOPHYSIOLOGY OF RVH

A. General

1. The **renin-angiotensin-aldosterone system** is important in maintaining blood volume, BP, and total body sodium.
2. Hemorrhage, sympathetic tone, posture, and renal artery sodium are known factors that alter renin release.

B. Function of the Renin-Angiotensin System (Figure 24-4)

1. Renin is a proteolytic enzyme that is released from the granules of the juxtaglomerular apparatus (JGA) in response to changes in the pressure of the afferent arteriole.

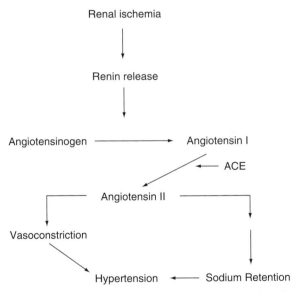

FIGURE 24-4. Renin-angiotensin system. Renin is released from the granules of the juxtaglomerular apparatus in response to changes in the pressure of the afferent vessels. Renin acts on angiotensinogen to produce angiotensin I, which is converted to angiotensin II (needs angiotensin-converting enzyme). Angiotensin II, a potent vasoconstrictor, releases aldosterone from the adrenal cortex potentiating sodium resorption and potassium excretion.

2. Renin is not a vasoconstrictor.
3. Renin acts on a protein in the plasma, angiotensinogen, to produce angiotensin I, which is then proteolytically converted by a plasma enzyme to angiotensin II, an extremely potent vasopressor.
4. Angiotensin II also affects the release of aldosterone from the adrenal cortex, which potentiates sodium reabsorption and potassium excretion in the distal renal tubule.
5. Compensatory mechanisms cause immediate vasoconstriction and enhance sodium reabsorption to expand the plasma volume in the face of decreasing afferent arteriolar pressure.
6. Local paracrine effects of increased endothelin production, renin-angiotensin-aldosterone activation, oxidative stress, and structural wall remodeling are responsible for sustained HTN.

C. Mechanisms of RVH (Figure 24-5)

1. There appear to be at least two mechanisms producing HTN in the setting of renal artery stenosis.
   a) **Renin-dependent HTN** is documented in 90% of patients with high BP and renal artery stenosis.
   b) **Renin-independent HTN.** It is well known that some individuals can become normotensive after surgical therapy even in the absence of elevated or lateralizing renin values. Current research is focusing on the role of prostaglandins as possible mediators of RVH in this small group of patients.
2. Renin activity is increased in the renal vein when the kidney is perfused through a stenotic renal artery. Moreover, in most patients peripheral blood renin levels are also increased.
3. Experiments reducing renal blood flow, but maintaining perfusion pressure, suggest that decreased renal flow per se will not elicit renin release.
4. Of greater significance is a large pressure gradient across the renal artery lesion or a low diastolic BP, both of which correlate well with renin release.
5. Pharmacologic therapy designed to lower the BP in patients with RVH interferes with this compensatory system designed to increase kidney perfusion pressure. This stimulates even more renin release and occasionally the HTN cannot be controlled.
6. In patients who respond to antihypertensive agents, the affected kidney may be inadequately perfused. This may explain the higher rate of renal failure and loss of renal mass in patients who are treated by medical therapy alone.

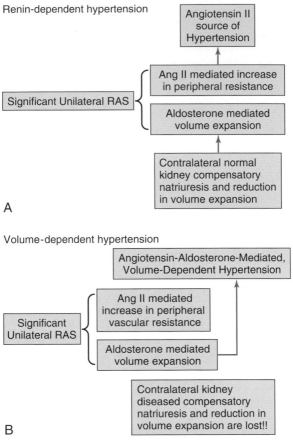

FIGURE 24-5. Mechanisms of renovascular hypertension. **A.** Renin-dependent hypertension. Unilateral renal artery stenosis activates angiotensin II and aldosterone resulting in increased peripheral resistance and hypertension. **B.** Volume-dependent hypertension. Volume expansion occurs due compensatory loss of the contralateral renal function.

V. CLINICAL PRESENTATION

Distinctive clinical features that enable the clinician to make the diagnosis of RVH do not exist and the presentation is often protean. However, the following findings in both the history and physical examination may lead one to suspect RVH.

- HTN in young women and children.
- Sudden onset of HTN.
- Severe HTN after age 55.
- Sudden difficulty controlling previously well-controlled HTN.
- Development of renal failure while on angiotensin-converting enzyme inhibitors.
- An abdominal bruit. This is audible in 40–50% of all patients with RVH.
- Acute flash pulmonary edema in the absence of acute coronary events.

VI. DIAGNOSTIC STUDIES

A. General

Despite immense research in the field of RVH, sound clinical judgment and radiologic imaging help identify renal artery stenosis. Duplex ultrasound and magnetic resonance angiography (MRA) are the most useful noninvasive tests. Digital subtraction angiography is still the most accurate method to detect renal artery stenosis. However, the demonstration of renovascular disease by angiography does not indicate whether the patient's HTN is of renovascular origin. Therefore, the focus of evaluation of these patients is on the functional significance of a stenosis before interventional therapy can be recommended.

B. Specific Tests

1. Laboratory Tests

a) Serum blood urea nitrogen (BUN), creatinine, sodium, potassium, bicarbonate, and chloride.
b) Urinalysis with electrolytes.
c) Peripheral plasma renin activity. Although often measured, it is not particularly reliable for identifying RVH. It is frequently normal in these patients and can be elevated in a large number of patients with essential HTN. However, when plasma renin activity is measured under strictly controlled conditions (salt and volume restriction, antihypertensive medications withdrawn), most patients who are known to have RVH will demonstrate an elevated secretion of renin.

2. Radiologic Evaluation

a) Rapid-sequence intravenous pyelography (IVP).

(1) Approximately 70% of patients with documented RVH will have a positive intravenous pyelogram by the following criteria.
  (a) A difference in length between kidneys of more than 1 cm.
  (b) Delayed pyelocalyceal appearance time (which reflects glomerular filtration).
  (c) Decreased concentration or prolongation in the early nephrogram (10–30 sec) on the involved side.
  (d) Underfilling of the collecting systems.
  (e) Segmental renal atrophy.
  (f) Notching of the upper ureter or renal pelvis by enlarged collateral vessels.
(2) The rapid-sequence IVP may appear to be normal in the presence of bilateral stenosis of the segmental renal arteries.
(3) The utility of the IVP is lessened because of a high false-negative rate. It is specifically for this reason that many clinicians advocate renal arteriography to identify patients with RVH. They believe that all patients with positive IVPs will need angiograms prior to surgery. Furthermore, patients should not be denied the benefit of cure based on a test with a poor specificity.

b) **Radionuclide scanning.** This study measures both renal perfusion and excretory function based on renal excretion of hippuran labeled with iodine 131. The addition of technetium 99m dimercaptosuccinic acid and technetium 99m diethylenetriamine penta-acetic acid (Tc-DMSA renogram) to the study allows calculation of differential renal excretory function for each kidney. In a patient with unilateral renal artery stenosis, the renogram demonstrates a decreased slope of isotope uptake in the ischemic kidney with delayed excretion, indicating impaired renal perfusion. This test has limited sensitivity in renal impairment and demonstration of bilateral renal artery lesions. Furthermore, any lesion that decreases renal inflow will give the renographic appearance of renal artery stenosis; thus, it is not a specific test. It has a 25–30% incidence of false-positive and false-negative results when used as a screening test for RVH. Its main use is as a noninvasive means of following renal function and identifying deterioration in renal function.

c) Duplex ultrasonography. Duplex ultrasound is the combination of B-mode ultrasound with pulsed Doppler ultrasound. This allows for imaging of anatomic details along with quantitative measurement of flow. As a screening test for renal artery stenosis, recent series have demonstrated a sensitivity of 84%, specificity of 97%, and overall accuracy of greater than 96%. This test is highly operator dependent and not all centers can duplicate these excellent results. However, as an **initial screening test, the benefit of duplex Doppler ultrasound is invaluable.** If the size of the kidney is less than 8 cm long, the patient will not benefit from surgical revascularization. Furthermore, the calculation of resistive index (RI = 1− [end diastolic velocity/maximal systolic velocity]) helps determine renal hemodynamics and the utility of any surgical intervention. Studies demonstrate that RI greater than 0.80 in a stenotic kidney indicates severe renovascular disease and will not likely respond to surgical intervention.

d) Captopril renal scintigraphy. Split renal function studies have shown a reversible decrease in renal function in renal artery stenosis patients, induced by the administration of captopril. The loss of glomerular filtration rate (GFR) due to captopril administration provides a provocative test for hemodynamically significant renal artery stenosis. If a captopril-induced change in the renogram is noted, revascularization of the affected kidney may be expected to significantly improve the patient's renal perfusion. However, the results may be affected by the volume status of the patient, underlying renal insufficiency, and concurrent medication. Furthermore, this study provides little data regarding the anatomy of the renovascular disease and therefore has limited clinical utility as a preliminary test.

e) MRA. The technique is noninvasive and non-nephrotoxic. Magnetic resonance arteriograms of the renal arteries, enhanced with the non-nephrotoxic contrast agent gadolinium, yield highly accurate images of the renal arteries when compared with contrast arteriography. Recent series report sensitivities and accuracy in the high 90% range. The main problem with MRA is overestimation of severity of renal artery stenosis. However, its noninvasive and non-nephrotoxic nature is highly desirable in patients with known renal impairment. New developments of combined MRA and phase-contrast magnetic resonance demonstrate accurate estimation of functional stenosis of renal arteries; however, it is experimental.

f) Computed tomography angiography (CTA). Multispiral computed tomography (CT) employs contrast agents to form three-dimensional arteriograms. These yield high-quality images of the abdominal aorta and its branch arteries, especially with the current multidetector scanners. However, the technique is very dependent on sophisticated image processing and requires contrast doses equivalent to that used for conventional arteriography, making this test undesirable as a screening tool.

g) Arteriography. Intra-arterial digital subtraction arteriography provides high-resolution arteriograms with less contrast material than standard arteriography. The value of arteriography, properly performed, is to evaluate the anatomy of the renal artery.

- Multiple arteries to both kidneys are frequent.
- Atherosclerotic stenosis can be differentiated from fibrodysplastic lesions.
- Although other tests alluded to may indicate the presence of a unilateral abnormality, they cannot specify the site or type of lesion present.
  (1) Atherosclerotic lesions are identified as stenotic areas in the proximal third of the artery.
  (2) Fibromuscular lesions occur in the distal two thirds of the vessel and may produce the "string of beads" sign.
  (3) The low morbidity and rare mortality of this test have led to its current widespread use.

VII. FUNCTIONAL RENAL STUDIES

A. General

Although angiography permits the diagnosis of renal artery disease in the presence of HTN, it does not confirm the diagnosis of RVH. Widespread use of angiography has shown that renal artery stenosis may be present in the absence of HTN. For this reason, functional assessment of the impact of the stenosis on the kidney must be performed. However, these tests are only infrequently used today but may be of value, especially in evaluating the viability of severely ischemic kidneys and the likelihood of salvaging them.

B. Differential Renal Function Studies

1. This test requires selective catheterization of ureters; prolonged collection of urine volumes; and multiple sample analysis of specimens for volume, sodium concentration, osmolality, and reabsorption of filtered sodium and water.

2. The test is based on the finding that tubular reabsorption of water is greater in the ischemic kidney than in the normal contralateral kidney. Thus, data can be affected greatly by changes in blood flow, perfusion pressure, and GFR.

3. A test result is considered positive if there is a reduction in urine flow rate and an increase in creatinine as well as an increase in para-aminohippuric acid concentration in the urine from the affected kidney when compared with the contralateral kidney.

4. Although this test may be positive in 80% of patients with unilateral main renal artery stenosis, it is negative in patients with RVH secondary to a segmental renal artery lesion.

5. It has been found that 73% of patients with positive tests were improved after surgical treatment, but 50% of patients with negative tests also improved after surgical treatment.

6. The combination of the test's low sensitivity and the relatively high rate of urologic complications (3–5%) have caused most clinicians to reserve this study for special situations.

C. Renal Vein Renin Assays

1. Most centers rely on the renal vein renin assay to select patients with HTN and renovascular disease for corrective treatment.

2. Renin samples are collected from the inferior vena cava and both renal veins by a catheter placed percutaneously in a retrograde fashion via a femoral vein.

3. The renal venous renin ratio is calculated by dividing the renin level of the ischemic kidney by the renin level of the contralateral kidney. A ratio of 1.5 to 1 is considered abnormal by most authors. This test is based on the notion that a unilateral stenosis opposite a normal contralateral kidney will result in unilateral hypersecretion of renin and contralateral suppression of renin secretion. More than 90% of patients meeting these criteria will respond to corrective interventions.

4. It is interesting that in the small group of patients with severe HTN and angiographically proven renal artery stenosis but normal renin values, approximately 50–80% will respond to surgical intervention. Speculation on the reason for this finding centers on the improper preparation of patients for the test. The lingering effects of the antihypertensive agents, inaccurately placed catheters, and failure to restrict sodium intake have all been described. Alternatively, the possibility of a non

renin-dependent mechanism for RVH remains consistent with current data.

5. When bilateral stenoses or contralateral parenchymal disease are present, the normal compensatory mechanisms are not active and HTN may be multifactorial rather than renin-mediated.

6. The renal vein renin ratio cannot be used as the sole criterion of selection for intervention due to the considerable number of false-negative results and the large number of these patients who benefit from interventions.

7. Confounding factors that may interfere with validity of assay include:
   a) Interference of antihypertensive medication with renin release.
   b) Suppression of renin release by volume expansion and salt loading.
   c) Variability of renin release from the kidney.
   d) Catheter placement error (lumbar vein, left renal vein proximal to gonadal or lumbar vein).

8. Some have stressed the importance of expressing the renal vein renin assay in relation to systemic renin activity rather than as a ratio of activities between the two renal veins. This renal-to-systemic renin index has been shown to reliably predict those patients who will be cured of RVH with intervention compared with those whose condition would only be improved.

D. Percutaneous Transluminal Angioplasty (PTA)

1. Recently it has been proposed that PTA should be performed routinely if angiography demonstrates a significant renovascular lesion amenable to angioplasty. This is based on the observation that a significant number of patients with RVH do not have demonstrable involvement of the renin-angiotensin system and that no tests or combination of tests yield a reliable diagnosis of RVH.

2. If the patient responds after a first dilation, this is taken as teleologic evidence that the patient's HTN was attributable to the angioplastied lesion.

VIII. MEDICAL THERAPY

A. General

The goal of medical therapy is good HTN control without deterioration of renal function.

B. Methods of Medical Control

1. Lifestyle modification including reduction of salt intake and weight loss is an integral part of HTN control.
2. Antiplatelets such as aspirin.
3. Statins if atherosclerosis is the etiologic factor.
4. Multidrug therapy including beta-blockers, α-blockers, calcium channel blockers, angiotensin II inhibitors, and vasodilators are often necessary to achieve BP control.
5. Angiotensin inhibitors help to control the BP of patients who are otherwise resistant to standard medical therapy. However, these drugs should be started in low doses and renal function should be assessed in 3- to 5-day intervals and the drug increased in gradual increments as they may reduce renal function in severe renal artery stenosis. The creatinine levels return to baseline when these drugs are stopped.

IX. PTA AND STENTING (FIGURE 24-6)

A. General

Historically, balloon dilation of vascular lesions was first performed in 1964. The first treatment of renovascular lesions by PTA was performed in 1978 by Gruntzig. Currently, increasing numbers of renal angioplasties have been performed for RVH with subsequent decrease in the use of open surgical techniques. The use of renal artery stents, particularly for ostial lesions, has further improved long-term patency rates.

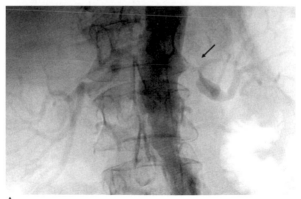

A

FIGURE 24-6. (Continued)

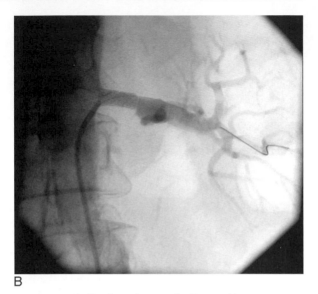

B

FIGURE 24-6. **A.** Renal arteriogram of a 66-year-old man demonstrating severe stenosis *(arrow)* of the left renal artery due to atherosclerosis. Note the post-stenotic dilatation. **B.** Angiogram showing the successful result after percutaneous angioplasty and stenting.

B. Patient Selection

Careful patient selection is important. Patients with extensive irreversible parenchymal damage, renal length less than 8 cm, and poor GFR will not benefit from revascularization. Patients with both arteriosclerotic and fibrodysplastic lesions treated by PTA/stent have improvement in BP.

C. Results

1. Endoluminal stenting of renal artery was introduced in the United States in 1988 as part of large multicenter trial.
2. Angioplasty is effective for treating RVH associated with atheromatous lesions. This has been indicated by a decreased rate of referrals for surgical renovascularization of atheromatous renovascular hypertensive nephropathy by the early 1980s (from 41% to 26%).
3. Technical success is achieved in more than 90% of patients, and patency rates are 90–95% at 2 years for FMD and 80–85% for atherosclerosis.

4. Restenosis requiring repeat angioplasty has been reported in fewer than 10% of patients with FMD and in 8–30% with atherosclerotic stenosis.

5. The recurrence rate after PTA has been reported to be between 12 and 23%. The rate is higher for atherosclerotic lesions than other types of stenoses.

6. Patients who have both aortic and renovascular disease respond poorly to PTA. Patients with lesions at the aortic ostium of the renal artery representing "spillover" atherosclerotic lesions as well as branch fibrodysplastic lesions and congenital stenoses also respond poorly to PTA and should have renal artery stenting (PTAS) or undergo primary surgical therapy.

7. Stenting of ostial renal artery stenoses has been demonstrated to improve the results with angioplasty of these lesions. The primary success rate was 57% for PTA compared with 88% for PTAS.

8. Recently, the use of filter devices to protect against renal embolization during renal artery stenting has shown to improve renal function to 95%.

9. Improvement in BP control with fewer antihypertensive medications is achieved in 30–35% of fibromuscular lesions and in 50–60% of atherosclerotic lesions.

10. Mortality rate is about 1%. The major complication rate is between 5 and 10%. The most common complications include acute renal failure, peripheral embolization, hematoma, pseudoaneurysm, and vessel damage at the femoral artery catheterization site.

11. There has never been a prospective randomized comparison of PTA and reconstructive procedures. However, all retrospective comparisons have found surgical results to be superior to PTA for patients with atherosclerotic lesions, whereas those with fibrodysplastic lesions responded well to either therapy.

12. Surgical intervention is indicated if PTA/stent fails.

X. SURGICAL THERAPY

A. General

The goals of surgical intervention include the cure of HTN and the preservation of functional renal tissue. Recent advances in endovascular and innovative surgical techniques combined with preoperative correction of cardiac and medical risk factors with improved anesthesia and monitoring have significantly reduced present-day morbidity and mortality. Criteria that predict salvageable renal function in a compromised kidney include:

1. Renal length greater than 8 cm.
2. Biopsy findings of greater than 80% viable glomeruli.
3. Angiographic evidence of a rich collateral circulation, a distal renal artery that reconstitutes via collaterals, and absence of severe intrarenal arterial disease.
4. Renal scan findings indicating more than 20% of total GFR attributable to the ischemic kidney.

B. Patient Selection

1. Failure of medical therapy.
2. Failure to tolerate medical regimens.
3. Deterioration of renal function in the presence of adequate BP control.
4. Young patients should undergo surgery to avoid medical treatment of long duration.
5. Simultaneous abdominal aorta aneurysm.
6. Renal artery aneurysm.
7. Renal artery occlusion (with unsuccessful thrombolysis).
8. Renal artery rupture.
9. RAS secondary to kinking.
10. Multiple branch lesions.
11. Renal artery lesions not amenable to angioplasty.

C. Surgical Procedures

1. Aortorenal bypass.
   a) Reversed or nonreversed vein grafts from the infrarenal or supraceliac aorta may be used to bypass a region of renal artery stenosis. The distal anastomosis is done in an end-to-end fashion, because end-to-side anastomoses have the potential for competitive flow as well as propagation of thrombus into the renal artery.
   b) Prosthetic grafts are reserved for patients who have no suitable autogenous vein, as these grafts have decreased patency rates compared with autogenous material.
   c) The supraceliac aorta, which is usually relatively spared of diffuse atherosclerotic disease, may be used for the proximal anastomosis if the infrarenal aorta is unsuitable.
2. Aortorenal endarterectomy may be performed through an aortic incision. This technique is suited to treatment of ostial lesions, directly removing the diseased intima and plaque.

3. Alternative renal artery reconstructive techniques may be used in specific clinical situations to avoid a diseased or otherwise unsuitable aorta as an inflow vessel.
   a) Hepatorenal bypass.
   b) Splenorenal bypass.
   c) Iliorenal bypass.
   d) Mesorenal bypass.
4. Heterotopic autotransplantation of the kidney to the iliac artery and vein relocating the kidney to the iliac fossa is an effective alternative method of renal revascularization.
5. Ex vivo arterial repair in which the kidney is removed from the patient allowing precise reconstruction of the renal vessels under ex vivo conditions of exposure, illumination, and magnification. This allows for precise reconstruction of complex lesions. The kidney may be replaced back into the renal fossa or autotransplanted to the iliac fossa.

E. Results

1. Most centers now achieve mortality statistics of less than 1% for fibrodysplastic lesions and less than 2% for atherosclerotic RVH.
2. Surgical cure of RVH is achieved in approximately 40% of atherosclerosis patients and 60% of fibrodysplasia patients.
3. Improvement in BP is noted in an additional 45% of atherosclerosis patients and 30% of fibrodysplasia patients, allowing adequate medical control of BP in these previously uncontrollable patients.
4. Overall, a beneficial BP response rate as high as 95% can be expected in surgically treated patients with RVH.
5. Preservation of renal function.
   - Untreated renal artery occlusive disease in patients with progressive renal deterioration has a poor prognosis.
   - Drug therapy of RVH, particularly in patients on angiotensin-converting enzyme inhibitors, has resulted in control of HTN, but often there is progressive loss of renal function.
   - Medical therapy of RVH does not inhibit the progression of renovascular disease.
   - Renal revascularization prevents or reverses chronic renal failure secondary to renovascular disease.
   - Ninety percent of patients can expect stabilization or improvement of renal function after revascularization. Additionally, there is some evidence that survival in revascularized patients is significantly improved when compared with an age-matched population.

XI. RECOMMENDATIONS

Prolongation of life due to better HTN control and preservation of renal function argue effectively for the interventional approach to patients with renovascular disease. Our approach to renovascular disease is outlined in the algorithm in Figure 24-7.

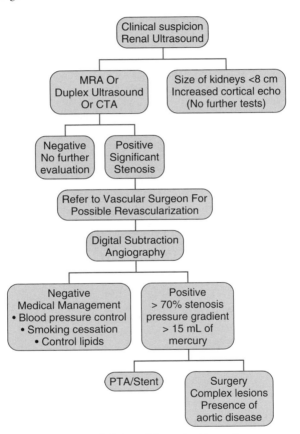

FIGURE 24-7. Strong clinical suspicion and evidence of sonogram demonstrating kidney larger than 8 cm with stenosis should be further evaluated with MRA or duplex ultrasound. If positive, the patient should be referred to a surgeon for possible revascularization. The surgeon typically performs a digital subtraction angiogram and if positive will balloon angioplasty (PTA) the lesion. If the lesion has functionally significant drop in pullback pressures of >15 mm Hg, it warrants PTA wall stent. Ostial lesions fare better with wall stents. If there is significant aortic disease or if the anatomy is complex, then open surgical revascularization is preferred.

XII. CONCLUSIONS

1. Failed medical management in new-onset HTN should be aggressively treated by enodovascular techniques or open surgery.
2. Surgical revascularization can improve BP control and renal function in selected patients in up to 90% of cases of renal HTN.
3. PTA provides success rates somewhat inferior to the results for atherosclerotic lesions but is the treatment of choice for RVH secondary to fibrodysplastic lesions.
4. PTA or PTAS has increased in popularity and is the current procedure of choice.
5. Open procedures are reserved for patients not amenable to percutaneous methods.

SELF-ASSESSMENT QUESTIONS

1. What is the most common cause of renovascular hypertension?
2. What is the workup for patients suspected of having renovascular hypertension?
3. What is the initial management?
4. What are the indications for referral to a vascular specialist?
5. What are the current revascularization techniques?

SUGGESTED READINGS

1. Connolly JO, Woolfson: Renovascular hypertension: Diagnosis and management. *BJU Int* 96:715–720, 2005.
2. Covit AB: Medical treatment of renal artery stenosis: is it effective and appropriate? *J Hypertens* 23(Suppl 3):S15–S22, 2005.
3. Holden A, Hill A, et al: Renal angioplasty and stenting with distal protection of the renal artery in ischemic nephropathy: early experience. *J Vasc Surg* 38:962–968, 2003.
4. The management of renovascular disorders. In Rutherford RB (ed): *Vascular Surgery*, 6th ed. Chapters 127–134.
5. Wierema T, Leeuw P: Renal artery stenosis: today's questions. *Curr Opin Pharmacol* 6:197–201, 2006.
6. Zalunardo N, Tuttle KR: Atherosclerotic renal artery stenosis: current status and future directions. *Curr Opin Nephrol Hypertens* 13:613–621, 2004.

C H A P T E R 25

Disorders of Sexual Development

Thomas F. Kolon, MD

Human sexual development occurs in an organized, sequential manner. Chromosomal sex is established at fertilization, which then directs the undifferentiated gonads to develop into testes or ovaries. Phenotypic sex results from the differentiation of internal ducts and external genitalia under the influence of hormones and transcription factors. When discordance occurs among these three processes (i.e., chromosomal, gonadal, or phenotypic sex determination), then disorders of sexual development (DSD) develop. This has previously been identified as "intersex" or "intersexualty," but the new nomenclature has ended the use of the term intersex and now refers to it as DSD. Sexual differentiation is regulated by more than 50 different genes on both the sex chromosomes and autosomes. These genes encode transcription factors, gonadal steroid and peptide hormones, and tissue receptors. The sex determination genetic cascade involves the *SRY* gene (sex-determining region on Y) as the testis-determining factor, although other upstream (*SF1*, *WT1*) and downstream (*DAX1*, *SOX9*, *Wnt4*, *AMH*, homeobox) genes are also likely involved (Figure 25-1).

In sexual development, the female phenotype represents the default pathway. Therefore, a failure of testis determination will usually result in the development of the female phenotype, whereas genetic alterations resulting in partial testicular development can give rise to a wide spectrum of masculinization. In addition to defects in peptide hormones and their receptors, timing of hormonal exposure is also critical to appropriate development. Although much work remains to be done, recent advances in our knowledge have begun to unravel of the molecular basis of DSD.

The first sections of this chapter provide a basic template for the etiology of DSD. However, it may be worthwhile to read the history, physical exam, and evaluation descriptions first and then begin again with the start of the chapter to keep this subject in perspective. The important issue with any DSD evaluation is not to get overwhelmed by the enormity of the

Genetic Etiology of DSD				
Syndrome	**Karyotype**	**Genital Phenotype**	**Gene**	**Locus**
21-Hydroxylase deficiency	XX	virilized	CYP21B	6p21.3
11-Hydroxylase deficiency	XX	virilized	CYP11 (B1,B2)	8q21-22
3BHSD deficiency	XX / XY	ambiguous	HSD3B2	1p13.1
17a-Hydroxylase or 17,20 lyase deficiency	XX / XY	ambiguous	CYP17	10q24-25
17BHSD deficiency	XY	ambiguous	17BHSD3	9q22
Lipoid adrenal hyperplasia	XX / XY	female, ovarian failure (XX)	StAR	8p11.2
Leydig cell failure	XY	ambiguous	hCG/LH receptor	2p21
Androgen insensitivity	XY	ambiguous (female- AIS 7)	AR	Xq11-12
5a-reductase deficiency	XY	ambiguous, pubertal virilization	SRD5A2	2p23
Persistent müllerian duct	XY	male	AMH / AMH II receptor	19q13.3 / 12q13
Gonadal dysgenesis:				
complete	XX	female, sexual infantilism	FSH receptor	2p16-21
	45X, 45X/46XX		X monosomy	paternal X loss
	XY		SRY	Yp53.3
			DSS (DAX-1)	Xp 21-22
			SOX9	17q24.3-25.1
			WT-1	11p13
Partial	45X/46XY / XY	ambiguous	unknown	unknown
XY Dysgenesis	XY	ambiguous	SRY	Yp53.3
	45X/46XY		DSS (DAX-1)	Xp 21-22
			XH-2	Xq13.3
			WT-1	11p13
			SOX9	17q24.3-25.1
			SF-1	9q33
Ovotesticular DSD	XX / XX/XY / XY	ambiguous	SRY / testis cascade / downstream genes	Yp53.3 / unknown
Klinefelter	47XXY / 46XY/47XXY	variable androgen deficiency	XY	sex chromosome nondisjunction
XX Testicular DSD	XX	ambiguous to normal	SRY	Y translocation to X

FIGURE 25-1. Genetic characteristics of DSD.

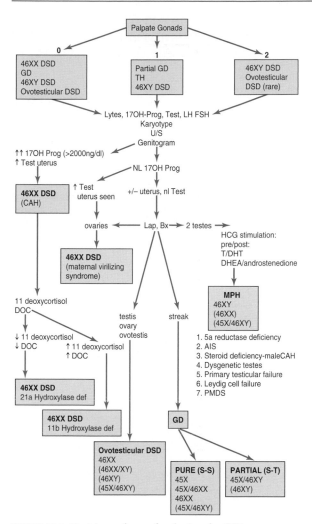

FIGURE 25-2. Decision pathway of evaluation for DSD.

differential diagnosis possibilities. Instead, work slowly through the differential diagnosis pathway (Figure 25-2) based on the physical exam and laboratory findings. Many possible diagnoses will remove themselves from contention in this manner.

46XX DSD (FORMERLY FEMALE PSEUDOHERMAPHRODITISM)

46XX DSD, previously known as female pseudohermaphroditism, is the most common DSD. The ovaries and müllerian derivatives are normal and the sexual ambiguity is limited to masculinization of the external genitalia. A female fetus is masculinized only if exposed to androgens, and the degree of masculinization is determined by the stage of differentiation at the time of exposure. Masculinization can occur secondary to exogenous maternal steroids as well.

Congenital adrenal hyperplasia (CAH) accounts for the majority of 46XX DSD patients. Inactivating or loss of function mutations in five genes involved in steroid biosynthesis can cause CAH: CYP21, CYP11B1, CYP17, HSD3B2, and StAR (Figures 25-2 and 25-3). Although all six of these biochemical defects are characterized by impaired cortisol secretion, only CYP21 and CYP11B1 are predominantly masculinizing disorders (HSD3B2 to a lesser extent). Although the female fetus is masculinized due to overproduction of adrenal androgens and precursors, affected males have no genital abnormalities. In contrast, HSD3B2, CYP17, and StAR deficiencies block cortisol synthesis and gonadal steroid production. Thus, affected males have varying degrees of 46XY DSD (formerly male pseudohermaphroditism), whereas females generally have normal external genitalia. Each of these genetic defects is inherited in an autosomal recessive pattern.

CYP21 (21α-Hydroxylase) Deficiency

Deficiency of CYP21 (cytochrome p450$_{c21}$) is the most common cause of genital ambiguity. The gene is located within the major HLA locus on the short arm of chromosome 6 (6p21.3). HLA types are codominantly inherited and can be used as a marker to distinguish homozygous, heterozygous, and unaffected individuals.

Two CYP21 genes are located on chromosome 6 between HLA-B and HLA-DR: a functional 10 exon CYP21B gene and a CYP21A pseudogene that are nonfunctional due to the presence of multiple stop codons. Recombination between CYP21B and the homologous but inactive CYP21A accounts for approximately 95% of 21α-hydroxylase deficiency mutations resulting in a variable decrease in 21α-hydroxylase activity. These conversions usually involve the transfer of inherent CYP21A mutations. Patients with simple virilizing 21α-hydroxylase deficiency have been noted to have a conversion

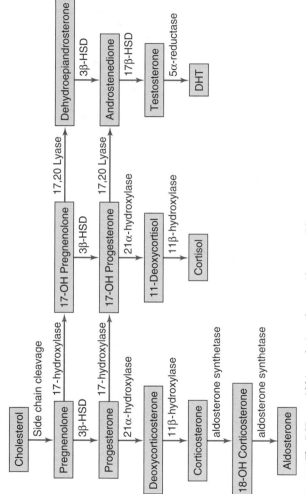

FIGURE 25-3. The DSD steroid biosynthetic pathways with responsible enzymes.

mutation (Ile-Asn) causing severely decreased enzyme activity but sufficient aldosterone production to prevent salt wasting. Nonclassical CAH conversion mutations have been shown to display 20–50% of normal activity.

Some centers have instituted screening for 17 hydroxy-progesterone levels at 3–5 days of life in conjunction with screening for other inborn metabolic diseases. HLA typing of amniotic fluid cells in mothers with a previously affected offspring has been used to identify a fetus with a *CYP21* deficiency. This has led to experimental prenatal treatment of CAH with good results of decreasing the masculinization. At issue is the controversy of initially treating one in eight fetuses who may not need the therapy.

CYP11B1 (11β-Hydroxylase) Deficiency

Cytochrome p450 is a terminal oxidase found on the inner mitochondrial membrane. Two distinct enzymes, *CYP11B1* and *CYP11B2*, are encoded by two tandem and homologous genes at 8q21–22. *CYP11B1* encodes 11β-hydroxylase, which converts 11-deoxycorticosterone (DOC) to corticosterone and 11-deoxycortisol to cortisol. This gene's protein is expressed in the adrenal zona fasciculata and is primarily under the influence of corticotropin. Alternatively, *CYP11B2* encodes for aldosterone synthetase, which converts DOC to corticosterone and 18-hydroxycorticosterone to aldosterone. It is expressed in the zona glomerulosa and is under the influence of angiotensin II and potassium. Cortisol deficiency results in increased secretion of 11-deoxycortisol, DOC, corticosterone, and androgen by the adrenal gland. Hypertension, which occurs in about two thirds of patients, is presumptively a consequence of excess DOC, with resultant salt and water retention. Excess androgen secretion in utero masculinizes the external genitalia of the female fetus. After birth, untreated males and females progressively masculinize and experience rapid somatic growth and skeletal maturation.

Although *CYP11B1* and *CYP11B2* are extremely homologous, both genes are functional. Thus, gene conversions are not the cause of impaired enzyme activity, as was described for 21α-hydroxylase deficiency. Similar to *CYP21*, alterations with less enzyme activity usually result in more severe phenotypes, but heterogeneity can occur. This disorder can be detected prenatally, and the masculinization of the fetus can be decreased following in utero dexamethasone treatment as previously described for 21α-hydroxylase deficiency. Other abnormalities such as 3β-hydroxysteroid dehydrogenase deficiency, CYP17 deficiency, and StAR deficiency are covered under disorders of 46XY DSD.

46XY DSD (FORMERLY MALE PSEUDOHERMAPHRODITISM)

46XY DSD is a heterogenous disorder in which testicles are present but the internal ducts and/or the external genitalia are incompletely masculinized. The phenotype ranges from completely female external genitalia to mild male ambiguity (such as hypospadias or cryptorchidism). 46XY DSD can result from eight basic etiologic categories: (1) testicular unresponsiveness to human chorionic gonadotrophin (hCG) and luteinizing hormone (LH) (Leydig cell aplasia/hypoplasia due to hCG/LH receptor defect); (2) enzyme defects in testosterone (T) biosynthesis, some of which are common to CAH (StAR, HSD3B2, CYP17, 17-βHSD3); (3) defects in androgen-dependent target tissues (androgen insensitivity syndrome [AIS]); (4) a defect in the enzymatic conversion of T to dihydrotestosterone (DHT) (5α-reductase deficiency); (5) defects in the synthesis, secretion, or response to anti-müllerian hormone (AMH) or müllerian inhibiting substance (MIS) resulting in persistent müllerian duct syndrome; (6) aberrations in testicular gonadogenesis (testicular dysgenesis); (7) primary testicular failure (vanishing testes); and (8) exogenous insults (maternal ingestion of progesterone/estrogen or environmental hazards).

Leydig Cell Aplasia/Hypoplasia

Leydig cell aplasia/hypoplasia is an autosomal recessive condition. In its complete form, these patients are 46XY but are cryptorchid and phenotypically female. Wolffian structures are present due to the secretion of MIS by intact Sertoli cells. However, the phenotypic presentation is variable. The underlying abnormality in this disorder is a failure of Leydig cell differentiation secondary to an abnormal LH receptor (LHR). LH is elevated, T is markedly decreased, and follicle-stimulating hormone (FSH) levels are unaffected. There is no T surge on hCG stimulation.

Testosterone Biosynthesis Enzyme Defects

Defects in four steps of the steroid biosynthetic pathway from cholesterol to T may produce genital ambiguity in the male (see Figure 25-3).

StAR Deficiency

Congenital lipoid adrenal hyperplasia, a rare autosomal recessive disorder, was once thought to arise from mutations in the gene encoding p450 scc (cholesterol side chain cleavage), *CYP11A*. However, studies have shown that such mutations are incompatible with survival, because these alterations would likely cause spontaneous abortions at the end of the first trimester from insufficient placental progesterone production, when corpus luteum secretion of progesterone wanes. Rather, lipoid CAH is a result of mutations in the *StAR* (steroidogenic acute regulatory) gene.[14] The StAR protein regulates the transfer of cholesterol from the outer mitochondrial membrane to the inner membrane, where it is metabolized by the *CYP11A* gene product, p450 scc.

These patients are often Asian and are born after an uneventful pregnancy. They subsequently present after a few days or weeks with severe adrenal insufficiency and will die from glucocorticoid and mineralocorticoid deficiency without hormone replacement. However, they can survive to adulthood if properly treated. 46XY males are born with female external genitalia, and the adrenal glands and testes are massively engorged with lipid deposits (cholesterol esters). Although 46XX females do experience feminization and cyclical vaginal bleeding at puberty, they invariably develop polycystic ovaries.

3β-Hydroxysteroid Dehydrogenase Deficiency

3β-hydroxysteroid dehydrogenase (3β-HSD) deficiency results in impaired adrenal aldosterone and cortisol synthesis as well as gonadal T and estradiol formation. In its complete form, severe mineralocorticoid and glucocorticoid deficiency in the first week of life are observed. Male infants exhibit variable degrees of 46XY DSD, whereas in females, clitoromegaly and mild masculinization are common. The masculinization is a result of conversion of the ?5 precursors to T via extragonadal (placenta and peripheral tissues) fetal 3β-HSD. Salt wasting may be present, depending on the severity of the 3β-HSD deficiency. Treatment involving glucocorticoids is similar to that of 21-hydroxylase deficiency and mineralocorticoids are added to treat the salt wasting forms. Sex steroid replacement may be necessary at puberty.

CYP17 Abnormality

The *CYP17* gene is located on chromosome 10q24.3 and contains eight exons. Its protein is absent from the placenta, ovarian glomerulosa cells, and the adrenal zona glomerulosa. The cytochrome p450 c17 protein catalyzes 17α-hydroxylase and 17,20 lyase (desmolase) activities. Therefore, mutations in *CYP17* would be expected to alter the activities of both enzymes. Although the existence of isolated 17,20 lyase deficiency has been questioned, two patients with hormonal and clinical findings consistent with isolated 17,20 lyase deficiency have been described.

Combined 17α-hydroxylase and 17,20 lyase deficiency causes deficient production of cortisol and sex hormones. Genetic females present with sexual infantilism due to a lack of ovarian estrogen synthesis at puberty, whereas genetic males often manifest a developmental spectrum ranging from a normal female phenotype to an ambiguous hypospadiac male. Overproduction of 11-DOC and corticosterone leads to hypertension, hypokalemic alkalosis, and carbohydrate intolerance. Genetic males with isolated 17,20 lyase deficiency also manifest variable degrees of incomplete masculinization. However, they do not suffer from the associated abnormalities in cortisol secretion and hypertension that occur in patients with combined 17α-hydroxylase/17,20 lyase deficiencies.

17β-Hydroxysteroid Dehydrogenase Deficiency

There are at least five known isoenzymes of 17βHSD.[7] The type 3 17βHSD catalyzes the reduction of androstenedione to T and is expressed only in the testis. Different isoenzymes catalyze the isoreduction of estrone to estradiol and androstenedione to T.

As expected, these patients have elevated plasma androstenedione (up to 10 times as high) levels, low plasma T (increased androstenedione-to-T ratio after hCG stimulation in prepubertal patients), elevated LH, and normal to high FSH levels. In these patients, more than 90% of plasma T is produced from the extragonadal conversion of androstenedione to T, compared to less than 1% in normal males. Plasma DHT may be normal in some patients, suggesting conversion from androstenedione.

These patients are usually 46XY males with ambiguous or female external genitalia and normal internal wolffian structures, including inguinal testes and a blind vaginal pouch. This occurs because there is little or no peripheral conversion of androstenedione to T and DHT during early gestation by the other 17βHSD isoenzymes. Additionally, increased aromatization of androstenedione to estrogen by the placenta may leave little substrate available for conversion to T and DHT. They are often raised as girls but may virilize at puberty and adopt a male gender role, similar to that seen in 5αRD-2 deficiency. At puberty, the expression of other 17βHSD isoenzymes in the peripheral tissues partially compensates for testicular 17βHSD-3 deficiency; however, the phenotype is variable. Some patients develop gynecomastia at puberty, depending on their T-to-estradiol ratio.

5α – Reductase Deficiency

5α-reductase deficiency, an autosomal recessive condition with alterations of the 5αRD-2 gene, was initially described as pseudovaginal perineoscrotal hypospadias because of the striking genital ambiguity/female external phenotype seen in these cases. These patients often have a clitoris-like phallus, severely bifid scrotum, and perineoscrotal hypospadias. Some patients may have less severe genital ambiguity, however. Normal wolffian structures, cryptorchidism, and a rudimentary prostate are other common findings.

At puberty, patients with 5α-reductase deficiency show signs of virilization with increased muscle mass, deepening of voice, substantial growth of phallus, rugation and hyperpigmentation of the scrotum, and normal libido. Migration of inguinal testis into the scrotum has been observed. They do not experience gynecomastia or male pattern balding, facial hair is decreased, and their prostates remain infantile. Although these patients are usually oligo- or azospermic, fertility via intrauterine insemination has been reported.

Androgen Insensitivity Syndrome

The broad phenotypic spectrum in these 46XY patients varies from normal female external genitalia (AIS7 or testicular feminization—Figures 25-4 and 25-5) to normal males with infertility (AIS1). Patients previously described by Lubs, Gilbert-Dreyfuss, Reifenstein, and others are now classified as AIS 1–7. This X-linked disorder affects 1 in 20,000 live male births. The androgen receptor (AR) gene is located in the pericentromeric region of the long arm of chromosome X at Xq11–12 and contains eight exons. The AR is a member of the nuclear receptor superfamily of transcription factors and has three major functional domains. The amino (NH_2) terminal domain is encoded by exon 1 and is critical to target gene transcription regulation. Exons 2 and 3 encode the DNA-binding domain and the 5′ region of exon 4 encodes the hinge region containing the nuclear targeting signal. The 3′ region of exon 4 and exons 5 through 8 encode the steroid-binding domain that confers ligand

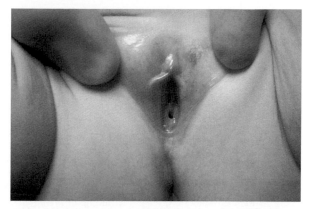

FIGURE 25-4. Normal introitus in 46XY patient with CAIS.

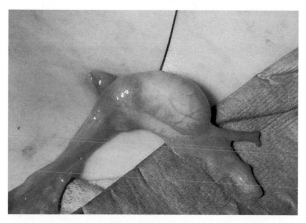

FIGURE 25-5. Abdominal testis identified at time of inguinal hernia repair in 46XY patient with CAIS.

specificity. Binding of DHT or T to this receptor ligand-binding domain results in "activation" of the receptor.

The NH_2 domain contains polymorphic glutamine (CAG) and glycine (GGC) repeats (i.e., the length of these repeats varies among individuals in the general population).[58] Hence, AR genes with different CAG and GGC repeat lengths represent different AR alleles. Interestingly, AR CAG repeat length varies by racial group: the most common Caucasian AR allele has 21 repeats, whereas the most common

African-American allele has 18 repeats. Deletion of the CAG repeat yields an AR with increased transcriptional activity, whereas an increase in the length decreases this activity. In men with spinal bulbar muscular atrophy and Kennedy's disease, the AR CAG repeat is at least twice as long as that of unaffected men.

Mutations in the DNA-binding region can produce a receptor that binds androgen normally but cannot induce transactivation due to faulty binding to DNA, destabilization of the protein structure, or lack of dimerization of the receptor.[15] The degree of impairment of transactivation correlates with the phenotype. The majority of AR gene mutations affect the steroid-binding domain and result in receptors unable to bind androgens or that bind androgens but exhibit qualitative abnormalities. Of note, however, is the finding of phenotypic variability in families with affected males with PAIS. This suggests that other factors in the sex differentiation cascade influence the phenotypic manifestations of gene mutations.

Persistent Müllerian Duct Syndrome (Hernia Uteri Inguinale)

Persistent müllerian duct syndrome (PMDS) is a rare (autosomal recessive) disorder that arises from a lack of MIS or AMH action on the müllerian ducts, resulting in the presence of müllerian structures in a normally masculinized XY male (Figure 25-6). PMDS is due to either a mutation in the AMH gene or a defect in the AMH type II receptor.

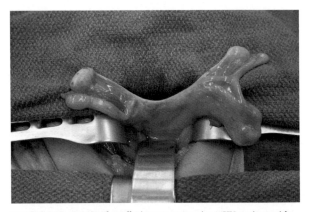

FIGURE 25-6. Retained müllerian structures in 46XY patient with persistent müllerian duct syndrome.

The AMH gene contains five exons and is located on chromosome 19p13.3. Alterations in the AMH gene were first reported in a Moroccan family and appear to occur mostly in Arab/Mediterranean countries, which have a high rate of consanguinity. They tend to be family specific and involve the entire length of the gene. The AMH receptor signals through two related but distinct receptors (type I and type II). The primary receptor (type II) binds MIS independently but requires the type I receptor for signal transduction. However, these mutations are not family specific and are more common in France and Northern Europe, and the mutations in the AMH type II receptor are not as variable.

The diagnosis is often made at surgery for cryptorchidism or inguinal hernia repair. Patients with type I PMDS will have low or undetectable levels of serum MIS, whereas those with type II PMDS secondary to a defective AMH receptor will have high normal or elevated serum MIS levels. Treatment consists of orchidopexy. Historically, hysterectomy was recommended, but recent reports suggest that leaving the uterus and fallopian tubes in situ may be optimal to avoid injury to the vas deferens. The retained müllerian structures should not be at risk for malignant degeneration.

46XY Gonadal Dysgenesis

Patients with dysgenetic gonads exhibit ambiguous development of the internal genital ducts, the urogenital sinus, and the external genitalia. Mutations or deletions of any of the genes involved in the testis determination cascade have been identified in dysgenetic MPH.

SRY is a single exon gene located on the short arm of the Y chromosome and is the "testis determining factor." SRY gene mutations generally result in complete gonadal dysgenesis (CGD) and sex reversal. Histologic analysis of dysgenetic gonads of XY males revealed that those with normal SRY had some element of rete testis and tubular function, whereas those with SRY mutations had completely undifferentiated gonads similar to those of 45X individuals. Thus, SRY may have a direct role in testicular formation in addition to its indirect role in initiating the male differentiation cascade.

Duplication of the DSS (dosage-sensitive sex reversal) locus has been associated with 46XY gonadal dysgenesis (GD) and other anomalies. It has been mapped to the Xp21 region, which contains the DAX1 gene. Mutations in DAX1 can cause X-linked congenital adrenal hypoplasia and hypogonadotropic hypogonadism. It is hypothesized that the duplicated gene escapes normal X inactivation, therefore disrupting testis formation despite *SRY* presence.

Male patients with Denys-Drash syndrome have ambiguous genitalia with streak or dysgenetic gonads, progressive neuropathy, and Wilms' tumor. Analysis of these patients revealed heterozygous mutations of the Wilms' tumor suppressor gene (*WT1*) at 11p13. Most *WT1* mutations in Denys-Drash syndrome occur de novo and act as dominant negative mutations.

The WAGR syndrome (Wilms' tumor, aniridia, genitourinary [GU] abnormalities, mental retardation) is also associated with *WT1* alterations (heterozygous deletions). The GU anomalies in the WAGR syndrome are usually less severe than in Denys-Drash syndrome.

The *SOX9* gene (17q24.3–25.1) has been associated with campomelic dysplasia, an often lethal skeletal malformation, and 46XY GD. Affected 46XY males have phenotypic variability from normal males to normal females, depending on the function of the gonads. The *SOX9* protein is expressed in the developing gonad, rete testis, and seminiferous tubules as well as skeletal tissue.

Vanishing Testes Syndrome

Vanishing testes syndrome (congenital anorchia) describes the spectrum of anomalies resulting from cessation of testicular function. Loss of testes prior to 8 weeks' gestation results in 46XY patients with female external and internal genitalia with agonadism or streak gonads. Loss at 8–10 weeks leads to ambiguous genitalia and variable ductal development. Loss of testis function after the critical male differentiation period (12–14 weeks) results in normal male phenotype externally and internally but anorchia.

Sex Chromosome Anomalies

46XX Testicular DSD (Sex-Reversed Males)

About 1 in 20,000 phenotypic males have a 46XX karyotype. Categories include classic XX male individuals with apparently normal phenotypes, nonclassic XX males with some degree of sexual ambiguity, and XX ovotesticular DSD. Eighty to 90% of 46XX males result from an anomalous Y to X translocation involving the *SRY* gene during meiosis. The amount of DNA material involved in the exchange varies, but, in general, the greater the amount of Y DNA present, the more masculinized the phenotype.

GONADAL DYSGENESIS

GD disorders comprise a spectrum of anomalies ranging from complete absence of gonadal development to delayed gonadal failure. Complete (pure) GD includes failed gonadal development in genetic males and females due to abnormalities of sex or autosomal chromosomes. Partial gonadal dysgenesis (PGD) refers to disorders with partial testicular formation at some point in development including partial GD, 46XY GD, and some forms of testicular regression.

Complete Gonadal Dysgenesis

The bipotential gonad differentiates into an ovary if testicular formation fails. However, if one X chromosome is present, the gonad develops into an ovary but then degenerates into a streak gonad with ovarian-like stroma and little or no germ cells.

XY GD (XY sex reversal or Swyer syndrome) occurs secondary to the absence of testes despite a Y chromosome. These patients appear female externally with internal müllerian ducts and bilateral streak gonads. They also display sexual infantilism at puberty. It is a heterogenous condition that can result from deletions of the short arm of the Y chromosome, SRY gene mutations, alterations in autosomal genes, or duplications of the DSS locus on the X chromosome. Other genetic alterations that may cause this type of GD (WT1, DAX1, SOX9) have been previously discussed in the section on XY GD.

Noonan syndrome patients (often referred to as male Turner syndrome) display Turner-like stigmata including short stature, webbed neck, and right heart disease. They have a normal sex chromosome constitution often with cryptorchidism of hypoplastic testes. Puberty is delayed and androgen deficiency can be seen. However, fertility may occur in the absence of cryptorchidism. Most cases are sporadic, but familial clusters are consistent with an autosomal dominant inheritance.

46XX pure GD is characterized by normal stature, normal external and internal female genitalia, sexual infantilism, and bilateral streak gonads. It is a heterogenous condition occurring sporadically or, when familial, as an autosomal recessive trait.

The cardinal features of 45X GD (Turner syndrome) includes webbed neck, shield chest, short stature, cardiac anomalies (coarctation of the aorta), and sexual infantilism. Although bilateral streak gonads are the rule, primary follicles have been described in the genital ridges of some 45X individuals correlating with the rare occurrence of menarche. Conceptions have been documented despite karyotyping revealing only 45X cell lines. A 45X constitution may be due to nondisjunction or chromosome loss during gametogenesis in either parent resulting in a sperm or ovum without a sex chromosome. 45X/46XX mosaicism may be present in up to 75% of Turner syndrome patients.

Partial Gonadal Dysgenesis

PGD is a result of impaired testicular determination in the presence of SRY resulting in PGD. The phenotypes vary including bilateral testicular dysgenesis (46XY GD), a testis and a streak gonad (partial or mixed GD), and absence of one or both testes (testicular regression). The majority of PGD patients have a 45X/46XY karyotype, but 46XY is also seen. In contrast to patients presenting with genital ambiguity and mosaicism, 95% of prenatally detected 45X/46XY mosaics have a normal male phenotype.[24] This contradiction may be related to separate cell lines in the streak gonad and the testis. Mutations in the pseudoautosomal region of the Y chromosome upstream of the SRY gene have been identified in PGD.[17] Many of the previously discussed mutations associated with CGD (WT1, DAX1, 10qdel) have also been reported in PGD, although the etiology of GD remains unknown in most cases.

OVOTESTICULAR DSD (FORMERLY TRUE HERMAPHRODITISM)

Ovotesticular DSD, previously referred to as true hermaphroditism, requires the presence of both ovarian and testicular tissue in the individual. This uncommon condition may be classified into three groups—lateral: testis and ovary (usually left); bilateral: ovotestis and ovotestis; unilateral (most common): ovotestis and testis or ovary. The genital development is ambiguous with hypospadias, cryptorchidism, and incomplete fusion of labioscrotal folds. Genital duct differentiation generally follows that of the ipsilateral gonad.

Ovotesticular DSD can result from sex chromosome mosaicism, chimerism, or Y chromosomal translocation. The most common karyotype is 46XX followed by 46XX/46XY chimerism/mosaicism and 46XY. Most 46XX ovotesticular DSD patients are SRY-negative, and the genes responsible have not yet been identified. A mutated downstream gene in the sex determination cascade likely allows for testicular determination.

Although sex chromosome mosaicism arises from mitotic or meiotic errors, 46XX/46XY chimerism is usually a result of double fertilization (an X sperm and a Y sperm) or, less commonly, fusion of two normally fertilized ova. Thus, chimeric patients have two distinct cell populations. The least common form of ovotesticular DSD, 46XY, may result from a cryptic 46XX cell line or gonadal mosaicism with a mutated sex determination gene.

HISTORY AND PHYSICAL EXAM

Patient history should include the level of prematurity, ingestion of exogenous maternal hormones such as those used in assisted reproductive techniques, and maternal use of oral contraceptives during pregnancy. A family history is also useful for any urologic abnormalities, neonatal deaths, precocious puberty, infertility, or consanguinity. Any abnormal masculinization or cushingoid appearance of the child's mother should also be noted. Abnormalities of the prenatal maternal ultrasound are also helpful, such as discordance of the fetal karyotype with the genitalia by sonogram (Figure 25-7).

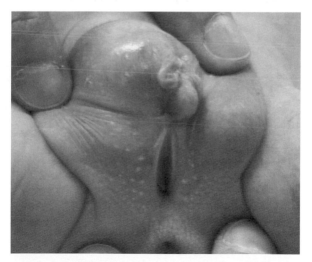

FIGURE 25-7. 46XY patient with severe hypospadias and bilateral cryptorchidism due to 46XY testicular dysgenesis.

On physical examination (see Figure 25-7), one should note any dysmorphic features including a short broad neck or widely spaced nipples. The patient should be examined in a warm room supine in the frog leg position with both legs free. An abnormal phallic size should be documented by width and stretched length measurements. I prefer to measure the penis by grasping the glans with a gauze pad, pressing down on the penopubic angle with a cotton tip applicator, and stretching the penis against the applicator to measure. One should describe the position of the urethral meatus and the amount of chordee (ventral curvature) and note the number of orifices: three in girls (urethra, vagina, and anus) or two in boys (urethra, anus). A rectal exam with your fifth finger should also be performed for palpation of a uterus. With warmed hands, one should begin the inguinal examination at the anterior superior iliac crest and sweep the groin from lateral to medial with a nondominant hand. Once a gonad is palpated, grasp it with the dominant hand and continue to sweep toward the scrotum with the other hand to attempt to bring the gonad to the scrotum. Occasionally, some soap or lubricant on the fingertips may aid in this examination. It is important to check size, location, and texture of both gonads if palpable. The undescended testis may be found in the inguinal canal; in the superficial inguinal pouch; at the upper scrotum; or rarely in the femoral, perineal, or contralateral scrotal regions. Also note the development and pigmentation of the labioscrotal folds along with any other congenital anomalies of other body systems.

For differential diagnosis and treatment purposes, the distinction needs to be made whether or not the gonad is palpable (see Figure 25-1). Unless associated with a patent processus vaginalis, ovaries and streak gonads do not descend, whereas testes, and rarely an ovotestis, may be palpable. If no gonads are palpable, any DSD diagnosis is possible. Of these, 46XX CAH is most commonly seen following by MGD. If one gonad is palpable, 46XX DSD (CAH) and PGD are ruled out, whereas MGD, ovotesticular DSD, and 46XY DSD remain possibilities. If two gonads are palpable, 46XY DSD and rarely ovotesticular DSD are the most likely diagnoses. In 46XY boys, hypospadias and cryptorchidism without an underlying intersex etiology would be diagnoses of exclusion after a full evaluation.

PATIENT EVALUATION

All patients require laboratory evaluation by karyotype, serum electrolytes, 17OH-progesterone, T, LH, and FSH levels. If the

17OH-progesterone level is elevated, 11-deoxycortisol and DOC levels will help differentiate 21α-hydroxylase deficiency from 11ß-hydroxylase deficiency. If the 17OH-progesterone level is normal, a T-to-DHT ratio along with androgen precursors before and after hCG stimulation will help elucidate the 46XY DSD etiology. During the period of 60–90 days of life, there is a normal gonadotropic surge with a resultant increase in the T level of the infant. During this specific time period, one can forego the hCG stimulation for the androgen evaluation. A failure to respond to hCG in combination with elevated LH and FSH levels is consistent with anorchia.

An ultrasound can identify a uterus or detect gonads in the inguinal region where they are also most easily palpable, but it is only 50% accurate in showing intra-abdominal testes. A computed tomography scan or a magnetic resonance imaging scan with gadolinium may also help to delineate the anatomy, although they are more expensive. A genitogram will evaluate a urogenital sinus including the entry of the urethra in the vagina. A cervical impression can be identified on the vaginogram. DSD infants, other than CAH, often require an open or laparoscopic exploration with bilateral deep longitudinal gonadal biopsies for histologic evaluation.

TREATMENT OPTIONS AND INDICATIONS

Much current research is aimed at understanding the influence of androgens on the fetal and newborn brain and its relationship to gender identity. Diagnosis and management of these children are very individualized and should always involve a "team approach," which includes the pediatric urologist, endocrinologist, geneticist, psychologist, and the child's parents immediately after birth.

46XX DSD (CAH)

Treatment of the newborn with CAH involves the correction of dehydration and salt loss by electrolyte and fluid therapy with mineralocorticoid replacement. Glucocorticoid replacement is then generally added on confirmation of the diagnosis. Infants who are going to be raised as girls usually undergo clitoral reduction and vulvovaginoplasty in early infancy, but controversy exists on the timing of surgery and all aspects must be weighed prior to decision making. Surgery can be performed for an infant, toddler, or adolescent. Many surgeons advocate early surgery for both technical and psychologic reasons realizing that vaginal revision may be needed after puberty. Surgery has three main aims: reducing the size of the enlarged masculinized clitoris, reconstructing the female labia, and increasing the opening and possibly length of the vagina. These procedures have gone through many changes during the history of surgery. Surgical technique continues to be revised to optimize the girl's external appearance and functional size while maintaining adequate sensation. Clitorectomy, which involves removing the entire clitoris, is long out of practice as is clitoral recession without reduction because it is associated with painful erections on stimulation. Reduction clitoroplasty is the operation of choice for most infants with severe clitoromegaly. The central portions of the corporal bodies are excised and the surgeon preserves the dorsal neurovascular bundles by incising Buck's fascia laterally at the 3 o'clock and 9 o'clock positions. The corporal bodies need to be dissected beyond the bifurcation to the inferior pubic rami where they are transected. The remaining proximal and distal portions of the bodies are then reapproximated and placed in the investing fascia. This optimizes future erectile function and sensation. A glansplasty is rarely required for an extremely large glans. A vulvoplasty is carried out by extending the incision for the clitoroplasty on either side of the midline strip of tissue down to the level of the vaginal orifice. Redundant labial scrotal skin is brought down as preputial flaps to form the labia minora.

The position of the vagina should be accurately determined preoperatively by the genitogram as part of the workup for intersex. There are four main types of vaginal repair: a simple "cut-back" of the perineum, a "flap" vaginoplasty, a "pull-through" vaginoplasty, or a more extensive rotation of skin flaps or segmental bowel interposition. Usually, a low vaginoplasty can be performed at the same time as the clitoroplasty. When the vagina opens very low, a simple cutback with a vertical midline incision may be all that is needed to open the introitus. Usually, however, a posterior based U-shaped flap is necessary for a tension free anastomosis reducing the risks of postoperative vaginal stenosis. Exposure of the high vagina requires either a perineal approach, a posterior vaginoplasty, or an anterior sagittal transanorectal vaginoplasty. When the vagina is extremely high and small, replacement with a bowel segment will be necessary usually with the sigmoid colon.

Gonadal Dysgenesis

A streak gonad does not descend but it may be palpable as a small remnant of tissue in an inguinal hernia sac. If a dysgenetic

847

testis is in the inguinal position, it can be removed using an incision in the groin as for a traditional orchiopexy or hernia repair. If the gonad is in the abdomen as is usually the case with the GD, then the treatment options include open abdominal exploration and removal of the gonads or laparoscopic gonadectomy, which is the usual preference. When a purely female anatomy exists, such as in Turner syndrome or Swyer syndrome, no treatment may be necessary. These girls have sexual infantilism at puberty marked by no onset of secondary sexual development. Some degree of female development, however, may be seen in up to 20–25%. Because gonadoblastoma can occur in the presence of Y chromosome material, removal of the streak gonads is required in these cases. Growth hormone is usually recommended early in childhood, and estrogen therapy is begun after puberty to optimize the patient's height. Although rare cases of spontaneous pregnancy have been reported, infertility usually occurs. Pregnancy may be possible using donor eggs and assisted reproductive techniques.

Ovotesticular DSD

Generally, a female sex has been assigned to most patients due to the presence of a vagina, uterus, and ovarian tissue. Less commonly, the patient has a 46XY karyotype with adequate penile development and without a uterus present, so a male sex assignment would be more appropriate. The decision of sex of rearing should always be deferred until the child has had an adequate evaluation of his GU system. Usually, the internal organs need to be visualized and the gonads biopsied. This can be done through an open abdominal exploration or accomplished with the use of the laparoscope. If raised as a female, the child should have dysgenetic testicular tissue removed due to the risk of malignancy. The possible need for vaginoplasty can be performed early or deferred until puberty. If the child is raised as a boy, he should have any hypospadias or cryptorchidism repaired as an infant. T supplementation may be needed if the amount of testicular tissue present is inadequate to begin or continue puberty. A persistent müllerian duct, such as a uterus and fallopian tubes, has usually not fully regressed and connects to the urethra near the bladder at the verumontanum. If there is a decision to rear the child as a boy, the structures are generally removed taking care not to injure the vas deferens, which usually runs along side the uterus. Extensive dissection behind the bladder neck and up to the area where the müllerian structures insert into the urethra is usually contraindicated to avoid damage to the sphincter mechanism risking incontinence. Both open and laparo-scopic excision has been reported. Arguments for removal of the müllerian structures include the possibility of cyclic hematuria post puberty or the formation of stones or chronic urinary tract infections if the continuity with the urethra is maintained and stasis occurs in a dilated müller-ian remnant. Arguments against removal maintain that complications from the structures are uncommon and their removal risks injury to the vas deferens, the bladder neck, and the urethral sphincter.

46XY DSD

Decreased masculinization (hypospadias with cryptorchidism or more ambiguous development) is seen in most patients with XY DSD. In untreated patients with 5α-reductase defi-ciency, significant virilization occurs at puberty as T levels increase into the adult male range, whereas DHT remains disproportionately low. Treatment is currently unclear for this enzyme deficiency when diagnosed in infancy. Male gender assignment has been recommended because the natural history of this deficiency is virilization at puberty with subse-quent change to male gender. However, this decision requires surgical hypospadias repair and orchiopexy with male hormo-nal replacement.

Rarely, do patients with dysgenetic testes have fully mas-culinized external genitalia. The surgical issues are very dependent on the degree of virilization in each individual case. This will also influence the decision process of sex assignment. If a 46XY infant with testicular dysgenesis is going to be raised as a male, he will need a hypospadias repair, orchiopexy, or possibly orchiectomy. Müllerian ducts have usually not fully regressed and may be fully or partially removed at the time of other repairs to facilitate orchio-pexies. As previously discussed, retained female structures have the potential for urinary tract infections, stones, or even cyclic hematuria at puberty. Dysgenetic testes may appear normal grossly but microscopically are disorganized and poorly formed; thus, a biopsy of the gonad is recom-mended in most children undergoing intersex evaluation. Currently, the recommendation is to remove an undes-cended dysgenetic testis because of the risk of malignancy. In 45X/46XY patients, if the biopsy is normal and the testis is scrotal or can be placed in the scrotum, it should not be removed, but a risk of malignancy correlates with the extent of testicular decent. Tumors have also been reported in scro-tal dysgenetic testes. A scrotal testis needs to be followed very closely for this reason. The possibility does exists of a male gender in these patients who would require a hypospadias repair yet would have removal of severely dysgenetic testis requiring replacement hormones. It would seem obvious that treatment in these cases needs to be individualized. The child's parents should discuss with the pediatric urologist, endocrinologist, geneticist, and psychiatrist the issues of T imprinting in utero, the need for hormones prepuberty and postpuberty, the degree of masculinization, the function of the testis, and the extent of surgery that is required.

Affected boys with errors in T production are undermasculinized with varied degrees of hypospadias, cryptorchidism, bifid scrotum, or a blind vaginal pouch. For the patient reared as a boy, T therapy may be indicated to augment penile size and to aid in the hypospadias repair. Some enzyme deficiencies require glucocorticoid and mineralocorticoid replacement and all of these patients need T replacement at puberty for masculinization. Gonadectomy is required in 46XY patients raised as girls to address the risk of tumor formation in the future.

Traditionally, a child with complete androgen sensitivity syndrome would be raised as a girl. Most of these children are not diagnosed until a workup is performed when amenorrhea occurs at puberty. Occasionally, it is discovered at the time of inguinal hernia repair or when a prenatal karyotype does not match the external phenotype of the newborn child. If the child is to be raised female, an orchiectomy is recommended for future cancer risk. The testes are at risk for cancer development and the incidence of malignant tumors is estimated to be 5–10%. Seminoma is the most common tumor seen but nonseminomatous germ cell tumors and other malignancies have also been reported. Tumor risks appears to be greater in older patients and in those with partial rather than complete androgen insensitivity and tumor formation appears to occur after puberty. Intratubular germ cell neoplasia has been identified in prepubertal boys with partial AIS but not complete AIS. Vaginal dilation or vaginal augmentation may or may not be needed. This usually is reserved until after puberty and a number of techniques are available. In patients with partial AIS, orchiectomy is recommended as soon as the diagnosis is made to avoid further virilization in patients who will be raised in the female gender. Male gender assignment is usually successful in patients with a predominantly male phenotype; however, predicting the adequacy of masculinization in adulthood may not be possible based on the maternal family history or characterization of the androgen receptor genetic defect. Some children do respond well to high-dose androgen therapy, but its durability is not yet clear.

Controversy exists concerning the best time to perform the orchiectomy. Traditionally, in an infant with complete AIS, the testes are left in place until after puberty to take advantage of the hormonal function, and in this way, natural female pubertal changes can occur by T conversion to estrogen, augmented by exogenous estrogen. After puberty is completed, the testes would be removed and replacement estrogen continued. Risks to be discussed include only one case of yolk sac tumor in an abdominal UDT in prepubertal CAIS children; carcinoma in situ (CIS), which has been uncommonly seen prepubertally; inguinal testes are easily injured; psychologic issues, including explaining to a mature postpubertal patient of the need to remove her testes; the risk of testis cancer increases if the patient is lost to follow-up care; and early orchiectomy requires full replacement hormones for pubertal changes.

Treatment of the child with DSD should not end with the first postoperative visit. A boy should be evaluated 1 year after orchiopexy for testes size, location, and viability. The parents should be made aware of the issues regarding cancer and infertility. Starting at puberty, the boy should be shown how to perform monthly testicular self-exams and offered a semen analysis check at age 18. Orchiopexy is not protective against testis cancer development, but it does allow easier palpation for subsequent physical exams. Although intra-abdominal testes comprise only 10–15% of all undescended testes, they account for almost 50% of those testes that develop cancer. The most common tumor in an undescended testes is a seminoma. Up to 35% of dysgenetic testes may develop cancer, most commonly a benign tumor called gonadoblastoma. Although this tumor does not spread, it can develop into a malignant form called a dysgerminoma. Patients with a 45X/45XY mosaic karyotype also have an increased risk of CIS. Some surgeons have recommended ultrasound and biopsy of a testis at puberty. Ultrasound is then performed yearly until age 20 when a repeat biopsy is performed. Absence of CIS at age 20 suggests that the risk of CIS is minimal.

The patient with hypospadias repaired as a child should remain in follow-up with his physician to identify and correct any long-term complications of the surgery. It is also important to document adequate control of voiding and the force of urinary stream. There appears to be no increase in infertility from a purely urethral point of view rather than that previously described for cryptorchidism.

Cosmetic and functional results improve yearly with advances in optical magnification, instrumentation and sutures, and tissue handling. Continuous research in this area allows the surgeon to refine the technique and provide the patient with the best repair possible. Girls who have undergone a feminizing genitoplasty again require long-term follow-up for issues of menstruation, intercourse, and sensation as previously described. With a proper assignment of sex of rearing and a continued management with continuity of care, DSD individuals should be able to lead well-adjusted lives and ultimately obtain sexual satisfaction. Simple, yet comprehensive, discussions with all physicians involved and the parents must take into account parental anxieties and social, cultural, and religious views to obtain appropriate gender assignment.

New molecular biology techniques have allowed genetic analysis to be commonplace for patient evaluation. As new genes have been described, a complex, yet specific pathway of sex determination and development has evolved that allows us to formulate clinical algorithms for both prenatal and postnatal diagnosis and treatment. The future holds great promise for the further definition of the genes involved in urogenital development and function.

SELF-ASSESSMENT QUESTIONS

1. What physical characteristic is most useful in the initial evaluation of the child with DSD?
2. How do children with congenital adrenal hyperplasia differ clinically among the various subsets of enzyme deficiencies (including male versus female)?
3. Describe the phenotypes seen in androgen insensitivity syndrome.
4. What gonadal tumors are most commonly seen in DSD and when is an orchiectomy recommended?
5. What laboratory tests (hormone levels) are used to evaluate abnormalities of androgen synthesis (including newborn versus 2 month old versus 4 month old)?

SUGGESTED READINGS

1. Donohue PA, Migeon CJ: Congenital adrenal hyperplasia. In: Scriver CR, Sly WS, Valle D (eds.): *The Metabolic and Molecular Basis of Inherited Disease*, 7th ed. New York, McGraw-Hill, 1995, pp 2929–2966.

2. Goodfellow PA, Lovell-Badge R: SRY and sex determination in mammals. *Ann Rev Genet* 27:71–92, 1993.
3. Hughes IA: Minireview: sex differentiation. *Endocrinology* 142:3281–3287, 2001.
4. Hughes IA, Houk C, Ahmed SF, Lee PA; LWPES/ESPE Consensus Group: Consensus statement on management of intersex disorders. *Arch Dis Child* 11:273–282, 2006.
5. Imperato-McGinley JL, Guerrero L, Gautier T, et al: Steroid 5α-reductase deficiency in man: an inherited form of male pseudohermaphroditism. *Science* 186:1213–1215, 1974.
6. Miller WL: Genetics, diagnosis and management of 21-hydroxylase deficiency. *J Clin Endocrinol Metab* 78:241–246, 1994.
7. Swain A, Narvaez V, Burgoyne P, et al: DAX1 antagonizes SRY action in mammalian sex determination. *Nature* 391:761–767, 1998.
8. Wiener JS, Marcelli M, Lamb DJ: Molecular determinants of sexual differentiation. *World J Urol* 14:278–294, 1996.

C H A P T E R 26

Pediatric Oncology

Michael C. Carr, MD, PhD and
Howard M. Snyder III, MD

I. WILMS' TUMOR

A. General

1. Characterized by Wilms in 1899, first described by Rance in 1814.
2. Seven new cases per 1 million children per year in the North America (450 cases per year).
   a) Eighty percent of all childhood solid tumors.
   b) Eighty percent of all genitourinary (GU) cancers in children younger than 15 years.
   c) Seventy-five percent in children between 1 and 5 years of age; peak incidence 3–4 years of age; 90% before 7 years of age.
   d) Male-to-female ratio equal, 1% familial; slightly higher rates in black population and lower in Asian children.

B. Pathology-Embryology

1. Gross pathologic features.
   a) Sharply demarcated, encapsulated.
   b) Usually solitary.
   c) Frequently hemorrhagic or necrotic.
   d) True cyst formation rare.
   e) Pelvis invasion rare; venous invasion 20%.
   f) Extrarenal sites (retroperitoneum, inguinal, mediastinal, sacrococcygeal) rare.
2. Microscopic features—wide spectrum.
   a) Triphasic: metanephric blastema, epithelium (glomerulotubular), and stroma (myxoid, occasionally differentiated into striated muscle, cartilage, or fat).
   b) Unfavorable histology (UH) in 10% of cases; two types:
      i) Anaplasia: threefold variation in nuclear size with hyperchromism and mitoses. Monomorphic sarcomatous-appearing tumors.
      ii) Rhabdoid: uniform large cells with large nuclei, prominent nucleoli, and eosinophilic cytoplasmic

853

inclusions (fibrils), metastasizes to brain, is probably not metanephric. Rhabdoid tumor of the kidney and clear cell sarcoma of the kidney have been reclassified and are now considered distinct entities from Wilms' tumor sarcoma.

   iii) Clear cell sarcoma, "bone metastasizing tumors of childhood": vasocentric spindle cell pattern, may be malignant version of congenital mesoblastic nephroma (pure blastemal origin) and not a true form of Wilms' tumor.

c) Favorable histology (FH) consists of all other types, tubular predominance being perhaps most favorable of all.

d) Cystic nephroma (CN) and cystic, partially differentiated nephroblastoma (CPDN) are benign neoplasms currently considered by many experts to be part of the spectrum of nephroblastoma; tumors occur in both adults and children, are generally asymptomatic, but may cause hematuria. CNs are all cystic, without solid component, with septa purely stromal without blastemal elements. CPDN is also cystic, but septae contain blastemal elements (or nephrogenic rests). It is important to note that nephroblastomas, clear cell sarcomas, and mesoblastic nephromas may also be predominantly cystic.

e) Congenital mesoblastic nephroma occurs in early infancy. It is associated with polyhydramnios, resembles leiomyoma grossly, and histologically exhibits sheets of spindle-shape uniform cells that appear to be fibroblasts. There is no capsule but when completely excised, it follows a benign course; it may be a hamartoma. The spindle cell variant may behave with a more malignant potential.

3. Genetics and associated anomalies.

a) 11p chromosomal deletion and sporadic, not congenital, aniridia associated with a 20% incidence of Wilms' tumors.

b) 11p deletion common in tumor genotype; 12q also reported.

c) Trisomy 8 and 18, 45 XO (Turner's), and XX/XY mosaicism associated.

d) Loss of heterozygosity for portion of chromosome 16q may portend poorer outcome.

e) Sporadic (nonfamilial) aniridia associated; full syndrome includes early tumor (less than 3 years), other GU anomalies. External ear deformities, retardation, facial dysmorphism, hernias, and hypotonia.

   f) Hemihypertrophy (1 in 14,000 general population, 1 in 32 in Wilms' patients) along with other malignancies (i.e., adrenal carcinoma, hepatoblastoma), as well as pigmented nevi and hemangiomas.

   g) Beckwith-Wiedemann syndrome: visceromegaly involving adrenal, kidney, liver, pancreas, often with hypoglycemia; gonads, with omphalocele, hemihypertrophy, microcephaly, retardation, macroglossia; 10% develop a neoplasm of liver, adrenal, or kidney.

   h) Musculoskeletal deformities exhibited in 2.9%, with 30-fold increase in neurofibromatosis incidence.

   i) GU anomalies exhibited in 4.4% including renal hypoplasia, ectopia or fusion, duplications, cystic disease, hypospadias, cryptorchidism, pseudohermaphroditism.

4. The neuroblastomatosis complex appears to be a precursor of Wilms' tumor and consists of persistent primitive metanephric elements beyond 36 weeks of gestation; occurs in three forms.

   a) Superficial infantile form in which entire kidney is replaced by blastema; infant presents with massive nephromegaly and dies shortly after birth; rarest form.

   b) Multifocal juvenile form or nodular renal blastema (NRB) consists of gross or microscopic NRB nodules that may be sclerotic or glomerulocystic and papillary, usually in the subcapsular region or along the columns of Bertin.

   c) Wilms' tumorlet exhibits triphasic histology and nodules between 1 and 3.5 cm.

   d) Some component of nephroblastomatosis is present in 100% of bilateral Wilms' patients, and in at least 40% of unilateral cases.

   e) May represent Wilms' tumor precursor in the "two-hit" theory of oncogenesis of Knudson and Strong.

   f) NRB should be sought, mobilizing and inspecting the contralateral kidney carefully. Any area of abnormal color or a cleft should be biopsied; it does respond to chemotherapy, but the best program and full therapeutic implications remain to be demonstrated.

C. Management of Wilms' Tumor

1. Diagnosis and management.

   a) Three fourths present with palpable abdominal mass, usually smooth and rarely crossing midline (in contrast to neuroblastoma).

Table 26-1:	Childhood Tumors

Malignant abdominal tumors
Renal: Wilms' tumor, renal cell carcinoma
Neuroblastoma
Rhabdomyosarcoma
Hepatoblastoma
Lymphoma, lymphosarcoma
Benign abdominal masses
Renal: renal abscess, multicystic dysplastic kidney,
    hydronephrosis, polycystic kidney, congenital mesoblastic
    nephroma
Mesenteric cysts
Choledochal cysts
Intestinal duplication cysts
Splenomegaly

b) One third present with abdominal pain, often associated with minor trauma and hemorrhage within tumor.

c) Hypertension accompanies 25–60% of cases.

d) Differential diagnosis includes other tumors and hydronephrosis or cystic disease (Table 26-1).

e) Abdominal ultrasound will diagnose most Wilms' tumors, as well as evaluate the retroperitoneum, liver, and vena cava for extension of disease.

f) Screening serial renal ultrasounds are needed for patients with aniridia, hemihypertrophy, and Beckwith-Wiedemann syndrome at an interval of every 3–4 months.

g) Four-view chest x-ray completes the metastatic workup.

h) Angiography and cavography are rarely indicated; computed tomography (CT) may be helpful with very extensive lesions, detecting bilateral disease and providing functional assessment of contralateral kidney.

   i) Complete blood count (CBC), urinalysis, serum creatinine, and urea nitrogen levels complete the preoperative testing; urine catecholamines help to rule out neuroblastoma.

2. Surgical treatment.

   a) Exploration is carried out as soon as the child is stable, the previously mentioned studies are completed, and the situation is no longer considered an emergency.

b) Transverse abdominal incision provides adequate exposure in most cases; from the tip of the 12th rib on the involved side to the lateral rectus border on the opposite side.

c) Exploration of the contralateral kidney with biopsy as needed should be carried out first; reflection of colon and complete mobilization of kidney are required for adequate visualization and manual inspection of front and back surfaces of the kidney.

d) Resectability depends largely on the degree of attachment to the liver, duodenum, pancreas, spleen, diaphragm, abdominal wall, or major vascular invasion into the vena cava. Heroic extirpation involving major resection of these organs or cardiopulmonary bypass to remove high caval or atrial tumors is not warranted.

e) Unresectable lesions should be treated with chemotherapy and re-explored; usually the tumor may then be removed. Pretreatment of large tumors reduces the rate of intraoperative rupture but does not influence and may alter histology (FH versus UH distinction). As the preoperative diagnostic error rate has been 5% in the United States, routine pretreatment has not been recommended.

f) Beginning the dissection along the posterior abdominal wall inferiorly and the great vessels medially, with early ureteral ligation, allows early exposure and ligation of renal vessels prior to mobilization of the mass.

g) Biopsy of the tumor or localized operative spill does not upstage the tumor unless it is massive, in which case, whole abdomen irradiation is needed to avoid an increased incidence of abdominal recurrence. Largest relative risk for local recurrence in National Wilms' Tumor Study (NWTS)-4 observed in patients with stage III disease, those with UH (especially diffuse anaplasia), and those reported to have major tumor spillage during surgery.

h) The adrenal is taken if the tumor involves the upper pole.

i) Gross assessment of nodes has a 40% false-positive and 0% false-negative rate, and thus routine biopsy of hilar and periaortic nodes is warranted; radical node dissection does not influence survival but does improve staging. The absence of lymph node biopsy is associated with an increased relative risk of recurrence, which was largest in children with presumed stage I disease due to understaging.

**Table 26-2:   Staging System of the National Wilms'
Tumor Study (NWTS)**

Stage	Description
I	Tumor limited to the kidney and completely excised. The renal capsule is intact and the tumor was not ruptured prior to removal. There is no residual tumor. The vessels of the renal sinus are not involved.
II	Tumor extends beyond the kidney but is completely excised. There is regional extension of tumor (i.e., penetration of the renal capsule, extensive invasion of the renal sinus). The tumor may have been biopsied or there may be local spillage of tumor confined to the flank. Extrarenal vessels may contain tumor thrombus or be infiltrated by tumor.
III	Residual nonhematogenous tumor confined to the abdomen; lymph node involvement, diffuse peritoneal spillage either before or during surgery, peritoneal implants, tumor beyond surgical margin either grossly or microscopically, or tumor not completely removed.
IV	Hematogenous metastases (lung, liver, bone, brain, etc.) or lymph node metastases outside the abdominopelvic region are present.
V	Bilateral renal involvement at diagnosis.

    j) Remaining tumor in nodes or other organs should be marked with surgical clips to facilitate direction of radiation therapy.

    k) NWTS investigators found a 20% incidence of surgical complications, with the most common being intestinal obstruction and hemorrhage.

3. Staging (Table 26-2).

    a) Histopathology and tumor stage are the most important predictors of survival in Wilms' tumor patients. The staging system has undergone refinement over the years as data have been examined with each NWTS study.

    b) In NWTS-3, the distribution by stage of FH tumors was stage I, 47%; stage II, 22%; stage III, 22%; and stage IV, 9%. Both the surgeon and pathologist have responsibility for determining local tumor stage.

Table 26-3: Protocol for National Wilms' Tumor Study (NWTS)-5

	Radiotherapy	Chemotherapy Regimen
Stage I, FH < 24 mo and < 550 gm tumor weight	None	None (surgery only for this group)
Stage I, FH > 24 mo and/or > 550 gm tumor weight	None	EE-4A (AMD plus VCR; 18 wk)
Stage II, FH		
Stage I, anaplasia		
Stage III-IV FH	Yes[a]	DD-4A (AMD, VCR, and DOX; 24 wk)
Stage II–IV, focal anaplasia		
Stage II–IV, diffuse anaplasia	Yes[a]	I (VCR + CPM + E; 24 wk)
Stage I–IV CCSK	Yes[a]	I as above
Stage I–IV RTK	Yes[a]	RTK (Carbo + E + CPM; 24 wk)
Stage V, bilateral: biopsy or limited surgery, both kidneys		
Stage I or II, FH		EE-4A as above
Stage III or IV, FH		DD-4A as above
Stage I–IV, anaplasia		I as above

aConsult protocol for details regarding radiation therapy.
FH, favorable histology; AMD, dactinomycin; VCR, vincristine; DOX, doxorubicin; CPM, cyclophosphamide; CCSK, clear cell sarcoma of the kidney; RTK, rhabdoid tumor of the kidney; E, etoposide; carbo, carboplatin.

4. Chemotherapy and radiation therapy are given in NWTS-5 according to Table 26-3.
   a) NWTS-4 demonstrated that a short administration schedule (6 months) of vincristine and dactinomycin is equally as effective as longer duration therapy (15 months) with respect to 4-year relapse-free survival (RFS).
   b) The use of single-dose (pulse-intensive) treatment with dactinomycin has an equivalent 2-year RFS to those treated with standard 5-day regimen. Pulse-intensive drug administration provides for equal efficacy, greater

administration dose intensity, and less severe hematologic toxicity.
   c) Patients with bilateral Wilms' tumor and/or nephrogenic rests should be managed with a nephron-sparing approach following primary chemotherapy. Those patients with anaplasia are at much greater risk for recurrence, so for them a renal-sparing approach is not beneficial.
5. Treatment of relapses.
   a) Variable prognosis based on initial stage, site of relapse, time from initial diagnosis to relapse, and prior therapy.
   b) Risk of tumor relapse in NWTS-3 at 3 years was 9.6, 11.8, 22, and 22%, respectively, for stages I through IV. Relapses occurred in 36% of stage I through III and 45% of stage IV patients with UH.
   c) Adriamycin, dacarbazine, cisplatin, or higher doses of vincristine and/or cyclophosphamide (Cytoxan) are used to treat relapses.
6. Complications of therapy.
   a) Bone marrow suppression, early or delayed radiation enteritis, bowel obstruction, hepatic dysfunction, scoliosis, radiation nephritis, interstitial pneumonitis, cardiomyopathy with congestive heart failure, and sterility.
   b) Secondary neoplasms are reported in 3–17% in 20- to 25-year survivors, especially in radiation fields.
7. Cooperative group trials.
   a) Prospective randomized trials have been necessary to answer questions about optimal treatment. The Children's Cancer Study Group and the Pediatric Oncology Group collaborated within the National Wilms' Tumor Study Group.
   b) Results of NWTS-3 summarized in Table 26-4.
   c) NWTS-5 is focusing on correlating biologic parameters with the outcome of treatment of Wilms' tumor. Genes on chromosome 11 may be responsible for induction of Wilms' tumor. Loss of heterozygosity for a portion of chromosome 16q in 20% of patients with Wilms' tumor has been noted.

II. NEUROBLASTOMA

A. Incidence

Represents 8–10% of all childhood malignancies and is the most common malignant tumor of infancy. Following brain

Table 26-4: Results of the National Wilms' Tumor Study 3

Stage	Histology	Four-Year Postnephrectomy Survival (%)
I	Favorable	97
II	Favorable	92
III	Favorable	84
IV	Favorable	83
I–III	Unfavorable	68
IV	Unfavorable	55
All patients		
Unfavorable		89
Clear cell sarcoma		75
Rhabdoid sarcoma		26

Adapted from D'Angio CJ, Breslow N, Beekwith JB, et al: *Cancer* 64:349–360, 1989. Reproduced from Snyder HM, D'Angio CJ, Evans AE, Raney RB: Pediatric oncology. In: Walsh PC, Retik AB, Stamey TA, Vaughan ED (eds): *Campbell's Urology*, 6th ed. Philadelphia, Saunders, 1992, p 1981.

tumors, it is the most common malignant solid tumor of childhood. One third of cases are diagnosed in first year of life and an additional quarter between 1 and 2 years of age.

B. Etiology

1. Arise from primitive, pluripotential sympathetic cells (sympathogonia) derived from neural crest.
2. Ganglioneuromas and ganglioneuroblastomas also arise from neural crest cells.
3. Characterized cytogenetically by deletion of the short arm of chromosome 1.

C. Pathology

Gross tumors are lobular, tend to be infiltrative, often associated with stippled calcification. Histologically, one of "small, round blue-cell tumors" of childhood. May form rosettes and exhibit neurofibrils if differentiation is good. Ultrastructure shows characteristic peripheral dendritic processes. Gradual degree of malignancy from neuroblastoma (most malignant) to ganglioneuroblastoma (intermediate) to ganglioneuroma (benign).

D. Location and Presentation

Can arise anywhere along the sympathetic chain from the head to pelvis. More than half arise in the abdomen and two thirds of these in the adrenal. Presents as an irregular, firm, nontender, fixed mass often extending beyond the midline. Abdominal paravertebral sympathetic ganglion origin has an increased incidence of dumbbell-shaped intraspinal extension, which may produce signs of cord compression. Presacral tumors may result in urinary frequency, retention, or constipation. Cervical sympathetic tumors can cause Horner's syndrome. Thoracic tumors may be asymptomatic or produce cough, dyspnea, or infection from airway compression. As many as 70% of patients have metastasis (liver is most common in younger children, bone in older children) at presentation. Unexplained fever, malaise, anorexia, weight loss, and irritability are common.

E. Diagnosis

Anemic if disease has disseminated. Bone marrow aspirate is indicated in all suspected cases: 50–70% positive. Ninety-five percent of patients have elevation of urinary catecholamines produced by tumor (vanillylmandelic acid and/or homovanillic acid). Can be checked on spot urine sample. Appropriate radiographic imaging will depend on site. For abdominal tumors, intravenous pyelography, ultrasound, CT, and magnetic resonance (MR) contribute to staging tumor and determining resectability. Chest x-rays, skeletal survey, and often, bone scan are routine. Table 26-5 depicts minimum recommended tests for determining extent of disease.

F. Staging and Prognosis

1. The current, favored staging system is based on clinical, radiographic, and surgical evaluation of children with neuroblastoma. The International Neuroblastoma Staging System (INSS or Evans classification) provides for uniformity in staging of patients, facilitating clinical trials and biologic studies around the world (Table 26-6).
2. A histologic-based prognostic classification (Shimada) is formulated around patient age and the following histologic features:
    a) Presence or absence of schwannian stroma.
    b) Degree of differentiation.
    c) Mitosis-karyorrhexis index (MKI).

Table 26-5: Minimum Recommended Tests for Determining Extent of Disease Neuroblastoma

Tumor Site	Tests
Primary	Three-dimensional measurement of tumor by CT scan or MR or ultrasound
Metastases	Bilateral posterior iliac bone marrow aspirates and core biopsies (4 adequate specimens necessary to exclude tumor)
	Bone radiographs and either scintigraphy (^{99m}Tc-diphosphonate or ^{131}I- or ^{123}I) meta-iodobenzylguanidine (MIBG) or abdominal and liver imaging by CT scan or MR or ultrasound
	Chest radiograph (AP and lateral) and chest CT scan
Markers	Quantitative urinary catecholamine metabolites (VMA and HVA)

AP, anteroposterior; CT, computed tomography; HVA, homovanillic acid; MR, magnetic resonance; VMA, vanillylmandelic acid.

3. Retrospective evaluation of the Shimada method demonstrated that histologic patterns were independently predictive of outcome, whereas stage was prognostically less important.

4. A simplified system has been devised, which predicts a favorable outlook based on presence of calcification and a low mitotic rate (less than 10 mitoses/10 high-power field). Grading system developed for finding tumors with both features (grade 1), the presence of only one of these features (grade 2), or absence of both features (grade 3). Combining grade with age (less than 1 or older than 1 year) and surgicopathologic staging, low- and high-risk groups emerge. Further evaluation will take into account histologic modifiers, such as level of serum ferritin, *N-myc* copy number, and tumor DNA content. *N-myc* amplification occurs in 25–30% of primary neuroblastomas from untreated patients and amplification is associated primarily with advanced stages of disease.

G. Treatment

1. Complete surgical removal is the most effective form of therapy, which also allows for diagnosis, provides tissue

Table 26-6:   International Neuroblastoma Staging System

Stage	Description
1	Localized tumor confined to the area of origin; complete gross excision, with or without microscopic residual disease; identifiable ipsilateral and contralateral lymph nodes negative microscopically
2A	Unilateral tumor with incomplete gross excision; identifiable ipsilateral and contralateral lymph nodes; identifiable contralateral lymph nodes negative microscopically
2B	Unilateral tumor with complete or incomplete gross excision; positive ipsilateral regional lymph nodes; identifiable contralateral lymph nodes negative microscopically
3	Tumor infiltrating across the midline with or without regional lymph node involvement; or unilateral tumor with contralateral regional lymph node involvement; or midline tumor with bilateral lymph node involvement
4	Dissemination of tumor to distant lymph nodes, bone, bone marrow, liver, and/or other organs (except as defined in stage 4S)
4S	Localized primary tumor as defined for stage 1 or 2 with dissemination limited to liver, skin, and/or bone marrow

for biologic studies and surgical stage of tumor, and allows for attempted excision of tumor. Based on INSS criteria, the operative protocol incorporates the following:

a) Resectability of primary or metastatic tumor determined in light of tumor location, mobility, relationship to major vessels, ability to control blood supply, and overall prognosis of patient.

b) Nonadherent, intracavitary lymph nodes should be sampled.

c) Routine biopsy of the liver in situations involving an abdominal neuroblastoma without evidence of metastatic disease has been advocated.

2. **Treatment of low-risk disease.** Treatment for patients with localized tumors consists most commonly of surgery

Table 26-7: Disease-Free Survival (Two-Year) Based on Risk Category and Age

Risk Category	Two-Year Disease-Free Survival (%)	Patient Age (Years)	INSS Stage
Low	>90	All	1
	85	All	2A
	87/89	<1	2B/3
	57–90	<1	4S
Intermediate	59	>1	2B/3
	75	<1	4
High	40/15[a]	>1	4

[a]Difference relates to complete versus partial surgical resection, respectively. INSS, International Neuroblastoma Staging System.

alone but in some cases surgery combined with 6–12 weeks of chemotherapy. Chemotherapy consists of carboplatin, cyclophosphamide, doxorubicin, and etoposide. Dose of agent is kept low to minimize permanent injury from chemotherapy regimen.

3. **Treatment of intermediate-risk disease.** Children with metastatic disease to regional lymph nodes and infants with INSS stage 4 tumors comprise this group. Chemotherapy occurs for 12–24 weeks of the same chemotherapy as described previously. In addition, radiation therapy is utilized to enhance disease-free survival.

4. **Treatment of high-risk disease.** Patients with disseminated disease require intensive treatment with multiagent therapy of various combinations, but overall survival has remained disappointingly low (below 15%). The use of high-dose chemotherapy (carboplatin, cyclophosphamide, doxorubicin, etoposide, and ifosfamide with high-dose cisplatin), surgery, intraoperative radiation, and bone marrow transplantation has resulted in improved 3-year survival rates (Table 26-7).

III. GU RHABDOMYOSARCOMA

Rhabdomyosarcoma arises from primitive totipotential embryonal mesenchyme. GU involvement occurs with the second greatest frequency after head and neck tumors. Sites include bladder, prostate, vagina, and cervix or paratesticular tissue. They comprise approximately 20% of all rhabdo-myosarcomas. The incidence of GU rhabdomyosarcoma is 0.5–0.7 cases per 1 million children younger than 15 years.

A. Pathology

1. Tumor arises from any site that develops from embryonic mesenchyme.
   a) Rhabdomyoblasts are the progenitor cell.
   b) Tumor subtypes differ based on extent of differentiation from mesenchymal progenitor.
   c) Classification system of Horn and Enterline based on primary histologic subtype: embryonal (60%); botryoid; alveolar (20%); spindle cell; and pleomorphic.
   d) New international classification system proposed by Intergroup Rhabdomyosarcoma Study (IRS) (Table 26-8).
   e) Desmin and actin stains sometimes useful in determining diagnosis.
   f) Genetic translocations between chromosome 1; 13 (favorable) and 2; 13 (very high risk) are prognostic markers for survival in patients with alveolar tumors with metastatic disease.

Table 26-8:	IRS-IV Staging				
Stage	N	M	Tumor Location	T	Size
1	N0 or N1	M0	Favorable sites	T1 or T2	a or b
2	N0	M0	Unfavorable site	T1 or T2	a
3	N1	M0	Unfavorable site	T1 or T2	a
	N0 or N1	M0		T1 or T2	b
4	N0 or N1	M1	Metastatic disease	T1 or T2	a or b

T1, confined to anatomic site of origin; T2, extension and/or fixation to surrounding tissue; Ta, tumor less than 5 cm in greatest diameter; Tb, tumor is 5 cm or larger; N0, regional lymph nodes are not clinically involved; N1, regional nodes are clinically involved by tumor; M0, no distant metastases; and M1, metastases are present. Genitourinary (GU) tumors considered to be favorable sites include the vulva and vagina. GU tumors considered to be unfavorable sites include the bladder, prostate, and uterus.

B. Presentation

1. Signs and symptoms dependent on organ of involvement and size of the primary at initial assessment.
   a) Bladder or prostate-irritative voiding symptoms, urinary retention, incontinence, or infection. Trigonal involvement leads to hydronephrosis and progressive obstruction. Hematuria and constipation are also seen.
   b) Vagina-visible mass, hemorrhage, and vaginal discharge.
   c) Paratesticular rhabdomyosarcoma presents as painless scrotal mass with two peak incidences at 3–4 months of age and again during teenage years.

C. Evaluation

1. Thorough assessment of both local and metastatic sites.
   a) CT and ultrasound scan of abdomen and pelvis.
   b) Lobulated soft tissue mass with homogenous echogenicity seen on ultrasound.
   c) Transrectal ultrasonography can document involvement of prostate and facilitate biopsies.
2. CT most widely used modality for GU rhabdomyosarcomas—employ oral, rectal, and intravenous contrast.
3. MR imaging with gadolinium-diethylenetriaminepentaacetic acid (DTPA) facilitates intravesical imaging and invasion into adjacent pelvic structures.
4. Accurate diagnosis based on histologic examination. Many GU tumors are amenable to endoscopic biopsy with cold cup forceps, either percutaneously, transvaginally, or transrectally.
5. Liver, lung, bone, bone marrow, and retroperitoneal nodes are most common sites for metastatic spread. Serum chemistries, including CBC and liver function tests, x-ray or CT of chest, bone scan, and bone marrow biopsy are needed to complete evaluation.

D. Staging

1. IRS represents collaborative efforts from multiple institutions. IRS staging is dependent on resectability of primary tumor and status of draining lymph nodes.
2. Group 1: local disease (without lymph node involvement) that has been completely removed both grossly and microscopically.
3. Group 2: tumors grossly removed but residual microscopic disease (2A), regional nodal involvement with no microscopic residual disease (2B), or both nodal involvement and residual disease (2C).

Table 26-9:   Intergroup Rhabdomyosarcoma Study
(IRS)-IV Staging and Treatment of Paratesticular
Rhabdomyosarcoma

Clinical Group	Tumor Status	Therapy
1	Tumor completely excised[a](not alveolar subtype)	Vincristine and actinomycin D for 1 year[b]
2	Tumor excised with microscopic residual disease at margin and/or positive lymph nodes involving ipsilateral hilar-para-aortic chain	Vincristine plus actinomycin D plus cyclophosphamide versus vincristine plus actinomycin D plus ifosfamide for 1–2 years plus radiation therapy to involved region[c]
3	Gross residual local and/or regional disease (retroperitoneal nodes) that is not surgically removable	Three- to 7-drug regimen plus radiation therapy to involved region[d]
4	Distant metastasis	Same as group 3

[a]If there has been scrotal contamination, hemiscrotectomy and relocation of the contralateral testis into the thigh are advised to avoid the effects of local radiation on the remaining gonad.
[b]No radiation for group 1 patients.
[c]Conventional radiation.
[d]Conventional or hyperfractionated radiation.

4. Group 3: incomplete removal of gross disseminated disease.
5. Group 4: distant metastatic involvement present.

This system is dependent on the extent of surgical resection. The IRS-IV staging system (TMN) has been designed to overcome some of these shortcomings. The most important change is the inclusion of pretreatment stage (Table 26-9), rather than surgical staging alone.

E. Intergroup Rhabdomyosarcoma Studies

1. The collective experience of a number of institutions was needed to assess a growing number of treatment options. IRS-I determined that:

a) Postoperative radiation therapy of the tumor bed was helpful in group 1 patients.
b) Chemotherapy with vincristine, actinomycin D, and cyclophosphamide (VAC) was superior to vincristine and actinomycin D alone (VA) in group 2 patients.
c) Pulse VAC following initial irradiation in groups 3 and 4 was beneficial.
d) Adriamycin provided additional benefit in those with advance disease (groups 3 and 4).

2. With the favorable results achieved in IRS-I, IRS-II (1978–1984) determined the feasibility of primary chemotherapy. Following biopsy-proven rhabdomyosarcoma, VAC therapy was initiated, response documented, and chemotherapy continued for 16 weeks. The residual mass was resected and chemotherapy continued for 2 years. Radiation therapy was added for gross or microscopic disease following resection.

3. IRS-III (1984–1988) addressed five specific issues regarding chemotherapeutic protocols and response to therapy. More aggressive chemotherapeutic protocols were used in patients with UH (alveolar, anaplastic, and monomorphous types). The use of second- and third-look surgery to assess response in groups 3 and 4 would lead to improved local control.

The results of IRS-III proved superior to IRS-I and II. There was a 60% salvage rate of functioning bladder at 4 years from diagnosis compared to only 22% and 25% in prior studies. Mortality in patients with disseminated disease (groups 1 through 3) declined to less than 10%.

F. Treatment

1. In IRS-IV, VAC was shown to be as effective as two other three-drug regimens (VIE/VAE-ifosfamide, etoposide). In IRS-V, low-risk patients are randomized to receive either VA or VAC, ± x-ray therapy (XRT). Intermediate-risk patients received chemotherapy and XRT and are randomized to VAC or VAC alternating with vincristine, topotecan, and cyclophosphamide. High-risk patients received CPT-11 (irinotecan, VAC, and XRT).

2. In IRS-IV, hyperfractionated radiation therapy did not achieve better results than conventional radiation therapy. For IRS-V, patients with group 1 embryonal pathology will not receive XRT. For other patients, the dose of radiation to residual primary will be higher than to microscopic residual disease, and metastasis will be irra-

diated as well. Surgery as treatment of gross residual disease after chemotherapy is still an option.

G. Relapse

Five-year survival after relapse is 64% for botryoid embryonal, 26% for other embryonal, and 5% for alveolar or undifferentiated pathology. Lower stage embryonal lesions portend improved survival after relapse: 52% stage I, 20% stage II and III, and 12% stage IV.

H. Complications

1. Hematologic complications similar to those seen with the same drugs in Wilms' tumor therapy occur.
2. The high radiation dose required to control this tumor often produces severe proctitis and fibrosing cystitis, which may destroy normal bladder function and complicate any subsequent surgery such as reconstruction.

IV. TESTIS TUMORS

Testis tumors are uncommon in children, accounting for approximately 1–2% of all pediatric solid tumors. Incidence in children is 1 per 100,000. Peak age incidence is 2 years of age; more benign tumors and fewer germinal testis tumors than in adults.

A. Classification

1. Classification has been debated (Table 26-10).
2. Germinal tumors constitute only approximately 77%, compared with 95% of testis tumors in adults.
   a) Yolk sac carcinoma (embryonal carcinoma, endodermal sinus tumor, orchioblastoma) comprises approximately 39–62% of all testis tumors in children. Rarely (4%) spreads to retroperitoneal nodes; more frequently (20%) spreads to lungs, especially if child is older than 1 year. Alpha-fetoprotein (AFP) elevated 90% of time. Average age of presentation is 3 years.
   b) Teratoma constitutes approximately 14%; uniformly benign tumor in children younger than 2 years, even when histology appears malignant.
   c) Seminoma is extremely rare before puberty and in essence should be considered a postpubertal tumor.

Table 26-10:	Classification of Prepubertal Testis Tumors	
I	Germ cell tumors	Yolk sac tumor Teratoma Mixed germ cell Seminoma
II	Gonadal stromal tumors	Leydig cell Sertoli cell Juvenile granulosa cell Mixed
III	Gonadoblastoma	
IV	Tumors of supporting tissues	Fibroma Leiomyoma Hemangioma
V	Lymphomas and leukemias	
VI	Tumor-like lesions	Epidermoid cyst Hyperplastic nodule attributable to congenital adrenal hyperplasia
VII	Secondary tumors	
VIII	Tumors of the adnexal	

3. Nongerminal tumors (stromal tumors); peak age of presentation is 4–5 years.
   a) Interstitial cell (Leydig cell) tumors are approximately 18% of all testis tumors, usually virilizing or virilizing with gynecomastia (rarely malignant). Must be differentiated from hyperplasia; nodules that develop in testes of boys with poorly controlled congenital adrenal hyperplasia. Leydig tumors are unresponsive to adrenocorticotropic hormone (ACTH) and dexamethasone and gonadotropin stimulation.
   b) Gonadal stromal (Sertoli cell) tumors: approximately 8% of all prepubertal testis tumors; usually present as painless mass and are rarely malignant.
   c) Paratesticular rhabdomyosarcoma constitutes approximately 4% of testis tumors in children.

Reticuloendothelial malignancy, primarily lymphomas and leukemias, may present with testicular secondary tumor in

2–3%. Patients with leukemias rarely present with a testicular mass and no evidence of systemic disease.

B. Examination

Although all boys with a testis mass will come to surgical exploration through the groin, a careful preoperative evaluation should be carried out. If it suggests a tumor is benign, the tumor may be removed with preservation of the gonad.

1. Scrotal ultrasound should be done in most cases; it helps to establish that the testis is abnormal with or without presence of hydrocele. If calcium and cysts are present, a benign teratoma is suggested. A hypoechoic pattern is characteristic of leukemia or lymphoma.
2. Four-view chest radiographs should be done; chest CT to follow any suspicious area.
3. CT is a mainstay of retroperitoneal evaluation, although ultrasound can also be useful.
4. All children should have AFP determined because it is a marker of yolk sac tumor.

C. Endocrine Evaluation

1. In cases of Leydig cell tumor, urinary 17-ketosteroids are evaluated. Chorionic gonadotropins, follicle-stimulating hormone (FSH), and luteinizing hormone (LH) are normal or low. Height, weight, bone age, and pubertal changes are advanced.
2. Sertoli cell tumors exhibit normal or elevated estrogens and androgens in urine and serum; 17-ketosteroids are normal, as are gonadotropins.

D. Management

1. Radical inguinal orchiectomy is standard unless preoperative evaluation suggests benign tumor with testis-sparing; local resection may be carried out.
2. Staging is similar to that of adult testis tumors (Table 26-11).
3. Yolk sac tumor.
   a) For those patients with organ-confined yolk sac tumor, AFP will fall rapidly to normal. If the CT scan is negative, close surveillance is the treatment of choice. Monitoring should include monthly AFP and chest x-ray for the first year, then bimonthly during the second year. CT scan of the chest and abdomen may also be obtained every 3 months for the first year and every 6 months for the second year (varies by institution).

Table 26-11: Intergroup Staging System for Testicular Germ Cell Tumors

Stage	Extent of Disease
I	Limited to testis (testes), completely resected by high inguinal orchiectomy: no clinical, radiographic, or histologic evidence of disease beyond the testis; tumor markers normal after appropriate half-life decline (AFP, 5 days; ß-hCG, 16 hours); patients with normal or unknown tumor markers at diagnosis must have a negative ipsilateral retroperitoneal node sampling to confirm stage I disease
II	Trans-scrotal orchiectomy: microscopic disease in scrotum or high in spermatic cord ($\leq$ 5 cm from proximal end); retroperitoneal lymph node involvement ($\leq$ 2 cm) or persistently elevated increased tumor markers
III	Retroperitoneal lymph node involvement ($\leq$ 2 cm), but no visceral or extra-abdominal involvement
IV	Distant metastases, including liver

AFP, alpha-fetoprotein; hCG, human chorionic gonadotropin.

b) Approximately 15% of children will present with metastatic disease. For those with stage II disease, both retroperitoneal lymph node resection (RPLND) and chemotherapy have been used alone and in conjunction. There is no clear consensus as to what is the optimal treatment because the number of cases is too few to draw valid conclusions.

c) Metastatic disease has been treated with VAC or cisplatin, bleomycin, and vinblastine. Children with hematogenous metastatic disease have been treated with combination regimens, with salvage rates approaching 100%.

d) RPLND should be reserved for patients with nonbulky tumor mass confined to the retroperitoneum or for persistently elevated AFP levels anytime following orchiectomy without evidence of disease elsewhere.

4. Mature teratomas in the prepubescent male warrant a partial orchiectomy in which the cord can be cross-clamped and the tumor shelled out for frozen section examination

with testicular preservation. Metastases from such a mature teratoma have never been reported in children.

5. Gonadal stromal tumors (Leydig, Sertoli) are thought to be benign in almost all cases and are treated with orchiectomy alone. Tumors have ultrasound appearance of an intraparenchymal homogenous, hypoechoic lesion. Enucleation of the tumor is a possible alternative to radical orchiectomy. Regression of virilizing signs is unpredictable.

6. Epidermoid cysts, which are hormonally inactive and usually present as a smooth, firm intratesticular mass, can be treated with testis-sparing surgery. The benign nature suggested by physical examination, serology, and ultrasound requires confirmation by a frozen section before organ sparing can be performed safely.

7. Reticuloendothelial tumors are managed by biopsy and systemic therapy.

E. Prognosis

1. More pediatric than adult testis tumors are benign.

2. Children younger than 2 years with yolk sac tumors have approximately a 90% chance of survival. The prognosis is worse in older children.

3. Tumor registry for pediatric testis tumor has been developed by the Urologic Section of the American Academy of Pediatrics. Therapy continues to evolve.

SELF-ASSESSMENT QUESTIONS

1. Describe the approach taken for a 2-year-old child who presents with bilateral Wilms' tumors.

2. Neuroblastoma involving the cervical ganglia can cause Horner's syndrome. How else can neuroblastoma present?

3. Prostatic rhabdomyosarcoma (RMS) can cause urinary retention or constipation. How would a 4-year-old child who is found to have a prostatic RMS be evaluated and managed?

4. Vaginal RMS can present in toddlers as blood noted in the diapers. What would you tell the family of a 2-year-old girl who is discovered to have sarcoma botryoides that is confined in her vagina?

5. What is your evaluation of an 8-month-old boy who presents with a scrotal mass that does not transilluminate? If a yolk sac tumor is diagnosed and there is no evidence of retroperitoneal involvement, what is recommended for treatment and follow-up?

SUGGESTED READINGS

1. Carr MC, Mitchell ME: Neuroblastoma. In Richie JP, D'Amico AV (eds): *Urologic Oncology.* Philadelphia, WB Saunders, 2005, pp 737–752.
2. Green DM: The treatment of stages I-IV favorable histology Wilms' tumor. *J Clin Oncol* 22:1366–1372, 2004.
3. Metcalfe PD, Bägli DJ: Prepubertal testicular tumors. In Richie JP, D'Amico AV (eds): *Urologic Oncology.* Philadelphia, Elsevier, 2005, p. 780.
4. Papaioannou G, McHugh K: Neuroblastoma in childhood: review and radiological findings. *Cancer Imaging* 5:116–127, 2005.
5. Raney RB, Stoner JA, Walterhouse DO, et al: Results of treatment of fifty-six patients with localized retroperitoneal and pelvic rhabdomyosarcoma: a report from The Intergroup Rhabdomyosarcoma Study-IV, 1991–1997. *Pediatr Blood Cancer* 42:618–625, 2004.
6. Ritchey ML, Coppes MJ: Wilms' tumor. In Richie JP, D'Amico AV (eds): *Urologic Oncology.* Philadelphia, Elsevier, 2005, p. 753.
7. Ross JH, Rybicki L, Kay R: Clinical behavior and a contemporary management algorithm for prepubertal testis tumors: a summary of the Prepubertal Testis Tumor Registry. *J Urol* 168(4 Pt 2):1675–1678, discussion 1678–1679, 2002.
8. Wu H-Y, Snyder HM III: Rhabdomyosarcoma of the pelvis and paratesticular structures. In Richie JP, D'Amico AV (eds): *Urologic Oncology.* Philadelphia, Elsevier, p. 773.

C H A P T E R 27

Pediatric Voiding Function and Dysfunction

Stephen A. Zderic, MD

BASIC EMBRYOLOGY

1. The urinary bladder and rectum arise from the primitive hindgut, which is partitioned by the urorectal septum.
2. The bladder and rectum share a substantial overlap in sensory innervation from the S2, S3, and S4 sacral segments.
   a) Clinical relevance—constipation is often seen in patients with voiding dysfunction.
3. The ureteral buds develop from the wolffian ducts and penetrate the blastema to start formation of the kidney.
4. In females, the ureteral bud takes off from the wolffian duct and may enter the lower urinary tract in an ectopic position that is distal to the urinary sphincter. Locations for such an ectopic ureter include the urethra, periurethral folds, or vagina along the lines of Gartner's ducts.

ANATOMY AND PHYSIOLOGY

1. The cortex is involved in the perception of bladder fullness and, in the mature child and adult, exerts volitional control over micturition by regulating the pontine micturition center.
2. The sensation of a full bladder has been localized to the pons, mid-cingulate cortex, and the bilateral prefrontal area using positron emission tomography (PET) scanning (although these studies were in adults and not in infants).
3. Coordination of micturition is centered in the brain stem in a cluster of neurons referred to as Barrington's nucleus.
4. Under conditions of bladder storage, neurons descending from Barrington's nucleus carry a stream of inhibitory signals to the reflex arc located in the sacral segments at S2, S3, and S4.
5. With bladder filling, afferent sensory nerves enter the posterolateral region of the sacral segments. These synapse with a short interneuron, which crosses the cord to synapse with the motor nuclei in the anterior horn.

877

6. The activity of this interneuron is modulated by descending influences from Barrington's nucleus in the brain stem. With the loss of the tonic inhibitory influences, the motor neuron is activated and voiding is initiated with the contraction of the detrusor.

7. The contraction of the detrusor is mediated by acetylcholine binding to muscarinic receptors. The M_3 and M_4 subtypes are found in bladder.

8. Concurrent with the rise in detrusor pressure, there must also be a funneling and opening of the bladder neck. This process is under autonomic control and this region of the bladder is rich in alpha-adrenergic receptors. It is also a region of the bladder that is rich in nitric oxide (NO) synthase implying that NO may serve as an important neurotransmitter in this area.

9. Concurrent with the rise in detrusor pressure, there must also occur a relaxation of the striated external sphincter located distal to the bladder neck. These striated muscle fibers are under voluntary control.

10. The striated external sphincter contractions are mediated by the neurotransmitter acetylcholine, which binds to nicotinic receptors.

THE NORMAL VOIDING CYCLE

1. Bladder filling proceeds under conditions of low storage pressures.
2. At a certain volume, the sensation of fullness is noted.
3. Barrington's nucleus removes its inhibitory influences.
4. The sacral reflex arc is activated.
5. With detrusor contraction, there is a rise in intravesical pressure.
6. This sustained rise in detrusor pressure is accompanied by a funneling of the bladder neck and a relaxation of the striated external sphincter.

Neonate and Infant

1. In the traditional view, neonates and infants voided to completion via activation of the sacral reflex arc, and it was assumed that there was no suprasacral control of micturition at this time.
2. Two lines of evidence demonstrate that neonates and infants have some degree of suprasacral control over micturition.
   a) Evidence for residual urine on voiding cystourethrography (VCUG).

b) Evidence of a contracting striated external sphincter on VCUG.

c) Evidence of post-void residuals following spontaneous voids.

3. Voiding in the neonate and infant is related to the sleep cycle. Sillen has shown that 90% of neonates and infants will awaken from sleep in the minute preceding micturition.

Transitional Phase

1. In time, the toddler begins to gain the sensation of bladder distention with filling.

2. The toddler begins to spend more time in the storage phase.
   a) Parents will report an increase in the number of dry diapers.
   b) Parents may note dry diapers in the morning.

3. Bladder capacity begins to increase.
   a) Increased urinary volumes.
   b) Increased time of storage.

4. Bowel continence appears.

5. The toddler expresses an interest in the commode.

6. A preference is expressed by the child for underwear.

Maturation

1. Even in the middle phases of the transition, a child may be dry by day, and yet the voiding cycle is incomplete.

2. The child has learned to fire the external sphincter to prevent an episode of incontinence.

3. Often the child is also contracting the external sphincter during voiding phase and thus fails to empty completely.

4. In time, there is better "fine tuning" of the voiding cycle by the child, and continence is achieved with a minimal post-void residual urine.

THE CLINICAL MANIFESTATIONS OF VOIDING DYSFUNCTION

Pediatric patients with voiding dysfunction present across a wide spectrum.

1. Urinary tract infections
   a) Cystitis
   b) Pyelonephritis
   c) Associated with reflux

2. Infrequent voider
3. Daytime incontinence
4. Diurnal incontinence
5. Nocturnal enuresis

The degree of symptoms span a spectrum from:
1. Mild dysfunctional voiding—occasional "accident"
2. Severe dysfunctional voiding—Hinman's syndrome

Hinman's Syndrome

1. Severe detrusor sphincter dyssynergia
2. Neurologically intact—normal clinical exam and magnetic resonance imaging (MRI) of spinal cord
3. Incontinence—often day and night
4. Fecal soiling
5. Recurrent cystitis
6. Pyelonephritis vesicoureteral reflux

THE CLINICAL APPROACH TO THE PATIENT

The efficient management of the pediatric patient with voiding dysfunction calls for a clear strategy that begins by gathering information, an assessment of severity, and the formulation of a therapeutic plan. Despite the technologic age we practice in, this process must begin with a careful history. In cases in which there is a failure of therapy, the history must always be revisited.

History

Physicians must approach such visits with ample time and patience. Time and again, families and patients will give us a first-rate history if we simply let them speak in their words and at their pace (Dr. Barry Belman has coined the term audio-uro-dynamics for this "procedure"). Simply giving the family and patient free reign and "letting them go" will provide many of the answers we seek. For some families, this may seem daunting, and a prompt, such as, "How does your child's bladder problem affect you on a car trip or a visit to the mall?" will get them to relay the information needed in their terms. This may at times be much easier said than done within a busy clinic. However, we all need to be reminded that an ounce of active listening validates the family's concerns far more than a pound of hastily given therapy no matter how accurate it may be. In managing these complaints, image is as valued as diagnostic acumen. All of us need to remember that among our seemingly endless stream of day and night wetters lurks the rare (1–3%) patient with an ectopic ureter or a posterior urethral valve whose cure and well-being can only be ensured by a surgical procedure.

Questions a Consulting Physician Must Consider

1. Gender.
2. Age of patient.
3. Age at which training was attempted.
4. Was the patient every dry?
5. Do parents ever remember a dry diaper?
6. Fluid intake—is your child thirstier than other children their age?
7. What is the child's maximal dry interval?
8. How frequently does your child void?
9. Does your child make a last minute rush to get to the bathroom (urgency)?
10. Does your child ever squat en route to the bathroom? (Vincent's curtsy—on occasion a parent will demonstrate this maneuver in which the child stops an episode of urgency by dropping down and tucking their heel into their perineum to create a compression.)
11. What does it sound like when your child is urinating? Many parents will relay the classic features of a starting and stopping staccato stream characteristic of detrusor sphincter dyssynergia.
12. Is your child constipated?
    a) Frequency of stooling.
    b) Are the stools hard or soft?
    c) Is defecation painful?
13. Is urination painful?
14. Has your child ever had a urinary tract infection?
    a) If yes, was this associated with a high fever?
    b) How was the urine specimen collected (bag, voided, or catheter)?
15. Have any radiology studies been done?
16. Was your child imaged with in utero sonography? Keep in mind that most (although not all) major congenital obstructive uropathies will be detected in utero. For many expectant mothers only one sonogram is performed at the 19- to 22-week time point. Although this screening sonogram will pick up major problems, hydronephrosis may be progressive, and prenatal sonography demands high-quality equipment and an experienced observer.
17. Is there a history of maternal diabetes? In such cases, the child is at risk for the development of sacral agenesis and may present some time later with a neurogenic bladder.

18. General social developmental questions should include:
    a) Any history of developmental delay.
    b) Grade in school.
    c) Scholastic performance.
    d) Social stressors (death of family member or friend, divorce).
19. What are the restrooms at school like?
    a) Does your child have unrestricted bathroom privileges?
    b) Are the restrooms safe?
20. Does your child wet the bed? How many nights within a week/month?
21. Is your child difficult to arouse from sleep?
22. Does your child snore? How loud? Does your child every stop breathing at night and awaken only to fall back into a deep sleep? Is your child falling asleep during the daytime hours?

Self and Family Assessment Tools

These are also critical measures at the time of intake. In some practices, a family whose child is being scheduled for a wetting complaint will be mailed an information packet that includes a voiding diary and a self-assessment tool that translates into a symptom score.

These additional self-reported data that should be reviewed by the physician include:

1. Voiding and elimination diaries.
   a) Times of voids.
   b) Volumes.
   c) Fluid intake.
   d) Bowel habits.
2. Voiding questionnaire with scoring system: At least two such questionnaires have been developed for voiding dysfunction and serve as a pediatric version of the AUA symptom score. These scales provide a practitioner with a sense of how many resources a patient will require during therapy. In addition, if a patient's score fails to improve, these scores may indicate the need for more advanced, expensive, and invasive testing.

The Physical Examination

1. General appearance—evidence of neurologic or developmental issues?
2. Unusual facies (downturn of smile)—Ochoa syndrome—described by Dr. Ochoa as an inherited syndrome of urinary and fecal incontinence. The pontine micturition

center is localized near the cranial nerves controlling facial expression. Autosomal recessive and localized to chromosome 10q23–24.

3. Gait and general neurologic assessment—Does the patient favor one limb over another? Do the shoes wear evenly?

4. Spine—a careful exam of the lumbar sacral region is crucial. Look for lipomas, hair tufts, or dimpling in this region. These are clues to the possible presence of a tethered cord.

5. Abdomen—distended from constipation?

6. Genitalia.

7. In female patients, check for continuous leakage—suspect ectopic ureter.

Observe the Patient Void

Direct observation of a void can be crucial. A patient who is voiding normally should be able to converse with ease. In contrast, a thin and weak yet steady stream with the patient unable to converse while applying a Valsalva maneuver would be indicative of a possible stricture. In contrast, a staccato stream with a start and stop pattern would be indicative of striated detrusor sphincter dyssynergia.

Laboratory Testing

The following lab studies are inexpensive and may be read from a dipstick analysis in the office and are always indicated:

1. Urinalysis
   a) Urine culture—if urinalysis is positive
2. Urine specific gravity

In severe cases with abnormal imaging, or recurrent pyelonephritis, a blood urea nitrogen (BUN)/creatinine (Cr) should be checked.

Imaging

In many instances, no imaging is needed. A well done history and physical followed by simple recommendations such as a timer watch and a voiding diary are all that are required to produce continence. However, in selected cases, imaging should be obtained beginning with the more simple, less invasive, and less expensive studies and proceeding to the more invasive and advanced studies only if required.

1. **Kidney ureter bladder (KUB) x-ray**—a simple and inexpensive study that demonstrates for physician, family, and patient alike the presence of significant constipation.

This is probably the most imaging the majority of these patients will need unless there is an associated history of urinary tract infections.

2. **Ultrasound**—increased expense but noninvasive. Offers the benefit of reassurance to physician, patient, and family that the anatomy is set correctly. It is okay to have a lower threshold for ordering an ultrasound given that it is profoundly frustrating for a family and patient to attempt behavioral management methods for a long time, only to discover after months of futility that the underlying problem was anatomic. Critical to order in situations in which one suspects anatomic incontinence in a female on the basis of ectopic ureter.

   a) Suspect ectopic ureter based on:
      i) Hydronephrosis most often in upper pole system.
      ii) Dilated ureter behind the bladder with ureter dropping below the level of the bladder neck.
   b) Must include renal *and* bladder views.
   c) Although rare, even a well done ultrasound may miss an ectopic ureter, and if the history is compelling enough, further imaging with intravenous pyelogram (IVP) or MRI-IVP is warranted.

3. **VCUG**—increased expense, invasive, and potentially traumatic to the child. Today there is a growing movement to limit the number of VCUGs being done except in those cases in which there simply is no alternative to searching for vesicoureteral reflux or excluding bladder outlet obstruction. The indications for a VCUG study in patients with voiding dysfunction:

   a) Febrile urinary tract infection.
   b) A male patient with a thick-walled bladder and upper tract changes to rule out the presence of posterior urethral valves or a urethral stricture.

Imaging That Is Less Frequently Indicated for Voiding Dysfunction

1. **IVP**—This study was the gold standard for detecting the presence of ectopic ureters and duplication anomalies. Certainly in the presence of adequately functioning renal parenchyma, there will be accumulation of contrast within a dilated system that provides a clue of possible ectopia. Delayed views are essential and this study must be monitored closely by the radiologist, as well as the urologist ordering the study. Failure to obtain the proper views will render the study worthless, hence the importance of communication between urologist and radiologist.

2. **Computed tomography (CT) scan or MRI-IVP**—In recent years advances in technology have expanded the use of rapid scanning using either the CT scan or MRI, and these have been applied to the search for ectopic ureters. For small, poorly functioning systems, the use of the CT with contrast or MRI with gadolinium will allow for detection of contrast within nondilated ureters that can escape detection with sonography or a conventional IVP.

3. **Lumbar-sacral MRI**—This study is indicated for any patient with focal neurologic signs (abnormal gait, foot drop) or findings on examination of the lumbar sacral spine (hair tuft, lipoma, abnormal dimple). In the absence of these findings, and in situations in which the patient is failing to improve, this study may also be considered to rule out a tethered cord.

Urodynamic Measurements

1. **Uro-flow and measurement of post-void residual with hand-held ultrasound unit.** This simple and easy to use technique is complementary to direct observation of the void. A sawtooth flow pattern suggests the firing and relaxation of the external sphincter seen with classic dysfunctional voiding. A slow, flat, and prolonged curve suggests outflow obstruction on an anatomic basis. For most patients, this is the only urodynamic study needed.

2. **Cystometrogram**—indicated to rule out uninhibited bladder contractions prior to initiating anticholinergic therapy.

3. **Videourodynamics**—indicated to rule out uninhibited contractions and also to assess the bladder neck in complex cases.

In our experience, cystometry and videourodynamics are rarely indicated in the assessment of pediatric voiding dysfunction. These studies will usually be limited to less than 5% of patients presenting to a pediatric voiding dysfunction clinic and should be restricted to those patients who fail the basic treatment protocols or anticholinergic therapy or those in whom internal sphincteric dyssynergia is suspected. This is in marked distinction to those patients in whom a clear-cut neurogenic bladder is present as in spina bifida patients, all of whom must undergo urodynamic testing. When urodynamic or videourodynamic studies are indicated, the best information will be obtained when the urologist ordering the study is present and communicates with the patient so as to best re-create in the laboratory setting the symptoms that the patient is experiencing.

TREATMENT OF DYSFUNCTIONAL VOIDING/ELIMINATION BY CATEGORY

Selection of the optimal treatment calls for an understanding of the cycle of failure (Figure 27-1). Based on this, one can begin to design a program for the patient that addresses the patient's unique needs.

Urinary Tract Infections

For many patients the sole manifestation of voiding dysfunction is recurrent cystitis. A careful voiding history often reveals a patient who is dry by day and night but who voids infrequently (2–3 times/day), has poor water intake, and is constipated. Treatment should consist of:

1. Timed voiding regimen (2-hour intervals)
2. Voiding logs
3. Timer watch
4. Antibiotic prophylaxis
5. Increased free water intake
6. Treat associated constipation

Infrequent Voider

These patients may void 2–3 times per day and often present with dampness as the primary complaint. In many instances, these are high-achieving children who just cannot break away from what they are doing to "listen to their bladder." In other instances, these children are reluctant to use the restrooms at school because of fear of sanitation and/or safety.

1. Timed voiding regimen (2-hour intervals)
2. Voiding logs
3. Timer watch
4. Treat associated constipation
5. Note to school nurse/teacher for unrestricted bathroom privileges

Constipation

Constipation is the enemy of continence. Time and again patients present with mild to moderate voiding dysfunction and/or urinary tract infections with significant constipation, and on institution of a bowel regimen all voiding complaints cease. Treatment should consist of:

1. Increase fruits and vegetable intake
2. Fiber-based cereals

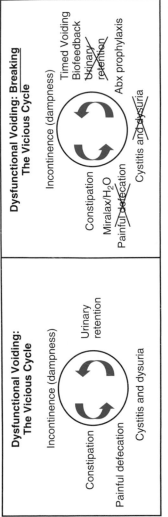

FIGURE 27-1. The cycle of dysfunctional voiding in which constipation leads to cystitis and dysuria, followed by retention and wetting, and the "menu" of choices by which the cycle is broken.

3. Increase water intake
4. Stool-softening regimens
   a) Lactulose
   b) Miralax
5. Enemas
   a) Administered per rectum
   b) Antegrade administration of enema via surgically cre-
      ated appendiceal access for medically refractory cases
      (antegrade colonic enema [ACE] procedure)

Dysfunctional Voiding with Detrusor Sphincter Dyssynergia

For patients in whom the diagnosis of detrusor sphincter
dyssynergia is suspected, confirmation with a uroflow may
be helpful to confirm the rising and falling flow rate. There
are two types of detrusor sphincter dyssynergia to consider,
and their treatments differ markedly.

Striated External Sphincter Dyssynergia

This is the most common form.

1. Timed voiding
2. Voiding diary
3. Timer watch
4. Treat constipation if present
5. Biofeedback therapy to coach the patient into relaxing the
   pelvic floor

Only if these less invasive means of treatment fail, would one
proceed to these remaining options, usually following a carefully performed videourodynamic assessment.

1. Clean intermittent catheterization
2. Cystoscopy and direct injection of botulinum toxin
   (Botox) into striated external sphincter

Internal Sphincteric Dyssynergia

This is the less common form—these patients demonstrate a diminished flow rate with a flattened curve. To make
this diagnosis accurately, videourodynamics are helpful. The
low flow rate, silent pelvic floor electromyogram (EMG),
and increased voiding pressures correlate with the closed
bladder neck on fluoroscopy to clinch this diagnosis.

1. Treat with alpha blocker to lower the resistance at the
   level of the bladder neck.

Hinman's Syndrome

These rare patients represent the extreme end of the dysfunctional voiding spectrum. The syndrome has also been labeled as the non-neurogenic neurogenic bladder. Hinman noted, in his original description of these patients, the presence of urinary incontinence, fecal soiling, urinary tract infections, and upper tract changes often associated with pyelonephritis, and, in some cases, renal failure developed. These patients will require imaging consisting of a renal bladder ultrasound, and a VCUG may be performed in conjunction with videourodynamics. Renal function must be assessed. In some instances, a lumbar-sacral MRI and neurologic consultation are warranted to completely exclude any spinal cord lesion. Treatment options for this complex group of patients may include:

1. Timed voiding.
2. Antibiotic prophylaxis.
3. Biofeedback.
4. An assessment of renal function.
5. Bowel regimen ranging from MiraLax to enemas. In the event that these simpler measures fail, more aggressive approaches may be indicated to preserve renal function.
6. Clean intermittent catheterization (CIC)—In many of these cases, the use of CIC will actually teach the child how to relax the external sphincter.

In rare instances, patients with Hinman's syndrome may become surgical candidates to preserve their renal function.

1. Vesicostomy—if the patient is noncompliant or the social situation is poor and the patient might be lost to follow-up.
2. Appendicovesicostomy with or without bladder augmentation.
3. ACE procedure for constipation.

Nocturnal Enuresis

This common problem often presents as a seemingly isolated finding. In fact, in taking a careful history, one can often elicit evidence for daytime voiding dysfunction. This is critical because more often than not addressing the daytime voiding dysfunction will result in nighttime dryness because the child is actually going to bed with an empty bladder.

Additional Background

1. Twenty percent of all 5-year-olds wet the bed.
2. This drops by 50% each year. By about age 10, 1% are still experiencing some degree of enuresis.

3. In a Swedish study, 90% of all neonates would awaken in the minute prior to urination, but 10% slept right on through their voiding. These investigators will ultimately tell us whether these 10% of neonates are the ones presenting at age 5 and beyond with persisting enuresis.

4. Consider the possibility of upper airway obstruction and sleep apnea; these patients need a sleep study and ear nose and throat (ENT) evaluation.

5. Consider the degree of thirst. Most children with enuresis will not get up to drink at night. If this is happening frequently, consider the possibility of diabetes insipidus (DI).

6. Measure the specific gravity (cheaply done via dipstick) and/or check an osmolality on the first morning urine if you suspect DI.

Treatments for This Condition

1. Triple void during the 1 hour before bedtime.
2. Limit fluids 1 hour before bedtime.
3. Alarm—This simple electrical circuit is placed in the pajamas and makes a buzzing sound if the contact is established by fluid.
4. Alarms work in 80% of cases after 3 months of work.
5. If the child sleeps through the alarm, the parent must awaken and arouse the child to void. Otherwise, the approach will fail.
6. Alarms work best in cases in which the child is a lighter sleeper.
7. Alarms function as a biofeedback tool—The child learns to associate the sensation of a full bladder during sleep with the need to arouse and then void.
8. Waking the child up at set hours during the night to void is not the same as using an alarm because the bladder may not be full at the time the child is awakened.

Pharmacologic Options for Enuresis

1. DDAVP—nasal spray (rarely used today) or tablet (0.2 mg tablets)
   a) 1–3 tablets at bedtime
2. Imipramine—25 up to 75 mg orally at bedtime (PO QHS)
   a) Rarely used today

Anticholinergic Therapy in Pediatric Voiding Dysfunction

The purpose of anticholinergic therapy is to enhance bladder capacity by eliminating the presence of uninhibited bladder contractions. Most children with dysfunctional voiding have excellent bladder capacity, and thus anticholinergic therapy is rarely indicated in this population. On occasion, we will identify children with severe urgency and frequency for whom a trial of oxybutynin (Ditropan) is indicated; however, this is a small number of patients. In these instances, empiric therapy is reasonable, although some might advocate urodynamic or videourodynamic studies prior to such therapy.

Voiding Dysfunction and Vesicoureteral Reflux

Many patients with vesicoureteral reflux will prove to have significant dysfunctional voiding.

1. Treating the dysfunctional voiding is also treating the reflux. Patients with dysfunctional voiding and reflux have a better prognosis for spontaneous than those with voiding dysfunction on a grade for grade basis.
2. Open reimplantation in the face of dysfunctional voiding has a higher complication rate and is to be avoided.

DIABETES INSIPIDUS

Rarely patients with DI will present to a urologist with voiding dysfunction. These patients have the following characteristics:

1. Thirsty
2. Crave cold water
3. Wake up at night to drink
4. Polyuric
5. Fabulous flow rates

In this setting, the following studies are indicated:

1. First morning urine for specific gravity
2. Water deprivation study with serum and urine osmolarities
3. Treated by endocrinologists with DDAVP

SELF-ASSESSMENT QUESTIONS

1. What is the embryologic explanation for the clinical association of constipation and voiding dysfunction?
2. What is the embryologic basis for why an ectopic ureter may lead to urinary incontinence only in females?
3. Can you explain the difference between striated external sphincter dyssynergia and internal sphincter

dyssynergia? How does the pharmacologic treatment for these two conditions differ?

4. Can you explain the rationale for use of biofeedback therapy for voiding dysfunction that is based on external sphincteric dyssynergia?

5. An 8-year-old child presents for evaluation of persistent urinary incontinence and during the course of the history, it is revealed that mom has been an insulin-dependent diabetic for 25 years. What diagnosis must you suspect is present in this child that might account for the urinary incontinence?

SUGGESTED READINGS

1. Cruz F, Silva C: Botulinum toxin in the management of lower urinary tract dysfunction: contemporary update. *Curr Opin Urol* 14:329–334, 2004.

2. Grafstein NH, Combs AJ, Glassberg KI: Primary bladder neck dysfunction: an overlooked entity in children. *Curr Urol Rep* 6:133–139, 2005.

3. Ochoa B: Can a congenital dysfunctional bladder be diagnosed from a smile? The Ochoa syndrome updated. *Pediatr Nephrol* 19:6–12, 2004.

4. Schulmann Sl: Voiding dysfunction in children. *Urol Clin North Am* 31:481–490, 2004.

5. Sillen U: Bladder function in infants. *Scand J Urol Nephrol Suppl* 215:69–74, 2004.

6. Upadhyay J, Bolduc S, Bagli DJ, et al: Use of the dysfunctional voiding symptom score to predict resolution of vesicoureteral reflux in children with voiding dysfunction. *J Urol* 169:1842–1846, 2003.

C H A P T E R 28

Congenital Anomalies

Pasquale Casale, MD and
Douglas A. Canning, MD

I. UPPER URINARY TRACT

A. Abnormalities of the Kidney Position and Number

1. Simple ectopia.
    a) Incidence is approximately 1 per 900 (autopsy) (pelvic, 1 per 3000; solitary, 1 per 22,000; bilateral, 10%). Left side favored.
    b) Associated findings include small size with persistent fetal lobations, anterior or horizontal pelvis, anomalous vasculature, contralateral agenesis, vesicoureteral reflux, Müllerian anomalies in 20–60% of females; undescended testes, hypospadias, urethral duplication in 10–20% males; skeletal and cardiac anomalies in 20%.
    c) Only workup, ultrasound, voiding cystourethrography.
2. Thoracic ectopia.
    a) Comprises less than 5% of ectopic kidneys.
    b) Origin is delayed closure of diaphragmatic angle versus "overshoot" of renal ascent.
    c) Adrenal may or may not be thoracic.
3. Crossed ectopia and fusion (Bauer).
    a) Incidence is 1 per 1000 to 1 per 2000; 90% crossed with fusion; 2:1 male, 3:1 left crossed; 24 cases solitary, five cases bilateral reported to date.
    b) Origin from abnormal migration of ureteral bud or rotation of caudal end of fetus at time of bud formation (Stephens, 1983).
    c) Associated findings include multiple or anomalous vessels arising from the ipsilateral side of the aorta and vesicoureteral reflux; with solitary crossed kidney only; genital, skeletal, and hindgut anomalies in 20–50%.
4. Horseshoe kidney.
    a) Incidence is 1 per 400 or 0.25%; 2:1 males.
    b) Origin is fusion of lower poles before or during rotation (4½ to 6 weeks' gestation).

    c) Associated findings include anomalous vessels; isthmus between or behind great vessels hindered by the inferior mesenteric artery; skeletal, cardiovascular, and central nervous system (CNS) anomalies (33%); hypospadias and cryptorchidism (4%), bicornuate uterus (7%), urinary tract infection (UTI) (13%); duplex ureters (10%), stones (17%); 20% of trisomy 18 and 60% of Turner's patients have horseshoe kidney.

    d) Excluding other anomalies, survival is not affected.

    e) Stones; infection may result from stasis; rarely is true obstruction present (see ureteropelvic junction obstruction [UPJO]).

5. Bilateral renal agenesis.

    a) Incidence is 1 per 4800 births or 1 per 400 newborn autopsies (75% are male) and typically lethal.

    b) Origin either ureteral bud failure or absence of the nephrogenic ridge.

    c) Associated findings include absent renal arteries, complete ureteral atresia in 50%, bladder atresia in 50%, Potter's syndrome (Potter, 1972). Also low birth weight, oligohydramnios, pulmonary hypoplasia, bowed limbs.

6. Unilateral renal agenesis.

    a) Incidence is 1 per 1100 in autopsy series, 1 per 1500 in radiographic series, 2:1 male, left kidney is more often involved than right kidney.

    b) Origin is probably ureteral bud failure; there is a familial trend.

    c) Associated findings include absent ureter with hemitrigone (50%), adrenal agenesis (10%), genital anomalies (20–40% in both sexes).

       i) Müllerian anomalies in females include uterovaginal atresia (Mayer-Rokitansky-Küster-Hauser syndrome), uterus didelphys, and vaginal agenesis.

      ii) In males, the vas and seminal vesicle are absent or atretic.

    d) If the single kidney is normal, no special precautions required and survival is not affected; management of the genital abnormalities.

7. Supernumerary kidney.

    a) Incidence is unknown.

    b) Origin a combined defect of ureteral bud and metanephros.

    c) Associated findings are hydronephrosis (50%), common ureter (40%), duplex ureter (40%), and ectopic ureter or one ending in the pelvis of the ipsilateral kidney (20%).

B. Cystic Abnormalities of the Kidney

1. Autosomal dominant polycystic kidney disease.
   a) Chromosome 16 and chromosome 4.
   b) Autosomal dominant transmission.
   c) Adult type is the most common cystic disease in humans, with an incidence of 1 per 1250 live births and accounts for 10% of all end-stage renal disease.
   d) Usually presents after between 30 and 50 years with pain, hematuria, and progressive renal insufficiency, but it is also seen in children. Rarely present in newborns.
   e) Intravenous urography (IVU) reveals irregular renal enlargement with calyceal distortion; ultrasound shows multiple cysts of variable sizes.
   f) Associated findings are liver cysts without functional impairment in one third of patients and berry aneurysms in 10–40%.
   g) Complications include uremia, hypertension, myocardial infarction, and intracranial hemorrhage (9%).
   h) Management involves control of blood pressure and urinary infection, relief of cardiac failure, and eventually dialysis or transplantation. Some of these patients encounter issues with pain typically from renal capsular stretching by the cysts.
   i) Pathology: rounded or irregular cysts located in all parts of the nephron.
2. Autosomal recessive polycystic kidney disease.
   a) Chromosome 6.
   b) Infantile type. Rare (1 per 10,000 live births), usually presents with bilateral flank masses in infancy but can present in childhood with renal or hepatic insufficiency.
   c) IVU shows huge (12–16 times normal) kidneys with a pronouncedly delayed nephrogram and characteristic streaked appearance ("sunburst" pattern).
   d) May be distinguished from hydronephrosis, renal tumor, and renal vein thrombosis by IVU and ultrasound. (Bright echoes on ultrasound.)
   e) Associated findings are congenital hepatic (periportal) fibrosis and dilation of bile ducts with the degree of hepatic insufficiency varying inversely with the severity of renal disease and directly with the age of presentation; cysts elsewhere are uncommon.
   f) Complications are renal and hepatic failure, hypertension, and respiratory compromise in the newborn; patients usually die within the first 2 months of life.

    g) Although respiratory support, blood pressure control, and dialysis can improve survival, patients will ultimately develop cirrhosis with all of the associated complications.

    h) Pathology is fusiform dilation of collecting ducts and tubules resulting in small subcapsular cysts.

3. Medullary sponge kidney (tubular ectasia) is an adult disease pathologically characterized by enlarged tortuous collecting ducts and occasional tiny cysts in the pyramids (75% bilateral; incidence, 1 per 20,000).

    a) Diagnosis: IVU shows collections of contrast adjacent to the calyces ("bristles on a brush" also called "blushing") often with calcifications in the medulla.

    b) Complications: infection, stones, distal renal tubular acidosis, and hematuria.

    c) Medical management of calculi and infections is often required.

    d) One third of patients with hypercalcemia.

4. Medullary cystic disease (juvenile nephronophthisis) refers to a group of disorders with various genetic patterns characterized pathologically by bilateral small kidneys, attenuated cortex, atrophic and dilated tubules, medullary cysts, and some interstitial fibrosis.

    a) Patients progress to end-stage renal disease by about age 20; juvenile form is responsible for 20% of childhood renal failure deaths.

    b) Medical management of renal failure can delay need for transplant.

    c) Polydipsia and polyuria in 80%, retinitis pigmentosa in 16%.

5. Unilateral multicystic dysplastic kidney is the most common cystic disease of the newborn and the second most common abdominal mass in infants after hydronephrosis, including UPJO.

    a) The left kidney is more commonly involved, but there is no sex predilection or familial tendency.

    b) Origin either (1) ischemic, from failure of the normal shift of vasculature as the kidney migrates, producing also the associated atretic ureter (Stephens, 1983), or (2) failure of ureteral bud to stimulate metanephric blastoma.

    c) Contralateral renal abnormalities are most common when the multicystic kidney is small and/or the ureteral atresia is low. Vesicoureteral reflux may be present in up to 20% of cases.

    d) Ultrasound is the most diagnostic study (multiple hypoechoic areas of various sizes without connections or dominant medial cyst and without identifiable parenchyma), as IVU or renal scan demonstrates ipsilateral nonfunction; IVU and voiding cystourethrography (VCUG) are done to evaluate the remainder of the urinary tract.

e) Histopathology includes atretic artery, cysts, some solid central stroma, low cuboidal epithelium, and some primitive nephrogenic structures, immature glomeruli occasionally.

f) Although the cystic kidney usually does not enlarge as the child grows and thus becomes relatively less conspicuous, a few adults have had problems related to multicystic kidneys (tumor, infection, pain) and it is not unreasonable to recommend removal of the multicystic kidney, although the risk of tumor is no greater than in normal kidneys.

C. Collecting System Abnormalities

1. Calyceal diverticulum occurs in 4.5 per 1000 urograms.
   a) Origin is failure of degeneration of third- and fourth-order branches of ureteral bud, leaving a pocket lined with transitional epithelium connected to the collecting system near the calyceal fornix.
   b) In approximately one third of patients, stones will form; some will become sites of persistent infection due to stasis; the rest remain asymptomatic.
   c) Treatment involves removal of stones, drainage of purulence, and marsupialization to the renal surface with closure of the collecting system and cauterization of the epithelium.
2. Hydrocalycosis is a rare lesion involving vascular compression, cicatrization, or achalasia of the infundibulum; it rarely requires any intervention.
3. Megacalycosis is a rare lesion involving all of one or both kidneys with dilated unobstructed calyces usually numbering more than 25 per kidney (normally 8–10 calyces per kidney). May be confused radiographically with obstructive uropathy.
   a) Results from combination of faulty ureteral bud division, hypoplasia of juxtamedullary glomeruli, and maldevelopment of calyceal musculature.
   b) Males 6:1 over females, only in Caucasians. X linked recessive gene.
   c) May be associated with stones or infection but in itself causes no deterioration of renal function.

4. Infundibulopelvic stenosis may involve part or all of one or both kidneys.
   a) The calyces become quite large but usually no progressive functional deterioration occurs. Pain difficult to manage when present.
   b) May be associated with dysplasia and lower tract anomalies (e.g., urethral valves).
   c) Commonly associated with vesicoureteral reflux.
5. UPJO is the usual cause of the most common abdominal mass in children (hydronephrosis).
   a) There is a 2:1 male predominance in children and left-sided predominance in all ages.
   b) Several possible causes, including segmental muscular attenuation or malorientation, true stenosis, angulation, and extrinsic compression. Crossing lower pole vessels are present in approximately 20–30% of cases, but an intrinsic lesion (either noncompliant or nonconducting) is common.
   c) Associated findings include reflux (5–10%), contralateral agenesis (5%), and contralateral UPJO (10%); rarely dysplasia, multicystic kidney, or other urologic anomaly.
   d) Symptoms and signs include episodic flank pain and/or mass, hematuria, infection, nausea and vomiting, and sometimes uremia. In infants, the flank mass may be the only sign, whereas the older child will exhibit any of the others; very often gastrointestinal distress and poorly localized upper abdominal pain are the only symptoms.
   e) Radiologic findings are delayed excretion on the affected side with variable dilation of pelvis and calyces or even no visualization on IVU; on ultrasound, multiple interconnected hypoechoic areas with dominant medial hypoechogenicity and identifiable cortical rim. There is usually some measurable function on renal scan. When function is good, the drainage is delayed even in the face of furosemide (Lasix) administration beyond 20 minutes.
   f) Prompt surgical repair by excision of the narrow segment and a spatulated anastomosis of the ureter to the tailored renal pelvis for symptomatic cases. Most are diagnosed antenatally and can be followed with serial renal scan and ultrasound.
   g) Follow-up consists of ultrasound at 1 month and renal scan at 3 months and ultrasound at 1 year postoperatively in most cases.

D. Ureteral Anomalies

1. Duplication of ureter occurs in 1 per 125 autopsies; 1.6:1 female, 85% unilateral.
   a) Autosomal dominant with incomplete penetrance.
   b) Seems to arise from two ureteral buds meeting the metanephros—in most cases, but may also be caused by a bud that bifurcates immediately after arising, before meeting the metanephros.
   c) Associated with reflux (42%), renal scarring and dilation (29%), ectopic insertion (3%), large kidneys with excess calyces, dysplasia/hypoplasia, infection, and ureteroceles.
   d) Duplication itself is of no clinical significance, but the associated anomalies may require intervention (see ureterocele, ectopia, etc.).
2. Atresia is usually associated with a multicystic dysplastic kidney; distal segment atresia is often associated with contralateral hydronephrosis or dysplasia (50%).
3. Megaureter has a 3:1 male and 3:1 left-sided predominance; the term is used loosely to describe any dilated ureter, but there are three distinct types.
   a) Refluxing megaureter originates because of the reflux, although some cases have an abnormal distal segment and some element of obstruction.
   b) A widened ureteral bud gives rise to a ureter dilated down to the orifice, which is in the normal position, and there is no obstruction (nonreflux, nonobstructed type).
   c) The primary obstructed type is the most common and results from a stenotic or aperistaltic distal short segment; the orifice is in the normal position.
   d) The refluxing type, with its laterally ectopic orifice, may be associated with a dysplastic kidney, one scarred by infection, or both; the other types drain normal or hydronephrotic kidneys.
   e) The ultrasound will show moderate to severe hydronephrosis and proportionately greater ureteral dilation; VCUG will diagnose the reflux type; a Lasix renogram would distinguish obstructed from nonobstructed types.
   f) There are mild primary obstructed megaureters with only a spindle-shape dilation of the distal ureter and normal (sharp) calyces; these require no treatment.
   g) Surgical correction is needed for some obstructed and refluxing megaureters. Refluxing megaureters more commonly require tailoring than obstructed ones,

which tend to decrease in caliber after excision of the aperistaltic distal segment.

h) Follow-up includes ultrasound at 1 month and renal scan at 3 months. An ultrasound is done 1 year postoperatively.

4. Vesicoureteral reflux (VUR) occurs in approximately 1 per 1000 in the general population but is 8 to 40 times more frequent in affected families; it can be found in 50% of infants and 30% of children with a UTI.

   a) It may occur because the ureteral bud arises ectopically leading to a laterally placed orifice and short submucosal tunnel or because the development of the intrinsic smooth muscle of the distal ureteral segment is delayed or incomplete. High intravesical pressures may cause a marginally competent ureterovesical junction to reflux, and evidence is growing that voiding dysfunction in the child may cause or exacerbate reflux.

   b) Duplicated ureters and renal hypodysplasia may be associated with refluxing ureters with laterally ectopic orifices. Infection and renal scarring are prominent findings with all types of refluxing ureters regardless of grade. Voiding dysfunction and urethral obstruction by valves are associated with an acquired form of reflux.

   c) Reflux is best graded I to V by the International Reflux Study system depending on the degree of dilation (Figure 28-1).

   d) All children with reflux should be placed on prophylactic antibiotics at one-fourth the therapeutic dose

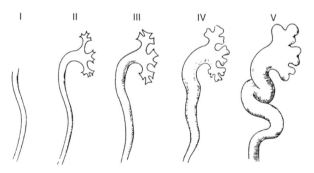

GRADES OF REFLUX

FIGURE 28-1. International classification of vesicoureteral reflux. (From Atala A, Keating M: Vesicoureteral reflux and megaureter. In Walsh PC, Retik AB, Vaughn ED, Wein AJ [eds]: *Campbell's Urology*, 8th ed. Philadelphia, Saunders, 2002, Fig. 59-3, p 2060.)

given once a day. Trimethoprim-sulfamethoxazole and nitrofurantoin are the most commonly used drugs after 2 months of age. Typically, amoxicillin is used in the newborn period until 2 months of age. Children require periodic upper tract radiographic assessment usually with ultrasound and re-evaluation of the reflux by VCUG or nuclear VCUG. Some advocate the use of dimercaptosuccinic acid (DMSA) to screen and follow for scarring in patients monitored with VUR because renal scarring is truly the detrimental effect of VUR and pyelonephritis.

e) Grades I–III (minimally dilated) are usually treated medically initially; grades IV–V usually require surgical correction. Low volume VUR (grades I–III) resolves at a rate of 17% per patient-year, whereas grade IV VUR resolves at a rate of 4% per patient-year.

f) Reimplantation of the refluxing unit by the Cohen technique is the standard surgical management, with nearly complete success; duplicated ureters are reimplanted in their common distal muscular sheath. Recently, subureteric injection as well as laparoscopic and vesicoscopic approaches have been used with good success in preliminary reports.

g) Breakthrough infections, failure to comply with the antibiotic prophylaxis regimen, persistent reflux into puberty in females, progressive scarring, and worsening renal function are all considerations that favor surgical intervention, but there are no absolute indications for surgery for reflux.

5. The incidence of ureteral ectopia is approximately 1 per 1900; ectopic ureters are duplex in 80% of females, more often single in males; there is a 3:1 female predominance, and approximately 10% are bilateral.

a) The cause is a failure of the ureteral bud to separate from the mesonephric duct, probably due to its ectopic origin on the duct.

b) Locations are shown in Figure 28-2.

c) Associated findings.

   i) Renal dysplasia correlates with the degree of ectopy.

   ii) Contralateral duplication accompanies single ectopic ureter in 80%.

   iii) Incontinence and ureteral obstruction are variable findings; incontinence may be due to an orifice located below the sphincter in females or to failure of bladder neck development.

Female

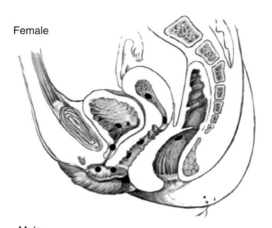

Male

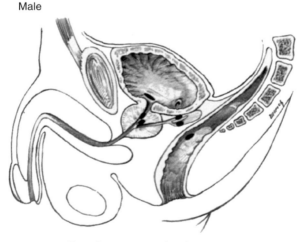

FIGURE 28-2. Sites of ectopic ureteral orifices in girls and boys. (From Schlussel R, Retik R: Ectopic ureter, ureterocele, and other anomalies of the ureter. In Walsh PC, Retik AB, Vaughn ED, Wein AJ [eds]: *Campbell's Urology*, 8th ed. Philadelphia, Saunders, 2002, Fig. 58-14, p 2014.)

iv) Bilateral single ectopic ureters in which the orifice is distal to the bladder neck lead to poorly developed bladder and incontinence due to outlet incompetence and failure of bladder cycling.

d) Management is most often removal of the renal segment and ectopic ureter; rarely the segment may be salvageable by ureteroureterostomy or reimplantation.

6. Ureterocele occurs with a frequency between 1 per 500 and 1 per 4000 in autopsies, accounting for approximately 1% of pediatric urologic admissions and is bilateral in 10–15% of cases. Females 4:1 over males.

   a) Develops due to a combination of an abnormal ureteral bud with either a stenotic orifice or involvement of the distal ureter in the expansion of the vesicourethral canal. The ureter is duplicated in children (80%), with the ureterocele draining the upper pole ureter. Presence of a simple ureterocele subtending a single ureter is less common in children.

   b) Associated anomalies include contralateral ureteral duplication in 50%; renal segmental dysplasia; renal fusion and ectopia; reflux (50%); and, rarely, incontinence.

   c) Classification is based on location of the orifice and is typically defined as intravesical or ectopic.

   d) Cecoureterocele, a subclassification of ectopic ureterocele, differs in that a "cecum" extends beyond the orifice down the urethra; it may be associated with poor bladder neck development and incontinence.

   e) Management is varied.

     i) Puncture of the ureterocele as newborn.

     ii) Upper pole nephrectomy with decompression of the ureterocele.

     iii) Same as ii with lower excision of the ureterocele with common sheath reimplantation and bladder neck reconstruction.

     iv) Same as i with delayed excision of ureterocele plus reimplant with bladder neck reconstruction if vesicoureteral reflux persists or occurs following i. It appears that whether one takes an approach that favors removal of the upper tract moiety only or puncturing the ureterocele, the development of de novo VUR is relatively the same (10–15%).

II. LOWER URINARY TRACT

A. Exstrophy/Epispadias—Spectrum of Anomalies

1. Origin is failure of the cloacal membrane to migrate toward the perineum at 4 weeks' gestation, preventing ingrowth of lateral mesoderm and coalescence of genital tubercles.

   a) The most consistent finding is some degree of separation of symphysis pubis.

b) Epispadias (30%) may be penopubic with incontinence in males (55%), penile (20%) with or without incontinence, or balanitic (5%) or may occur in females with incontinence (20%). It consists of a dorsal meatus with a distal mucosal groove, flattened glans, or bifid clitoris; in males, there is a variable dorsal chordee with shortening of the corporal bodies in severe forms (penopubic).

c) Nearly all cases of epispadias require complete disassembly with or without complete separation of the distal urethra from the glans (Mitchell) technique.

d) Classic exstrophy (60%) occurs in 1 per 50,000 births with 3:1 male predominance; the bladder and the urethra are open dorsally, and the penis is short or the clitoris is bifid.

e) Cloacal exstrophy (10%) results from the condition of failure of the urorectal septum to descend. It occurs approximately 1 per 200,000 births, about equally in males and females.

2. Associated findings.

   a) In classic exstrophy, undescended testes and inguinal hernias are common; often the infraumbilical rectus fails to develop; vaginal stenosis and/or bifid uterus may be present; the upper urinary tract is usually normal, or may be duplex.

   b) In cloacal exstrophy, there are a vesicointestinal fissure opening into the center of the exstrophied bladder, short blind distal colon, absent or duplicated appendix, and often omphalocele. Two thirds of females have an absent or duplex and stenotic vagina; nearly all have a tethered spinal cord with 50% having myelomeningocele. The penis or clitoris is bifid or may be absent.

3. Exstrophy may be managed in stages or by primary single repair. A staged closure begins with bladder closure in the newborn period.

   a) Penile lengthening by freeing corpora from pubic bone attachments and tubularization of the bladder neck is accomplished during the first stage.

   b) In cloacal exstrophy, the omphalocele and vesicoenteric fissure must be dealt with by lateral closure of the bowel end colostomy and omphalocele repair. The bladder halves are approximated in the first stage.

4. The second stage is epispadias repair, in most cases at approximately 1–2 years of age.

5. The third stage in those with functioning, sufficiently large bladders is achieving continence by bladder neck tubularization (60% success).
   a) Those who fail this are candidates for augmentation plus intermittent catheterization.
   b) Most cloacal exstrophy patients have undergone early ileal loop diversion, but a few may be reconstructed along the same principles.
6. Second option is complete penile disassembly with bladder closure and bladder neck and epispadias repair all done at a single stage (Mitchell repair).
7. All patients require careful follow-up throughout life with survey of the upper tracts by IVU or ultrasound, monitoring of acid base balance, renal function tests, and supportive counseling.

B. Urachus

Patent urachus and persistence of portions of the urachus as cysts result from failure of fibrosis of the cranial embryonic bladder segment; they are excised when symptomatic. If infected, primary drainage, antibiotic coverage, and secondary resection are appropriate. In a few cases, the urachal segment may undergo malignant transformation (adenocarcinoma).

C. Posterior Urethral Valves (Type I)

1. Incidence. In boys, 1 per 5000 to 8000; >50% are diagnosed in the first year of life, generally with more severe obstructions.
2. Proposed cause is failure of regression of the terminal segment of the mesonephric duct, which is normally represented by the plicae colliculi. Type II valves are nonobstructing normal folds in the prostatic urethra; type III valves represent either more marked anterior fusion of the valve leaflets or congenital urethral membrane (a separate embryologic entity). Recent observations suggest that types II and III are variations of type I valves.
3. Associated findings.
   a) Vesicoureteral reflux (40%, approximately one half bilateral) resolves in approximately one third of cases generally within 2 years. Persistent unilateral reflux is usually associated with a nonfunctioning kidney, most commonly the left one.
   b) Severe renal dysplasia is common in those with severe obstruction.
   c) Severe hydroureteronephrosis.

d) Acute renal failure and acidosis in the newborn are obstructive phenomena; chronic renal insufficiency from dysplasia may occur.

4. Diagnosis.
   a) Antenatal diagnosis.
   b) UTI or poor stream in an infant or older child; incontinence occasionally in an older child.
   c) A newborn with palpable bladder and kidneys and urinary ascites.
   d) VCUG is the diagnostic study; ultrasonography and renal scan are employed to assess the extent of upper tract damage and postoperative recovery.

5. Management.
   a) In the sick infant, bladder drainage with a small feeding tube (6 F) per the urethra is maintained while acidosis and sepsis are treated; VCUG may be done with this catheter in place.
   b) The healthy infant or older child may undergo transurethral incision of valves initially; the sick infant when creatinine stabilizes and sepsis resolves.
   c) Cutaneous vesicostomy can be used as a temporizing measure in a very small infant but is rarely required with today's endoscopic equipment.
   d) Nonfunctioning kidneys with refluxing ureters should be preserved. The ureters may be used as tissue for augmentation of the bladder if needed at the time of renal transplant.
   e) Ureteral tailoring and reimplantation are almost never indicated and are often fraught with failure.
   f) Antibiotic prophylaxis is maintained as long as reflux persists or upper tract emptying is slow (usually through adulthood).

6. Results.
   a) Children whose creatinine levels stabilize below 0.7 mg/dL after relief of obstruction generally do well, whereas those with creatinine levels above 1.0 mg/dL often "outgrow" their renal function by puberty and require transplantation.
   b) Continence is eventually achieved in virtually all who undergo valve incision. Bladder volume increases. Some children must practice double voiding or intermittent catheterization to ensure complete bladder emptying.

D. Megalourethra

1. This rare lesion is usually associated with prune belly syndrome.

2. Occurs in two types.
   a) Scaphoid type is a deficiency of corpus spongiosum allowing ballooning of the urethra during voiding; it can be repaired with hypospadias techniques.
   b) Fusiform type involves deficiency of corpora cavernosa as well as corpus spongiosum, resulting in elongated flaccid penis with redundant skin. This form is seen usually in stillborn infants with other cloacal anomalies and is difficult to correct because of the lack of adequate corporal tissue.

E. Miscellaneous

1. Anterior urethral valve or diverticulum is a rare obstructing lesion with a large saccular outpouching and obstructing distal lip of mucosa. The diverticulum is excised with careful attention to prevent the distal flap from obstructing.
2. Enlarged utriculus masculinus is a dilated müllerian remnant, usually asymptomatic, associated with hypospadias or an intersex state; it can be excised retrovesically or transvesically if stasis leads to UTI or the full utricle interferes with bladder emptying. These rarely require surgical intervention.
3. Aphallia and diphallia are exceedingly rare failure of fusion of the genital tubercles or failure of differentiation of the phallic mesenchyme.
4. Micropenis is often associated with CNS lesions or an intersex state; gender conversion, practiced in some cases in the past, is almost never considered currently.

III. EXTERNAL GENITAL MALFORMATIONS

A. Hypospadias

Hypospadias occurs in 1 in 300 live boys; there is a 14% incidence in siblings and an 8% incidence in offspring.

1. Caused by failure of the mesodermal urethral folds to converge in midline; chordee results from failure of urethral plate disintegration or fibrosis of inner genital folds (which form the spongiosum and dartos fascia).
2. Associated findings.
   a) Blunted human chorionic gonadotropin response to gonadotropin releasing hormone and low androgen receptor levels in a few cases.
   b) Undescended testes in 9.3% (30% with penoscrotal or more proximal meatus). Up to one third of boys with hypospadias and undescended testes have an intersex state, usually genetic mosaicism.

   c) Inguinal hernia in 9%.
   d) Upper tract anomalies in 46% when associated with
      imperforate anus, 33% when meningomyelocele is pre-
      sent, 12–50% when one other system anomaly is present,
      5% with isolated hypospadias (screening intravenous
      pyelogram [IVP] not needed for simple hypospadias).
3. Classification (simplified) (Figure 28-3).
   a) Hypospadias without chordee (straight erections,
      meatus between midshaft and corona).
   b) Hypospadias with chordee.
      i) Meatus penile or penoscrotal after release of chordee.
      ii) Meatus scrotal or perineal.
   c) Chordee with hypospadias.
      i) With normal urethra.
      ii) With short or hypoplastic urethra.
4. Management.
   a) One-stage correction between 4 and 12 months of age
      is preferred.
   b) Glanular hypospadias may be corrected by meatal
      advancement and glanuloplasty (MAGPI) (Figure 28-4).
      For coronal repairs, the Snodgrass or TIP (Figure 28-5)

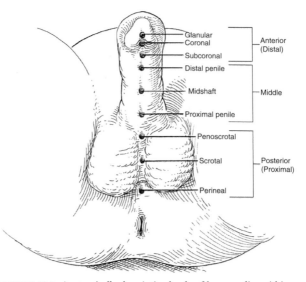

FIGURE 28-3. Anatomically descriptive levels of hypospadias within
the three major categories, based on the level of the meatus
following orthoplasty. (From Retik A, Borer J: Hypospadias.
In Walsh PC, Retik AB, Vaughn ED, Wein AJ [eds]: *Campbell's
Urology*, 8th ed. Philadelphia, Saunders, 2002, Fig. 65-3, p 2287.)

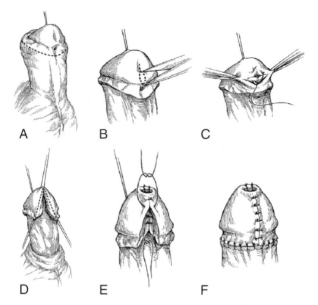

FIGURE 28-4. Meatoplasty and glanuloplasty (MAGPI).
A. Circumferential subcoronal incision is marked. Longitudinal incision (**B**) and transverse approximation (**C**) (Heineke-Mikulicz procedure) of transverse glanular "bridge" in urethral plate.
D. Ventral edge of meatus is pulled distally and medial glands "trimming" incisions are marked. **E.** Deep suture approximation of the glands. **F.** Superficial approximation of the glans and skin.
(From Duckett JW: Hypospadias. In Walsh PC, Retik AB, Vaughan ED Jr, Wein AJ [eds]: *Campbell's Urology,* 7th ed. Philadelphia, Saunders, 1998, pp 2093–2119.)

    or onlay island flap (Figure 28-6) procedure, depending on meatal position as well as surgeon preference are most commonly employed.

c) Penile shaft or more proximal hypospadias may be managed by inner preputial transverse island flap (Figure 28-7).

d) Severe penoscrotal hypospadias may require combined island flap and primary (Duplay) closure of the proximal urethra and may need secondary scrotoplasty to improve the cosmetic result.

e) Degloving the penis and mobilizing the urethra may treat skin chordee without urethral involvement.

f) Chordee with hypoplastic urethra requires island flap urethroplasty after chordee release due to bowstring effect of short urethra.

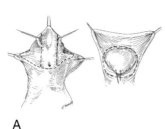 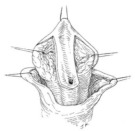

A   B

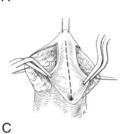 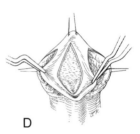

C   D

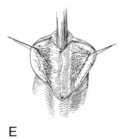 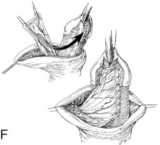

E   F

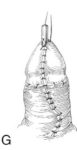

G

For legend see opposite page

FIGURE 28-5. Tubularized incised plate (TIP) urethroplasty in distal, primary hypospadias repair. **A.** Stay sutures are placed, and proposed urethral plate demarcating and circumferential incisions are marked. **B.** Parallel longitudinal and circumferential incisions have been made. **C.** Proposed longitudinal line of incision in the midline of the urethral plate. **D.** Urethral plate has been incised. **E.** Urethral plate tubularized over a 6-F Silastic catheter with care not to close the distal extent (meatus) of the incised urethral plate too tightly. **F.** Subcutaneous (dartos) tissue flap is harvested from lateral or dorsal penile shaft and repositioned over the neourethra as a second layer of coverage. **G.** Glans penis has been approximated in two layers, redundant skin excised and indwelling bladder catheter secured. (From Retik AB, Borer JG: Primary and reoperative hypospadias repair with the Snodgrass technique. *World J Urol* 16:186, 1998.)

---

    g) Urinary diversion for 2 weeks in all but very distal repairs, with a small Silastic urethral stent ensures adequate bladder drainage.

    h) Compressive dressing for 2–3 days is commonly used.

5. Results and complications.

    a) Small urethrocutaneous fistulae are the most common complication. These may be closed in layers with 90% success.

    b) Postoperative bleeding can usually be stopped with compression.

    c) UTI occurs in less than 10% of cases and can be treated with the usual oral agents.

    d) Strictures are rare and usually occur at the meatus or the proximal end of the repair and are treated by Y-V meatoplasty or excision; direct vision urethrotomy is sometimes successful for short strictures.

    e) When carefully done, the procedures outlined provide functional and cosmetically nearly normal penis and meatus even in the most severe hypospadias cases.

B. Cryptorchidism

1. Incidence is 1% of boys.

2. Origin: aberrant testicular descent; possible failure of pituitary-gonadal axis in late gestation, that is, absent luteinizing hormone (LH) surge or blunted testicular response.

3. Associated findings.

    a) Patent processus vaginalis 90%; symptomatic hernia rarely occurs.

    b) Infertility is doubled in untreated unilateral undescended testis, may be as high as 35% in bilateral cryp-

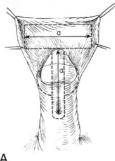

A

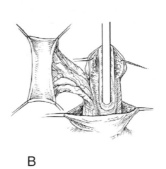

B

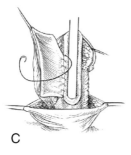

C

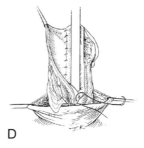

D

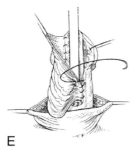

E

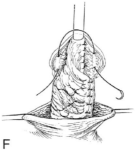

F

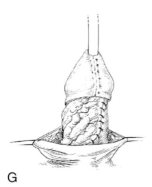

G

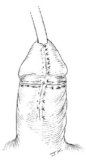

H

For legend see opposite page

FIGURE 28-6. Onlay island flap repair. **A.** Proposed incisions for urethral plate and preputial skin onlay. **B.** Pedicled preputial skin onlay with stay sutures. **C.** Initial full-thickness suture approximation of onlay flap and urethral plate. **D.** Approximation at proximal extent. **E.** Completion of anastomosis with running subcuticular technique. **F.** Inferolateral border of onlay pedicle has been advanced as a second layer coverage of proximal and longitudinal suture lines. **G.** Approximated glans. **H.** Completed repair. (From Atala A, Retik AB: Hypospadias. In Libertino JA [ed]: *Reconstructive Urologic Surgery*, 3rd ed. St. Louis, Mosby, 1998, p 467.)

torchidism. Surgery before age 2 and treatment with an analogue of LH releasing hormone may improve fertility.

   i) Ectopic testis is normal histologically and not usually associated with infertility.

   c) Testicular malignancy is 10–100 times more common than in the general population.

   d) Undescended testis is part of many syndromes, for example, prune belly, exstrophy, genetic disorders, and intersex states (when associated with even mild hypospadias).

4. Diagnosis.
   a) Careful examination will discriminate retractile from truly undescended testis.
      i) A testis that can be manipulated into the scrotum with gentle stretch of the cremaster that does not retract into the canal is retractile and requires no surgery.

5. Management.
   a) Inguinal exploration at 4–6 months of age (spontaneous descent is rare after 3 months).
   b) Most undescended testes are palpable; 85% are canalicular even if impalpable and can be brought down with conventional orchiopexy.
   c) If the canal is empty, the peritoneum is opened; either a testis or blind ending vas deferens and gonadal vessels are found overlying the psoas above the internal inguinal ring. Only identification of the vessels proves testicular absence and constitutes sufficient exploration, as the vas may be embryologically separate from the testis.
   d) Fowler-Stephens orchidopexy will bring down an intra-abdominal testis by dividing the spermatic vessels. In this case, collateral flow to the testis via the artery to the vas deferens or the vessels running with the cremasteric muscle will provide adequate perfusion in more than 70%.
   e) A testis that cannot be brought into the scrotum should be removed if the contralateral one is normally descended.

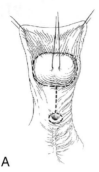

A

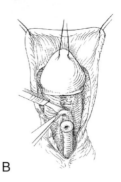

B

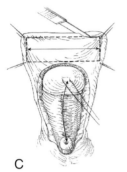

C

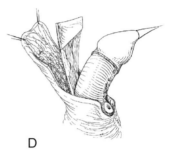

D

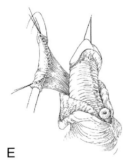

E

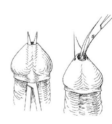

F

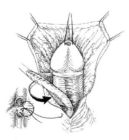

G

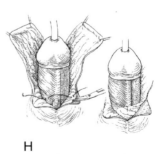

H

For legend see opposite page

FIGURE 28-7. Transverse preputial island flap repair. **A.** Proposed initial incisions for proximal shaft/penoscrotal hypospadias. **B.** Release of tethering urethral plate and "dropping" of meatus proximally. **C.** Incision of preputial skin of appropriate dimensions for length of defect and width for desired luminal diameter. **D.** Harvested transverse preputial island flap. **E.** Running subcuticular suture tubularization has been performed over a Silastic catheter to be followed by a second layer running Lembert suture. **F.** Generous glans channel is fashioned for neourethral passage. A core of glans tissue is excised to achieve sufficient caliber. **G.** Native urethral meatus is fixed to corpora cavernosa prior to performing proximal anastomosis with the neourethra. **H.** Subcutaneous (dartos) tissue coverage of anastomosis. (From Atala A, Retik AB: Hypospadias. In Libertino JA [ed]: *Reconstructive Urologic Surgery*, 3rd ed St. Louis, Mosby, 1998, p 467.)

6. Results.
   a) The Fowler-Stephens procedure in our experience has been 70% successful, as judged by palpation of a normal-feeling testis in the scrotum.
   b) Results of conventional orchidopexy are better.

C. Hernia/Communicating Hydrocele

1. Incidence is 1–4% of mature infants and 13% of premature infants.
2. Origin is failed closure of processus vaginalis after testicular descent or may be associated with incomplete descent.
3. Only associated findings may be frank hernia (sac containing bowel or other organ) or undescended testis.
4. Principle differential diagnosis is with a congenital scrotal hydrocele associated with a closed processus vaginalis. Neonatal scrotal hydroceles are present half the time in infants and will usually be reabsorbed by 12–15 months of age. No surgery is required. A communicating hydrocele is suggested by changing volume of fluid surrounding the testicle. It is important not to confuse contraction of the dartos muscle of the scrotal wall with a change in hydrocele size.
5. Unlike a true hernia, which is repaired promptly in infants due to risk of incarceration, a communicating hydrocele may be fixed electively, usually before the first birthday.

D. Appendages

1. Testicular and epididymal appendages are present usually at the upper pole of the testis or epididymis, represent

müllerian or wolffian duct remnants, and are only bothersome when torsion of the appendage occurs.

2. Torsion of the appendix can sometimes be differentiated from testicular torsion by point tenderness and swelling at the upper pole or the "blue dot" sign in which the infarcted tissue is apparent beneath the scrotal skin as a dark spot. Boys with torsion of the appendix testis may have a visible cremaster reflex. Cremasteric contraction almost never occurs with torsion of the spermatic cord.

3. When doubt exists, and risk of spermatic cord exists, scrotal exploration is essential. If the diagnosis is certain, treatment is symptomatic; pain will usually resolve in 3–5 days. If pain persists, trans-scrotal excision usually results in complete resolution of pain.

IV. CLOACAL DYSGENESIS/PERSISTENT CLOACA

A. Cloaca Anomaly

Cloaca anomaly represents failure of the urorectal septum to descend, resulting in a single perineal opening or a sinus into which the rectum, vagina, and urethra enter.

1. The upper urinary tract is usually normal but should be evaluated with ultrasonography.

2. Genitosinography, VCUG, if possible, and cystovaginoscopy are necessary to assess the anatomy. Diverting colostomy is usually done early, as in an imperforate anus, and this assessment can be performed under the same anesthetic.

3. Reconstruction via a midline posterior approach (Pena-DeVries) is carried out at age 4–12 months and consists of:
   a) Rectal tapering and pull through.
   b) Combined mobilization of the vagina and urethra as a unit with longitudinal separation of the urogenital sinus for cloacas that are shorter than 3 cm. Longer cloacas may need abdominal and perineal mobilization of the bladder, vagina, and rectum.
   c) Spinal anomalies and neurogenic bladders are common.

B. Vaginal Atresia and Mayer-Rokitansky-Küster-Hauser Syndrome

1. Hormonal assays can be used to distinguish primary vaginal atresia from a short vagina in girls with testicular feminization. Girls with primary vaginal atresia have

normal LH and follicle-stimulating hormone (FSH) levels and low testosterone levels.

a) Failure of müllerian duct to penetrate the urogenital sinus.

b) Vascular accident.

c) Isolated anomaly.

d) Often presents at puberty with amenorrhea.

e) Usually atretic or absent uterus.

f) Vaginoplasty performed using a 10 cm loop of colon, which is reversed and brought to the perineum at the introitus.

2. Rokitansky syndrome.

a) Combination of müllerian duct abnormality, often duplication with vaginal atresia with ipsilateral renal agenesis.

b) Abnormality of the müllerian ducts may be associated with absence of the mesonephric duct because both structures are closely associated during early embryonic differentiation.

c) May present in newborn period with hydrocolpos but commonly presents with amenorrhea or hematocolpos at puberty; some discovered during investigation of a solitary kidney.

d) Those with complete uterovaginal agenesis are managed as primary vaginal atresia; some have normal or septate uteri above the level of obstruction. Girls with uterine obstruction require vaginoplasty.

e) A special case is the patient with complete uterovaginal duplication and unilateral vaginal atresia.

i) Because one uterine horn drains normally, these girls have normal menstrual periods, cyclic abdominal pain, and pelvic mass.

ii) These girls may be managed by transvaginal marsupialization thereby establishing drainage of the obstructed segment or by resection of the blocked segment if the uterus is atrophic.

f) Ultrasound is the study of choice for the evaluation of these genital anomalies; VCUG is used to evaluate for reflux. Cystovaginoscopy helps to delineate the introital anatomy.

SELF-ASSESSMENT QUESTIONS

1. Discuss the incidence and pathophysiology of kidney fusion anomalies and give three examples.

2. Name three subtypes of cystic abnormalities of the kidneys and their pathophysiologies.

3. Discuss the incidence of ureteral duplications and describe the association with vesicoureteral reflux and obstruction.
4. Describe the grading system for vesicoureteral reflux and why it is important to the practicing urologist.
5. Describe anomalies that are associated with hypospadias and create an algorithm for surgical correction of hypospadias depending on the location of the meatus.

SUGGESTED READINGS

1. Bauer SB: Anomalies of the upper urinary tract. In Walsh PC, Retik AB, Vaughn ED, Wein AJ (eds): *Campbell's Urology,* 8th ed. Philadelphia, Saunders, 2002, pp 1885–1913.
2. Canning DA, Koo HP, Duckett JW: Anomalies of the bladder and cloaca. In Gillenwater JY, Grayhack JT, Howards SS, Duckett JW (eds): *Adult and Pediatric Urology,* 3rd ed. St. Louis, Mosby, 1996, pp 2445–2488.
3. Gearhart JP: Exstrophy, epispadias, and other bladder anomalies. In Walsh PC, Retik AB, Vaughn ED, Wein AJ (eds): *Campbell's Urology,* 8th ed. Philadelphia, Saunders, 2002, pp 2136–2196.
4. Glassberg KI: Renal dysgenesis and cystic disease of the kidney. In Walsh PC, Retik AB, Vaughn ED, Wein AJ (eds): *Campbell's Urology,* 8th ed. Philadelphia, Saunders, 2002, pp 1925–1994.
5. Grady RW, Mitchell ME: Complete primary repair of exstrophy. *J Urol* 162:1415–1420, 1999.
6. Park JM: Normal and anomalous development of the urinary tract. In Walsh PC, Retik AB, Vaughn ED, Wein AJ (eds): *Campbell's Urology,* 8th ed. Philadelphia, Saunders, 2002, pp 1737–1764.
7. Retik AB, Borer JG: Hypospadias. In Walsh PC, Retik AB, Vaughn ED, Wein AJ (eds): *Campbell's Urology,* 8th ed. Philadelphia, Saunders, 2002, pp 2284–2333.
8. Snyder HM: Anomalies of the ureter. In Gillenwater JY, Grayhack JT, Howards SS, Duckett JW (eds): *Adult and Pediatric Urology,* 3rd ed. Chicago, Mosby, 1996, pp 2197–2231.
9. Stephens FD: *Congenital Malformations of the Urinary Tract.* New York, Praeger, 1983, p 195.

C H A P T E R 29

Geriatric Urology

George W. Drach, MD

UROLOGY AND AGING PATIENTS

Our growing geriatric population will affect urology in major
ways over the next 2–3 decades. General urologists will see in
their offices nearly 50% of their patients within the older than
65 age group (Table 29-1). Urologists will also face difficult
management decisions opting for or against major surgery
in these patients. This is especially true for patients with bladder and prostatic cancer, because they often do not reach the
stage of invasive cancer until older than age 70 years
(Figure 29-1). Some of these surgical candidates remain relatively healthy. Others demonstrate poor surgical risk because
of their general condition and comorbidities.

   Should we in urology approach these elderly patients differently from our younger, healthier patients? Yes, but the
response to this question comes in modification of three elements of our usual "evaluation and management" algorithm:
steps in initial evaluation of the elderly patient differ, decision
processes regarding further evaluation and recommendation
for treatment require alteration, and decisions on management
of definitive therapy require additional thought integrated with
the milieu of aging. Several excellent sources of help exist
for geriatric urology. Throughout this chapter, I refer to a
small text, *Geriatrics at Your Fingertips* (GAYF), which is of
great assistance in management of all geriatric patients.
Another source is the text *Geriatrics Syllabus for Specialists.*
Both are available from the American Geriatrics Society (see
later), and both should be on the office bookshelf of every
urologist.

SPECIAL ASPECTS OF APPROACH TO
THE GERIATRIC PATIENT

Initial Evaluation

Of course, one begins with the usual history and physical
examination, but several additional inquiries and examinations are needed. A first caution **includes careful attention**

Table 29-1: Outpatient Visits by Medicare Patients (2001)

Specialty	%
Cardiology	58.4
Ophthalmology	48.5
Urology	47.9
General internal medicine	42.7
General surgery	35.8
Neurology	28.6
Dermatology	28.1
Otolaryngology	22.5
Orthopedic surgery	25.0
Family practice	25.9
Psychiatry	9.9
Gynecology	7.1

Adapted from Drach GW, Forciea M: Geriatric patient care: basics for urologists. AUA Update Series 24:286–296, 2005.

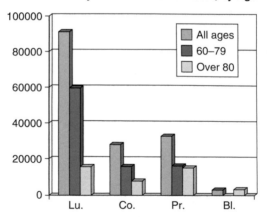

FIGURE 29-1. Most prostate cancer deaths occur after age 60. Bladder cancer deaths do not become noticeable until after age 80. *Lu, lung; Co, colon; Pr, prostate; Bl, bladder.* (Adapted from Hollenbeck BK, Miller DC, Taub D, et al: Aggressive treatment for bladder cancer is associated with improved overall survival among patients 80 years old or older. *Urology* 64:292, 2004.)

to the medication regimen and the patient's adherence to it. Elderly patients often do not take medications as prescribed. They may take only half-doses or take daily doses only once weekly. In other cases, they may not take the medication at all, perhaps because of excessive expense or their perception of side effects. In addition, one must ask them about their intake of all over-the-counter medications and herbal or other supplements that can affect their health. The average person older than age 70 takes 4–5 prescription medications and also 2–4 supplemental medications. These all must be recorded so that all personnel know what is actually taken.

One risk buried below this problem is that one must avoid the routine rewriting on admission of all medications "in the record." What happens if you give an α-blocking agent such as terazosin to a patient who has not in reality taken this prescribed medication? One risks side effects such as postural hypotension and falls. On admission, administer only those necessary drugs that the patient actually takes, and those needed for procedural preparation (e.g., antibiotics).

Another challenge is the **recovery of information specific to prior treatment.** Older people tend to forget details of treatments received years ago. If the patient has received radiation, what was the total dose and area of the field(s)? If surgery, what was actually done? Did the prior surgeon take out more than 4 feet of small bowel? Even though chasing down such information can be difficult, it is very necessary.

Another significant addition to the geriatric evaluation is an assessment of the cognitive, flexibility, and mobility functions. These three elements can be combined to give an estimate of the patient's overall functional ability. First, it is extremely important to develop your own opinion of the patient's mental abilities and to enter that assessment into the record. If the patient seems to be a poor historian or defers the history to a caretaker, perform a simple mental evaluation such as the "Mini-Cog and Clock-Drawing" tests (found in GAYF) and record the results. This determination is very important if you are to obtain informed consent for any medical therapy or surgical procedure. Second, if mobility seems limited, do a brief mobility test (again found in GAYF). Third, as a component of your physical examination, evaluate the flexibility of the limbs and back. A full range of motion (ROM) of every joint is not needed for adequate function, but severe restrictions will indicate the need for supplemental help and/or rehabilitative services before and after treatment.

All the previously mentioned factors contribute to your assessment of the "functional capacity" of the patient. No element of your initial geriatric evaluation predicts less risk of postchemotherapy or perioperative morbidity and mortality than a high level of functional ability. As an example of the importance here, it is wonderful to successfully repair stress urinary incontinence in the older female but begets a failure if you do not realize that because of limited mobility she cannot get to the bathroom in time to void anyway.

At this point, also, urologists must learn of the social status and living capabilities of their patients. Do they live alone (as do more than 60% of U.S. females older than age 70)? Does their home have stairs? Do they have adequate toileting facilities? Do they have adequate heat or air conditioning? Who assists them when necessary? Can they perform fully all the activities of daily living (ADLs) and instrumental activities of daily living (IADLs) (again see GAYF). This type of survey will indicate to you whether the patient will need assistance when undergoing chemotherapy or following discharge after surgery.

Another important part of initial evaluation should include your estimate of the nutritional status of the older person. About one fourth of all elderly patients show evidence of malnutrition when first seen. Certain findings hint at such a problem: body mass index (BMI) <22, serum albumin <3.5 g/dL, total cholesterol <160 mg/dL, involuntary weight loss of >10 lb in the last 6 months.

THERAPEUTIC DECISIONS

At this point, having performed a more global evaluation, one reaches an overall assessment of the health status of the patient. Comorbidities are noted and evaluated also. One then decides to pursue further evaluation and/or treatment based on the physiologic health and functional ability rather than an arbitrary chronologic age. **This avoids two great errors that can be made in care of the geriatric patient: withholding adequate care because of chronologic age alone or providing overaggressive care in spite of physiologic frailty.** This contrast in care becomes evident in decisions about aggressive surgery in treatment of, for example, bladder cancer. Such a patient at 78 years in reasonable health with only one comorbidity (diabetes mellitus type II) can expect to live at least 10 years and can definitely be offered cystectomy and diversion for potential cure. However, to

Table 29-2: Mean Life Expectancy of the Older Patient

Present Age (yr)	65	70	75	80	85	90	95	100
Men								
White	16	13	10	7	5	4	3	2
Black	14	12	9	7	6	4	4	3
Women								
White	20	15	12	9	7	5	3	2
Black	17	14	11	9	6	5	4	3

From *National Vital Statistics Reports* 51:30, 2002.

use this knowledge effectively, the physician must know the brackets of life expectancy for the aged patient (Table 29-2).

Another example of the use of this approach to really helping the patient is summarized in Table 29-3, which provides recommendations about administering chemotherapy to elderly patients with advanced cancer. The same recommendations should apply to radical surgical approaches. Most authorities agree that presence of more than two serious comorbidities (such as coronary or peripheral artery disease, diabetes mellitus, chronic obstructive pulmonary disease) should lead one to more conservative treatments in most instances (see Table 29-3). This is especially true when deciding on chemotherapy or radical surgery for urologic malignancies. The decision to administer chemotherapy or surgery to an

Table 29-3: Geriatric Urology: Oncology and Decisions

Algorithm: (treat elderly patients within each group according to their health, functional ability, and degree of comorbidity):

Group 1: Healthy and fit = standard treatment

Group 2: Partially dependent and 2 or fewer comorbidities = would life expectancy with treatment be better, or could treatment be tolerated?

Group 3: Frail, dependent, 3 or more comorbidities = treat palliatively only

Adapted from Cancer Control, Moffit Cancer Center 8:2–26, 2001.

Table 29-4: Decisions Needed in Moving Forward in Elderly Patient's Evaluation	
Screening?	PSA, cytology
Imaging?	KUB, CT, MRI, ultrasound, other
Biopsies?	Prostate, penile, renal, bladder, other
Procedures?	Cystoscopy, percutaneous approaches

CT, computed tomography; KUB, kidney, ureters, and bladder; MRI, magnetic resonance imaging; PSA, prostate-specific antigen.

individual who has a life expectancy of only 2 years seems ludicrous if that person would face significant risk of complications and death from chemotherapy or surgery alone. On the other hand, chemotherapy, radiotherapy, or even surgery may be clearly indicated for the severely ill patient if it will provide additional comfort and daily functioning (palliation) for the remaining days of the patient's life.

If indeed the geriatric patient appears to have a high degree of health for his or her age, then one proceeds with additional evaluative steps (Table 29-4). The admonition at this point remains the well-known statement: "If you are not likely to treat the patient (or the patient will not accept treatment) even if the test/biopsy is positive, then why do the test/biopsy?" This quandary has become very important in the context of the age at which we should cease prostate-specific antigen (PSA) screening for prostate cancer. At a recent conference that I attended in the state of Iowa, the consensus recommendation for cessation of PSA testing after age 75 did *not* include an age limit. Rather, it proposed that PSA testing should continue as long as the patient had an expectation of 5–10 years of functionally productive life and would be a candidate for definitive therapy.

THE PERIOPERATIVE PERIOD

If one decides to proceed with operative treatment of some disease process, then several steps become more important for the geriatric patient.

Preoperative Patient Optimization

These steps include any additional preoperative evaluation and improvement of comorbidities. Experience and literature emphasize that **special attention must be paid to cardio-vascular status, renal function, and gastroenteric function.** Our geriatric medicine colleagues may assist with improvement in cardiac and renal functions. If nutrition is inadequate, studies have shown that intense brief measures, such as "hyperalimentation" seldom have benefit. The best program, if time allows, is that developed for the patient by a dietitian, who also monitors compliance in some way over the several months that are needed to improve nutritional status.

There is also need for re-verification of informed consent with comments again on mental capacity of the patient, review of or initiation of living will and advance directives, confirmation of overall functional capacity, analysis of social conditions that will apply on discharge, and early discharge planning. Because most of these older patients will be covered by Medicare or similar insurance, your plans must include attention to necessary financial constraints. Table 29-5 summarizes approaches to sites for discharge based on Medicare concepts. In addition, a specific additional category exists for those patients needing rehabilitative services.

Perioperative Problems

Some specific postoperative complications of the elderly require mention. The first regards changes in mentation: delirium, dementia, or depression. **Postoperative delirium is especially common in the elderly and must be a part of the postoperative daily evaluation (see *Geriatric Syllabus*).**

Second, geriatric patients remain at **high risk for falls** while in the hospital. Restraints actually increase this risk and should not be used. Any use of psychiatric medications greatly increases the risk of falls, so they should be avoided. Finally, **pain control for the elderly must be managed carefully** with special attention to age-related peculiarities (e.g., meperidine increases risk of seizures).

To summarize, for our geriatric urology patients, one must alter the initial evaluation to include careful drug history, obtain necessary old records, and evaluate functional abilities. Therapeutic decisions must be based on presence or absence of comorbidities along with total functional capacity, rather than chronologic age. Finally, the perioperative period must include concern for optimization of comorbidities, attention to pain control, fall prevention, and early discharge planning. All possible steps to prevent or ameliorate mental status change are necessary. With these details accomplished, care of our aged patients will be more beneficial.

Table 29-5: Functional Abilities Required for Living Accommodation Level

ADL/IADL	Home	Senior Housing	Assisted Living	Nursing Home
Mobility	Independent or assisted	Independent or assisted	Independent or assisted	Dependent
Toilet	Independent	Independent	Independent	Dependent
Chew/swallow	Independent	Independent	Independent	Dependent
Dressing	Independent	Independent	Independent	Independent, assisted, or dependent
Bathing	Independent	Independent	Independent	Independent, assisted, or dependent
Transportation	Independent	Independent	Assisted or dependent	Assisted or dependent
Finances	Independent	Independent	Assisted or dependent	Assisted or dependent
Telephone	Independent	Independent	Assisted or dependent	Assisted or dependent
Shop/cook	Independent	Independent	Assisted or dependent	Dependent
Laundry/clean	Independent	Independent	Assisted	Dependent

ADL, activity of daily living; IADL, instrumental activity of daily living.
Adapted from Drach GW, Forciea M: Geriatric patient care: basics for urologists.
AUA Update Series 24:286–296, 2005.

SELF-ASSESSMENT QUESTIONS

1. Initial evaluation of the geriatric urology patient requires what three steps in addition to the usual history and physical examination?
2. What single factor in the evaluation of the elderly patient gives the best estimate of how the patient will respond to the challenges of chemotherapy or surgery?
3. What history, signs, or laboratory findings point to the possibility of poor nutrition in the elderly?
4. How do we separate the three groups of the elderly in our algorithm for advising advanced treatment, such as chemotherapy or surgery?
5. When performing discharge planning, what elements must be met to place the patient into senior housing?

SUGGESTED READINGS

1. Diokno A (ed): Geriatric urology. *Urol Clin North Am* 23:1–163, 1996.
2. Drach G, Griebling T: Geriatric urology. *J Am Geriatr Soc* 51:S355, 2003.
3. Krouse RS, Jonasson O, Milch RA, et al: An evolving strategy for surgical care (palliative care). *J Am Coll Surg* 149–155, 2004.
4. *Geriatrics at Your Fingertips.* New York, American Geriatrics Society, 2005.
5. *Geriatrics Syllabus for Specialists.* New York, American Geriatrics Society, 2002.
6. O'Donnell PD (ed): *Geriatric Urology.* Boston, Little, Brown, 1994.

Index

Note: Page numbers followed by t refer to tables and f refer to figures.